P9-DDN-448

Control of Communicable Diseases Manual

David L. Heymann, MD, Editor

Nineteenth Edition

2008

An official report of the American Public Health Association

American Public Health Association
800 I Street, NW
Washington, DC 20001-3710

American Public Health Association
800 I Street, NW
Washington, DC 20001-3710

Georges C. Benjamin, MD, FACP
Executive Director

Nina Tristani
Director of Publications

Terence Mulligan
Production Manager

Printed and bound in the United States of America

Cover Design: Ellie D'Sa and Jennifer Strass
Typesetting: Cadmus
Set in: Garamond
Printing and Binding: United Book Press, Inc., Baltimore, Md

Notes on the cover design: The cover illustrates four basic
aspects of communicable disease control. Grain—proper
nutrition; microscope—research; syringe—prevention and
treatment; hand and soap—sanitation

ISBN 978-0-87553-189-2 soft cover
ISBN 978-0-87553-190-8 hardcover
20M/04/11

Johan Giesecke, MD, Professor
Chief Scientist, European Centre for Disease Prevention and Control
SE-17183, Stockholm, SWEDEN

Dr. Donato Greco
Capo Dipartimento della Prevenzione e Comunicazione
Ministero della Salute
Via G.Ribotta, 5, 00144 – Roma, ITALY

Paul R Gully, MB, ChB, FRCPC, FFPH
Senior Adviser to ADG/HSE
World Health Organization
Avenue Appia, CH 1221 Geneva 21, SWITZERLAND

Margaret Hamburg, MD
Senior Scientist, Global Health and Security Initiative
Nuclear Threat Initiative
1747 Pennsylvania Ave, NW, Washington DC, USA

Dr Zuhair Hallaj
Special Adviser to the Regional Director for Communicable Diseases
World Health Organization
2 El Koba Street, Heliopolis, Cairo, EGYPT

Professor David R Harper
Director General
Health Improvement and Protection
Department of Health
London, UNITED KINGDOM

James M. Hughes, MD
Professor of Medicine and Public Health
Senior Advisor for Infectious Diseases, International Association of
National Public Health Institutes, and Center for Global Safe Water
Director, Program in Global Infectious Diseases
Rollins School of Public Health
Emory University
1462 Clifton Road NE, Atlanta, GA 30322, USA

Nyoman Kandun, MD
Director General of the Centre for Disease Control
Ministry of Health
Jakarta JL, Percetakan Negara No. 29, INDONESIA

Rima F. Khabbaz, MD
Director, National Center for Preparedness, Detection, and Control of Infectious Diseases
Centers for Disease Control and Prevention
1600 Clifton Road NE, Mailstop C12, Atlanta, GA 30333, USA

Omar A. Khan, MD MHS FAAFP
Assistant Professor & Attending Physician, University of Vermont College of Medicine
Attending Physician, A.I. duPont Hospital for Children
Program Chair, International Health, American Public Health Association
800 I Street NW, Washington DC 20001-3710, USA

Ann Marie Kimball, MD, MPH, FACPM
Director, Asia Pacific Economic Cooperation Emerging Infections Network
Professor, Epidemiology, Health Services
Adjunct Professor, Biomedical and Health Informatics and Medicine
School of Public Health and Community Medicine, University of Washington
BOX 357236, Seattle, 98195, USA

Mary Ann Lansang, MD, MMSc
Professor of Medicine and Clinical Epidemiology
College of Medicine
University of the Philippines, Manila
547 Pedro Gil St., Manila 1000, PHILIPPINES

James W. LeDuc, PhD
Professor, Microbiology and Immunology
Robert E. Shope Chair in Global Health
Director, Program in Global Health
Institute for Human Infections and Immunity
Associate Director
Galveston National Laboratory
University of Texas Medical Branch
301 University Blvd, Galveston, TX 77555-0610, USA

Professor Rose G. F. Leke
Head of Department of Infectious Diseases, Hematology and Immunology
Faculty of Medicine and Biomedical Sciences
The University of Yaounde
Yaounde, CAMEROON

Professor John S Mackenzie
Premier's Fellow and Professor of Tropical Infectious Diseases and
Deputy CEO
Australian Biosecurity CRC
Curtin University of Technology
GPO Box U1987, Perth, WA6845, AUSTRALIA

Tatsuo Miyamura, MD, PhD
Director General, National Institute of Infectious Diseases
1-23-1 Toyama, Shinjuku-ku, Tokyo 162-8640, JAPAN

Professor Angus Nicoll, CBE
Senior Expert, Influenza Coordination
European Centre for Disease Prevention and Control
SE-17183, Stockholm, SWEDEN

Guenael Rodier, MD
Director, International Health Regulations Coordination Programme
Health Security & Environment
World Health Organization
Avenue Appia, CH 1221 Geneva 21, SWITZERLAND

Michael Ryan, MD
Director, Epidemic and Pandemic Alert and Response
Health Security and Environment
World Health Organization
Avenue Appia, CH 1221 Geneva 21, SWITZERLAND

Bijan Sadrizadebh
Senior Adviser to the Minister
Ministry of Health & Medical Education,
Islamic Republic of Iran
Tehran, 11365, ISLAMIC REPUBLIC OF IRAN

Prof. K. Srinath Reddy
President, Public Health Foundation of India
PHD House, Second Floor 4/2, Sirifort Institutional Area
August Kranti Marg, New Delhi, INDIA

Ronald Waldman, MD, MPH
Professor of Clinical Population and Family Health
Mailman School of Public Health
Columbia University
New York, NY, USA

Dr. Suwit Wibulpolprasert
Senior Advisor on Disease Control
Thailand Ministry of Public Health
5th Floor, Building 1
Office of Permanent Secretary, Ministry of Public Health
Tiwanond Road, Nonthaburi 11000, THAILAND

CHAPTER AUTHORS AND REVIEWERS

Centers for Disease Control and Prevention
1600 Clifton Road NE, Mailstop C12, Atlanta, GA 30333, USA

Ballard R
Barton Behravesh C
Barzilay E
Belay E
Bern C
BooreA
Brandt M
Bridges C
Buff A
Damon I
Dasch G
Eberhard M
Eremeeva M
Fry A
Gage K
Glynn K
Gottlieb S
Griffin P
Hayes E
Henao O
Herwaldt B
Hicks L
Holmberg S
Iwamoto M
Johnson R
Jones J
Joyce MP
Jumaan A
Kamb M
Kilmarx P
Klevens M
Lammie P

Lynch M
Massung R
Mintz E
Mody R
Moore M
Newman L
Nicholson W
O'Reilly C
Olson C
Patrick M
Peterman T
Reef S
Richards F
Rollin P
Rupprecht C
Schantz P
Seward J
Sheth A
Slutsker L
Sodha S
Spradling P
Staples JE
Sun W
Swerdlow D
Tiwari T
Unger E
Van Beneden C
Visvesvara G
Watson J
Ye Tun
Yu P

World Health Organization
Avenue Appia, CH 1221 Geneva 21, SWITZERLAND

Antal G
Aylward R
Barbeschi M
Bertherat E
Chu M
Connolly M
Cosivi O
Daumerie D
Dayal-Drager R
Decock K
Duclos P
Dziekan G
Engels D
Fontaine O
Fukuda K
Gabrielli A
Hardiman M
Hemachuda T
Karam M
Kindhauser MK
Lavanchy D
Lim M

Lo Fo Wong D
Mendis K
Merianos A
Meslin FX
Mohammadi A
Ndowa F
Otaiza F
Perea W
Pessoa Da Silva C
Previsani N
Qazi S
Raviglione M
Remme J
Resnikoff S
Rietveld A
Roth C
Savioli L
Schlundt J
Shindo N
Simarro P
Strebel P
Thompson D

Chapter reviewers and authors affiliated to other organizations

Arrowood M
Chokephaibulkit K
Chomel B
Chotipanich T
Halperin S
Hartskeel R
Kern P
Knight R
Ko A
Mackenzie J
Mead P
Nielsen HV

Nimmannitr S
Parkin D
Severo L
Sjöstedt A
Smith D
Sylla B
Turnbull P
Ungchusak K
Wattanagoon Y
Wilde H
Yeoh EK

TABLE OF CONTENTS

FOREWORD

Communicable diseases continue to represent a formidable challenge to efforts to ensure the public's health by the professionals who track and contain them. These diseases are a leading cause of morbidity and mortality around the world and remain an enigma to many. The new threats caused by climate change and bioterrorism represent emerging problems that raise the specter of an explosion of new and reemerging infectious diseases. They also represent an opportunity for the global community to work collectively to mitigate this risk.

This new version of *Control of Communicable Diseases Manual* (CCDM), the 19th revision of this 90-year-old favorite of the health community, is available to address these important concerns. The text was initially written in the early 20th century, as a pamphlet for New England health officials, by Dr. Francis Curtis, then the health officer of Newton, Massachusetts. Later, Dr. Robert Hoyt, a health officer from Manchester, New Hampshire, recognized its importance and convinced the American Public Health Association (APHA) at its annual convention in Cincinnati to review, edit, and adopt the text as its own. In 1917, it was published in *Public Health Reports* (32:41:1706–1733), by the United States Public Health Service. Its 30 pages contained disease control measures for the 38 communicable diseases that were then reportable in the United States. It was available from the Government Printing Office for a modest five cents. This manual is now the classic by which all other infectious disease manuals are measured. CCDM has undergone several rewrites over the years. Even the last word in the title was changed from "Man" to "Manual" to remove the perception of gender bias. This text remains a global treasure and continues to be translated into multiple languages.

The five people that have served as editors for the CCDM over the years are to be saluted for their efforts:

Haven Emerson: 1st–7th editions
John Gordon: 8th–10th editions
Abram S. Benenson: 11th–16th editions
James Chin: 17th edition
David L. Heymann: 18th & 19th editions

This updated edition of the CCDM strengthens the value of this text as a global resource. The current editor Dr. David Heymann and his team of experts from around the world continue to maintain the high quality of this text and I thank them for their work. I also want to thank the many men and women who work silently behind the scenes and on occasion have given their lives to contain the threat of infectious disease.

Finally, I would be remiss in not acknowledging the death during the updating of this edition of CCDM of our Director of Publications for the

APHA Press, Mrs. Ellen Meyer. Ellen loved books and CCDM was one of her favorites. As a dedicated professional, mother, wife and community member we honor her memory through this important work.

Georges C. Benjamin, MD, FACP, FACEP(E)
Executive Director
American Public Health Association

PREFACE TO THE NINETEENTH EDITION

This 19th edition of the Control of Communicable Diseases Manual (CCDM) sticks to a tried and tested structure that has been developed over the years since 1916, when Dr Haven Emerson edited the first edition for the American Public Health Association, entitled *Control of Communicable Diseases in Man*.

For this new edition, parallel updates have been carried out on most chapters by experts at both the Centers for Disease Control and Prevention (Atlanta, USA) and the World Health Organization (Geneva, Switzerland), the better to ensure its global relevance. New disease variants are included, and some chapters have been entirely reworked—the chapter on influenza, for example, includes separate sections on seasonal influenza and human influenza of avian/animal origin. New chapters have been added, following feedback from previous editions, in order to keep the manual as relevant as possible in the face of ever-changing public health needs. These new chapters include some topics fundamental to public health, such as infection control and responding to an outbreak report; others that are concerned with public health security in a globalized world, and encompass the International Health Regulations and deliberately-caused infectious disease outbreaks; and still others that provide practical guidance in communicable disease control at mass gatherings, after natural disasters, or in complex emergency situations.

At time of writing, approximately 46% of all deaths in low-income countries are due to communicable diseases. Most occur from just six infectious processes: diarrheal diseases, acute respiratory infections, malaria and measles among children, and AIDS and tuberculosis among adults. These diseases cause severe short- or long-term disability, and are major obstacles to economic development. The chapters that deal with them have been carefully updated by some of the world's best public health experts; and we see that while vaccine development has lagged, anti-infective drugs are available as treatment, as are preventive measures such as bed nets and condoms. Internationally accepted prevention and treatment strategies are presented for these diseases, as they are in each of the book's disease chapters.

The disability-causing communicable diseases, which include polio, leprosy, lymphatic filariasis, Guinea worm, and onchocerciasis, can affect people on every continent. Those most at risk are the less advantaged who often live in economic poverty, and these diseases cause a double economic burden—a burden on the work force, depleted by long-term disability, and a burden on the families and societies upon which the disabled must often depend for support. Anti-infective drugs and vaccines are available for some of these diseases, and the challenge for global public health is to get them to each person in need. The chapters addressing these conditions have been updated to ensure that they represent the most current international consensus on strategies to prevent, control, eliminate, or eradicate.

Finally, the entire world is at risk of the unexpected communicable diseases, those that have been labelled emerging and re-emerging infections during the early 1990s. These are often unpredictable because risk factors for transmission or for change in epidemiology are not clearly understood, or because they are newly identified organisms in humans whose infection is the result of a breach in the animal/human species barrier. Included in this category are communicable diseases that have the potential to occur because of a deliberate attempt to cause harm, as was the case with the outbreak of human anthrax in the United States during 2001, when spores were sent through the United States postal system.

The cause of emerging infections is often viral—as with Ebola and Marburg hemorrhagic fevers, severe acute respiratory syndrome (SARS), and avian influenza (H5N1). In addition to causing human suffering and death, emerging and re-emerging infections place health workers at great risk—not only to their own health, but to that of their families and close contacts, who can serve as the link of communicable disease between hospitals and communities. Like other communicable diseases, emerging and re-emerging infections can cause a heavy economic burden—the costs to countries of the outbreaks of Bovine Spongiform Encephalopathy and the associated new variant of Creutzfeldt Jakob Disease (vCJD) in Europe, and that of avian influenza (H5N1) in Asia, are stark reminders of their impact. Chapters for emerging and re-emerging infections have been updated for this edition the better to reflect international understanding, making them more useful in today's globalized world.

For many of the communicable diseases in this manual, science has given us vaccines and anti-infective drugs that help keep them under control. Nothing demonstrates the effectiveness of vaccines better than the successful eradication of smallpox, and the more recent decreases in polio and measles as mass vaccination campaigns continue to supplement routine immunizations. Likewise, the effectiveness of anti-infective drugs is clearly demonstrated through prolonged life and better health in those infected with viral diseases such as AIDS, bacterial diseases such as tuberculosis, and parasitic diseases such as malaria. But anti-infective drugs are rapidly losing their effectiveness as resistance continues to develop, and a short new chapter on anti-infective drug resistance provides a preview of this increasing public health problem—as do the disease-specific chapters, which are updated with the most recent developments in anti-infective drug use.

It has been a privilege to work with the world's experts in communicable diseases and public health to update this 19th edition of the Control of Communicable Diseases Manual. It has also been a very great sadness to learn of the deaths of two of our colleagues since the 18th edition was published. Dr Aileen Plant, a true field epidemiologist with an immense dedication to public health, died on an assignment in Indonesia while working on issues related to avian influenza. Ellen Meyer, our constant point of reference at the American Public Health Association for work on this Manual, died just as efforts on this edition began to gather momentum. Both represent a huge loss to the world of public health, and we hope to some degree that this Manual will bear testament to the lasting value of their work.

It is my hope—and that of the editorial board and the many experts who have contributed time and effort to updating and writing the new chapters in this 19th edition—that the tradition begun by Dr Haven Emerson in 1916, and continued by editors John Gordon, Abram Benenson and James Chin, has been respected in this latest incarnation of the Manual. It has been our wish throughout the editing process that it remain as relevant and useful as ever to public health professionals around the world.

David L Heymann, M.D.

USER'S GUIDE TO CCDM19

Each disease chapter in CCDM19 is presented in a standardized format that includes the following information:

Disease name: Each disease is identified by the numeric code assigned by the WHO *International Classification of Diseases*, 9th Revision, Clinical Modification (ICD-9 CM) and 10th Revision, ICD-10.

Disease names recommended by the Council for International Organizations of Medical Sciences (CIOMS) and WHO in the *International Nomenclature of Diseases*, Volume II (Part 2, Mycoses, 1st edition, 1982, and Part 3, Viral Diseases, 1st edition, 1983) have been used unless the recommended name has become significantly different from that in current use. In that case, the recommended name is shown as first synonym.

1. **Identification** presents the main clinical features of the disease, and differentiates the disease from others that may have a similar clinical picture. Also noted are those laboratory tests most commonly used to identify or confirm the etiological agent.

2. **Infectious agent** identifies the specific agent or agents causing the disease; classifies the agent(s); and may indicate its (or their) important characteristics.

3. **Occurrence** provides information on where the disease is known to occur and in which population groups it is most likely to occur. Information on past and current outbreaks may also be included.

4. **Reservoir** indicates any person, animal, arthropod, plant, or substance—or combination of these—in which an infectious agent normally lives and multiplies, on which it depends primarily for survival, and where it reproduces itself in such a manner that it can be transmitted to a susceptible host.

5. **Mode of transmission** describes the mechanisms by which the infectious agent is spread to or among humans.

6. **Incubation period** is the time interval between initial contact with the infectious agent and the first appearance of symptoms associated with the infection.

7. **Period of communicability** is the time during which an infectious agent may be transferred directly or indirectly from an infected person to another person; from an infected animal to humans; or from an infected person to animals, including arthropods.

8. **Susceptibility** (including immunity) provides information on human or animal populations at risk of infection, or that are resistant to either infection or disease. Information on immunity subsequent to infection is also given.

9. **Methods of control** are described under the following headings:

A. **Preventive measures:** for individuals and groups.

B. **Control of patient, contacts and the immediate environment:** measures designed to prevent further spread of the disease from infected persons, and specific best current treatment to minimize the period of communicability and to reduce morbidity and mortality.

- Recommendations for isolation of patients depend first on standard (universal) precautions, with specific measures cited from CDC and WHO guidelines available on the internet, and described in more detail in the new *Infection control and antimicrobial resistance* chapter.

- CCDM19 is not intended to be a therapeutic guide. However, current clinical management is presented in section 9B7 in each disease chapter. Specific dosages and clinical management are indicated primarily for those diseases where delay in instituting therapy might jeopardize the patient's life.

- Some of the licensed drugs needed for treatment of rare or novel diseases are available at no cost from WHO, and those which are not licensed may at times be available from CDC as Investigational New Drugs (IND).

- Relevant details, including telephone numbers and e-mail addresses, are entered in section 9B7 for those diseases where such drugs or biologics may be available.

C. **Epidemic measures:** describes those procedures of an emergency character designed to limit the spread of a communicable disease that has developed widely in a group or community, or within an area, state or nation.

D. **Disaster implications:** given a disaster, indicates the likelihood that the disease might constitute a major problem if preventive actions are not initiated.

E. **International measures:** outlines those interventions designed to protect populations against the known risk of infection from international sources. The WHO Collaborating Centres, the CDC, and many national institutions can provide national authorities with the following services: laboratory diagnosis, consultation, analysis of information, production and distribution of standard and reference materials and reagents, training, organization of collaborative research, and provision of further information on specific diseases. WHO can be approached directly for further details about these Collaborating Centres, listed at:

<http://www.who.int/collaboratingcentres/database/en/>

Outbreaks can be electronically reported 24 hours a day by e-mail to:

outbreakwho.int

F. Measures in case of deliberate use of biological agents to cause harm: this section provides information and guidelines for public health workers who may be confronted with a threatened or actual deliberate use of a specific infectious disease agent to cause harm.

The relevant telephone numbers are as follows:

WHO:

- (+41) 22 791 2111

CDC:

- (+1) 770 488 7100
- (+1) 404 639 3311
- (+1) 404 639 2888

The relevant websites are:

WHO:

- <http://www.who.int/csr/delibepidemics>
- <http://www.cdc.gov/>

Outbreaks can be electronically reported 24 hours a day at:

outbreak@who.int

REVIEWING PROCESS

Updating

To update CCDM19 from the 18th edition, a literature review was carried out to identify publications during the preceding five-year period for each disease in that edition. These publications were provided to the chapter reviewers and authors for use in updating the chapter for CCDM19 (2008). For most chapters, parallel updates were carried out by different experts from more than one institution, with the intention of making the CCDM even more internationally relevant and useful than it has been in the past. Additionally, a number of new chapters were added (see below).

The names of the reviewers/authors for each chapter are provided in square brackets at the beginning of the chapters, along with those of the reviewers/authors for CCDM18 on whose work the current update is most recently based. Where they are different, reviewers for the 18th and 19th editions are differentiated by the acronyms CCDM18 and CCDM19 respectively. Disease chapters that did not undergo major updating for the 18th edition but were updated for the 19th will only show the names of the later reviewers. Disease chapters that did not undergo major updating for either edition were reviewed by the Editorial Board for this edition, and are accredited accordingly.

New chapters

Several new chapters have been added for this edition of the Control of Communicable Diseases Manual. These aim to provide an overview of several themes and areas significant for the control of communicable disease—and, where relevant, to point the reader to sources of further information. The new chapters are arranged as follows:

Section I: overarching concerns for surveillance, monitoring, prevention and control of communicable disease outbreaks

1. Communicable disease control and the International Health Regulations (2005)
2. Reporting of communicable diseases
3. Response to an outbreak report
4. Risk assessment and risk management
5. Risk communication during a communicable disease outbreak
6. Communicable disease alert and response during mass gatherings
7. Outbreak response in case of deliberate use of biological agents to cause harm

INTRODUCTION TO NEW CHAPTERS

The following section is new for this edition of the Control of Communicable Diseases Manual. It aims to provide an overview of several themes and areas significant for the control of communicable disease—and, where relevant, to point the reader to sources of further information. The new chapters are arranged as follows.

Section I: overarching concerns for surveillance, monitoring, prevention and control of communicable disease outbreaks

1) Communicable disease control and the International Health Regulations (2005).
2) Reporting of communicable diseases.
3) Response to an outbreak report.
4) Risk assessment and risk management.
5) Risk communication during a communicable disease outbreak.
6) Communicable disease alert and response during mass gatherings.
7) Outbreak response in case of deliberate use of biological agents to cause harm.

Section II: important cross-cutting issues in communicable disease control
8) Infection prevention and control.
9) Mass vaccination in public health.
10) Communicable disease control in humanitarian emergencies.
11) Handling of infectious materials.

COMMUNICABLE DISEASE CONTROL AND THE INTERNATIONAL HEALTH REGULATIONS (2005)

[M. Hardiman]

Background

The 1969 International Health Regulations (IHR 1969) were the principal legally binding global agreement addressing the risks of the international spread of infectious disease. They were implemented by the World Health Organization (WHO), but were limited in scope, as they concerned only four infectious diseases: cholera, plague, yellow fever, and smallpox prior to certification of its eradication. To address these and other shortcomings, the IHR were updated by WHO in 2005 in line with current needs and communication technology, and broadened in scope to address the challenges presented by an increasingly globalized world. At time of writing in early 2008, the newly revised IHR (2005) have entered into force for 194 of the world's countries—all the Member States of WHO.

The IHR (2005) provide broad new mandates and obligations both for participating countries and for WHO, with the following goal:

> ***To prevent, protect against, control, and provide a public health response to the international spread of disease in ways that are commensurate with, and restricted to, public health risks, and which avoid unnecessary interference with international traffic and trade.***

The IHR (2005) are designed to take into account environmental factors that increase the risk from infectious disease including:

- Intensified human encroachment on natural environments.
- Increasing urbanization and crowding of human populations.
- Habitat and climatic alterations that lead to changes in vector density and geographical distribution.
- The continuing extension of international travel and global trade, including food products.
- Changing animal husbandry practices.
- The changing patterns of drug resistance.

The IHR (2005) depend heavily on global surveillance, alert and response activities, which aim to support countries and the international community in identifying and responding to emerging public health risks. In this respect, the IHR (2005) now recognize and mandate the use of outbreak information from a variety of sources, and not only the information officially reported by the country in which the outbreak may be occurring.

The IHR (2005) aim to avoid the stigmatization of particular diseases or of the countries in which they are occurring—factors that proved significant barriers to compliance with the previous regulations.

Finally, the IHR (2005) support the strengthening or re-establishment of public health infrastructures designed to facilitate early recognition of, and rapid response to, emerging disease threats—which, for a variety of reasons, have either never been established or have declined in effectiveness in some parts of the world over recent decades.

The text of IHR (2005) consists of 66 articles and 9 annexes. This chapter addresses only those articles and annexes most directly relevant to the detection of, and response to, communicable disease outbreaks.

Surveillance Under IHR (2005)

The process of global surveillance involves the systematic collection of information from many different sources, its assessment, and taking prompt public health action based on the conclusion. When an event is assessed as a potential public health emergency of international concern (PHEIC), then verification and further information are sought from the affected country. On the basis of the information thus obtained, events may be discarded from consideration, or may undergo continuous risk assessment to monitor ongoing need for further information or response activities. The surveillance-related provisions of the IHR (2005) provide a firm institutional mandate and legal framework for key elements of this process within WHO.

The provisions of the IHR do not of themselves create the basis for any international system of surveillance for specific diseases. Instead, the regulatory requirements—including those for notification to WHO and obligations to respond to WHO requests for verification—aim to identify any public health event that may constitute a public health emergency of international concern (or PHEIC, see below), as determined through a standard decision protocol.

National IHR Focal Points and WHO IHR Contact Points

Under the IHR (2005), urgent communications, including those concerning country reporting, are transmitted to WHO through specific National IHR Focal Points. Each of the six WHO Regional Offices has established an IHR Contact Point for the countries within its respective Region; and as of early 2008, almost all WHO member states have identified National IHR Focal Points.

Notification

A central reporting obligation under the IHR (2005) is the mandatory duty for countries to carry out an assessment of public health events occurring within their territories, in accordance with the decision protocols and criteria found in Annex 2 of the regulations, and then to notify WHO of all qualifying events within 24 hours of the assessment. The events that are to be notified are effectively defined by four criteria in the decision protocol:

1) Whether the event has a serious public health impact.
2) Whether the event is unusual or unexpected.
3) Whether the event risks spreading internationally.
4) Whether the event risks resulting in restrictions on international trade and/or travel.

If an event within a country fulfils two of the four listed criteria, it qualifies as an event that may constitute an international emergency, and so must be notified by that country to WHO, through the National IHR Focal Point. In addition to these criteria, there are a number of sub-questions, and indicative examples of factual contexts, to guide use of the decision protocol.

Consistent with the broad scope of the IHR (2005), the decision protocol—and hence notification—does not require that the event involve a particular disease or type of causative agent (i.e. biological, chemical, or nuclear). The decision protocol was designed to allow the assessment of events where the nature of any disease or agent is still undefined at the time of assessment, and does not exclude events based upon whether they are or may be accidental, natural, or intentional in nature.

While the decision protocol and Annex 2 of IHR (2005) require that all events remain subject to assessment as indicated above, they also specifically require that certain events, involving a limited number of specific diseases that have demonstrated the ability to cause serious public health impact and to spread rapidly internationally, must always be analyzed utilizing the decision protocol. These must be notified if they fulfill the requirements.

The diseases in this category are:

1) Cholera.
2) Pneumonic plague.
3) Yellow fever.
4) Viral hemorrhagic fevers (e.g. dengue hemorrhagic fever, Ebola, Marburg).
5) West Nile fever.
6) Other diseases of special national or regional concern (e.g. dengue fever, Rift Valley fever, and meningococcal disease).

Finally, the IHR (2005) identify four specific disease entities that are always considered unusual or unexpected, and which may have serious public health impact, and hence which always may constitute a public health emergency of international concern. Accordingly, even one case of these diseases must be notified to WHO.

These diseases are as follows:

1) Smallpox.
2) Poliomyelitis due to wild-type poliovirus.
3) Human influenza caused by a new subtype (e.g. H5N1 in humans).
4) Severe Acute Respiratory Syndrome (SARS).

Other Types of Reporting

As a complement to the obligation to notify, the IHR (2005) provide an option for countries to keep WHO informed, on a confidential basis, about events within their territories that are not notifiable as described above, and to consult with WHO on the appropriate responsive health measures. This provision focuses in particular on those events for which there is insufficient available information to complete the decision protocol.

In addition to notification of events within their territories, countries are required to inform WHO within 24 hours of receipt of evidence of a public health risk identified outside their territory that may cause international disease spread, as manifested by exported or imported:

1) Human cases.
2) Vectors carrying infection or contamination.
3) Goods that are contaminated.

The IHR (2005) do not include any provision referring explicitly to reporting suspected intentional or deliberate releases of harmful agents. However, they stipulate that where a country has evidence of an unexpected or unusual public health event within its territory—irrespective of origin or source—that may constitute a public health emergency of international concern, it must provide to WHO all relevant public health information.

Response Under IHR (2005)

The IHR (2005) require WHO to collaborate with countries in the risk assessment and response to public health events whenever they request WHO to do so. Such collaboration can include the provision of technical guidance, assessment of the effectiveness of control measures, and mobilization of international teams either for risk assessment or for control purposes.

WHO's event detection and verification activities provide risk assessment support needed by member states to protect the health of their populations during certain public health events. This support can take the form of different types of assistance to countries already affected by the event, as well as the provision of information regarding the event to countries as yet unaffected. This is so that the latter can take action to prevent their populations from becoming affected, or prepare themselves to take effective response actions should they become affected.

WHO ensures that countries have rapid access to the most appropriate experts and resources for risk assessment and outbreak response, through the Global Outbreak Alert and Response Network (GOARN) of institutions able to provide support and expertise. The GOARN partnership was formalized in April 2000 to improve the coordination of international outbreak responses, and to provide an operational framework to focus the delivery of support to countries. The network's primary aims are as follows:

- To support countries with disease control efforts by ensuring rapid and appropriate technical expertise to affected populations.
- To investigate and characterize events and assess risks of rapidly emerging epidemic disease threats.
- To support national outbreak preparedness by ensuring that responses contribute to sustained containment of epidemic threats.

Since 2000, WHO and GOARN have responded to over 50 events worldwide, with over 400 experts providing field support to some 40 countries. More information can be found on the WHO website at:
<http://www.who.int/csr/outbreaknetwork/en/>

Provision of Information

Providing authoritative information on public health events that have particular international significance is an important part of an effective public health response. WHO manages the information provided by an affected country in ways that both protect that country from unjustified over-reaction by other countries and ensure that other countries are provided with the information they need to protect their populations— including citizens who travel to the affected country/countries.

As part of an incentive to State Parties to notify and report events to WHO, the IHR (2005) guarantee that information in notifications, reports and consultations under the IHR is not made generally available to other countries unless circumstances arise that justify dissemination in order to address the risk of international spread. The contexts that justify communication of the information to other State Parties are clearly specified, and include situations where the Director-General has declared a public health emergency of international concern (see below), where international spread has been confirmed, where control measures are not likely to succeed, and/or where implementation of international control measures is required immediately.

When WHO intends to make such information available to other countries, it has an obligation to consult with the country experiencing the event. WHO may also make information available in the public domain, if other information about the event is already public, and if a need exists for public availability of information that is authoritative and independent.

Public Health Emergencies of International Concern (PHEIC)

The experience gained during the international collaboration to respond to the emergence of Severe Acute Respiratory Syndrome (SARS) led to the inclusion within the IHR (2005) of specific provisions governing actions in response to rare and serious events, which are called Public Health Emergencies of International Concern (PHEIC). The responsibility of determining whether a potential PHEIC falls into this category lies with the Director-General of WHO, acting on the advice of her staff, and requires the convening of a committee of health experts (the IHR Emergency Committee). These experts advise WHO on recommended control measures on an emergency basis, as well as the determination or otherwise of an event as a PHEIC in circumstances where there is inconsistency between the assessment of the Director-General and that of the affected country. The Emergency Committee continues to advise the Director-General throughout the period of the PHEIC, including advising on necessary changes to the recommended measures for control and on the termination of the PHEIC.

Development and Maintenance of Core Surveillance Capacities

One of the most important elements of the IHR (2005) is the requirement for all participating countries to develop and maintain core public health capacities for surveillance and response, in accordance with the functions described in Annex 1 of the Regulations. These core public health capacities must be developed within 5 years of entry into force of the IHR (2005) for each country. For more on surveillance, see the relevant sections in the *Response to an outbreak report* chapter.

Through these requirements, the IHR (2005) seek to ensure that all countries have the basic infrastructure needed in order to undertake the identification and risk assessment of, and response to, outbreaks of disease and other public health events when and where they occur, so that their threat of international spread can be minimized.

Note

This chapter concentrates on those elements of the IHR (2005) that are of relevance to the control of communicable disease, and particularly the recognition of and response to public health events such as disease outbreaks. The IHR (2005) also contain provisions for the routine application of health measures in the context of international travel and transportation in the absence of such events. Where these measures have relevance to a specific communicable disease (such as, for example, those pertaining to the international certificate of vaccination), they are mentioned in the relevant chapter of this book.

The main web page for the International Health Regulations can be found at:
<http://www.who.int/csr/ihr/en/>

REPORTING OF COMMUNICABLE DISEASES
[Editorial Board]

Reporting of selected communicable diseases is required within countries, and in some instances reporting is also required internationally to WHO. Reporting usually takes the form of either a case report or infection reports (some countries only require aggregate reporting), or an outbreak or event report.

> 1) **Case reports:** Case reporting provides diagnosis, age, sex and date of onset for each person with the disease. Sometimes it includes identifying information, such as the name and address of the person with the disease. Additional information, such as treatment provided and its duration, are required for certain case reports.

National legislation or guidelines often indicate which diseases must be reported, who is responsible for reporting, the format for reporting, and how case reports are to be entered into and forwarded within the national system. If there is a requirement for international case reporting (see below), national governments report to WHO.

> 2) **Outbreak or event reports:** Outbreak reporting provides information about an increase in the number of cases above the expected of persons with a communicable disease that may be of public concern. The specific disease causing the outbreak may not be included in the list of diseases officially reportable, or it may be of unknown etiology if it is newly recognized or emerging.

National legislation or guidelines may indicate which types of outbreak must be reported, who is responsible for reporting, the format for reporting, and how case reports are to be entered into and forwarded within the national system. In general, outbreak reporting is required by the most rapid means of communication available. When there is a requirement for outbreak reporting internationally (see below), national governments report to WHO. The diseases listed in CCDM19 are distributed among 5 classes of reporting, referred to by class number throughout the text under section 9B1 of each disease.

Class 1: Case report required internationally to WHO by the International Health Regulations (2005), or as a disease under surveillance by WHO

International Health Regulations (2005)
For more information about the IHR, see the chapter on *International Health Regulations (2005)*.

Diseases under surveillance by WHO
Diseases under surveillance by WHO include:

- Louse-borne typhus fever
- Relapsing fever
- Meningococcal meningitis
- Paralytic poliomyelitis
- Malaria
- Tuberculosis
- HIV/AIDS
- Influenza
- SARS.

For both subcategories in Class 1, case report is required to the WHO through the national health authority. Collective outbreak reports including the number of cases and deaths may be requested on a daily or weekly basis for diseases with outbreak potential, such as influenza.

Class 2: Case report regularly required wherever the disease occurs

Diseases of relative urgency require reporting either because identification of contacts is required, or because the source of infection must be known in order to begin control measures.

National health authorities generally require reporting of the first recognized case in an area, or the first case outside the limits of a known affected local area, by the most rapid means available, followed by weekly case reports— examples include diseases under surveillance by WHO (see above), typhoid fever and diphtheria. National health authorities may also require reports of infectious diseases caused by agents that may be used deliberately, such as anthrax or tularemia.

Class 3: Selectively reportable in recognized endemic areas

Many national health authorities do not require case reporting of diseases of this class. Reporting may be required in instances of undue frequency or severity, in order to stimulate control measures or acquire essential epidemiological data. Examples of diseases in this class are scrub typhus, schistosomiasis and fasciolopsiasis.

Class 4: Obligatory report of outbreaks only—no case report required

Many countries require reporting of outbreaks to health authorities by the most rapid means available. Information required often includes number of cases, date of onset, population at risk and apparent mode of spread. Examples are staphylococcal foodborne intoxication and outbreaks of an unidentified etiology.

Class 5: Official report not ordinarily justifiable

Diseases in this class occur sporadically or are uncommon, often not directly transmissible from person to person (chromoblastomycosis), or of an epidemiological nature that offers no practical measures for control (common cold).

RESPONSE TO AN OUTBREAK REPORT
[Editorial Board]

The response to an outbreak report must include the case management of those infected, and the containment or mitigation of the outbreak by interrupting or reducing transmission of the infectious agent. Public and political reaction, urgency and the local situation may make it difficult, but steps in an outbreak response should be systematic and based on epidemiological evidence. The following provides a minimal list of the steps essential for responding to outbreaks. Often these are undertaken concurrently.

- Verify the diagnosis and establish a case definition.
- Confirm the existence of an outbreak.
- Establish an outbreak control team with a defined role. This team should meet regularly, with minutes of meetings recorded.
- Identify affected persons and their epidemiological characteristics.
- Record typical case histories.
- Identify additional cases.
- Define the population at risk.
- Investigate the outbreak and formulate a hypothesis as to its source and spread.
- Determine the likely control measures.
- Contain or mitigate the outbreak through measures to prevent spread.
- Manage cases.
- Implement control.
- Establish regular communications including with the affected population.

- Conduct ongoing disease surveillance (also called active surveillance).
- Prepare a report and audit the response.

Verify the Diagnosis and Establish a Case Definition

Initial notification of an outbreak is often made by a health worker, who must collect as detailed a history as possible from the initial cases. A tentative differential diagnosis may be made, for example, food poisoning or cholera, that enables the investigator to anticipate the diagnostic specimens required and the kind of equipment to be used during the investigation. The laboratory that will analyze the specimens should be alerted at this stage. If initial cases have died, the extent and need for autopsies should be considered. For surveillance and control purposes, investigators must agree on a common *surveillance case definition* that may not always correspond to the clinical case definition.

Confirm the Existence of an Outbreak

Outbreaks must be confirmed as soon as possible after being reported. Some diseases, although long endemic in an area, remain unrecognized; then new cases may come to light—for instance, when new treatments attract patients who previously relied on traditional medicines. Such "false outbreaks" must be excluded, through attempts at determining the previous incidence or prevalence of the disease.

An outbreak can be demonstrated on a graph of incidence over time, or by a map of geographical extension, or both. For endemic diseases, an outbreak is said to have begun when incidence rises above the normally expected level. For diseases showing a cyclical or seasonal variation, the average incidence rates over particular weeks or months of previous years, or average high or low levels over a period of years, may be used as baselines.

Syndromic Surveillance

"Syndrome" in the context of syndromic surveillance is NOT synonymous with the word "syndrome" in the clinical context: syndromic surveillance is a method of detecting possible outbreaks using health-related information and wide clinical descriptions (e.g. "acute respiratory infection," "bloody stools," and so on) instead of laboratory-confirmed clinical diagnoses. It is based on statistical analysis of short-term data and any deviation from previously determined baseline definitions of what is considered "normal." Case definitions have low specificity but are highly sensitive, and the trigger threshold must be set precisely: too low and resources run the risk of being diverted into investigating false-positives; too high and events could be detected late, or not at all. A good syndromic surveillance system will have the capacity to alter thresholds over time to adapt to different contexts.

Syndromic surveillance is designed to detect outbreaks more quickly than monitoring that is confined to clinically confirmed cases. The advantages offered thereby are speed and sensitivity, and therefore the ability to detect very quickly the possibility of a developing problem, and its broad nature. What syndromic surveillance cannot do is define problems with precision, and its sensitivity means it can produce misleading results, especially in instances where the "syndromes" it picks up can be caused by different infectious agents.

Syndromic surveillance is also useful for eliminating potential problems from consideration. If no further increases occur in the areas highlighted by a syndromic surveillance system once it has resulted in an alert, it can be said that according to this approach no such problem exists, even without laboratory testing and confirmation.

Because of its limitations, syndromic surveillance is really no more than an early warning system: it must be seen as a system to precipitate more thorough investigation of the potential problems it reveals.

Establish an Outbreak Control Team with a Defined Role and Meet Regularly, with Minutes of Meetings Recorded

Once the local responsible person has determined that an outbreak is occurring, they should rapidly establish a team that will investigate and control the outbreak. This team should meet regularly and formally until the outbreak is over, and proceedings should be recorded.

Identify Affected Persons and Their Epidemiological Characteristics

Record Case Histories

Information about each confirmed or suspected case will be recorded to obtain a complete understanding of the outbreak. Depending on the disease, this information includes name, age, sex, occupation, place of residence, recent movements, details of symptoms (including dates and time of onset), and dates of previous childhood immunizations or immunizations against other diseases. Other details will vary with the differential diagnosis. If the incubation period is known, information on possible source contacts may be sought. This information is best recorded on specially prepared record forms called line lists. The logistics of printing forms, data entry and verification must be worked out in relation to reporting (see *Reporting*).

Identify additional cases

Initial notification of an outbreak may come from a single clinic or hospital; enquiries in health centers, dispensaries and villages in the area may reveal other cases, sometimes with a range of additional symptoms.

Define and Investigate the Population at Risk

The population at risk of infection must be identified; this provides the denominator required and ensures that remaining cases can be identified, and defines where surveillance and control measures should be implemented. Overall or specific attack rates (age-specific, village-specific) can then be calculated. These calculations, and the areas of higher incidence (or "hot spots") they reveal, may lead to new hypotheses requiring further investigation and development of study designs. In addition the population at risk may require laboratory investigation (e.g. rate of nasal meningococcal carriage in the population). Microbiological typing and susceptibility to antibiotics can then be used to develop appropriate control measures.

Investigate the Outbreak and Formulate a Hypothesis as to Its Source and Spread

Determine why the outbreak occurred when it did, and what set the stage for its occurrence. Whenever possible, the relevant conditions before the outbreak should be determined. For example, with food-borne outbreaks it is necessary to determine source, vehicle, predisposing circumstances and portal of entry. If transmission is widespread, this may prove difficult. All links in the process must be considered:

1) Disease-causing agent in the population and its characteristics.
2) Existence of a reservoir.
3) Mode of exit from this reservoir or source.
4) Mode of transmission to the next host.
5) Mode of entry.
6) Susceptibility of the host.

Determine the Control Measures

Based on the investigations, the outbreak control team has to decide rapidly on the control measures that need to be implemented, which will depend on the suspected cause and mode of spread. For example, a food-borne infection will require withdrawal of the contaminated food source, and a vaccine preventable disease will require rapid immunization of those at risk.

Contain or Mitigate the Outbreak

The key to effective containment of an outbreak is a coordinated response by the control team and those they represent, including clinicians, epidemiologists, microbiologists, health educators, the public health authority, and the local community. Depending on the nature of the outbreak this can involve a number of other bodies, such as those producing foods (food-borne outbreaks), or the travel industry (an outbreak involving travelers).

Manage Cases

Health workers, including clinicians, must assume responsibility for treatment of diagnosed cases. The nature of this will depend on the infections concerned. In outbreaks of meningitis, plague or cholera, emergency accommodations may have to be found and additional staff may require rapid essential training. Outbreaks of diseases such as sleeping sickness and cholera may require special treatment and recourse to drugs not normally available. The control team must estimate requirements and obtain supplies urgently. Outbreaks such as poliomyelitis will leave in their wake patients with an immediate need for physiotherapy and rehabilitation; timely organization of these services will lessen the impact of the outbreak.

Implement Control Measures to Prevent Spread

Once understanding of the epidemiological characteristics of the outbreak has improved, it is possible to implement control measures to prevent further spread of the infectious agent. However, from the very beginning of the investigation, the investigative team must attempt to limit the spread and the occurrence of new cases.

A number of communicable diseases can be prevented by chemoprophylaxis or vaccination. Immediate isolation of affected persons can prevent spread, and measures to prevent movement in or out of the affected area may be considered. Universal precautions in patient care are essential.

If supplies of vaccines or drugs are limited, it may be necessary to identify the groups at highest risk for initial control measures. Once these urgent measures have been put in place, it is necessary to initiate more permanent ones, such as health education, improved water supply, vector control or improved food hygiene. It may be necessary to develop and implement long-term plans for continued vaccination after an initial campaign.

Establish Regular Communications Including
with the Affected Population

Whatever the urgency of the control measures, they must also be explained to the community at risk. The willingness of the population to engage in such activities as reporting new cases, attending vaccination campaigns, and improving standards of hygiene is critical for successful containment. Equally, there will need to be official reports to the authorities, and through them to regional and international bodies including WHO (see the *Risk communication* chapter).

Conduct Ongoing Disease Surveillance (Active Surveillance)

During the acute phase of an outbreak, it may be necessary to keep persons at risk (e.g. contacts) under surveillance for disease onset. Fever surveillance—daily temperature monitoring—is often a useful form of surveillance to detect cases early in the course of disease. After the outbreak has initially been controlled, continued community surveillance may be needed in order to identify additional cases and to complete containment. Sources of information for surveillance include:

1) Notifications of illness by health workers, community chiefs, employers, school teachers, and/or heads of families.
2) Certifications of deaths by medical authorities.
3) Data from other sources, such as public health laboratories and entomological and veterinary services.

It may be necessary to maintain estimates of the immune status of the population when immunization is part of control activities, by relating the amount of vaccine used to the estimated number of persons at risk, including newborns.

Prepare a Report and Audit the Response

The outbreak control team should record its meetings and update the responsible authority at intervals while control measures are being undertaken. After the outbreak is over, a final report should be prepared, and the response audited. Reports may be:

1) A popular account for the general public, so that members of the public understand the nature of the outbreak and what is required of them to prevent spread or recurrence.
2) An account for planners in the Ministry of Health/relevant local authority, to ensure that the necessary administrative steps are taken to prevent recurrence.
3) A scientific report for publication in a medical journal or epidemiological bulletin (reports of recent outbreaks are valuable aids when teaching staff about outbreak control).

Undertake Experimental Verification of Agent and Mode of Transmission

The verification of hypotheses about an outbreak may at times require experimental evidence of biological feasibility. For example, it may be necessary to show that sliced foodstuffs can be contaminated by an infected slicing machine if this has not been proven during the outbreak investigation. Such verification requires more laboratory facilities than are available in the field, and is often not completed until long after the outbreak has been contained.

RISK ASSESSMENT AND RISK MANAGEMENT
[A. Merianos]

Effective prevention and control of communicable disease outbreaks requires risk assessment, risk management, and risk communication.

Risk assessment is the process of evaluating the probability and consequences of a communicable disease outbreak arising from exposure to identified hazards, and of characterization of the risk to human health. Risk assessment can be qualitative and/ or quantitative, and consists of the following aspects:

1. Hazard and exposure assessments
2. Vulnerability assessment
3. Risk characterization
4. Risk analysis.

Risk management is an iterative process that continues from the identification of a risk before or at the onset of an outbreak, until the point that the risk is controlled. The goal of risk management is to prevent disease transmission, to reduce morbidity and mortality resulting from a communicable disease outbreak, and to reduce the disruptive social and economic effects and political consequences of such an outbreak. The risk management process consists of the following aspects:

1. Options analysis
2. Response to a potential threat or an outbreak
3. Monitoring
4. Response modification.

Risk communication is the provision of information required for decision making to the public, governments, and politicians, before an outbreak occurs or during an event. It is an integral part of the risk management process, and can reduce the social, political and economic turbulence that often occurs when a threat is identified, or during outbreaks. Risk communication is covered more fully in the *Risk communication* chapter, which follows immediately after this one.

I. RISK ASSESSMENT

Risk assessment identifies hazards and the conditions under which transmission of infection and disease can occur, and characterizes the likelihood that these hazards will cause a communicable disease outbreak.

Effective risk assessment allows early identification and proactive management of risk. It also allows public health planners to balance resources —for example, between preparedness for high-probability, low-impact events, and preparedness for low-probability, high-impact events.

Risk assessment can be described as the consideration of "what if" scenarios including the analysis of: what can happen; where, when, why and how could it happen; what will be the impact when it happens; and who can contribute to prevention and/or control.

Identifying disciplines and individuals that need to be involved in an assessment ensures that key information, including that from the "gray" literature or other informal sources, is captured. It also ensures that a good risk assessment team includes the right mix of technical experts and decision-makers.

Although the terminology referring to communicable disease prevention and control varies, all risk assessment approaches include the following elements:

Hazard and Exposure assessments

Hazard assessment is the recognition, characterization and analysis of an infectious agent, and necessitates an understanding of the biological characteristics of that agent. For example, to be effective, such an understanding might have to include the following:

- Virulence
- Transmissibility
- Pathogenesis
- Environmental conditions influencing the growth and survival of the agent, including pH, temperature, humidity, rainfall and vegetation cover
- Data on incidence, prevalence, morbidity and mortality.

Exposure is the potential to become infected, and exposure assessment requires an understanding of such key factors such as:

- The distribution of an infectious agent in the human population, animal population and/or environment of interest. In particular this relates to the threat posed by emerging infectious diseases moving into new ecological niches and the possibilities of trans-boundary movement, in addition to such factors influencing the likelihood of exposure as the presence of disease vectors and animal reservoirs, the extent of human encroachment into animal habitats and vice versa, environmental degradation, and climate change
- Modes of transmission
- Information from previous outbreaks of unknown etiology, which may prove instructive
- Information from outbreaks caused by novel infectious agents, which may also be useful.

Vulnerability assessment involves analyzing the context of disease transmission, focusing on factors that can promote, prevent or mitigate transmission. Such factors can be divided into a number of categories:

Host factors include, but are not limited to, the following:

- Underlying medical conditions causing immunodeficiency
- Malnutrition
- Pregnancy
- Frequency, intensity, nature and duration of past or on-going exposure
- Social factors such as occupation, travel history and population density
- Behavioral factors such as hand washing, respiratory hygiene, sexual behavior and drug use.

Organizational factors include, but are not limited to, the following:

- Effectiveness of health care systems
- Legal requirements (and enforcement) for disease prevention and control services
- Quality and standards for therapeutic agents and biologics
- Water and sanitation measures
- Air quality
- Chemical safety
- Presence, and nature, of vermin
- Food safety standards
- Event-based and indicator-based surveillance systems
- Availability of quality laboratory diagnosis and laboratory biosafety and biosecurity
- Provision for case isolation and quarantine
- Safety of health care workers
- Linkages between human, animal and wildlife health services (given that an estimated 75% of emerging infectious diseases of humans have a zoonotic origin)
- Routine immunization programs for humans and animals
- Vector control.

Societal factors include, but are not limited to:

- Conflict
- Population displacement and migration
- Breakdown of curative and public health services
- Intensive animal husbandry and farming practices.

Risk characterization provides an overall picture of risk based on the hazard, exposure and vulnerability assessments. The level or character of risk can be described either qualitatively, using categories such as 'high', 'medium' or 'low'; or quantitatively, using numerical estimates generated by risk modeling and/or changes in disease incidence, prevalence, morbidity, and mortality.

Risk characterization involves, but is not limited to, the following procedures:

- Developing "problem trees" that identify the pathways between hazard, exposure and vulnerability
- Determining how risks apply to individuals and populations in terms of the types of risk, their extent, and the severity of potential adverse health effects
- Determining the degree of confidence in the assessments
- Scenario consideration and testing when the degree of uncertainty is high.

II. RISK MANAGEMENT

Options analysis and response

Options analysis includes the comparison of risks, setting risk priorities, and deciding on the most appropriate responses. Depending on whether the options analysis aims to identify the best preventive or responsive strategies, the risk management team may choose to:

- Accept low-impact risks (e.g. transmission of common respiratory infections of low virulence)
- Focus preventive and early response activities on managing the reducible component of risks that cannot be completely avoided
- Reduce transmission by decreasing exposure to the infectious agent (e.g. through food or product recalls)
- Decrease community susceptibility to infection and disease by active or passive immunization
- Enhance surveillance by active case finding, and by contact tracing to ensure early identification of those who are exposed
- Communicate about risks in order to promote behavior change
- Focus responses on consequence management and impact mitigation once the outbreak has occurred or spread, by measures such as case management, mass chemoprophylaxis, and social mobilization.

Options analysis should take into account all relevant science, sociopolitical drivers, financial and logistic considerations, and risk communication needs. Scenario building should consider the potential effects of uncertainty arising from missing or incomplete data, variable data quality, and the limitations of the risk model used to inform the risk assessment.

Monitoring and response modification

Monitoring preventive and response measures provides information needed for modifying strategies and activities in mid-course if necessary, and for longer-term program planning and capacity building. Depending on the resources available to undertake monitoring, some or all of the following indicators may be included:

- Cost of, and skills required for, response activities, including human, financial and material resource costs (input indicators)
- Effectiveness of activities such as clinical case management, contact tracing, training, and enhancing surveillance (process indicators)
- Effectiveness of response activities, such as quality of guidelines developed and number of health care workers trained (output indicators)
- Quality of enhanced surveillance, defined by criteria such as number of new cases that occurred after disease control interventions were implemented and appropriateness of any outbreak response (outcome indicators)
- Estimated number of cases prevented, and social, economic and political consequences caused or averted (impact indicators).

In addition, the monitoring process should also consider possible unintended consequences of intervening, consequences of failing to intervene, and ethical considerations of the impact of public health measures (such as case quarantine, for example) on the population at risk.

RISK COMMUNICATION DURING A COMMUNICABLE DISEASE OUTBREAK
[M. K. Kindhauser, D. Thompson]

THE OUTBREAK COMMUNICATION ENVIRONMENT

Uncertainty

Communication with the public during a communicable disease outbreak is critical not only for the rapid control of the outbreak, but also for reducing the social, political and economic turbulence that often attend outbreaks. The uncertainty that surrounds many communicable disease outbreaks breeds speculation, and a public eager for explanations may turn for information to those who are informed or those who are not.

Such outbreaks are unfolding events. Initially, their cause may be uncertain, and the geographical region of harm may not be known for weeks or months. They unfold in ways that are unpredictable. Setbacks and surprises are common in outbreaks—among other things, treatments may fail if drug resistance develops, or reluctance to take drugs or vaccines may occur among populations thought to be at risk; new risk groups are often identified; and methods of transmission may change, or appear to do so. As has been learned in many events concerning Ebola or other less common pathogens, even when outbreaks seem to be coming under control, new foci of disease can suddenly emerge as cases escape contact tracing, or through lapses in hospital infection control.

Consequently, the information provided to the public may have to be modified one day and corrected the next. In 1999, for example, initial information led public health authorities in New York City to identify the source of a mosquito-borne outbreak as St. Louis encephalitis; shortly afterwards, it was determined to be the first appearance of West Nile virus. Shifting information can undermine the public's confidence in authorities — but this does not have to be the case.

It must be remembered that if communication is not carried out with uncertainties in mind, public health workers may be held accountable unfairly when their communications are found to be wrong in light of evolving information and changing circumstances.

Anxiety

Anxiety can run high in the speculative and unpredictable environment of a communicable disease outbreak. Public reaction to anxiety can result in social and economic disruptions that are out of proportion to the true degree of risk faced. For example, during the SARS outbreak in 2002–2003, the widespread unnecessary wearing of masks and cancellation of travel to unaffected but neighboring countries was observed in many situations, as was stigmatization of certain ethnic groups. In an environment of anxiety, stigmatization can magnify existing social discord. Another consequence of public anxiety can be seen in the significant shifts in consumer consumption patterns such as those caused by avoiding chicken in the diet during recent outbreaks of avian influenza in poultry; these shifts have in turn caused enormous and unfounded economic damage to farmers and the food industry.

Less well appreciated by risk communicators is the "fear of fear" among outbreak managers and policymakers themselves—that is to say, the fear of triggering or exacerbating economic and/or social damage. This reluctance can profoundly influence those making decisions on whether and when to communicate.

Information Management

Uncertainty and anxiety often turn outbreaks into high-profile media events. With intense attention from the press magnifying threats to the economy, international relations and even social stability, outbreaks often take on a powerful political dimension. Communication decisions are frequently erroneously transferred from health authorities to political leaders or their media advisers.

Outbreaks are complex communication environments. Information at the start of an outbreak is often incomplete, and sometimes wrong, and decisions must sometimes be made with inadequate information. Perceived risks may be high for economies, affected populations and politicians, and those making decisions about public health communication may not have a background in communicable diseases, or even in public health.

Impact

The impact of most communicable disease outbreaks can be thought of much like a hurricane, with a relatively limited damage zone, but with knock-on impacts that reach a much broader area. The center is the outbreak itself, and the wider damage is inflicted through negative economic impact, social turbulence and political upheaval. When severe acute respiratory syndrome, or SARS, killed 800 people in 2003, it caused around $30 billion worth of economic damage, fear and panic in certain communities, and the forced change of a number of political leaders. The outbreak of bovine spongiform encephalopathy (BSE) in the UK in the early 1990s cost billions and led to a major public enquiry. A confirmation of BSE in the United States—one single cow confirmed with the infection—was estimated to cost the economy US $2 billion. Outbreaks of cholera in Peru and Tanzania resulted in embargoes on trade in seafood and decreases in tourism that likewise caused severe economic impact in the millions of dollars.

All this collateral damage, or the fear of it, can wrongly drive communications during outbreaks. In these circumstances, messages are frequently aimed at avoiding the damage associated with the outbreak rather than communicating about the outbreak itself. As a result, decision-makers might wait too long to announce further details about an outbreak, and when finally forced to comment, might provide overly reassuring comments or choose to conceal troubling aspects of the situation. All these factors have been shown to later exacerbate the impact of an outbreak.

OUTBREAK COMMUNICATION GUIDELINES

Five elements are strongly associated with successful communication when they are present, and strongly associated with failure when they are not:

1) Trust
2) Early announcement
3) Transparency
4) Listening
5) Operational planning.

Trust

The overarching goal during an outbreak is for public health experts dealing with the outbreak, and those communicating with the public, to communicate in ways that build, maintain or restore trust. This is a fundamental issue that applies across cultures, economies, and different types of outbreaks. Behavioral research confirms that the less trust there is in public health experts dealing with communicable disease outbreaks, the more concerned the general public becomes. The best time to build trust is before it is needed: prior to outbreaks.

Trust in outbreak communication impacts directly on the public perception of the motives, honesty and competence of public health experts managing an outbreak, and the political officials on whom they depend for support. Important questions related to the following factors may be asked by those affected by, or at risk from, the outbreak:

- **Motives** – Are the outbreak responders acting first and foremost to safeguard my health and the health of my family?
- **Honesty** – Are the outbreak responders holding back information or downplaying information to reduce anxiety?
- **Competence** – Are the outbreak responders skilled enough to do the job?

If the public does not trust the source, they will not trust the message. There is compelling evidence demonstrating that when authorities are trusted, the public perceives lower levels of threat. More importantly, when trust is high, so is public acceptance of official advice.

Trust, then, is the currency of outbreak communication. It is either earned or spent with each public communication during an outbreak. The goal is to have a reservoir of trust, because mistakes will almost inevitably be made in communicating during an outbreak, and it will be necessary to draw on that reservoir.

Announce Early

The parameters of trust are established in the first official announcement of an outbreak. The timing, candor and completeness of this announcement will play a role in how much trust the public subsequently places in public health officials.

There are many advantages to announcing early, in addition to laying the foundation for trust, including the following:

- Early announcement can encourage correct protective behaviors.
- It can stimulate greater or more effective surveillance and generate more information about the outbreak.
- It demonstrates leadership.
- It fills the information vacuum, which will otherwise be filled by less informed sources.
- It helps officials to frame the outbreak before others do.
- If it leads to effective action it will reduce the size of the incidence.

A good example of best practice was provided in 2001 by the response of the authorities in New York City, USA, to an anthrax attack. City Hall was notified of the laboratory confirmation of the city's first attack at 10 pm; after a brief consultation, the authorities opted for early announcement of the results at an 11:30 pm press briefing.

New York's anthrax announcement was a rarity, however. In the age of 24-hour news coverage and text messages, governments are often caught unaware by media reports of an outbreak, and it must be borne in mind that the first official announcement may not necessarily be the first the public has heard of an outbreak. Nevertheless, the public will still decide how much trust to place in officials according to the timing, candor and completeness of the official response.

Public health officials and their technical staff are often understandably reluctant to make announcements based on information that is incomplete and subject to change. In other words, unfortunately, the kind of information that is characteristic of the early stages of an outbreak. There are, however, communication techniques that allow officials to deal with uncertainties in public announcements.

Quick Release

In considering how quickly to release the first information about an outbreak, it should be remembered that the longer public health officials withhold worrisome information, the more frightening the information will seem to be when it is revealed, especially if it is first revealed by an outside source. Delay contributes to decreasing public trust, which reduces public acceptance of eventual recommendations for outbreak management. The desire for certainty should not become an excuse for delayed warning.

Accurate Reassurance

A further common communication pitfall associated with first announcements is over-reassurance. In the early days of an outbreak, when anxiety is running high and speculation abounds, public health officials sometimes provide unjustified reassurance to the public, to mitigate the impact of the first announcement. While this reassurance can ring hollow, officials will suffer no loss of trust if the outbreak produces no surprises; but outbreaks often produce surprises, and unfounded assurances will undermine trust as the outbreak unfolds.

Assessing Information Quality

It is a mistake to be overly confident about the quality of tenuous information. It should be explained clearly when communicating that the information made public is likely to change as more is learned. As that information does change, changes should be announced quickly, with acknowledgment of previous reports.

Transparency

Transparency is a widely recognized method for building trust, while a lack of transparency will undermine trust. Transparent communication means communication that is easily understood, complete, and free of misleading information. Outbreak communicators should aim for complete openness, and should provide good reasons for those instances in which they cannot be totally candid.

Total transparency will not, however, automatically lead to trust: for example, informing passengers on an aircraft that a member of the cockpit crew has just died may not instill trust in the remaining members of the crew. Transparency builds trust best when it reveals that the people managing the outbreak are competent.

Total transparency is a theoretical goal. In practice, transparency is a balancing act: there are some things that, it is broadly agreed, should not be made public in an outbreak or public health setting. Such things include confidential data about patients, information that could lead to discrimination against patients and their families, and information that has no public health benefit.

Transparency may also be difficult in meetings, including those meetings focusing on risk analysis and policy development. To enhance confidence in these critical processes, it is vital to ensure that clear records are maintained, to justify decisions reached and to describe where and how differences of opinion have arisen. The record should also note where assumptions and uncertainties have shaped conclusions. Participants in these meetings should be informed that their discussion will be on the record, and that that record may be used later in a "lessons to be learnt" analysis of the how the outbreak was managed.

Probably the most significant barrier to transparency is fear on the part of public health officials that they, or those for whom they are responsible, will be punished as a result of having been transparent. Indeed, this is often the case: During recent outbreaks of avian influenza, many countries suffered harsh economic losses in their poultry industries when outbreaks were reported.

While reasonable lines may be drawn to limit transparency, they should not become excuses for secrecy. One method for identifying reasonable limits is to inform the public of those things that they will not be told, explaining why certain information is kept confidential, such as information that identifies individuals. If the public disagrees, it will soon become apparent, and a measured reaction can be formulated.

As far as early announcement is concerned, there is a very compelling argument for transparency in the fact that, in this age of instant communication, it is nearly impossible to conceal threatening information for long anyway. Once hidden information is revealed, officials are left not only to explain the threat, but also to explain why they have tried to cover it up. Such forced admissions are difficult, embarrassing, and damaging to public trust.

Transparency may play a special role when resources are limited. During an influenza pandemic, for example, large populations will be at risk while resources such as vaccines and antivirals may not be sufficient to cover an entire population (or, in many countries, may not be available at all). Furthermore, certain measures, including home quarantine or cancellation of mass gatherings, may heighten public concern about response efforts. Under such circumstances there is a clear need for transparency—to demonstrate fairness in allocation of scarce resources—and for maintaining trust, to ensure that response control measures are followed.

To summarize, transparency is essential in order to ensure public acceptance of important information, and as a practical measure for ensuring trust. It should be the default option for all decisions about communication, and any instances where transparency is inadvisable must be clearly explained.

Listening (Communication Surveillance)

A survey of outbreak literature indicates that some approaches have been shown clearly to have failed in the past. The first of these is the so-called "decide and announce" method whereby, essentially, experts tell the world that something is, or is not, important. This approach has failed in numerous situations, and it was initially assumed that the failure was because the public was scientifically illiterate. The approach was therefore modified to include an education component, but this also proved less than effective in convincing the public, and it became apparent that the "decide and announce" model was flawed in a more fundamental way.

This one-way risk communication model has been replaced by dialogue, changing from a model of one-way information transfer to one of discussion: listening to the public, understanding its objections, identifying points of confusion, and responding to public concerns. Best practice assumes it is impossible to build public trust—particularly with an audience that may be wary of messages and/or the institutions they come from—if it is not known what the public is thinking and hearing.

One of the hardest parts of risk communication is **listening without judgment**. In a technical world filled with rational scientists and other experts, the reaction of the public after hearing troubling news may be considered irrational, and perceived as a challenge. Approaching public dialogue by attempting to address such a perceived irrational audience is wrong and paternalistic. It is also generally ineffective. The concerns and assessments of the public must be viewed as legitimate. Listening must be a major task of the public health communicator. Also known as **communication surveillance**, this is mainly done through monitoring of media reports. In some instances, though, communication surveillance may need to reach out directly to concerned audiences—particularly critics—in order to understand their concerns more accurately.

Listening to the public expands the role of outbreak communicators. Communication becomes a task not only of understanding what the public is thinking, but of bringing that understanding into communication strategy.

Operational Planning

Communication

Those making critical communication decisions during an outbreak are rarely communicators themselves; therefore, it is essential that decision makers have time to evaluate their decisions. While methods like announcing early or aiming for total transparency can increase trust, they may seem counterintuitive to some decision-makers; therefore, communicators should be able to explain clearly why these methods should be supported. It is much easier to do, and will seem much less risky, if thorough analysis and discussion can take place when an outbreak is still only a theoretical possibility.

Training and Procedures

Operational planning should ensure that people are trained and procedures established before they are needed. Guides and checklists on effective communication during a pandemic can be obtained at:
    <http://www.who.int/csr/resources/publications/WHO_CDS_2005_31/en/index.html>

Summing Up

The components of successful public health communication can be summed up by the acronym TOTAL which encompasses the five elements strongly associated with successful risk communication:

Trust
Operational planning
Transparency
Announce early
Listening.

Based on current information, TOTAL represents best communication practice for communicable disease outbreaks. Public health officials must report, fully and rapidly, what they know, what they suspect, and what they are doing; and they must listen to the responses of the public. In the high-risk environment of an outbreak, they must strive to ensure that these best practices are not bypassed by politicians wishing to control the press. Outbreak communicators are many things: they are ears, listening to subtle public conversation; they are the representatives of the public in internal meetings; they are trainers and planners; they are lobbyists for transparency; and, most of all, they are the guardians of trust. The work of outbreak communicators must ensure that each public message, even in times of calm, strengthens the public's trust.

COMMUNICABLE DISEASE ALERT AND RESPONSE DURING MASS GATHERINGS

[M. Barbeschi]

Introduction

Mass gatherings are events in which large numbers of people come together for a common goal or purpose. A communicable disease outbreak at a mass gathering has the potential to overwhelm the public health system of the community or country in which the mass gathering is occurring. Even when public health and other support services are adequate to detect and respond to communicable disease outbreaks in the community, they may not be able to provide adequate support when there is an influx of large numbers of people (national and/or international). Planning for mass gatherings should therefore include risk assessment for communicable disease outbreaks, and planning for management of those risks.

Risk Asessment

Gatherings of people from within the same country may increase the risk of outbreaks from communicable diseases caused by indigenous pathogens. Gatherings that draw visitors from different nations, regions and cultures, however, have the potential for importation of communicable disease pathogens that are not present in the host community, and which may require public health expertise not normally available. In addition, responses to such outbreaks may require accommodating the needs of populations with differing languages, social norms and customs.

Systematic risk assessment helps identify potential outbreak risks and guides the establishment of realistic risk management goals. Sporting events or rock concerts, for example, may have risks associated with alcohol abuse, drug abuse leading to acute blood-borne infections from unsafe injecting practices, or increased transmission of sexually transmitted infections. The risk management goal in such instances would be reduction of risk by ensuring that prevention measures and counseling services are made available, and that those who are infected receive treatment and support.

Religious and/or faith healing gatherings might attract a significant number of the ill and infirm, some of whom could have communicable diseases with the potential to spread to others. Large religious gatherings place pilgrims in very close contact with one another for days, and can impose potential additional risks (such as sleeping outside and increasing risk of hypothermia or hyperthermia if held in inclement circumstances). These may require *ad hoc* risk communication strategies (teenagers are generally reluctant to absorb strict guidance); for more information, see the *Risk communication* chapter. Likewise, gatherings of senior citizens may increase the risk and seriousness of respiratory or other communicable disease outbreaks. Risk management goals at such events would be for the provision of facility-based health care in addition to preventive measures.

Of particular concern are mass gatherings at which food is available. These may require special food services to prevent outbreaks caused by contaminated food, along with—as at all mass gatherings— considerations of water safety and sanitation.

Finally, in addition to assessing the risk of naturally occurring outbreaks, systematic risk assessment will also help identify vulnerabilities that could increase the potential for deliberately caused public health risks that require interaction with security and other government agencies (for more information, see the chapter on *Deliberate use of biological agents to cause harm*).

The risk assessment framework and methodology for communicable disease outbreaks are provided in the *Risk assessment and risk management* chapter. Some of the specific information required for successful risk analysis in advance of a mass gathering could take the form of a checklist including the following considerations:

General Features of the Gathering

- Age and sex of those likely to participate.
- Likely number of participants and countries of provenance.
- Season in which the gathering will occur.
- Potential insect and animal vectors present.
- Quality of water and sanitation services.
- Likely food vendors, if any.
- Features of the hosting location and venues (e.g. geographic/regional features, climate and weather, relevant language(s), population/ethnic groups, customs/traditions, social considerations, security).
- Movement of population and visitors, accommodation, displacement or overcrowding.
- Political, systemic or other vulnerabilities that could lead to deliberately-caused communicable disease outbreaks.

Specific Communicable Disease Information

- Indigenous infectious agents circulating in local populations, and in other populations likely to participate, including relevant animal data (epizootics with human cases).
- Potentially imported infectious agents.
- Health intelligence obtained by reviews of available health information (at regional and international level), and from history of outbreaks during previous mass gatherings.
- Vaccine coverage/immunity levels for common infections controllable by vaccination.

Diseases that are important causes of outbreaks at mass gatherings, based on past experience, include those that are highly infectious and have modes of transmission likely to be enhanced by close person-to-person contact and breaks in safe water supply or sanitation and unsafe foods. Diseases with these characteristics should be considered of high priority during risk assessment.

If risk assessment has suggested political or other vulnerability to deliberately caused outbreaks, links should be planned and operationally tested with agencies dealing with criminality (for more information, see the list of agents with potential for deliberate use in the chapter on *Deliberate use of biological agents to cause harm*).

Risk Management and Planning

Effective management of risks of communicable disease outbreaks in mass gatherings requires advance planning. The *Risk communication* chapter describes the risk management process for outbreaks and the importance of identifying outbreaks early, and the importance of responding in a timely manner in order to decrease the size of the outbreak and its consequent morbidity and mortality, and to reduce its social, economic and political costs. For outbreaks in mass gatherings the same requirements hold true, and risk management activities should be planned in order to ensure that the necessary services and resources are available. Risk management during a mass gathering is complicated by high event visibility, which may result in political and media pressure that affects the decision-making process.

In particular, planning for mass gatherings should ensure the following:

- Surveillance and outbreak alert systems, including a system to manage surveillance information, are established to identify risks or actual outbreaks. If these surveillance systems are not in place before the events occur, interpretation of information will be difficult, because of the lack of baseline data.
- Health services are adequately equipped to offer preventive services and to deal with an outbreak should it occur, and linked with other services, such as those responsible for personal security, food safety, sanitation and water.
- Contact tracing/quarantine measures are planned well in advance.
- Provisions are made for management of dead bodies (see the chapter on *Communicable diseases in humanitarian emergencies*).
- Outbreak communications and counseling capacity are adequate to cope with projected needs (see the *Risk communication* chapter).
- A set of standard operating procedures has been developed that ensures that all involved in outbreak management understand their roles so they can work closely together during the mass gathering.
- Ensure support to outbreak control after the end of the mass gathering, including assistance to the sick after the event is concluded, and providing information on the risks/outbreaks to relevant other countries and to transport hubs and airline/transport companies taking attendees home.

Finally, a budget should be prepared for any necessary reinforcement in infrastructure or health manpower, and training should be provided to health staff and others as required, in order to ensure adequate detection, investigation and response capacity for potential outbreaks.

Legacy of Planning

Care should be taken to ensure that planning maximizes the *legacy* of the mass gathering: while some investments made during the planning phase may be beneficial only for the duration of the mass gathering, others will provide permanent benefit to public health infrastructure.

Since the investments may be costly, decision makers should clearly understand which lasting benefits will result, and ensure that investment in advance will prevent greater, non-necessary cost in future, should an outbreak occur.

Surveillance and Outbreak Alert

Planning for communicable disease surveillance should preferably build on pre-existing routine systems for infectious diseases surveillance and notification. Surveillance should already be in place to provide baseline data, and systems should be based on case definitions of the indigenous and/or potential imported disease risks identified, while at the same time ensuring detection of other events should they occur. It should be pro-active, and preferably based on an electronic platform so that communication can occur as rapidly as possible.

A major component of alert systems is an event management system that provides the electronic platform, electronic tools, and procedures required to manage information about communicable diseases in a format permitting verification, risk assessment, and data management in a single, reproducible process. Processing of information during the daily routines of the mass gathering, including information protection and its necessary distribution, should also be planned and tested.

Public health laboratory support is vital to surveillance. Laboratories should be capable of identifying known pathogens, especially those circulating in the country where the mass gathering is held and among populations that may travel to the mass gathering from other geographic and climatic areas. They should also maintain valid internal and external quality control, and have provisions for safe and reliable transport and storage of samples, with a capacity that exceeds normal demands.

In the absence of suitable national laboratories, an international laboratory should be identified that can provide the relevant training and/or services, and guidelines for the transfer of specimens between laboratories.

The international transit of large numbers of travelers may require the host nation to report under the International Health Regulations (2005). Instances in which this may be necessary include:

- Those concerning relevant domestic and international detection and reporting requirements for the host nation.
- Those concerning the quarantine, surveillance, inspection and medical examination rights and reporting obligations of other states that

may be receiving international travelers or transport from the host nation.

For more information on the International Health Regulations, see the dedicated chapter.

Health Services

The tasks of ensuring prevention and patient management services require robust health services. Some of the specific aspects required in such services could take the form of a checklist including the following considerations:

- Quality first line prevention and patient management services, including counseling.
- Number of emergency medical staff.
- Geographical proximity to the mass gathering site.
- Sufficient surge capacity.
- Transport to other medical facilities.
- Supplies for prevention.
- Medicines or vaccines that correspond to potential risks.
- Reliable diagnostic laboratory support.
- Safety of water supplies, sanitation and food.
- Sustainability for the duration of a potential outbreak or during a prolonged period of heightened alert.
- Availability of language interpreters/experts on other cultures if gathering is international.
- Capacity for rapid mobilization of equipment, infection control messages and use of fact sheets and tools (these may need translation).
- Capacity to supply and quickly distribute potentially large quantities of supplies (e.g. blankets, food, clothing) safely and securely.

Functions that the health services should provide in addition to outbreak investigation include patient management and outbreak containment, and are described more fully in other chapters. Certain of these functions—such as infection control, contact tracing, quarantine, management of dead bodies and outbreak communication—are, however, of a different magnitude and complexity when outbreaks occur in a mass gathering. The following section describes these functions more fully in the context of mass gatherings.

Infection Control

Increased numbers of people seeking medical care during a mass gathering may result in breakdowns in infection control procedures and capacities, especially when personnel resources are stretched. Infection control measures (see also the chapter on *Infection prevention and control*) may be necessary at health posts, venues, accommodations, hospitals and other medical facilities where large-scale isolation of patients may potentially be required following an outbreak of infectious disease, as well as in transport hubs, at airports, on buses and trains, and so on.

It is important for public health professionals in such scenarios to protect uninfected patients and contacts housed in common settings. Demographic factors such as language and culture also impact infection control at medical facilities when visitors seek and/or receive care. A vital part of control of disease outbreaks in mass gatherings is the provision of information about the outbreak and disease avoidance procedures to those visitors who are uninfected or asymptomatic, and the problems of language and culture should be taken into account when planning this part of the process.

Contact Tracing/Quarantine

Contact tracing and quarantine measures such as fever surveillance (daily checking for temperature by contacts) require close links with the following:

- Air and other types of public transport systems, and their hubs.
- Hotels, hostels, boarding houses and camping grounds.
- Diplomatic missions and embassies if participants or other patients have come from other countries.
- Law enforcement authorities, to help locate and identify contacts.
- Systems and records detailing people's movements.

As part of the planning process, all these should be linked together, with agreements prepared in advance for their mutual operation in the event of an outbreak.

Contact tracing could in some instances lead to the need for mass drug or vaccine prophylaxis, and plans and supplies for mass prophylaxis should also be developed based on the outcome of the risk assessment (see the chapter on *Mass vaccination in public health* for further information).

Management of Dead Bodies

Dead bodies should be handled as described in the Management of dead bodies section of the *Communicable disease control in humanitarian emergencies* chapter, and according to the rites and customs prescribed by the relevant religions or cultures. Religious or other leaders who could perform these rites should be identified during the planning process. Emergency mortuary facilities may be required, and should likewise be identified during the planning process, as should the availability of pathologists, including those with forensic skills, especially if bodies are not readily recognizable. Some dead bodies will require repatriation involving international transport carriers, and planning should include relevant consultations and agreements in advance.

Outbreak Communication

Outbreak communication at a mass gathering follows the normal procedures described in the *Risk Communication* chapter. Multiple language capability may be required for international mass gatherings, and this should be planned for in advance. Communication may be especially important in assuring populations at the mass gathering that risks are being dealt with in an effective and rapid manner. Past experiences have shown the need to arrange the feeding of pre-determined routine risk management-related information to the press once or twice daily.

Counseling

A disease outbreak or other health emergency occurring during a mass gathering may lead to an increased demand for psychological support services from those who are affected, and also those who fear they are at risk. Such demand may be magnified if the outbreak is particularly widespread, has severe health impact, or is the result of a deliberate act. Counseling services need to be planned for persons who have been directly affected by disease, or who have been identified as potentially exposed or otherwise at risk; and also for persons not directly affected but nonetheless having an emotional or mental health response that requires psychological support. Examples of the latter group may include friends and family of patients at home, participants not at any known risk, and medical and/or other staff responding to the outbreak.

Religious leaders, counselors and social workers who are available to provide counseling may need to respond by telephone, and may require assistance from organizations such as the International Federation of Red Cross and Red Crescent Societies.

Standard Operating Procedures

Because many different public health and other community/government services are required for a response to a communicable disease outbreak at a mass gathering, planning should include a mechanism to ensure that preparation and response are well-coordinated. In most large gatherings, several operational units and command posts operate contemporaneously, and many of the necessary public health tasks during an outbreak may require decision-making at a level with authority over all of them.

Carefully prepared and tested standard operating procedures that clearly outline the role of each of the required services are a good way of assuring coordination, and a pre-established operations center can provide the necessary coordination and command/control required for these procedures. A network of liaison officers in each command post facilitates the information sharing necessary for decision-making in operations centers.

For further information and guidance on the issues contained in this chapter, see:

<http://www.who.int/csr/mass_gathering/en/index.html>

OUTBREAK RESPONSE IN CASE OF DELIBERATE USE OF BIOLOGICAL AGENTS TO CAUSE HARM
[BIOTERRORISM, BIOLOGICAL WARFARE]
[M. Barbeschi]

Intentional releases of biological agents remain a threat in many contexts, and are a public health risk of potential importance both nationally and internationally. The sociopolitical implications of deliberate events may require national health agencies to collaborate with security agencies in response, because of the change in the context in which public health services are to be delivered due to widespread fear, the potential for multiple attacks, high visibility of the event, and co-investigation with law enforcement. Capacity for managing the health risks of potential outbreaks involving the deliberate use of pathogens or toxins is based on the capacity of the health care system, emergency management, security and other sectors to coordinate planning, and should be built into the planning for outbreak alert and response.

The risk of deliberate use cannot be quantified or predicted, but the importance of the public health response is enormous—as was shown in the USA in October 2001, when anthrax spores were deliberately distributed through the postal system, causing 22 infections and five deaths. The public health response included identifying all those at risk of infection through the postal system, and prescribing antibiotics to over 32 000 persons identified as potentially in contact with envelopes contaminated with anthrax spores. It also involved emergency and law enforcement services in the USA and around the world, where numerous false alarms occurred simultaneously, and the event and associated hoaxes caused unprecedented demands on public health laboratory services. Several nations had to recruit private laboratories to deal with the overflow.

Public health security efforts will facilitate the assessment of public health risks during an outbreak, and will contribute to keeping countries' health and emergency policies in line with actual or perceived threats. By leveraging the public health security role, national and international organizations will find solutions that do not compromise the traditional impartiality and independence of the public health and medical sectors.

The approach to international public health security anticipates future challenges, in particular in relation to the implementation of the revised International Health Regulations (IHR 2005) and the WHO Strategy for Global Health Security (which can be found in the WHO World Health Report 2007 on Global Health Security, available directly from WHO).

Key Issues to Consider

A deliberately caused outbreak at a mass gathering or event of other significance has the potential to overwhelm the public health system of the community or country in which the event is occurring (for more information, see the chapter on *Communicable disease alert and response during mass gatherings*). If the biological agent in question is widely dispersed and/or easily transmissible, capacity may be required to cope with large numbers of patients, and systems must be available for the rapid mobilization and distribution of medicines or vaccines according to the agent released. In certain types of outbreaks, alternative models of response should be considered: for example, should a stadium host an outbreak of a highly communicable disease, it may be necessary to bring clinical capacity to the location of the outbreak rather than transporting contaminated and infectious people and substances through the transport systems of a major city and into a health care facility, the capacity of which could thus be compromised or overwhelmed. An inappropriate response runs the risk of multiplying the infection rather than controlling it.

In the event that the agent is transmissible, additional capacity will be required for contact tracing and active surveillance. Incubation period, period of communicability and susceptibility are agent-specific. Some of the infectious agents of concern include bacteria and rickettsia (anthrax, brucellosis, melioidosis, plague, Q fever, tularemia, and typhus), fungi (coccidioidomycosis) and viruses (arboviruses, hemorrhagic fever viruses and variola virus). International threat analysis considers that deliberate use of biological agents to cause harm is a real threat that can occur at any time. Such risk analysis is not, however, generally considered a public health function. A more complete illustrative list of agents with potential for deliberate use follows later in this chapter.

Prevention of the deliberate use of biological agents presupposes accurate and up-to-date intelligence about deliberate users and their activities. The agents may be manufactured using equipment necessary for the routine manufacture of drugs and vaccines, and the possibility of dual use of these facilities adds to the complexity of prevention. This has led many analysts to regard a strong public health infrastructure, with rapid and effective detection and response mechanisms for naturally occurring infectious diseases of outbreak potential, as an essential part of a society's response to the threat of deliberately caused outbreaks of infectious disease.

The deliberate release of a biological agent may occur overtly or covertly. If the release of a biological event is perpetrated overtly in the setting of an "announced event," it may result in immediate mass hysteria. Such an occurrence, whether related to a real event, to a hoax or to a perceived event, could quickly overwhelm and incapacitate an entire health care system if not managed quickly and appropriately.

The first indication of a covert biological attack could be the inexplicable and rapid onset of respiratory distress and incapacitation of victims—and early response should take into account the possibility of the accidental release of a toxic agent. Symptoms may be masked in the first instance if the release is accompanied by an explosion and attendant trauma and panic. Alternatively, if the biological agent has been administered to food or beverage supplies at a mass gathering, the first symptoms will be more typical of rapid onset food poisoning. It is unlikely that the sequelae of a deliberate attack at a short duration mass gathering will manifest themselves before the attendees depart, so symptoms are more likely to develop in a disseminated population. Exposure would most likely manifest itself some time after the event—not sooner than 1–2 days later—through the victims or clusters of victims developing atypical symptoms and conditions detected by clinical observation supported by hospital laboratory diagnosis and/or epidemiological surveillance.

Key considerations related to the health risks of deliberate use of pathogens or toxins include:

- The fact that the alert and response mechanism for dealing with suspected or confirmed deliberate events is a specific contextual use of the alert and response plans covering any significant naturally occurring event (e.g. SARS, avian influenza).
- The need to enhance epidemiological and laboratory capacities in order to cope with their duties in such an event, which includes coordination with security/investigative agencies (e.g. carrying out forensic epidemiology, ensuring chain of custody, safeguarding confidentiality, carrying out sample collection and preservation of evidence).

Standard Operating Procedures (SOP)

Organizations that would respond to deliberately caused outbreaks should consider developing, testing and implementing standard operating procedures that identify roles and responsibilities, and should set out the key tasks to be undertaken by specific staff in the first 48 hours following the onset of the emergency of deliberate nature. Aspects of the response that need to be clarified, and their operation rehearsed in simulation exercises, include:

- Multi-agency working protocols and procedures to establish the roles of the medical services in preparedness and response in the event of a covert or overt deliberately-caused outbreak, including command, control and co-ordination procedures at strategic, tactical and operational venues/levels.
- Means of informing the local and national public and media, of interacting with local and national governments, and of informing and/or seeking assistance from the key regional and international organizations (e.g. WHO, and the OIE [the World Organization for Animal Health] in the case of biological agents that could affect or be transmitted by animals).

- Infection control because of the risk of the deliberate release of chemical/biological/radiological/nuclear (CBRN) agents that could affect medical personnel if adequate infection control procedures (e.g. those regarding the use of specialized PPE and decontamination) are not followed rigorously.

Routine national and global surveillance systems for naturally occurring outbreak-prone and emerging infectious diseases enhance capacity to detect and respond to deliberately caused infectious diseases, because the public health detection and response mechanisms are similar. Adequate background information on the natural behavior of infectious diseases will facilitate recognition of an unusual event, and help determine whether suspicions of deliberate use should be investigated.

Outbreak plans should contain elements to cope with suspected or confirmed deliberate release, and indications of actions to be taken should such release be suspected.

Most health workers will have little or no experience in managing illness arising from several of the infectious agents with the greatest potential for deliberate use to cause harm; training in clinical recognition and initial management may therefore be needed for first responders. This training should include methods for infection control, safe handling of diagnostic specimens and body fluids, and decontamination procedures. One of the most difficult issues for the public health system is to decide whether preparedness should include stockpiling of drugs, vaccines and equipment.

NB: Outbreaks of international importance, whether naturally occurring or thought to have been deliberately caused, should be reported electronically by national governments to:
    < outbreakwho.int >

For further information on reporting obligations, see the chapters on the *International Health Regulations (2005)* and *Reporting*.

For further information on preparedness for deliberate outbreaks, please see the relevant WHO website: <http://www.who.int/csr/en>

Illustrative List of Agents with Potential for Deliberate Use

With current movement toward an all-hazard, all pathogens approach, proscriptive lists of this type are losing meaning. There are a number of lists of infectious agents more or less suited to different contexts and threat assessments, and meaningful preparedness for deliberate use must take fully into account the specific nation/space/time for which it is considered.

Generalized lists (for example, those generated by CDC, the EU or ASEAN) are useful for budgeting and planning but are by no means all-inclusive. They should be considered as illustrative lists, the relevance of which is affected by changing targets, pathogens (natural or genetically modified), the means/path of delivery, and other factors.

In addition, such lists change quickly over time, as more is understood about the agents in question and their potential for use in a deliberate attack.

The following is an illustrative list of a number of pathogens thought potentially suitable for deliberate attacks, or which have been or are being developed in biological offensive programs, or which have been deliberately used in the past to cause outbreaks.

BACTERIA, such as:

- Anthrax (*Bacillus anthracis*)
- Brucellosis (*Brucella abortus, Brucella suis* and *Brucella melitensis*)
- Glanders (*Burkholderia mallei*)
- Melioidosis (*Burkholderia pseudommallei*)
- Tularemia (*Francisella tularensis*)
- Plague (*Yersinia pestis*)
- Q Fever (*Coxiella burnetii*)
- Typhus Fever (*Rickettsia prowazeki*).

FUNGI, such as:

- Coccidioidomycosis (*Coccidiodes immitis*).

VIRUSES, such as:

- SARS
- Ebola, Marburg and other viral hemorrhagic fevers (VHFs)
- Venezuelan equine encephalomyelitis
- Smallpox (*Variola* virus).

BACTERIAL TOXINS, such as:

- Staphylococcal enterotoxins
- Botulinal neurotoxins.

For more information and illustrative examples of more comprehensive lists, please see the following lists from CDC:
    <http://www.bt.cdc.gov/agent/agentlist.asp>
- and from WHO:
    <http://www.who.int/csr/delibepidemics/annex3.pdf>

Illustrative List of Indicators That an Outbreak/Incident is Potentially a Deliberate Event

The following criteria constitute an illustrative list of potential indicators for deliberate events, based on pathogens/toxins that have been or are being developed in biological offensive programs, or which have been deliberately used in the past to cause outbreaks (to be considered also in relation to Annex 2 of the International Heath Regulations [2005] reporting mechanisms, if appropriate):

- Large or multiple simultaneous outbreaks of an infectious disease.
- Recognition of infectious diseases that are not endemic to an area.

- Presentation of multiple patients with infectious diseases that may be endemic to an area, but which rarely infect humans.
- A cluster of 2 or more cases, related in time and space, of the following syndromes (single cases of severe illness in a previously well person may also be considered):
- Neurological syndrome—meningitis, encephalitis, encephalopathy or neurological disturbance.
- Respiratory syndrome—pneumonia, infiltrates, pneumonitis, ARDS.
- Acute fulminating septicemia or shock.
- Fulminant hepatitis or hepatic failure.

Illustrative List of Alert and Surveillance Signals

(To be integrated in the routine surveillance and alert systems)

- Overt threat of deliberate use.
- All rumors and reports of smallpox-like illness.
- All rumors and reports of disease with test results confirming a specific agent with potential for deliberate use in a non-endemic area (e.g. pulmonary anthrax, tularemia, or plague).
- Previously well persons presenting with severe unexplained disease or syndrome, or death.
- Disease of known etiology occurring in an unusual setting, population or season, or with an atypical clinical presentation/higher morbidity and mortality.
- Multi-centric outbreaks—same syndrome or confirmed disease in non-contiguous areas.
- Illness or deaths among animals that precede or accompany illness or death in humans.
- Suspected or known deliberate or accidental release in another country.
- Illness affecting a key sector of the community (e.g. political, financial) or a mass gathering event.

Illustrative List of Indicators Based on Clinical and Epidemiological Findings

- Failure of a common disease to respond to usual therapy/prophylaxis.
- Unusually short median/mean incubation period for a known disease.
- Previously unknown modes and/or routes of transmission.
- Infectivity (the number of people infected by a single person, or a high value) significantly higher than expected (increased transmissibility).
- Case-fatality rate significantly higher than expected (increased virulence).
- Dose response, e.g. lower attack rates among people who had been indoors, especially in areas with filtered air or closed ventilation systems, compared with people who had been outdoors.
- An unusual increase in the number of people seeking health care,

especially if presenting with fever, respiratory, neurological or gastrointestinal symptoms.

Suggestive Laboratory Findings

- Confirmed atypical, genetically engineered, or antiquated strain of an agent.
- Laboratory confirmed case/cluster of specific agent with no known risk factors for a natural infection.
- Indistinguishable molecular and genetic characteristics of agents detected in temporally or spatially distinct sources.

INFECTION PREVENTION AND CONTROL

I. HEALTH CARE FACILITIES
[F. Otaiza, C. Pessoa Da Silva]

Health care associated infections occur as a result of health care, in facilities or in the community. Infections can take place in all types of facilities, independent of resources, and are a major cause of death and increased morbidity in hospitalized patients worldwide. The most severe health care associated infections are found where very ill patients are being treated.

At any one time, over 1.4 million people worldwide suffer from infectious complications of health care. In developed countries, about 5–10% of patients admitted to acute care hospitals develop an infection that they had acquired before or after admission while they are in the health care facility; while in resource-poor countries, the burden of health care associated infections may be even greater.

Health care workers may also be infected, and therefore prevention and control measures increase safety for them as well as for patients. Special measures may be required to reduce risk for visitors to health care facilities.

Health care settings can act as amplifiers of infection, resulting in outbreak, with an impact on both hospital and community health. For example, at time of writing, nosocomial transmission accounts for 55% to 72% of recorded probable cases of Severe Acute Respiratory Syndrome (SARS). In outbreaks of Ebola and Marburg viral hemorrhagic fevers in Africa, health care workers have accounted for up to 10% of all cases, and have served as sources of infection in their families and communities.

Epidemiology

The most frequent sources of health care associated infections are patients. The modes of transmission of infections in health care settings and in the community are alike, but processes in health care settings may facilitate the spread of community-acquired infections after admission. During health care procedures, an infectious agent may reach a new site in a patient—for example, the bloodstream—when transported from a site where it is normally contained—such as the intestine—or from a site where it causes a different type of infection, such as on the skin. In health care facilities, opportunities for contact between infected and susceptible patients are increased, particularly when health care workers manipulate infectious materials and then touch susceptible patients without proper hand hygiene, or when they reuse equipment involved in patient care.

Infectious agents causing health care associated infections may vary greatly from one facility to another, depending on the predominant sites of infection, the type of patient (e.g. adults or children), the scope of health services provided, and the incidence of infections in the community. Most health care associated infections are caused by bacteria from the normal or transitory flora of the skin, the intestine, the upper respiratory tract and the upper digestive tract. Viral agents are less frequent, and are mostly associated with infections in children such as acute respiratory or intestinal infections—the exception being blood-borne viral infections, such as hepatitis B & C, and HIV. Fungi are infrequent pathogens, with the exception of *Candida* spp., which can cause bloodstream infections in patients with central venous catheters or parenteral nutrition, and *Aspergillus* spp., which is involved in pulmonary infections of immunocompromised hosts.

The majority of health care associated infections are sporadic, but a small proportion is associated with outbreaks. Outbreaks can originate from community-infected patients (e.g. acute respiratory infections with adenovirus), from the contamination of a common source within the facility (e.g. contamination of antiseptic solutions or intravenous medications), or as a result of systematic breaks of the aseptic technique for a given procedure.

Host risk factors, such as age and severity of underlying disease, are a major influence on the incidence of most types of health care associated infections. Some practices, such as use and manipulation of invasive devices (e.g. urinary and central vascular catheters, naso/orotracheal tubes and mechanical ventilation) and procedures (e.g. surgery) are also associated with infections, and high rates can be observed when adequate infection prevention and control practices are not observed. Contamination of air, water or equipment surfaces plays a minor role in most health care associated infections.

While host factors cannot easily be modified, health care practices and procedures may be successfully modified, using various preventive strategies. Environmental risk factors can be modified, but the impact of such interventions may be limited to reduction of risk of only certain very specific infections (e.g. airborne viruses, *Aspergillus* spp., and vancomycin-resistant enterococcus).

Health care workers with infections or who are colonized with transmissible microbial agents—particularly those workers treating patients—are a risk for patient infection. These infections may be minor (e.g. skin infections, conjunctivitis, and upper respiratory tract infections), but can severely affect certain patients, such as the immunocompromised. At times, health care workers must be treated and/or removed from certain direct patient care procedures until the risk of transmission is over.

Health care workers are frequently exposed to injuries and infectious agents through occupational activities, particularly infections that are blood-borne (e.g. hepatitis B virus) and airborne (e.g. *M. tuberculosis*). Health care workers must therefore be evaluated periodically for infections and risk of infections, as must the procedures they perform. Preventive measures such as vaccination of staff against hepatitis B, use of personal protective equipment, and effective post-exposure management or treatment must be practiced in all health care facilities.

Prevention and Control

The most frequent prevention and control measures are intended to reduce the presence of microbiological agents in a health care facility through the use of Standard (Universal) Precautions during patient care, in order to prevent cross infection, and to ensure prompt and effective treatment of infected patients.

Standard Precautions are a series of procedures that must be performed when dealing with all patients, independent of their infectious status. The key elements of Standard Precautions are:

- Hand hygiene with soap and water or the use of alcohol-based preparation before and after patient contact, and after contact with contaminated environmental surfaces or equipment.
- Use of personal protective equipment (e.g. gloves, gowns, masks and eye protection) based on the risk assessment of the procedure (see table at the end of this section).
- Respiratory hygiene, by covering the nose and mouth with a tissue when coughing or sneezing, disposing of the tissue after use, and performing hand hygiene afterwards.
- Promotion of safe injection practices, by ensuring that only disposable needles and syringes are used, and never re-used.
- Handling and disposal of sharp equipment and materials in such a way as to prevent injuries to the handler or others, particularly if the equipment has been in touch with blood or any body fluid, secretion or excretion.
- Waste management in accordance with local regulations.
- Cleansing, disinfection and sterilization of patient care equipment and of the patient—particularly when performing an invasive procedure or one that may require access to a normally sterile tissue.
- Isolation measures for infected patients in accordance with known means of transmission, such as placing a patient in single room with proper ventilation for active pulmonary tuberculosis, or maintaining

separation of at least one meter between patients when infectious
agents are present which can be propelled by aerosolization, as is the
case for some respiratory viruses.
- Use of aseptic technique whenever natural host barriers are breached,
e.g. any incision or puncture, or during manipulation of a port of
entry, such as hubs of intravenous lines or the site of catheter
insertions.

Adherence to infection control measures should be monitored, with
feedback of results to health care workers and supervisors, and there
should be formal liaison with public health services, especially when
infections involve the community.

Prompt and effective treatment is sometimes complicated by the
presence of infectious agents, mainly bacteria, that are resistant to
anti-infective drugs. Health facility associated infections with anti-infective
drug resistant organisms are more frequently observed in intensive care
units and other settings containing severely ill patients or those hospitalized for the long-term.

The dissemination of resistant strains throughout a health care facility is
by the same routes as with any other infectious agent. Asymptomatic
carriers—both patients and health care workers—are of special importance in the dissemination of resistant strains, since they may not be
recognized, and preventive measures may therefore not be in place.

For effective control, it may be necessary to place infected or colonized
patients with the same known pathogen in the same designated unit (in
same space, and with the same staff working on the unit), to which
patients without the infection cannot be admitted. This is sometimes
referred to as "cohorting."

Antimicrobial resistance is dealt with more fully in the second section of
this chapter.

Infection Control Programs

Infection control programs must compile Standard Precautions and
ensure prompt patient management. The efficacy of good infection
prevention and control programs in reducing the risk of infections in
hospitals has been clearly demonstrated, and hospitals with an ongoing
culture of safe practices are better prepared to control sporadic infections,
and to avoid outbreaks. Most of the successful models of infection control
programs in health care facilities include:

- Specialized infection control staff, with appropriate training
- Policies and guidelines for health care practices
- Supervision of clinical procedures
- Surveillance.

Infection control programs require trained medical and nursing professionals with time allocated to perform the necessary functions, and an
infection control committee that sets policies and monitors the impact of

infection control activities. To be effective, senior management of a facility must support the committee by ensuring that infection control activities are routinely integrated into hospital policies, training strategies and supervision of patient care practices.

Surveillance is required to provide data to describe the incidence, trends, risk factors and etiology of health care associated infections; to identify high-risk patients; to detect outbreaks early; and to assess the impact of interventions.

There are several surveillance models, and all require standard case definitions and systematic active case finding procedures. Surveillance must be designed in such as way as to satisfy information needs while allowing health care workers the necessary time to implement prevention and control measures.

Health care workers themselves will often be the first to notice the emergence of a new disease, or of changes in the epidemiology of an existing disease in the community—i.e. changes in incidence and/or prevalence, mode of transmission, severity and/or susceptibility to treatment. Timely reporting to community-based public health services is required. On the other hand, community outbreaks or other communicable disease emergencies should be reported directly to health care facilities by community public health services in order to ensure best possible outbreak management and prevention of spread to other patients, visitors and health care workers.

Over the past decades, the field of infection control has accumulated a large body of evidence-based recommendations to prevent health care associated infections, but significant gaps still exist between knowledge and implementation of infection control practices.

II. ANTIMICROBIAL RESISTANCE
[G. Dziekan]

Introduction

Antimicrobial resistance reduces the options and effectiveness of anti-infective therapy in all infectious disease areas: bacterial, viral, fungal and parasitic. The emergence of antimicrobial resistance is a natural phenomenon, but can be promoted by the use of anti-infective drugs. The evolution of antimicrobial resistance is greatly accelerated when anti-infective drugs are used inappropriately.

Antimicrobial resistance costs money and human lives. It leads to increased morbidity and mortality, and the need for prolonged treatment, sometimes with more expensive and toxic combination therapies. It also prolongs the periods during which patients are infectious and can spread disease.

Evolution of Antimicrobial Drug Resistance

The emergence of antimicrobial resistance is the result of constant evolutionary selection in infectious diseases: bacterial, viral, fungal and parasitic. Microbes reproduce rapidly, mutate frequently, are able readily and freely to exchange genetic material, and therefore easily develop or acquire resistance to anti-infective therapy. Anti-infective drugs eliminate susceptible pathogens while selecting resistant ones, providing them with an evolutionary advantage that enables them to develop further and pass on their resistance-encoding genes to the next generation. Resistance genes encode various mechanisms that allow micro-organisms to resist specific anti-infective drug therapy. These mechanisms offer resistance to other antimicrobials of the same class, and sometimes to several different antimicrobial classes. The prevalence of resistance varies between geographical regions and over time, but it has become clear that sooner or later resistance will emerge to almost every antimicrobial drug.

By increasing selective pressure, both by over-use and under-use of anti-infective drugs in the treatment of human or animal illness, the natural phenomena that cause the development of drug resistance are exacerbated and amplified.

Several reasons have been identified for the incorrect use of drugs in developing countries: inadequate or inconsistent access leading to truncated treatment or failure to take a full course of therapy; the purchase of drugs on the open market in the absence of legislation or enforcement of the law; and the sale of counterfeit, often sub-standard drugs. Among 46 recent reports of counterfeit drugs from 20 countries, 32% of the drugs in question contained no active ingredient, and the rest contained either incorrect quantities of active ingredients, or impurities.

In industrialized countries, over-prescribing of anti-infective treatment by health care workers and excessive demand by the general population contribute to increased selection pressure. Antibiotics are often prescribed empirically in the absence of laboratory confirmation of infection. Estimates suggest that up to 50% of all antibiotic consumption may be unnecessary, both in hospitals and in ambulatory settings. Antibiotic treatment is also often too broad, failing to target specifically the infection-causing pathogen.

Over and under-use of anti-infective drugs occurs in most countries, and is often linked to socio-economic status: those patients who are economically better-off tend to consume significantly more antibiotics than patients who are less easily able to obtain them.

Increased selection pressure amplifying the selection and survival of resistant microbes does not only occur in humans. Anti-infective drugs are vital in the treatment of infections in animals: up to 50% of all anti-infective drug production is for animal use. Antibiotics are also added to animal feed as prophylaxis against infections or as growth promoters, mainly in the mass production of poultry and pigs, and to water to treat fish diseases. Several antibiotics used in animal husbandry are also used in humans, resulting in the selection of cross-resistance in pathogens that are important in human medicine, or of resistant organisms that can be passed from animals to humans. Furthermore, anti-infective drugs are often used as pesticides in agriculture products. Development and transfer of drug resistance to other organisms may be caused by such agricultural use, but the mechanisms are less well understood. Once drug-resistant, organisms can then spread rapidly throughout the world in humans, animals, vectors or food.

Reduced investment in research and development of new classes of anti-infective drugs contributes to the seriousness of antimicrobial resistance and its impact on public health. The decline in remaining treatment options is not only a threat to individuals, but to entire populations.

Measures to Reduce Selective Pressure for Anti-Infective Drug Resistant Microbes

To reduce the selective pressure of anti-infective drugs, all aspects of drug use in humans, animals and agriculture must be addressed. The lack of scientific and medical evidence makes it difficult to prioritize interventions, but the components of a broad strategy include the following:

- More prudent use of anti-infective drugs in human medicine, animal medicine, and animal husbandry/agriculture
- Measures to prevent the spread of anti-infective-drug-resistant organisms, including better patient diagnosis and management
- Hand hygiene and avoidance of unnecessary injections in health care facilities, especially if there is a chance that syringes and needles will be re-used
- Development and use of clinical treatment guidelines containing dosage and duration of treatment
- Targeted campaigns with clear messages designed to educate the general population about when anti-infective drugs are necessary, and when they are not necessary
- Education of farmers and policy-makers about appropriate use of antimicrobials in animal husbandry and agriculture
- Legislation to regulate sale of, and where appropriate enforce the banning of, certain anti-infective drugs used as growth-promoters in livestock
- Vigilance against counterfeit drugs.

Finally, the use of infection-preventing interventions (such as bed-nets, condoms and vaccines) prevents infections, therefore obviating the need to use anti-infective drugs.

Global Trends in Antimicrobial Drug Resistance Development— Some Examples

Tuberculosis

Tuberculosis is estimated to cause 1.7 million deaths globally per year, 95% of which are in developing countries. It is further estimated that an average of 5.3% of all acute pulmonary tuberculosis is multi-drug resistant TB (MDR-TB), representing approximately 500 000 cases and 110 000 deaths each year.

MDR-TB does not respond to a standard six-month treatment course using first-line drugs: MDR-TB strains show resistance to isoniazid and rifampicin. Treating resistant strains can take years, using drugs that are more toxic and more than 100 times more expensive than first-line drugs.

Extensively drug-resistant TB (XDR-TB) is caused by bacteria resistant to all of the most effective drugs—an MDR-TB resistance pattern plus resistance to any fluoroquinolone and any of the second-line anti-TB injectable drugs: amikacin, kanamycin and capreomycin. XDR-TB had been reported from 47 countries at time of writing in early 2008, and in countries of the former USSR, the proportion of XDR-TB among MDR-TB ranges from 4% to 24%. It is estimated that approximately 40 000 XDR-TB cases emerge every year.

For more information on TB, see the *Tuberculosis* chapter.

MRSA

Infections with methicillin-resistant *Staphylococcus aureus* (MRSA) have long been associated with health care facilities causing adverse patient outcomes, and significantly increased health care costs. Since the 1980s, the frequency of isolates of MRSA among *S. aureus* has increased to almost 70% in health care facilities in Japan and the Republic of Korea, and around 40% in facilities in the USA. Within Europe, an increasing trend is seen, with MRSA rates around 40% in health care facilities in many countries. A greater number of MRSA strains are susceptible only to vancomycin and other glycopeptides, and decreased vancomycin susceptibility has emerged within most MRSA lineages.

MRSA is of growing concern outside of health care facilities, with the rate of invasive community-acquired MRSA approaching 10% in some countries. Most often, it causes skin and soft tissue infections, but recent studies suggest that a growing number of community-acquired MRSA strains may cause invasive infections such as necrotizing pneumonia. Community-acquired MRSA strains are genetically different from hospital-associated strains, and in contrast to most health care associated MRSA, are usually sensitive to a wider range of anti-infectives, except beta-lactam antibiotics.

Influenza

Various seasonal influenza-causing strains (e.g. A/H3N2) have been found to show high levels of resistance to both amantadine and rimantadine, two drugs regularly used in the past to treat seasonal influenza. Resistance of seasonal influenza viruses has also recently developed to oseltamivir. In the 2007-2008 influenza season, levels of resistance to oseltamivir in seasonal influenza virus A/H1N1 were reported to be highly variable in Europe, ranging from almost zero up to 70%. In Thailand, resistance to oseltamivir has been shown in H5N1 human infections – causing concern should H5N1 develop into a human pandemic influenza strain.

For more information on influenza, see the *Influenza* chapter.

HIV

HIV is a highly mutant virus that easily develops drug resistance. In industrialized countries, where antiretroviral therapy (ART) has been widely accessible for over a decade, studies suggest that between 5% and 20% of persons diagnosed with HIV show resistance to at least one class of ART drugs. In developing countries, where ART is based on an effective three-drug regimen and adherence rates are generally good, studies indicate that the development of drug-resistance has been minimized. This is in part due to the advantage these countries have had over those that started treatment programs earlier, when only mono-therapy or two-drug regimens (which are more likely to lead to resistance) were available.

For more information on HIV, see the *Acquired Immunodeficiency Syndrome* chapter.

Malaria

Chloroquine resistance of *Plasmodium falciparum* malaria is now prevalent worldwide. Mortality estimates from public health records in Africa indicate a two- to eleven-fold increase in malaria-associated mortality among children when drug resistance develops, with hospital attendance showing similar increasing trends. Following the global occurrence and spread of high-level resistance against two second-line antimalarials, sulfadoxine-pyrimethamine and mefloquine, the recommended treatment of malaria relies on combination therapy with artemisinin and its derivatives as one component. Currently, resistance is developing to antimalarial drugs with increasing rapidity, and it is recommended that multi-drug combinations be used exclusively, in an effort to slow the development of resistance, and to better preserve the effectiveness of existing antimalarial drugs. This is especially true for the newer drugs, such as artemisinin derivatives. However, resistance against artemisinin has recently been demonstrated *in vitro*, and it is feared that growing selection pressure will increase the likelihood of artemisinin-resistance development *in vivo* as well.

Table: Summary of IC precautions

Individual barriers: Standard, Contact, Droplet and Airborne Precautions

Measures	Occasion for use	Hand hygiene	Gloves	Gown	Medical mask	Filtering face piece*	Eye wear
Standard precautions	Before and after patient contact, and after contact with contaminated environmental surfaces or equipment	Always	✔				
	In cases of direct contact with patient blood and body fluids, secretions, excretions, mucous membranes or non-intact skin	Based on risk assessment	✔	✔	✔		
	If there is a risk of spills of infectious material onto the health care worker's body and face	Based on risk assessment	✔	✔	✔		✔
Contact precautions	Always**, on entering patient room***	✔	✔	✔			
Droplet precautions	Always**, on entering patient room***	✔			✔		
Airborne precautions	Always**, on entering patient room***	✔				✔	

* Filtering face pieces for use in health care are particulate respirators with high filtration efficiency (e.g. EU FFP2, US NIOSH-certified N95)

** Whenever entering the patient room or whenever providing care for the patient

*** Single room facilitates the application of specific contact and droplet precautions, and is obligatory for the application of airborne precautions. In addition, the room for airborne precautions should be adequately ventilated.

MASS VACCINATION IN PUBLIC HEALTH
[D. Heymann, R. Aylward]

Mass vaccination campaigns, conducted over short time periods, continue to play an important role in the control of vaccine-preventable diseases, in both industrialized and developing country settings. Mass vaccination is particularly important for:

- Preventing or containing emerging outbreaks of vaccine-preventable diseases.
- Rapidly boosting population immunity in emergency settings.
- Optimizing the impact of a new vaccine.
- Achieving very high herd immunity levels to attain international disease control goals (especially eradication).
- Supplementing routine immunization of young children in some settings.

Mass vaccination and routine immunization are a necessary alliance for attaining both national and international goals in the control of vaccine-preventable diseases.

Mass Vaccination to Prevent or Contain Infectious Disease Outbreaks

The most widely accepted reason for using mass vaccination is to increase population (herd) immunity rapidly in the setting of an existing or potential communicable disease outbreak, thereby limiting the morbidity and mortality that might result. The rationale for using a mass vaccination approach is particularly strong when the incidence of an epidemic-prone disease is beginning to rise; when it is suspected that community immunity is sub-optimal; and/or when there has been no routine vaccination because vaccines are unsuitable for routine use, or because populations have been displaced and routine immunization services disrupted.

Some disease examples follow.

Meningitis

Meningococcal meningitis is one of a number of diseases for which mass vaccination is a standard, proven element of epidemic control. Although meningococcal meningitis occurs throughout the world, the largest epidemics occur in the semi-arid areas of 12 sub-Saharan African countries, designated the "African meningitis belt." Most countries within the meningitis belt experience increased transmission each year during the dry season, with large epidemics occurring every 8–12 years during the past 50 years, particularly in regions with extensive communication and mixing of populations.

Meningitis epidemics in sub-Saharan Africa are generally caused by sero-group A organisms, though W135 serogroups have also recently played an important role. Meningococcal vaccines based on capsular polysaccharide antigens are often then deployed. They are not routinely used in early child-hood, because of their general lack of efficacy in infants and young children, those at greatest risk of infection and disease.

When increased transmission of meningitis occurs in sub-Saharan Africa, epidemiological surveillance is important in order to determine when the threshold of transmission that leads to epidemics has been reached. Once that threshold is reached, mass vaccination should be started, targeted at a broad age range, and sometimes at the whole population. Rapidly organized and conducted mass vaccination cam-paigns effectively protect susceptibles, and can often interrupt epidemic transmission within two or three weeks. Mass vaccinations are usually provided by mobile vaccination teams or by fixed vaccination stations at health centers or other community facilities. If newly developed menin-gococcal conjugate vaccines are shown to be protective in infants and young children, meningococcal vaccination could eventually be included in national immunization programs in areas at high risk of meningococcal disease.

Influenza

Influenza vaccines are not included in routine immunization programs in many poorer countries because of the need to alter the vaccine composi-tion each year, making it necessary to routinely but rapidly vaccinate populations at risk before the annual epidemic of seasonal influenza begins. Each year, seasonal influenza occurs during the winter months in both the Northern and Southern Hemispheres. WHO estimates that up to 500 000 persons die each year from seasonal influenza, mainly those over the age of 60 years or with other underlying medical conditions. The influenza virus is highly unstable, and constantly mutates through a process called antigenic drift. At times, when there is an influenza pandemic, a major antigenic shift occurs as a new influenza virus enters human populations. Because antigenic drift and shift decrease the efficacy of the influenza vaccine, the recom-mended antigenic composition of the vaccine is altered annually, based on prevalent virus strains: once in February for the Northern Hemisphere influenza season that will begin roughly eleven months later, and again in August for the influenza season in the Southern Hemisphere.

As soon as new vaccines become available each year, they are provided to the populations at risk (usually the elderly, and in some countries to health care workers as well), through mass vaccination at fixed health facilities, mainly in industrialized countries. At time of writing in early 2008, the provincial government of Ontario in Canada has recently recommended vaccination of populations of all ages with influenza vaccine; this experience will provide a comparative evaluation of that approach against the "risk-group" approach being used in most other countries. Although it is known that seasonal influenza epidemics occur in developing countries, further study is needed to understand the target populations and vaccination strategy required to optimize the impact of mass vaccination in these settings.

Yellow Fever

The yellow fever vaccine is integrated into routine immunization programs in some countries at risk, but not all. Yellow fever occurs sporadically in 33 countries in Africa and 11 countries in South America. A severe epidemic of human-to-human transmission is most likely to occur when conditions allow the density of mosquito vector populations to increase substantially, as often happens during the rainy season. Epidemiological surveillance is a key strategy for limiting yellow fever epidemics by rapidly identifying human infections when they occur. Mosquito control is also an effective supplemental prevention strategy. However, the most effective means of preventing yellow fever epidemics is through vaccination at 9 months of age, using the vaccine as part of routine immunization programs.

If routine immunization at 9 months does not reach the level needed for herd immunity in the general population, epidemic transmission is a risk, and mass vaccination is required to fill the gap in immunity. The target population for mass vaccination, once yellow fever has been identified in human populations, is the entire population living or working in the area from which the infection has been identified.

When financial resources or vaccine supply are limited, the primary target population is usually children aged between nine months and 14 years. Vaccinations are generally provided through house-to-house campaigns, during which there is active questioning to determine whether additional human infections are occurring. As with any epidemic, planning and implementation of mass vaccination must begin as soon as possible after an outbreak is confirmed, and emergency supplies of 17D yellow fever vaccine must be ordered immediately.

Displaced Persons

Sudden and large or massive influxes into a single area of people with varied backgrounds and immunization status can occur during civil disturbance, war and natural disasters. In such situations, routine immunization activities are often not available. Where displaced populations live in close proximity, and where sanitation and water supplies may be compromised, an environment is created that is particularly conducive to epidemics of vaccine-preventable diseases.

Major vaccines used in mass campaigns among displaced persons are those for measles, meningococcal meningitis, and yellow fever. Mass vaccination for measles is usually conducted immediately after displaced persons congregate, particularly if vaccine coverage rates are estimated to be less than 80%. The target population is often extended, to a lower age limit of 6 months and an upper limit of 14 years, with re-vaccination of infants when they reach 12 months of age. Mass vaccination for meningitis and yellow fever is conducted if risk factors for epidemics are present, while studies of the applicability of the new cholera and typhoid vaccines in displaced populations are under way at time of writing in several geographic areas, to evaluate their usefulness in mass campaigns among displaced persons.

Threat of Deliberately Caused Outbreaks

There are a variety of circumstances under which public health authorities gauge the risk of a deliberately caused epidemic or biologic threat. Mass vaccination campaigns are then sometimes conducted as a deterrent, and to prevent or limit a deliberately caused outbreak should one be planned or occur. Some countries perceive a particular threat from disease such as smallpox and/or anthrax, and have begun to stockpile vaccines against these perceived threats that would be used for mass vaccination of entire populations should such a threat be realized.

Strategies for the use of these vaccines vary, but most countries state as the first priority mass vaccination of primary responders, followed by mass vaccination of the general population if the deliberately used infectious agent has the potential to spread from person to person. The strategies for mass vaccination may, however, be much more complex than for other indications, due to the deterrent nature and the need to be as safe as possible. For example, because infection with HIV has been associated with generalized vaccinia and death after smallpox vaccination, strategies of preventive mass vaccination using smallpox vaccine need to incorporate the ability to avoid vaccination of HIV infected persons, and to provide them with protection by other means, such as passive immunization with vaccinia immune globulin.

For more information on planning for, and reaction to, the deliberate use of infectious agents, see the chapter on *Outbreak response in case of deliberate use of biological agents to cause harm*.

Mass Vaccination to Accelerate Disease Control

A second important use of mass vaccination strategies is to accelerate disease control to rapidly increase coverage with a new vaccine at the time of its introduction into routine immunization programs, and to attain the herd immunity levels required to meet international targets for eradication and mortality reduction. Since the late 1980s, international accelerated disease control targets have been established for eradication, for mortality reduction, and for heightened control of infectious diseases. Reaching these targets requires rapidly increasing population immunity, usually with the goal of interrupting human-to-human transmission of the causative infectious agent. Mass vaccination campaigns are a particularly important element of these efforts as the vaccination coverage levels required to achieve herd immunity, especially in densely populated areas, often exceed the coverage rates from routine immunization programs.

Mass Vaccination to Prevent Outbreaks and Resurgence

Even with well-managed immunization programs, numbers of susceptible individuals can slowly accumulate to the point where there are enough
to sustain outbreaks and ongoing transmission. This phenomenon can be
accelerated by primary vaccine courses waning in effectiveness in older
children, influxes of unvaccinated migrants, and temporary or sustained
vaccination scares affecting groups of children, often in age cohorts. Such
situations can be detected through sero-epidemiology or administrative
surveys indicating that there are growing numbers of susceptible individuals; modeling is then applied to indicate the risk of outbreaks, and mass
vaccination "catch-up" campaigns are used to head off resurgence, targeting susceptible groups or whole populations. This has been done successfully—for example, to prevent resurgence of measles.

Introduction of New Vaccines

During the past sixty years, over 20 new vaccines have become
available. Mass vaccination is a key element of new vaccine introduction,
the goal being quickly to reduce the proportion of susceptible persons at
risk at the time the new vaccine is introduced into the routine immunization program. The impact of the mass campaign is to equalize population immunity levels, thus preventing a potential exacerbation of the targeted disease due to a sudden change in its transmission patterns or other
epidemiological characteristics, which might occur as a result of vaccinating only a portion of the susceptible population through routine immunization programs.

At the time of new vaccine introduction, persons considered at risk of
infection are vaccinated in mass vaccination campaigns to "mop up" or
protect all those who are susceptible. Mass vaccination is then ended, and
the vaccines remain incorporated in routine immunization programs to
vaccinate susceptible persons as they enter the cohort of susceptibility
(usually at birth). A first clear example of this strategy occurred in the
1950s, when the Salk inactivated polio vaccine was first licensed. Initially
it was offered in mass campaigns to all populations considered at risk of
polio, and then it was incorporated into routine childhood immunization
programs to ensure that children entering the birth cohort were fully
protected.

Although routine childhood immunization against rubella is now a
standard component of vaccination programs in industrialized countries,
the vaccine has until recently seen limited uptake in developing countries.
Decision-making on whether or not to introduce rubella vaccine has been
complicated by concern that routine childhood immunization against the
disease can shift the average age of infection to older girls, inadvertently
increasing, at least transiently, the risk of disease in pregnant women, and
thus the incidence of congenital rubella syndrome. Consequently, the introduction of routine childhood immunization against rubella is sometimes

accompanied by a one-time mass campaign, targeting all girls less than 15 years of age, and in some countries targeting all women of childbearing age.

It is likewise recommended standard practice to accompany the introduction of yellow fever vaccine into routine childhood immunization programs with a one-time mass vaccination campaign. In these campaigns, children aged less than 15 years are targeted in order to prevent yellow fever epidemics, which could continue to occur because of the immunization gap that would exist until immunized childhood cohorts reach adulthood.

Eradication

Polio vaccination has been included in routine immunization programs since the licensing of the Salk and Sabin vaccines. In 1988, when the goal of eradicating polio was set, an increasing number of countries had already interrupted human-to-human transmission of wild poliovirus by using oral poliovirus vaccine (OPV) in routine immunization programs. In many countries in Latin America, where routine immunization programs had not ever achieved high-level control, it was demonstrated that by supplementing routine immunization with mass vaccination, these tropical and semi-tropical developing countries could rapidly interrupt transmission.

The mass vaccination strategy currently used in polio eradication targets all children under the age of 5 years, during National Immunization Days or Weeks in which OPV is administered to children through fixed sites, with house-to-house mop-up campaigns that sometimes target a broader age group—if required—to interrupt the final chains of transmission. In some densely populated areas, interrupting poliovirus transmission has required well over 90% coverage in up to nine or ten mass vaccination campaigns each year. Areas with low standards of sanitation and high population densities have required the greatest number of campaigns.

Prior to conducting mass vaccination, district level micro-planning is used to identify areas where children under the age of 5 years may be living, and to prepare maps that are used by social mobilizers and vaccinators as they pass from community to community and house to house. The oral route of OPV administration allows the widespread use of health care workers, schoolteachers and community volunteers trained in short courses to administer polio vaccine during the campaigns. At time of writing in early 2008, mass vaccination was being further intensified in the four countries that remained polio-endemic, the countries that had re-established polio transmission due to imported virus, and other countries where it was necessary to control outbreaks following polio importation.

Despite the impact of the global polio eradication initiative to date, the use of mass vaccination strategies with the endpoint of eradication remains in uneasy alliance with routine immunization programs, largely due to the massive marginal and opportunity costs associated with eliminating the final chains of human-to-human transmission. This debate has led to the establishment of careful and comprehensive criteria for considering future eradication programs, particularly the need for explicit and appropriate cost-benefit analysis in advance, and the establishment of capacity to sustain sufficient societal and political support throughout the process.

Mortality reduction

Measles

Although measles vaccine is universally included in routine immunization programs in developing countries, targeting children between the ages of 9 and 12 months, there is frequent failure of children to seroconvert to measles vaccine, because of the presence of maternal antibody to measles. Once maternal antibody disappears, the window of opportunity to vaccinate children effectively before natural infection is short, and operationally difficult to exploit. Mass vaccination campaigns are a frequently used strategy for overcoming this problem.

Based on the age profile of measles susceptibility (and therefore duration of protection from maternal antibody), a one-time nationwide catch-up campaign is conducted in Latin America each year to reduce population susceptibility and interrupt transmission. Usually all children aged less than 15 years are targeted, regardless of prior measles immunization status. Follow-up mass vaccination campaigns, targeting children aged less than 5 years, are then conducted every 3-5 years thereafter, giving those who have not previously seroconverted a second opportunity. Countries achieving very high coverage through routine immunization programs generally provide this second opportunity prior to school entry.

Maternal and neonatal tetanus

To prevent maternal and neonatal tetanus, mass vaccination campaigns are conducted in high-risk areas delineated using surveillance data, and data on the prevalence of clean birth and delivery practices. In most countries with the explicit goal of eliminating maternal and neonatal tetanus, districts are now ranked from highest to lowest risk of these diseases. Multiple rounds of mass vaccination, targeting young girls and women of childbearing age, are often required for rapid boosting of immunity against tetanus.

COMMUNICABLE DISEASE CONTROL IN HUMANITARIAN EMERGENCIES

[M.A. Connolly]

Background

Communicable diseases are a major cause of mortality and morbidity in humanitarian emergencies.

Humanitarian emergencies include natural disasters (e.g. floods and earthquakes) and conflict situations, which have been defined as war or civil strife leading to large-scale population displacement. In this chapter, the generic term "emergencies" will be used to encompass all situations in which populations are in need of humanitarian assistance.

The communicable disease burden after an emergency depends on the type of emergency, its geographical location, baseline health of the population, and the level of development and accessibility of the affected area. Diarrheal diseases, acute respiratory infections, measles and malaria in endemic areas are the major killers. Other communicable diseases, such as epidemic meningococcal disease, tuberculosis, relapsing fever and typhus, have also caused large epidemics among emergency-affected populations.

Following an emergency, there may be an increase in epidemic diseases such as cholera, bacillary dysentery or meningitis, or endemic diseases such as malaria and acute respiratory infections. Natural disasters rarely cause large-scale outbreaks unless there is significant population displacement. However, conflict and post-conflict circumstances are associated with an increased risk of both outbreaks and endemic diseases. Emergencies occur in both industrialized and developing countries, but the impact is often much greater in the latter, where essential services may not be available, and inadequate shelter, water and sanitation, along with overcrowding in camps, lead to high risk of communicable disease.

People who are displaced across national borders are termed "refugees," whereas those who have been displaced within their country are called "internally displaced persons" (IDPs). There are an estimated 40 million refugees and IDPs worldwide, but non-displaced populations living in conflict-affected countries can also be at increased risk of communicable diseases. At time of writing in early 2008, there are over 25 conflict-affected countries that require humanitarian assistance, the majority of which are in sub-Saharan Africa.

COMMUNICABLE DISEASE RISK IN HUMANITARIAN EMERGENCIES

In natural disasters, most deaths occur in the immediate aftermath of the disaster and are primarily due to trauma and drowning. There may be population displacement after the disaster, and breakdowns in essential services such as shelter, water, sanitation and health care provision. The communicable disease risk depends on the extent of the displacement and the baseline health status of the affected population. Specific risks may be influenced by the type of disaster—for example, flooding often leads to the increased risk of water-related diseases.

In conflict and post-conflict situations, the magnitude of population displacement is often greater and more prolonged. These populations often have poor health status in advance of the emergency, and children are at particular risk. Highest excess mortality and morbidity most commonly occur during the first few weeks after acute conflict. Death rates of over 60 times the baseline have been recorded in refugee populations, with over three-quarters of these deaths caused by communicable diseases.

The factors determining the communicable disease risk in both natural disaster and conflict situations are as follows:

1) Population displacement.
2) Baseline health status including prevalence of malnutrition.
3) Lack of access to shelter, food, water and sanitation.
4) Overcrowding in temporary settlements or camps.
5) Lack of access to basic health services—e.g. primary health care and immunization.

Major Pathogens

Water-Related Diseases

Diarrheal diseases are a major cause of mortality and morbidity in emergencies. These diseases result mainly from inadequate quality and quantity of water, substandard and insufficient sanitation facilities, overcrowding, poor hygiene and scarcity of soap. In camp situations, diarrheal diseases have accounted for more than 40% of deaths in the acute phase of an emergency, with over 80% of these deaths occurring in children aged less than two years. The common sources of diarrheal disease outbreaks include polluted water sources (by fecal contamination of surface water entering incompletely sealed wells), contamination of water during transport and storage (through contact with hands soiled by feces), shared water containers and cooking pots, scarcity of soap, and contaminated foods.

In the USA, diarrheal illness was noted after Hurricanes Allison and Katrina, and norovirus, *Salmonella*, and toxigenic and non-toxigenic *V. cholerae* were confirmed among Katrina evacuees. In contrast, in developed parts of Europe, diarrheal diseases are less often a feature of flooding. However, the risk of diarrheal disease outbreaks following an emergency is much higher in developing countries. After the influx of 800 000 Rwandan refugees into North Kivu, Democratic Republic of the Congo (DRC), in 1994, 85% of the 50 000 deaths that were recorded in the first month were caused by diarrheal diseases, of which 60% were a result of cholera and 40% were caused by shigellosis. In Aceh Province, Indonesia, a rapid health assessment in the town of Calang two weeks after the tsunami in December 2004 found that 100% of the survivors drank from unprotected wells, and that 85% of the town's population reported diarrhea in the previous two weeks.

An outbreak of diarrheal disease after flooding in Bangladesh in 2004 led to over 17 000 cases; *V. cholerae* (O1 Ogawa and O1 Inaba) and enterotoxigenic *Escherichia coli* were isolated. A large cholera epidemic (O1 Ogawa) with over 16 000 cases occurred in West Bengal in 1998 following floods. In a study of risk factors for infection with *Cryptosporidium parvum* in Indonesia in 2001–2003, cases were four times more likely than controls to have been exposed to flooding.

Hepatitis A and E are also transmitted by the fecal-oral route, in association with lack of access to safe water and sanitation. Hepatitis A is endemic in most developing countries, and most children are exposed and develop immunity at an early age. As a result, the risk for large outbreaks is usually low in these settings. In hepatitis E-endemic areas, outbreaks frequently follow heavy rains and floods; the illness is generally mild and self-limited, but for pregnant women case-fatality rates can reach 25%. After the 2005 earthquake in Pakistan, sporadic hepatitis E cases and clusters were common in areas with poor access to safe water.

Leptospirosis is an epidemic-prone zoonotic bacterial disease that can be transmitted by direct contact with contaminated water. Flooding facilitates spread of the organism, because of the proliferation of rodents and the proximity of rodents to humans on shared high ground. Outbreaks of leptospirosis occurred in Taiwan, Republic of China, associated with Typhoon Nali in 2001; in Mumbai, India, after flooding in 2000; in Argentina after flooding in 1998; and in the Krasnodar region of Russia in 1997. After flooding in Brazil in 1996, incidence rates of leptospirosis doubled in the flood-prone areas of Rio de Janeiro.

Diseases Associated with Crowding

Crowding is common in populations displaced by natural disaster or conflict situations, and can facilitate the transmission of communicable diseases.

Measles risk in an emergency is dependent on baseline immunization coverage among the affected population, and in particular among children aged less than 15 years. Overcrowding is associated with the transmission of higher doses of measles virus, resulting in more severe clinical disease; in eastern Sudan and Somalia in 1995, measles accounted for 53% and 42% of deaths in refugees, respectively. A measles outbreak in the Philippines in 1991 among persons displaced by the eruption of Mount Pinatubo involved over 18 000 cases. Case-fatality rates are estimated at 3–5% in developing countries, but may be as high as 10–30% in displaced populations, particularly where the prevalence of malnutrition is high. However, the large-scale epidemics reported in the 1980s and 1990s are not presently reported as frequently, probably due to the prompt implementation of mass measles immunization campaigns in emergencies as part of humanitarian responses, and to global measles control efforts that have markedly decreased incidence while increasing vaccination coverage and protection.

Acute respiratory infections (ARIs) are a major cause of illness and death among displaced populations, particularly in children aged less than five years. Lack of access to health services and to antimicrobial agents for treatment further increases the risk of death from ARIs. Risk factors among displaced persons include crowding, exposure to indoor cooking using open flames, inadequate shelter, lack of blankets (especially in cold climates), and poor nutrition. The reported incidence of ARIs increased fourfold in Nicaragua in the 30 days after Hurricane Mitch in 1998, and ARIs accounted for the highest number of cases and deaths among those displaced by the tsunami in Aceh in 2004 and by the 2005 earthquake in Pakistan. In Kabul, Afghanistan, in 1993, 30% of deaths in residents aged less than 5 years and 23% of deaths in displaced people were as a result of ARIs.

Meningitis is transmitted from person to person, particularly in situations of crowding. Large outbreaks of meningococcal meningitis are well documented in populations displaced by conflict, but have not been recently reported following natural disasters. Serogroup A and C *Neisseria meningitidis* are the main causes of epidemic meningococcal meningitis, although serogroup W135 is becoming increasingly prevalent in sub-Saharan Africa. Epidemics are occurring beyond the traditional meningitis belt, to include east, southern and central Africa (e.g. Burundi, Rwanda, and Tanzania, from June to October 2002). Cases and deaths from meningitis among those displaced in Aceh and Pakistan have been documented.

Vector-Borne Diseases

Natural disasters, particularly cyclones, hurricanes, and flooding, can affect vector breeding sites and vector-borne disease transmission. While initial flooding may wash away existing mosquito breeding sites, standing water caused by heavy rainfall or overflow of rivers can create new breeding sites. This situation can result (typically with some weeks delay) in an increase of the vector population and potential for disease transmission, depending on the local mosquito vector species and its preferred habitat. The crowding of infected and susceptible hosts, inadequate access to health services preventing early and appropriate treatment, a weakened public health infrastructure, and interruptions of ongoing control programs all increase vector-borne disease transmission.

Malaria outbreaks in the wake of flooding are a well-known phenomenon. For example, an earthquake in Costa Rica's Atlantic Region in 1991 was associated with changes in habitat that were beneficial for mosquito breeding and preceded an extreme rise in malaria cases. Additionally, periodic flooding linked to El Niño/Southern Oscillation has been associated with malaria epidemics in the dry coastal region of northern Peru.

Populations moving from areas of low endemicity (including non-immune people) to hyperendemic areas are exposed to high malarial transmission. A large malaria epidemic occurred in Burundi between October 2000 and March 2001 affecting 7 of 17 provinces, and causing over 2.8 million cases in a country with a population of 7 million.

Other Diseases Associated with Emergencies

Tetanus is caused by a toxin released by the anerobic tetanus bacillus *Clostridium tetani*. Contaminated wounds, particularly in populations where vaccination coverage levels are low, are associated with illness and death from tetanus. A cluster of 106 cases of tetanus, including 20 deaths, occurred in Aceh in 2004, peaking 2 ½ weeks after the tsunami. Cases were also reported in Pakistan following the 2005 earthquake.

Methods of Control in Emergency Response

A systematic approach to the control of communicable diseases is a key component of emergency and humanitarian response, and is crucial to protecting the health of affected populations.

The main methods of control are as follows:

A. Preparedness measures

Many emergencies, while not predictable, are more likely to occur in areas predisposed to natural phenomena—such as earthquake zones, or regions liable to flooding or seasonal severe weather events—and preparedness is therefore a possibility. Even in the case of war or conflict, there is often a long period in advance of hostilities where preparations can be made to ensure a more functional and rapid response. Activities include risk mapping, contingency planning, stockpiling, training, development of surge capacity in health facilities, improving the physical resilience of health facilities and undertaking simulation exercises. Such disaster or emergency planning is vital to ensure a smooth, multi-sectoral response that will reduce deaths and disease.

1) Identify emergency risks, population vulnerabilities and likely impact/consequences.
2) Engage in multi-sectoral contingency planning.
3) Develop readiness plans for prevention, detection and control of priority communicable diseases and undertake desktop simulation exercises.

B. Rapid assessment after onset

Identify the communicable disease threats faced by the emergency-affected population, including those with epidemic potential. Define the health status of the population by conducting a rapid assessment.

1) Identify main disease threats, including potential epidemic diseases and their geographic distribution.
2) Obtain data on the host country and countries of origin of displaced persons, and on the areas through which they may have passed.
3) Identify priority public health interventions.
4) Identify the lead health agency.
5) Establish health coordination mechanisms.

C. Preventive measures

Prevent communicable disease by maintaining a healthy physical environment and good general living conditions.

1) Select and plan campsites.
2) Ensure adequate water and sanitation facilities.
3) Ensure availability of food.
4) Provide essential clinical services.
5) Control insect vectors and infection reservoirs, such as rodents.
6) Implement immunization campaigns (e.g. measles).
7) Provide basic laboratory facilities.

D. Control of patient and contacts

The use of standard treatment protocols in health facilities with agreed upon first-line drugs is crucial in order to ensure effective diagnosis and treatment. Simplified drug regimens are particularly important in emergencies.

1) Identify target diseases likely to occur.
2) Develop simple treatment protocols (e.g. for cholera, meningitis, ARIs, malaria).
3) Train health care workers in management of major diseases.
4) Ensure supply of drugs and other supplies.
5) Develop clear systems of referral for management of severe cases.

E. Surveillance/early warning system

Set up or strengthen a disease surveillance system with an early warning mechanism to ensure the early reporting of cases, to monitor disease trends, and to facilitate prompt detection and response to outbreaks.

1) Identify target diseases/syndromes.
2) Develop simple case definitions for reporting.
3) Establish simple and robust reporting mechanisms (including a rapid alert system).
4) Ensure adequate laboratory confirmation services.
5) Monitor disease trends and carry out continuous risk assessment.
6) Feed information back to participating sites.

F. Epidemic measures

Ensure outbreaks are rapidly controlled through understanding and use of preparedness measures (i.e. stockpiles of medical supplies, establishment of standard treatment protocols and staff training) and rapid response (i.e. rapid confirmation, investigation and implementation of control measures).

1) Identify and train epidemic response teams.
2) Ensure adequate supplies of vaccines, drugs and equipment.
3) Establish standard operational procedures for verification, investigation and implementation of control measures.
4) Ensure appropriate risk communication with partners, government and media.

Management of Dead Bodies

Deaths associated with natural disasters are overwhelmingly caused by blunt trauma, crush-related injuries or drowning. Violence in a conflict situation can also lead to large numbers of deaths due to deliberate injury. The sudden presence of large numbers of dead bodies (corpses) in an emergency-affected area can fuel fears of outbreaks.

There is no evidence that dead bodies pose a risk of epidemics following natural disasters or acute conflict situations where deaths are due to violence, though they may cause personal communicable disease risks to relief workers who have direct contact. The source of infection is more likely to be survivors than those killed by the natural disaster or acute conflict. Even when deaths are due to communicable diseases, pathogenic organisms generally do not survive longer than a few hours in the human body following death (with the exception of HIV, which can survive in the body up to 6 days after death).

Corpses posing a risk of outbreak in a small number of situations that may require specific precautions are those from persons who died from cholera, shigellosis or hemorrhagic fevers. Despite such exceptions, the risk of outbreaks from corpses after natural disasters and acute conflict is frequently exaggerated by both health officials and the media.

On the other hand, however, emergency relief workers who routinely handle corpses may be at considerable risk of contracting tuberculosis, blood-borne viruses (such as hemorrhagic fevers, hepatitis B, hepatitis C and HIV), and gastrointestinal infections (such as rotavirus diarrhea, salmonellosis, *E. coli*, typhoid/paratyphoid fevers, hepatitis A, shigellosis and cholera).

- Tuberculosis can be acquired if the bacillus is aerosolized (via exhalation of residual air in lungs, or fluid from lungs spurted up through nose/mouth during handling of the corpse).
- Exposure of relief workers to blood-borne viruses can occur from direct contact of blood or body fluid of the corpse with non-intact skin; injury from bone fragments and other sharp body protrusions; or exposure of the mucus membranes and splashing of blood or body fluids.
- Gastrointestinal infections can occur when dead bodies leak feces. Transmission occurs via the fecal-oral route through direct contact

with the body and soiled clothes, or contaminated vehicles or equipment. Dead bodies contaminating the water supply may also cause gastrointestinal infections.

The management of dead bodies is often based on the false belief that they represent an epidemic hazard if they are not buried or burned immediately. Immediate burial or cremation, however, does not constitute an essential public health measure, and may violate important social norms.

When managing dead bodies in a humanitarian emergency, best practices are the following:

1) Burial is preferable to cremation in mass casualty situations.
2) Every effort should be made to identify all corpses.
3) Mass burials should be avoided if at all possible.
4) Families should have the opportunity to conduct culturally appropriate funerals and burials according to social custom, on the understanding that any practices that could transmit disease from the corpse to the family members should be avoided.
5) Where customs vary, separate areas should be available for each social group to exercise their own funerary traditions with dignity.
6) Where existing facilities such as graveyards or crematoria are inadequate, alternative locations or facilities should be provided.
7) The affected community should also have access to materials to meet their needs for culturally acceptable funeral pyres and other funeral rites.

Additional procedures/guidelines for emergency relief workers who routinely handle dead bodies:

1) Ensure universal precautions for blood and body fluids.
2) Ensure use and correct disposal of gloves.
3) Use body bags if available.
4) Wash hands with soap after handling bodies.
5) Disinfect vehicles and equipment.
6) Dead bodies do not need disinfection before burial (except in the case of deaths due to cholera, shigellosis or hemorrhagic fever).
7) The bottom of any grave must be at least 1.5 meters above the water table, with a 0.7 meter unsaturated zone.

Conclusion

Much of the excess mortality and morbidity due to communicable diseases that occur in emergency-affected populations is avoidable through appropriate planning, understanding and preparedness. Effective interventions are usually available, and if rapidly implemented along with preventive measures as part of the humanitarian response, can significantly reduce the impact of these diseases on the population. Coordination between governments, UN agencies and non-governmental agencies working at local, national and international levels, and collaboration between all sectors providing emergency relief—health, food and nutrition, shelter, water and sanitation—is crucial in order to protect the health of emergency-affected populations.

HANDLING OF INFECTIOUS MATERIALS
[N. Previsani]

I. BIOSAFETY/BIOSECURITY

Laboratory Biosafety

Laboratory biosafety, as defined by WHO, describes "the containment principles, technologies and practices that are implemented to prevent unintentional exposure to pathogens and toxins, or their accidental release".

Good biosafety practice is essential for the protection of laboratory workers, the environment and the wider population from contamination with infectious substances. Its foundation is a combination of good work practices, proper containment facilities and equipment, effective design and ergonomics of work environments, regular maintenance and competent operation of equipment, and logistical competence to reduce or eliminate the risk of contamination. Additionally, before working with any infectious agent in a laboratory, proper facility-specific risk assessment must be undertaken to determine whether it is sensible to work on that particular agent in that particular facility, taking into account the following:

- Pathogenicity and mode of transmission of the agent in question.
- Local availability of effective preventive measures in case of a possible outbreak.
- Local availability of treatment for infection.
- Equipment and procedures necessary for safe work with the agent in question.
- Capacity of available laboratory facilities.

Laboratory Biosecurity

Laboratory biosecurity, as defined by WHO, describes "the protection, control and accountability for valuable biological materials within laboratories, in order to prevent their unauthorized access, loss, theft, misuse, diversion or intentional release." Valuable biological materials (VBM) are defined as "Biological materials that require (according to their owners, users, custodians, caretakers or regulators) administrative oversight, control, accountability, and specific protective and monitoring measures in laboratories to protect their economic and historical (archival) value, and/or the population from their potential to cause harm". VBM may include pathogens and toxins, as well as non-pathogenic organisms, vaccine strains, foods, genetically modified organisms (GMOs), cell components, genetic elements, and extraterrestrial samples.

WHO recommends the establishment of national standards that recognize and address the responsibility of countries and institutions to protect specimens, pathogens and toxins from misuse.

Guidance on issues pertaining to both laboratory biosafety and biosecurity is available at:

<http://www.who.int/csr/bioriskreduction/biosafety/en/index.html>

II. TRANSPORT AND TRANSFER OF INFECTIOUS SUBSTANCES

Diagnostic specimens collected from humans and/or animals suspected of infection with a communicable disease must at times be shipped from one location to another. In these situations, they must be transported safely, efficiently and legally, and packaged and transported in such a way as to protect those engaged in their transportation from the risk of infection.

This risk can be kept to a minimum by ensuring proper packaging. Damage to packaging means that samples are unlikely to arrive at their destination on time, and that people involved in the shipping process have been placed at risk. Packaging of specimens of potentially infectious materials is highly regulated to ensure appropriateness and consistency, and to make sure that materials are accompanied with adequate information.

Specimens that potentially contain communicable disease agents are divided into two categories:

- **Category A** specimens potentially contain infectious agents capable of causing permanent disability and/or life-threatening or fatal disease in otherwise healthy humans or animals.
- **Category B** specimens are those infectious materials that do not meet the criteria for inclusion in Category A.

For transport of specimens of both Categories A and B, standard consensus recommendations have been developed by the United Nations.

For Category A specimens, triple packaging must be used consisting of the following three layers:

1) A watertight and leak-proof primary receptacle containing the specimen, packaged with sufficient absorbent material to absorb all fluid in case of breakage
2) Secondary durable, watertight, leak-proof packaging to enclose and protect the primary receptacle(s). Several primary receptacles may be placed in one secondary packaging, but sufficient additional absorbent material must be used to absorb all fluid in case of breakage of all primary receptacles
3) An outer packaging.

The packaging must meet strict performance criteria and must be shipped with documents certifying that it has passed the necessary testing. Tests for compliance include a 9-meter drop test, a puncture test, and a pressure test. The outer packaging must bear the United Nations packaging specification marking, which indicates that the packaging has passed the performance tests to the satisfaction of the competent authority. UN-specific packages for the shipment of Category A infectious substances must be purchased from authorized providers.

For Category B specimens, the same three layers of packaging are required, but documents certifying testing are not required. Tests for Category B packaging include a 1.2-meter drop test and a pressure test. Packaging may be sourced locally rather than through authorized suppliers, provided the packaging manufacturer and shipper comply fully with testing and packaging requirements.

Specific markings and labeling requirements apply for Category A and Category B specimens, as well as for the dry ice and liquid nitrogen that are used to keep the samples frozen. Shipping documents accompanying the consignments must include completed *pro forma* invoices, air waybills, and appropriate import/export permits if required.

A shipper's Declaration for Dangerous Goods is required for shipments of Category A specimens. It is the responsibility and full liability of the shipper to ensure the correct classification, packaging, labeling and documentation of all potentially infectious substances destined for transport. Non-compliance may lead to civil penalties and/or prosecution.

Transfer

Shipments of specimens across borders require import/export permits from the countries of departure, transit and destination, in order to allow the tracking of the transfer. The details of the required documentation are dictated by the characteristics of the agents being transported. Generally, transfer issues are addressed by national health, agriculture and/or customs authorities.

Efficient transport and transfer require coordination between the shipper, the carrier and the receiver of the materials, in order to ensure that they are transported safely, and that they arrive on time and in good condition. Such coordination depends upon well-established communication and the existence of a good working relationship between all three parties. It is recommended that such a working relationship be developed in advance of shipping.

Shippers, carriers and receivers have specific responsibilities in ensuring successful transportation. Compliance with the rules in the execution of these responsibilities will reduce the likelihood that packages will be damaged and leak, thereby reducing exposure and possible infections, and improving the efficiency of package delivery.

Carriers not wishing to carry particular goods are under no legal obligation to do so. They have the right to refuse to carry goods, or to add additional requirements for their passage.

Some regions are not regularly covered by commercial transport services, and some countries may not have specific transport regulations in place, further adding to the difficulty of shipping specimens. Only through focused efforts to address any issues that are an impediment to transport will suitable conditions be developed and maintained that ensure the efficient, timely and legal transport and transfer of infectious substances.

Further substantive information on transport of infectious substances, including guidelines, diagrams and checklists for packaging, international regulations and spill clean-up procedure, are available at:

<http://www.who.int/csr/resources/publications/biosafety/WHO_CDS_EPR_2007_2/en/index.html>

❖

ACQUIRED IMMUNODEFICIENCY
SYNDROME ICD-9 042-044, 279.5; ICD-10 B20-B24
(HIV infection, AIDS)
[CCDM19: P. Kilmarx]
[CCDM18: T. Boerma]

1. Identification—Acquired Immunodeficiency Syndrome (AIDS) was first recognized in 1981 in a cluster of diseases associated with loss of cellular immunity in adults who had no obvious reason for presenting such immune deficiencies. AIDS was subsequently shown to be the late clinical stage of infection with the human immunodeficiency virus (HIV). Within several weeks after infection with HIV, many persons develop an acute self-limited mononucleosis-like illness lasting for a week or two. They may then be free of clinical signs or symptoms for years before other clinical manifestations develop. The frequency and severity of subsequent HIV-related opportunistic infections or cancers is, in general, directly correlated with the degree of immune system dysfunction.

According to CDC and WHO, HIV infection is defined by laboratory criteria, usually based on detection of HIV antibody, but may also include virological tests for HIV or one of its components. The CDC surveillance AIDS case definition was last revised in 1993, and includes presence of at least one of 23 clinical conditions, provided other causes of immunodeficiency are ruled out. The presence of one of three other clinical conditions or a CD4+ cell count of under $200/mm^3$ or a CD4+ T-lymphocyte percentage of total lymphocytes under 14%, regardless of clinical status, are also regarded as AIDS cases if laboratory tests showed evidence of HIV infection. The WHO case definition of AIDS is based on laboratory-confirmed HIV infection plus the presence of any of 22 "stage 4" clinical conditions or a CD4+ lymphocyte count of under $200/mm^3$ or a CD4+ percentage of less than 15. WHO and CDC also have published pediatric AIDS case definitions.

The proportion of HIV-infected persons who, in the absence of anti-HIV treatment, will ultimately develop AIDS has been estimated at over 90%. In the absence of effective anti-HIV treatment, the AIDS case-fatality rate is high: survival time in many developing country studies is often under 1 year; in industrialized countries 80%–90% of untreated patients used to die within 3–5 years after diagnosis. Routine use of prophylactic drugs to prevent *Pneumocystis* pneumonia and other opportunistic infections, seen in most industrialized countries before effective anti-HIV treatment had become widely available, significantly postponed the development of AIDS-defining clinical conditions and death.

Serological tests for antibodies to HIV have been available commercially since 1985. The most commonly used screening tests (EIA or ELISA) are highly sensitive and specific. Testing strategies depend on the purpose of testing. For surveillance purposes, different strategies are recommended according to the expected level of HIV prevalence in the population tested: a single test is recommended in populations with a prevalence rate above 10%, but lower prevalence levels require a minimum of 2 different tests for reliability. For diagnostic purposes, a 3-test strategy for asymptomatic persons is recommended in populations with an HIV prevalence rate under 10%, and a 2-test strategy in populations with higher rates. Selection of tests depends on such factors as accuracy and local operational characteristics. Different combinations of testing formats, EIA and rapid tests can be used. Confirmatory testing may include the Western blot or indirect fluorescent antibody (IFA) tests. A non-reactive supplemental test negates an initial reactive EIA test; a positive reaction supports it; and an indeterminate result in the Western blot test calls for further evaluation. Rapid testing techniques on blood or oral mucosal transudate facilitate delivery of testing and counseling services.

Most persons infected with HIV develop antibodies detectable with modern tests within one month after infection. The vast majority of people have positive antibody tests by three months after infection. Other tests to detect HIV infection during the period after infection but prior to seroconversion are available; these include tests for circulating HIV antigen (p24) and PCR tests to detect viral nucleic acid sequences. The window period between the time of infection and seroconversion is short, an average of 3-4 weeks with currently available antibody tests. DNA PCR testing plays an important role in pediatric HIV diagnosis, because the presence of passively transferred maternal antibody can result in positive HIV antibody tests in the absence of HIV infection before 18 months of age.

The absolute T-helper cell (CD4+) count or percentage is used most often to evaluate the progression of HIV infection and to help clinicians make treatment decisions. Viral load tests serve as a marker of disease activity and response to treatment. The differential window periods of EIA and tests such as p24 antigenemia have served to identify recent infections for surveillance purposes. A person reacting positively on the sensitive test and negatively on the less sensitive is likely to have been infected recently. When HIV testing and treatment history are known, the prevalence of recently infected persons may be used to estimate population-level HIV incidence.

2. Infectious agent—Human immunodeficiency virus (HIV), a retrovirus. Two serologically and geographically distinct species, HIV-1 and HIV-2, have been identified. The transmissibility and pathogenicity of HIV-2 may be lower than that of HIV-1. This chapter refers to HIV-1 except where specified. Three groups of HIV-1 have been identified—M, N and O. Group M is the most prevalent and is subdivided into seven subtypes or clades. Circulating recombinant forms, initially derived from co-infection with different subtypes, are also prevalent. There may be differences between HIV-1 subtypes in rates of disease progression and possibly in transmissibility.

3. Occurrence—AIDS was first recognized as a distinct clinical entity in 1981. In retrospect, however, isolated cases appear to have occurred during the 1970s, and even earlier in several areas (Africa, Europe, Haiti, USA). Of the estimated 33 million persons (95% confidence interval, 31–36 million) worldwide living with HIV infection or AIDS (HIV/AIDS) in 2007, the largest elements were estimated at 22.5 million in sub-Saharan Africa, 4.0 million in south and southeastern Asia, 1.6 million in Latin America, 1.6 million in eastern Europe and central Asia, and 1.3 million in North America. Globally, AIDS caused an estimated 2.1 million deaths in 2007 (1.9–2.4 million); the epidemic has continued growing, with estimates of 2.5 million new infections (1.8–4.1 million) and 2.1 million children under 15 years (1.9–2.4 million) living with HIV/AIDS. AIDS is now the leading cause of death in persons aged 15 to 59 years old. HIV-1 is the most prevalent HIV species throughout the world; HIV-2 has been found primarily in western Africa, with cases also in countries linked epidemiologically to western Africa.

Sub-Saharan Africa is the most affected region; southern Africa is the worst affected. Unlike other regions, the majority of people (61%) living with HIV in sub-Saharan Africa are women. Prevalence has stabilized or is decreasing in most countries, along with some evidence of decreasing risk behavior. In Asia, prevalence is highest in southeast Asia, with considerable variation in trends – declining in some countries while continuing to grow in others. The Caribbean region has the second-highest prevalence worldwide after sub-Saharan Africa, with two countries, the Dominican Republic and Haiti, accounting for most people with HIV infection in the region. In eastern Europe and central Asia, Russia and Ukraine account for most new HIV diagnoses, but rates are also rising in other countries. Injection drug use is a major factor in the region. Latin America's HIV epidemics are generally stable, with transmission largely in higher-risk populations such as sex workers and men who have sex with men. In North America, Western, Central Europe, Australia and New Zealand, HIV continues to be transmitted mainly through unprotected sex between men.

4. Reservoir—Humans. HIV-1 evolved from chimpanzee simian immunodeficiency viruses (SIVcpz) that crossed over to humans, presumably from bites or from hunting, butchering, or consumption of bush meat. HIV-2 evolved from cross-species transmission events of sooty mangabey SIV (SIVsm).

5. Mode of transmission—Person-to-person transmission through unprotected penile-vaginal or penile-anal intercourse; the use of HIV-contaminated needles and syringes, including sharing by intravenous drug users; vertical transmission from mother to infant during pregnancy, delivery, or breastfeeding; transfusion of infected blood or its components.

Less common modes of transmission include contact of abraded skin or mucosa with infectious body secretions; and the transplantation of HIV-infected tissues or organs. Transmission though pre-mastication (pre-chewing) of food by HIV-infected pediatric caregivers has also been reported.

The approximate transmission risk per 10 000 exposures with an infected partner for receptive penile-vaginal sex is 10; for insertive penile-vaginal sex, 5; receptive penile-anal sex, 50; insertive penile-anal sex, 6.5; injection drug use with shared injection equipment, 67; and contaminated blood transfusion, 9 000.

The risk of sexual HIV transmission is increased by the presence of other sexually transmitted diseases, especially genital ulcerative disease. Lack of male circumcision also substantially increases the risk of female-to-male HIV transmission. At the population level, the frequency of concurrent sex partners (multiple partners in the same time period) is an important determinant of HIV infection rates.

In the absence of prevention interventions, the transmission rate of HIV from infected mothers to their children is about 25% in the absence of breastfeeding and about 35% in breast feeding populations.

After direct exposure of health care workers to HIV-infected blood through injury with needles and other sharp objects, the rate of seroconversion is less than 0.5%, much lower than the risk of hepatitis B virus infection after similar exposures (about 25%). Unsafe injections may account for up to 5% of HIV transmission. The risk to health care workers after mucous membrane exposure has been estimated to be 0.09%; the risk after exposure of non-intact skin has not been quantified, but is estimate to be lower than for mucous membrane exposure.

Carriers are usually asymptomatic; they—and their potential partners—are usually therefore unaware of their potential infection status in the absence of HIV testing.

While the virus has occasionally been found in saliva, tears, urine and bronchial secretions, transmission after contact with these secretions in the absence of blood has not been reported. The risk of transmission from oral sex is not easily quantifiable, but is presumed to be low. No laboratory or epidemiological evidence suggests that biting insects have transmitted HIV infection.

6. Incubation period—Variable. Although the time from infection to the development of detectable antibodies is generally less than one month, the time from HIV infection to diagnosis of AIDS has an observed range of less than 1 year to 15 years or longer. The median time to development of AIDS in infected infants is shorter than in adults. The increasing availability of effective anti-HIV treatment since the mid-1990s has reduced the development of clinical AIDS, especially in developed countries. Before effective treatment was available, about half of all HIV-infected adults and adolescents in developed countries died within 11 years following infection.

There is some evidence that disease progression from HIV infection to AIDS is more rapid in developing countries than in other populations. The only factor that has been consistently shown to affect progression from HIV infection to the development of AIDS is age at initial infection: adolescent and adults (males and females) who acquire HIV infection at an early age progress to AIDS more slowly than those infected at an older age. Disease progression may also vary by viral subtype.

7. **Period of communicability**—Not known precisely; begins early after onset of HIV infection and presumably extends throughout life. Infectiousness is related to viral load. The risk of transmission may be high in the first months after infection when viral load is high, before immune suppression has occurred, and while the high-risk behaviors that led to infection may still be ongoing. Viral load also increases in late symptomatic infection. The presence of STIs has been shown to increase HIV viral load in genital secretions. While use of antiretroviral drugs reduces HIV viral load in blood and genital secretions, individuals on treatment should still be considered infectious.

8. **Susceptibility**—Unknown, but presumed to be general: race, gender and pregnancy status do not appear to affect susceptibility to HIV infection or AIDS. There is increasing evidence of host factors such as chemokine-receptor polymorphisms that may reduce susceptibility. Lack of male circumcision also increases susceptibility to female-to-male transmission. The presence of other STIs, especially if ulcerative, increases susceptibility.

While HIV infection increases the risk of many opportunistic infections, interactions between HIV and several infectious disease agents have caused particular medical and public health concern. An interaction of major public health importance is with *Mycobacterium tuberculosis* infection. Persons with latent tuberculous infection who are also infected with HIV develop clinical tuberculosis at an increased rate, with a lifetime risk of developing tuberculosis that is multiplied by a factor of 6–8. This increased risk and the resulting increased transmission have contributed to a parallel pandemic of tuberculosis: in some urban sub-Saharan African populations where 10%–15% of the adult population have dual infections (*Mycobacterium tuberculosis* and HIV), annual incidence rates for tuberculosis increased 5- to 10-fold during the latter half of the 1990s.

HIV infection may increase rates and severity of malarial infection, and anti-malarial treatment may be less effective in HIV-infected individuals. Other adverse interactions with HIV infection include genital herpes, pneumococcal infection, non-Typhi salmonellosis, and visceral leishmaniasis.

In the other direction, infections such as tuberculosis, malaria, and genital herpes may increase HIV viral load and the rate of decline of CD4+ cells. However, the long-term clinical implications of these laboratory findings are less well understood.

9. **Methods of control** – Global resources for HIV/AIDS prevention, care and treatment have ramped up considerably in the last several years. An estimated US$10 billion was available for HIV/AIDS worldwide in 2007 with ongoing substantial increases in prevention programs, prevention of mother-to-child transmission, antiretroviral treatment, and other care and support for people with HIV/AIDS, orphans and vulnerable children.

A. **Preventive measures:** HIV/AIDS prevention programs can be effective only with full community and political commitment to change and/or reduce high HIV-risk behaviors. Health education efforts should include both broad-based campaigns to raise awareness of risk, modes of transmission, and prevention measures, and to reduce stigmatization, as well as targeted programs to educate and reduce risk among high-risk groups such as sex workers, injection drug users, and men who have sex with men.

Abstaining from sexual intercourse, while not practical for many, is an absolutely effective way of preventing transmission. Engaging in sex with an uninfected, mutually monogamous partner is also effective, although ensuring mutually monogamy and absence of infection may be challenging. In other cases, correct and consistent use of male condoms is highly effective in preventing transmission. Female condoms, although more costly, are also effective.

Prevention and treatment of injection drug use reduces HIV transmission, as do programs that provide clean injection equipment or instruct users on decontamination of equipment between uses.

Post-exposure prophylaxis with combination antiretroviral drugs is available and recommended in some settings after occupational exposure or non-occupational exposure to HIV infection. If indicated and available, treatment should begin within hours of exposure and is usually recommended to continue for 28 days.

HIV testing and counseling is important to identify infected individuals for referral for care and treatment, and, for pregnant women, to prevent vertical transmission. Risk behavior for HIV-infected persons decreases when infection is identified. HIV testing also provides a setting for condom distribution and delivery of prevention messages for HIV-negative persons. In many settings, the emphasis is on universal, opt-out testing for all individuals, especially in high-prevalence communities.

Mother-to-child HIV transmission can be minimized through primary prevention of HIV infection in women of child-bearing age, prevention of unintended pregnancy in HIV-infected women, and universal screening of pregnant women. An additional HIV test in the third trimester of pregnancy may identify women who seroconverted during pregnancy. With use of maternal and infant antiretrovirals in accordance with national guidelines, vertical transmission rates can be reduced by 50-90% or more. Transmission by breastfeeding may be avoided through use of infant formula, but only where it is acceptable, feasible, affordable, sustainable, and safe. Elective cesarean section may also play a role in resource-rich settings, where use of multiple preventive measures results in transmission rates of under 2%.

Blood donations should be sought from unpaid, volunteer donors. All donated units of blood must be tested for HIV antibody; only donations testing negative can be used. Testing for HIV antigen or nucleic acid can further reduce the risk of contamination. People who have engaged in behaviors that place them at increased risk of HIV infection should not donate plasma, blood, organs for transplantation, tissue or cells (including semen for artificial insemination). Organizations that collect plasma, blood or other body fluids or organs should inform potential donors of this recommendation and test all donors. When possible, donations of sperm, milk or bone should be frozen and stored for 3-6 months before use. Donors who test negative after that interval can be considered not to have been infected at the time of donation. Only strictly medically necessary transfusions should be given. The use of autologous transfusions should be encouraged. Only clotting factor products that have been screened and treated to inactivate HIV should be used.

Only medically necessary injections should be given. Care must be taken in handling, using and disposing of needles or other sharp instruments. Medical waste should be safely stored and destroyed. Health care workers should be provided with and instructed on the proper use of latex gloves, eye protection and other personal protective equipment as needed in order to avoid contact with blood or with fluids. Universal precautions must be taken in the care of all patients and in all laboratory procedures.

WHO recommends immunization of asymptomatic HIV-infected children with the EPI vaccines; those who are symptomatic should not receive BCG vaccine. Live Measles-Mumps-Rubella and Polio vaccines are recommended for all HIV-infected children. CDC does not recommend use of OPV for HIV-infected children.

B. Control of patient, contacts and the immediate environment:

1) Report to local health authority: Official reporting of AIDS cases is obligatory in most countries. Official reporting of HIV infections is required in some areas, Class 2 (see *Reporting*). Whether or not name-based reporting is the rule, care must be taken to protect patient confidentiality.

2) Isolation: Isolation of the HIV-positive person is unnecessary, ineffective and unjustified. Universal precautions apply to all hospitalized patients. Observe additional precautions appropriate for specific infections that occur in AIDS patients.

3) Concurrent disinfection: Of equipment contaminated with blood or body fluids, and with excretions and secretions visibly contaminated with blood and body fluids according to universal precautions guidelines, by using bleach solution or germicides effective against *M. tuberculosis*.

4) Quarantine: Not applicable. Patients and their sexual partners should not donate blood, plasma, organs for transplantation, tissues, cells, or breast milk for human milk banks. Although not widely recommended, some centers have reported safe impregnation of women by HIV-infected male partners through semen processing or viral suppression in the men with antiretroviral treatment.

5) Immunization of contacts: Not applicable.

6) Notification of contacts and source of infection: Sex and needle-sharing partners should be notified of their exposure. Notification may be done by the index patient or by health staff with strict confidentiality.

7) Specific treatment: Early diagnosis of infection and referral for medical evaluation are indicated. Consult current sources of information for appropriate drugs, schedules and doses, including WHO and UNAIDS websites. Ongoing education and counseling to maintain the patient's health, adherence to treatment, and prevention of transmission are indicated.

a) Prophylaxis of opportunistic infections. Prophylactic use of oral cotrimoxazole is recommended to prevent *Pneumocystis* pneumonia and other infections. Isoniazid preventive treatment is given in some settings, with our without use of tuberculin skin tests. Other primary or secondary prophylactic medications may be recommended in specific situations.

b) AIDS must be managed as a chronic disease; antiretroviral treatment is complex, involving a combination of drugs: resistance will rapidly appear if only one or two effective drugs are used. The drugs may have toxic side effects, and treatment must be life-long. Adherence is critical for the success of the treatment. A successful treatment is not a cure, although it results in suppression of viral replication. Ideally, decisions to initiate or change antiretroviral treatment should be guided by the laboratory parameters of both plasma HIV RNA (viral load) and CD4+ T cell count where available, and by assessing the clinical condition of the patient. Laboratory results provide important information about the virological and immunological status of the patient and the risk of progression to AIDS. Once the decision to initiate anti-retroviral treatment has been made, treatment should be aggressive with the goal of maximal viral suppression. In general, two nucleoside reverse transcriptase inhibitors and either a non-nucleoside reverse transcriptase inhibitor or protease inhibitors should be used initially. Special considerations apply to pediatric patients and pregnant women, with specific treatment regimens for these patients.

C. *Epidemic measures:* HIV is currently pandemic, with large numbers of infections reported in Africa, Asia, Americas, and Europe. See 9A (*Preventive measures*) for recommendations.

D. *Disaster implications:* Emergency personnel should follow the same universal precautions as health workers. If latex gloves are not available and skin surfaces come into contact with blood, this should be washed off as soon as possible. Surgical masks, visors and protective clothing are indicated when performing procedures that may involve spurting or splashing of blood or bloody fluids. Emergency transfusion services should use blood donations screened for HIV antibody; when it is not possible to test donated blood, donations should be accepted only from donors who have engaged in no HIV-risk behaviors, and preferably from donors who have previously tested negative for HIV.

E. *International measures:* Neither the United Nations Joint Program on HIV/AIDS (UNAIDS, the body that coordinates HIV- and AIDS-related UN activities) nor WHO endorse measures such as requirements for AIDS or HIV examinations for foreign travelers prior to entry into a country.

ACTINOMYCOSIS   ICD-9 039; ICD-10 A42

1. **Identification**—A chronic bacterial disease, most frequently localized in the jaw, thorax or abdomen. The lesions, firmly indurated areas of purulence and fibrosis, spread slowly to contiguous tissues; eventually, draining sinuses may appear and penetrate to the surface. In infected tissue, the organism grows in clusters, called "sulfur granules."

Diagnosis is made by demonstrating slim, non-spore-forming, Gram-positive bacilli, with or without branching, or "sulfur granules" in tissue or pus; and by isolating microorganisms from samples of appropriate clinical materials not contaminated with normal flora during collection. Clinical findings and culture allow distinction between actinomycosis and actinomycetoma, which are very different diseases (for more information, please see *Mycetoma*).

2. Infectious agents—*Actinomyces israelii* is the usual human pathogen; *A. naeslundii*, *A. meyeri*, *A. odontolyticus* and *Propionibacterium propionicus* (*Arachnia propionica* or *Actinomyces propionicus*) are reported to cause human actinomycosis. Rarely, *A. viscosus* has been reported, but it is more reliably established as contributing to the etiology of periodontal disease. All species are Gram-positive, non acid-fast, anerobic to microaerophilic higher bacteria that may be part of normal oral flora.

3. Occurrence—An infrequent human disease, occurring sporadically worldwide. Men and women of all races and age groups may be affected; frequency is maximal between 15 and 35 years; the M:F ratio is approximately 2:1. Cases in cattle, horses and other animals are caused by other *Actinomyces* species.

4. Reservoir—Humans are the natural reservoir of *A. israelii* and other agents. In the normal oral cavity, the organisms grow as saprophytes in dental plaque and in tonsillar crypts, without apparent penetration or cellular response in adjacent tissues. Sample surveys in Sweden, the USA and other countries have demonstrated *A. israelii* microscopically in granules from crypts of 40% of extirpated tonsils, and by anerobic culture in up to 48% of specimens of saliva or material from carious teeth. *A. israelii* has been found in vaginal secretions of approximately 10% of women using intrauterine devices. No external environmental reservoir, such as straw or soil, has been demonstrated.

5. Mode of transmission—Presumably the agent passes by contact from person to person as part of the normal oral flora. From the oral cavity, the organism may be aspirated into the lung or introduced into jaw tissues through injury, extraction of teeth or mucosal abrasion. Abdominal disease most commonly originates in the appendix. The source of clinical disease is endogenous.

6. Incubation period—Irregular; probably many years after colonization in the oral tissues, and days or months after precipitating trauma and actual penetration of tissues.

7. Period of communicability—How and when *Actinomyces* and *Arachnia* species become part of normal oral flora is unknown; except for rare instances of human bite, infection is unrelated to specific exposure to an infected person.

8. Susceptibility—Natural susceptibility is low. Immunity following infection has not been demonstrated.

9. **Methods of control—**

A. **Preventive measures:** Maintenance of oral hygiene, particularly removal of accumulating dental plaque, will reduce risk of oral infection.

B. **Control of patient, contacts and the immediate environment:**

1) Report to local health authority: Official report not ordinarily justifiable, Class 5 (see *Reporting*).
2) Isolation: Not applicable.
3) Concurrent disinfection: Not applicable.
4) Quarantine: Not applicable.
5) Immunization of contacts: Not applicable.
6) Investigation of contacts and source of infection: Not beneficial.
7) Specific treatment: No spontaneous recovery. Prolonged administration of penicillin in high doses is usually effective; tetracycline, erythromycin, clindamycin and cephalosporins are alternatives, though tetracycline cannot be used in children less than eight years of age. Surgical drainage of abscesses is often necessary.

C. **Epidemic measures:** Not applicable, a sporadic disease.

D. **Disaster implications:** None.

E. **International measures:** None.

AMEBIASIS
(Amoebiasis)

ICD-9 006; ICD-10 A06

[CCDM19: M. Eberhard, A. Gabrielli, L. Savioli, G. Visvesvara]
[CCDM18: L. Savioli]

1. **Identification**—A protozoan parasite (*Entamoeba histolytica*) infection that exists in 2 forms: the hardy infective cyst and the more fragile, potentially pathogenic trophozoite. The parasite may act as a commensal, or invade the tissues and give rise to intestinal or extraintestinal disease. Most infections are asymptomatic, but may become clinically important under certain circumstances. Intestinal disease varies from acute or fulminating dysentery with fever, chills and bloody or mucoid diarrhea (amebic dysentery) to mild abdominal discomfort with diarrhea containing blood or mucus, alternating with periods of constipation or remission. Amebic granulomata (ameboma), sometimes mistaken for carcinoma, may occur in the wall of the large intestine in patients with intermittent

dysentery or colitis of long duration. Dissemination via the bloodstream may occur and produce abscesses of the liver, less commonly of the lung or brain. Ulceration of the skin, usually in the perianal region, occurs rarely by direct extension from intestinal lesions or amebic liver abscesses; penile lesions may occur in active homosexuals.

Amebic colitis is often confused with forms of inflammatory bowel disease such as ulcerative colitis; care should be taken to distinguish the two, since corticosteroids may exacerbate amebic colitis. Amebiasis can also mimic numerous noninfectious and infectious diseases. Conversely, the presence of amebae may be misinterpreted as the cause of diarrhea in a person whose primary enteric illness is the result of another condition.

Diagnosis is by microscopic demonstration of trophozoites or cysts in fresh or suitably preserved fecal specimens, smears of aspirates, scrapings obtained by proctoscopy, or aspirates of abscesses or sections of tissue. The presence of trophozoites containing red blood cells is indicative of invasive amebiasis. Examination should be done on fresh specimens by a trained microscopist, since the organism must be differentiated from nonpathogenic amebae and macrophages. Examination of at least 3 specimens will increase the yield of organisms from 50% in a single specimen to 85-90%. Stool antigen detection tests have recently become available, but do not distinguish pathogenic from nonpathogenic organisms. Available assays specific for *Entamoeba histolytic* are also available, such as EIA and PCR (fresh, unpreserved stool is required for EIA and PCR testing), but reference laboratory services may be required. Many serological tests are available as adjuncts in diagnosing extraintestinal amebiasis, such as liver abscess, where stool examination is often negative. Serological tests, particularly immunodiffusion and ELISA, are very useful in diagnosis of invasive disease. Scintillography, ultrasonography and CAT scanning are helpful in revealing the presence and location of an amebic liver abscess, and can be considered diagnostic when associated with a specific antibody response to *E. histolytica*.

2. Infectious agent—*Entamoeba histolytica*, a parasitic organism not to be confused with *E. hartmanni*, *E. dispar*, *E. moshkovskii*, *E. coli* or other intestinal protozoa. In isolates, 9 potentially pathogenic and 13 nonpathogenic zymodemes (classified as *E. dispar*) have been identified. Most asymptomatic cyst passers carry strains of *E. dispar*. Immunological differences, isoenzyme patterns, and PCR permit differentiation of pathogenic *E. histolytica* from the morphologically identical, nonpathogenic *E. dispar*.

3. Occurrence—Amebiasis is ubiquitous. Invasive (symptomatic) amebiasis is mostly a disease of young adults. Liver abscesses occur predominantly in males. Amebiasis is rare below age 5, and especially below age 2, when dysentery is due typically to shigellae. Asymptomatic carriers are common in endemic areas. The proportion of cyst passers who have clinical disease is usually low. Published prevalence rates of cyst passage, usually based on cyst morphology, vary from place to place, with rates generally higher in areas with poor sanitation, in mental institutions, and among sexually promiscuous male homosexuals (probably *E. dispar*). In areas with good sanitation, amebic infections tend to cluster in households and institutions.

4. Reservoir—Only humans, usually a chronically ill or asymptomatic cyst passer.

5. Mode of transmission—Mainly through ingestion of fecally contaminated food or water containing amebic cysts, which are relatively chlorine resistant. Cysts can survive in moist environmental conditions for weeks to months. Transmission may occur sexually by oral-anal contact with a chronically ill or asymptomatic cyst passer. Patients with acute amebic dysentery probably pose only limited danger to others because of the absence of cysts in dysenteric stools and the fragility of trophozoites.

6. Incubation period—Variable, from a few days to several months or years; commonly 2–4 weeks.

7. Period of communicability—During the period in which *E. histolytica* cysts are passed, which may continue for years.

8. Susceptibility—Susceptibility to infection is general; those harboring *E. dispar* do not develop disease. Susceptibility to reinfection has been demonstrated but is apparently rare.

9. Methods of control—

   A. Preventive measures:

   1) Educate the general public in personal hygiene, particularly in sanitary disposal of feces and in handwashing after defecation and before preparing or eating food. Disseminate information regarding the risks involved in eating uncleaned or uncooked fruits and vegetables, and in drinking water of questionable purity.
   2) Dispose of human feces in a sanitary manner.
   3) Protect public water supplies from fecal contamination. Sand filtration of water removes nearly all cysts and diatomaceous earth filters remove them completely. Water of undetermined quality can be made safe by boiling for 1 minute (at least 10 minutes at high altitudes). Chlorination of water as generally practiced in municipal water treatment does not always kill cysts; small quantities of water are best treated with prescribed concentrations of iodine, either liquid (8 drops of 2% tincture of iodine or 12.5 ml of a saturated aqueous solution of iodine crystals per liter or quart of water), or as water purification tablets (1 tablet of tetraglycine hydroperiodide per liter or quart of water). Allow for a contact period of at least 10 minutes (30

minutes if cold) before drinking the water. Portable filters with less than 1.0 micrometer pore sizes are also effective.

4) Treat known carriers; stress the need for thorough hand-washing after defecation to avoid reinfection from an infected domestic resident.

5) Educate high-risk groups to avoid sexual practices that may permit fecal-oral transmission.

6) Health agencies should supervise the sanitary practices of people who prepare and serve food in public eating places and the general cleanliness of the premises involved. Routine examination of food handlers as a control measure is impractical.

7) Disinfectant dips for fruits and vegetables are of unproven value in preventing transmission of *E. histolytica*. Thorough washing with potable water and keeping fruits and vegetables dry may help; cysts are killed by desiccation, by temperatures above 50°C (122°F), and by irradiation.

8) Use of chemoprophylactic agents is not advised.

B. *Control of patient, contacts and the immediate environment:*

1) Report to local health authority: In selected endemic areas; in many countries not reportable, Class 3 (see Reporting).

2) Isolation: For hospitalized patients, enteric precautions in the handling of feces, contaminated clothing and bed linen. Exclusion of individuals infected with *E. histolytica* from food handling and from direct care of hospitalized and institutionalized patients. Release to return to work in a sensitive occupation when chemotherapy is completed.

3) Concurrent disinfection: Sanitary disposal of feces.

4) Quarantine: Not applicable.

5) Immunization of contacts: Not applicable.

6) Investigation of contacts and source of infection: Household members and other suspected contacts should have adequate microscopic examination of feces.

7) Specific treatment: Asymptomatic carriers should be treated with a luminal amebicide in order to reduce the risk of transmission and protect the patient from symptomatic amebiasis. Common luminal amebicides are: diloxanide furoate, clefamide, etofamide, paromomycin and teclozan. Symptomatic amebiasis should be treated with a systemically-active compound such as metronidazole (30 mg/kg daily in 3 divided doses for 8-10 days), followed by a luminal amebicide to eliminate any surviving organisms in the colon. Tinidazole and ornidazole are also systemically-active compounds that are an alternative to metronidazole (but which are not available in some countries, including the USA).

If a patient with a liver abscess remains febrile after 72 hours of metronidazole treatment, non-surgical aspiration may be indicated. Chloroquine is sometimes added to metronidazole for treating a refractory liver abscess. Abscesses may require surgical aspiration if there is a risk of rupture or if the abscess continues to enlarge despite treatment.

Metronidazole is not recommended for use during the first trimester of pregnancy; however, it may be a life-saving drug in case of fulminating amebiasis in late pregnancy, and there has been no proof of teratogenicity in humans.

C. **Epidemic measures:** Any group of possible cases requires prompt laboratory confirmation to exclude false-positive identification of *E. histolytica* or other causal agents, and epidemiological investigation to determine source of infection and mode of transmission. If a common vehicle is indicated, such as water or food, appropriate measures should be taken to correct the situation.

D. **Disaster implications:** Disruption of normal sanitary facilities and food management will favor an outbreak of amebiasis, especially in populations that include large numbers of cyst passers.

E. **International measures:** None.

ANGIOSTRONGYLIASIS ICD-9 128.8; ICD-10 B83.2
(Eosinophilic meningoencephalitis, Eosinophilic meningitis)
[CCDM19: M. Eberhard, A. Gabrielli, L. Savioli]
[CCDM18: L. Savioli]

1. Identification—A parasitic disease of the CNS (Central Nervous System) caused by a zoonotic nematode, with predominantly meningeal involvement. Invasion may be asymptomatic or mildly symptomatic; it is commonly characterized by severe headache, neck and back stiffness, and various paresthesias. Temporary facial paralysis occurs in 5% of patients. Low-grade fever may be present. The worm has been found in the CSF (Cerebral spinal fluid) and lung, and, rarely, in the eye. CSF usually exhibits pleocytosis with over 20% eosinophils; blood eosinophilia is not always present, but has reached 82%. Illness is usually self-limiting, and may last a few days to several months (usually 4 weeks). Deaths have rarely been reported.

Differential diagnosis includes cerebral cysticercosis, paragonimiasis, echinococcosis, gnathostomiasis, tuberculous, coccidioidal or aseptic meningitis, and neurosyphilis.

The presence of eosinophils in the CSF and a history of eating raw mollusks suggest the diagnosis, especially in endemic areas. Immunodiagnostic tests are presumptive; demonstration of worms in CSF or at autopsy is confirmatory.

2. Infectious agent—*Parastrongylus* (*Angiostrongylus*) *cantonensis*, a nematode (lungworm of rats). The third-stage larvae in the intermediate host (terrestrial or marine mollusks) are infective for humans.

3. Occurrence—The nematode is widely distributed, found as far north as Japan; as far south as Brisbane, Australia; in Africa as far West as Côte d'Ivoire; and also in Egypt, Madagascar, the USA and Puerto Rico. The disease is endemic in China (including Taiwan), Cuba, Indonesia, Malaysia, the Philippines, Thailand, Viet Nam, Pacific islands including Hawaii and Tahiti, and much of the Caribbean.

4. Reservoir—The rat (*Rattus* and *Bandicota* spp.).

5. Mode of transmission—Ingestion of raw or insufficiently cooked mollusks (snails, slugs or land planarians), which are intermediate or transport hosts harboring infective larvae. Prawns, fish and land crabs that have ingested snails or slugs may also transport infective larvae. Lettuce and other leafy vegetables contaminated by small mollusks may serve as a source of infection. The mollusks are infected by first-stage larvae excreted by an infected rodent; when third-stage larvae have developed in the mollusks, rodents (and people) ingesting the mollusks are infected. In the rat, larvae migrate to the brain and mature to the adult stage; young adults migrate to the surface of the brain and through the venous system to reach their final site in the pulmonary arteries, where they become sexually mature and mate. After mating, the female worm deposits eggs that hatch in terminal branches of the pulmonary arteries; first-stage larvae enter the bronchial system, pass up the trachea, are swallowed, and are passed in the feces.

In humans, young adults are not able to leave the brain, do not reach maturity, and do not complete the life cycle. This explains the typical neurological symptomatology, which is mainly attributable to the death of young adult worms in the CNS.

6. Incubation period—Usually 1–3 weeks; may be longer or shorter.

7. Period of communicability—Not transmitted from person to person.

8. Susceptibility—Susceptibility to infection is general. Malnutrition and debilitating diseases may contribute to an increase in severity, and even (rarely) to a fatal outcome.

9. **Methods of control**

A. *Preventive measures:*

1) Educate the general public in the preparation of raw foods and snails, both aquatic and terrestrial.
2) Control rats.
3) Boil snails, prawns, fish and crabs for 3–5 minutes, or freeze at 15°C (5°F) for 24 hours; this effectively kills the larvae.
4) Avoid eating raw foods that may be contaminated by snails or slugs; thorough cleaning of lettuce and other greens to eliminate mollusks and their products does not always eliminate infective larvae. Radiation pasteurization would be effective.

B. *Control of patient, contacts and the immediate environment:*

1) Report to local health authority: Official report not ordinarily justifiable, Class 5 (see *Reporting*).
2) Isolation: Not applicable.
3) Concurrent disinfection: Not necessary.
4) Quarantine: Not applicable.
5) Immunization of contacts: Not applicable.
6) Investigation of contacts and source of infection: Investigate source of food involved and its preparation.
7) Specific treatment: Treatment is controversial; no anthelminthic drug is proven effective, and some patients have worsened with therapy. Mebendazole or albendazole may shorten course of infection; steroid cover is recommended. The usefulness of any treatment is debated because of the fact that the infection is usually self-limiting, and because the pathology associated with the infection is attributable to dead worms rather than to live ones.

C. *Epidemic measures:* Any grouping of cases in a particular geographic area or institution warrants prompt epidemiological investigation and appropriate control measures.

D. *Disaster implications:* None.

E. *International measures:* None.

ABDOMINAL
ANGIOSTRONGYLIASIS   ICD-9 128.8
INTESTINAL
ANGIOSTRONGYLIASIS   ICD-10 B81.3

1. **Identification**—A parasitic disease caused by a zoonotic nematode, with predominantly intestinal involvement. Common findings include

abdominal pain and tenderness in the right iliac fossa and flank, fever, anorexia, vomiting, abdominal rigidity, a tumor-like mass in the right lower quadrant, and pain on rectal examination. Fever, anorexia, vomiting, constipation or diarrhea are frequent in children. Leukocytosis is usually present, with eosinophils ranging from 20% to 60%.

Adult worms and eggs in the mesenteric arteries damage the endothelium, causing inflammation, thrombosis and necrosis. On surgery, the whole wall of the intestine is thickened and hardened, with yellow granulations in the subserosa of the intestinal wall; adult worms are found in the small arteries, generally in the ileocecal area, while eggs and larvae are found in lymph nodes, intestinal wall and omentum.

Since its first description in Costa Rica in 1967, human infections have been reported—mainly in children—in several central and south American countries, and in the USA.

Differential diagnosis includes malignant tumors, appendicitis, Crohn's disease and Meckel's diverticulum.

The presence of the above symptoms with a high eosinophilia suggests the diagnosis, especially in children living in endemic areas. Clinical diagnosis may be aided by X-ray. Serological diagnostic techniques are also available. Parasitological diagnosis by biopsy or resective surgery is confirmative. In humans, eggs are not found in feces.

2. Infectious agent—*Parastrongylus* (*Angiostrongylus*) *costaricensis*, a nematode. The third-stage larvae in the intermediate host (slugs) are infective for humans.

3. Occurrence—The nematode is common in rodents in the Americas. Human cases occur mostly in children, and have been reported in Argentina, Brazil, Colombia, Costa Rica, Dominican Republic, Ecuador, El Salvador, Guadeloupe, Guatemala, Honduras, Martinique, Nicaragua, Panama, Peru, USA, and Venezuela. Transmission in other continents is debated.

4. Reservoir—The cotton rat (*Sigmodon hispidus*) is the natural host. Several species of rodents and other mammals, such as marmosets, dogs and coatimundis, can act as final hosts.

5. Mode of transmission—Ingestion of raw or insufficiently cooked slugs, which are intermediate or transport hosts harboring infective larvae. Also ingestion of slug's slime (mucus) on lettuce and other leafy vegetables, or following playing with slugs (in children). Slugs are infected when they ingest first-stage larvae excreted with feces by an infected rodent; when third-stage larvae have developed in the slugs, rodents (and people) ingesting the slugs are infected. In the rat, larvae penetrate the intestinal wall and migrate to the lymphatics of the intestinal wall and mesentery. After molting into young adults, they migrate to the mesenteric arteries, where they mature and release eggs that hatch and are excreted with feces by 24 days after infection.

In humans, eggs laid by adult worms in the mesenteric arteries are not able to hatch into larvae, and the cycle is interrupted.

6. Incubation period—Usually 2-4 weeks; may be longer or shorter.

7. Period of communicability—Not transmitted from person to person.

8. Susceptibility—Susceptibility to infection is general. Malnutrition and debilitating diseases may contribute to an increase in severity.

9. Methods of control

 A. Preventive measures:

   1) Educate the general public in the preparation of raw foods and slugs.
   2) Control rats.
   3) Boil slugs for 3-5 minutes, or freeze at 15°C (5°F) for 24 hours; this effectively kills the larvae.
   4) Avoid eating raw foods that may be contaminated by slugs; thorough cleaning of lettuce and other greens to eliminate slugs and their products does not always eliminate infective larvae. Radiation pasteurization is effective.

 B. Control of patient, contacts and the immediate environment:

   1) Report to local health authority: Official report not ordinarily justifiable, Class 5 (see *Reporting*).
   2) Isolation: Not applicable.
   3) Concurrent disinfection: Not necessary.
   4) Quarantine: Not applicable.
   5) Immunization of contacts: Not applicable.
   6) Investigation of contacts and source of infection: Investigate source of food involved and its preparation.
   7) Specific treatment: thiabendazole, albendazole and diethyl-carbamazine have shown some effect. The usefulness of any medical treatment is debated, however, because the infection is usually self-limiting in a few weeks to many months; death of adult worms following chemotherapy causes acute inflammation in the surrounding tissues; and surviving worms might wander erratically and cause further lesions.

      In advanced stages of disease, surgery is a common form of treatment; in light infections only the appendix might be involved, but in heavy infections the terminal ileum, cecum and ascending colon might require excision.

 C. Epidemic measures: Any grouping of cases in a particular geographic area or institution warrants prompt epidemiological investigation and appropriate control measures.

D. Disaster implications: None.

E. International measures: None.

ANISAKIASIS   ICD-9 127.1; ICD-10 B81.0
[CCDM19: M. Eberhard]
[CCDM18: D. Engels]

1. Identification—A zoonotic parasitic disease of the human GI tract usually manifested by cramping, abdominal pain and vomiting, acquired through ingestion of uncooked or under-treated marine fish containing larval ascaridoid nematodes. The motile larvae burrow into the stomach wall, producing acute ulceration with nausea, vomiting and epigastric pain, sometimes with hematemesis. They may migrate upwards and attach in the oropharynx, causing cough. In the small intestine, they cause eosinophilic abscesses, and the symptoms may mimic appendicitis or regional enteritis. At times they perforate into the peritoneal cavity; rarely, they involve the large bowel.

Diagnosis is made by recognition of the 2-cm-long larvae invading the oropharynx, or by visualizing the larvae through gastroscopic examination or in surgically removed tissue.

2. Infectious agents—Larval nematodes of the subfamily Anisakinae, genera *Anisakis* and *Pseudoterranova*.

3. Occurrence—The disease occurs in individuals who eat uncooked and inadequately treated—e.g. frozen, salted, marinated or smoked— salt-water fish, squid or octopus. This is common in Japan, where over 12 000 cases have been described (sushi and sashimi); Scandinavia (gravlax); on the Pacific coast of Latin America (ceviche); and, less commonly, in the Netherlands (herring). With growing consumption of raw fish, cases are seen with increasing frequency throughout western Europe and the USA.

4. Reservoir—Anisakinae are widely distributed in nature, but only some of those parasitic in sea mammals constitute a major threat to humans. The natural life cycle involves transmission of larvae through predation from small crustaceans to squid, octopus or fish, then to sea mammals, with humans as incidental hosts.

5. Mode of transmission—The infective larvae live in the abdominal mesenteries of fish; after death of the fish host they often invade body muscles. When ingested by humans and liberated through digestion in the stomach, they may penetrate the gastric or intestinal mucosa.

6. Incubation period—Gastric symptoms may develop within a few hours of ingestion. Symptoms referable to the small and large bowel occur within a few days or weeks, depending on the size and location of the larvae.

7. Period of communicability—Direct transmission from person to person does not occur.

8. Susceptibility—Apparently universal susceptibility.

9. Methods of control—

A. Preventive measures:

1) Avoid ingestion of inadequately cooked marine fish. Larvae are killed by heating to 60°C (140°F) for 10 minutes; blast-freezing to −35°C (−31°F) or below for 15 hours; or freezing by regular means at −23°C (−9.4°F) for at least 7 days. The latter control method is used with success in the Netherlands. Irradiation effectively kills the parasite.

2) Cleaning (evisceration) of fish as soon as possible after they are caught reduces the number of larvae penetrating into the muscles from the mesenteries.

3) Candling (exposure to a light source) is useful for fishery products where parasites can be visualized.

B. Control of patient, contacts and the immediate environment:

1) Report to local health authority: Not ordinarily justifiable, Class 5 (see *Reporting*). A case or cases recognized in an area not previously known to be involved, or where control measures are in effect, must be reported.

2) Isolation: Not applicable.

3) Concurrent disinfection: Not applicable.

4) Quarantine: Not applicable.

5) Immunization of contacts: Not applicable.

6) Investigation of contacts and source of infection: Examination of others possibly exposed at the same time may be productive.

7) Specific treatment: Endoscopic removal of larvae; surgical excision of lesions.

C. Epidemic measures: None.

D. Disaster implications: None.

E. International measures: None.

ANTHRAX   ICD-9 022; ICD-10 A22
(Malignant pustule, Malignant edema, Woolsorter disease,
Ragpicker disease)
[CCDM19: K. Glynn, O. Cosivi, P. Turnbull]
[CCDM18: R. Diaz]

1. **Identification**—An acute bacterial enzootic disease that can occur in three forms: pulmonary, cutaneous, or gastrointestinal, depending on the route of exposure. Anthrax has been associated with state biological weapons programs and bioterrorism. More than 95% of naturally acquired human cases worldwide are cutaneous anthrax, manifested by initial itching of the affected site, followed by a lesion that becomes papular, then vesicular, developing in 2–6 days into a depressed black eschar. Moderate to severe and very extensive edema invariably surrounds the eschar, sometimes with small secondary vesicles. Pain is unusual and, if present, is due to edema or secondary infection. The head, neck, forearms and hands (exposed areas of the body) are common sites of infection. The lesion has been confused with human Orf (see Orf virus disease), early boils, arachnid bites, ulcers (especially tropical), and a variety of other infections, such as vaccinia, clostridial infection and more. Obstructive airway disease due to associated edema may complicate cutaneous anthrax of the face or neck, and tracheotomy may be needed. Untreated infections may spread to regional lymph nodes and the bloodstream with overwhelming septicemia. The meninges can become involved. Untreated cutaneous anthrax has a case-fatality rate of between 5% and 20%; with effective treatment, however, deaths from cutaneous anthrax are very rare. The lesion evolves through typical local changes even after the initiation of antimicrobial therapy.

Initial symptoms of inhalation anthrax are mild and nonspecific and may include fever, malaise, and mild cough or chest pain; acute symptoms of respiratory distress, including stridor, severe dyspnea, hypoxemia, diaphoresis, shock and cyanosis, and X-ray evidence of mediastinal widening, follow in 3–4 days, with death shortly thereafter. Pleural effusion is common, and infiltrates can sometimes be seen on chest X-ray. Maximum case fatality rate is estimated to be >85%, and early aggressive antimicrobial therapy along with supportive care may considerably reduce mortality. Anthrax is treatable in the early prodromal stage, but mortality remains high despite antimicrobial treatment if it is initiated after the onset of respiratory symptoms. In poor endemic countries, where the value of the meat from an animal that has died unexpectedly outweighs the perceived risks of illness that might result from eating it, ingestion anthrax is not uncommon and may take the form of oropharyngeal anthrax or, more commonly, gastrointestinal anthrax. In the former, the lesion is in the oral cavity, on the buccal mucosa, tongue, tonsils, or posterior pharynx wall. Sore throat and regional lymphadenopathy in the neck, with extensive edema that may lead to tracheal obstruction, are the predominant early features. In gastrointestinal anthrax, the lesion may lie at any point along the intestinal tract and is ulcerative and massively edematous, leading to hemorrhage, obstruction, perforation and extensive ascites. Ingestion anthrax is not invariably fatal, but, even with treatment mortality can be high, with development of septicemia, shock, coma and death. The incubation period is generally 3 to 7 days.

Gastrointestinal anthrax is rare and difficult to recognize; it tends to occur in explosive food poisoning outbreaks, where abdominal distress characterized by pain, nausea and vomiting is followed by fever, signs of septicemia, and death in typical cases. A rare oropharyngeal form of primary disease, characterized by edematous lesions, necrotic ulcers and swelling in the oropharynx and neck, has been described. Systemic illness, including fever, shock and dissemination to other organs, can occur with any form of anthrax, and may include meningitis that is usually fatal.

Laboratory confirmation is through demonstration of the causative organism in blood, lesions or discharges by direct polychrome methylene blue (M'Fadyean)-stained smears, or by culture on sheep blood agar. Animal inoculation (mice, guinea-pigs or rabbits) is discouraged due to increased risk of human exposure. Standard diagnosis remains culture of the organism from clinical specimens, but this may be difficult to achieve after antimicrobial treatment is initiated. Rapid detection can be achieved by PCR, and through immunodiagnostic testing; antigen detection methods include direct fluorescence antibody test (DFA), time-resolve fluorescence assay (TRF), and Immunohistochemistry (IHC). Most rapid assays are available only at reference laboratories, including laboratories participating in the laboratory response network. Commercially produced ELISA is available for antibody testing. Suspicion of anthrax in the case of both ingestion and inhalation depends on knowledge of the patient's history.

2. Causative agent—*Bacillus anthracis*, a Gram-positive, encapsulated, spore forming, non-motile rod. Specifically, the anthrax spores of *B. anthracis* are the infectious agent; vegetative *B. anthracis* rarely establish disease.

3. Occurrence—Primarily a disease of herbivores; humans are incidental hosts. In most industrialized countries, anthrax is an infrequent and sporadic human infection, and is primarily an occupational hazard of workers who process hides, wool, hair (especially from goats), bone and bone products imported from endemic regions; and of veterinarians and agriculture and wildlife workers who handle infected animals. Human anthrax is endemic in the agricultural regions of the world where anthrax in animals is common, such as sub-Saharan Africa and Asia, south and central America, and southern and eastern Europe. New areas of infection in livestock may develop through introduction of animal feed containing contaminated bone meal.

Environmental events such as floods, or disruption of soil over previous burial sites of infected carcasses, may provoke epizootics. Anthrax has been deliberately used to cause harm; as such, it could present in epidemiologically unusual circumstances, exemplified by the recent deliberate spread of *B. anthracis* spores through the postal system in USA. In non-endemic countries in the past, effluent from tanneries processing imported hides from endemic countries have been notorious as sources of incidents and outbreaks. However this has become rare with the implementation of appropriate veterinary controls and good factory hygiene.

4. Reservoir—Animals (normally herbivores, both livestock and wildlife) shed the bacilli in terminal hemorrhages or blood at death. On exposure to the air, vegetative cells sporulate and the *B. anthracis* spores, which resist adverse environmental conditions and disinfection, may remain viable in contaminated soil for years. The spores may be redistributed passively in the soil and adjacent vegetation through the action of water, wind and other environmental forces. Flies and scavengers feeding on infected carcasses may also disperse anthrax spores beyond the site of death, either through blood and viscera adhering to their fur, feathers or skin, or through excretion of viable anthrax spores in fecal matter. *B. anthracis* is not usually an invasive organism, however, and is not highly infectious even for herbivores, so there is a complex relationship between the number of spores a vector is likely to carry from a carcass and deposit at another site and the chance of another animal becoming infected from contact with that site. Dried or otherwise processed skins and hides, bones, etc. from infected animals may harbor spores for years, and are the fomites by which the disease is spread worldwide.

5. Mode of transmission—Contact with tissues of any parts of livestock or wild animals (cattle, sheep, goats, horses, pigs and others) dying of the disease, and/or hair, wool, hides or bone material taken for trade and products made from them (e.g. drums, brushes, and rugs); possibly also through biting flies that have fed on such animals; contact with soil contaminated by infected animals; or contact with contaminated bone meal used in gardening. Cutaneous infection requires a pre-existing lesion, and so is mostly seen on exposed areas of the body (hands, wrists, neck, face). Intestinal and oropharyngeal anthrax may arise from ingestion of inadequately cooked meat from such animals; there is no evidence that milk from infected animals transmits anthrax. Inhalation anthrax results from inhalation of *B. anthracis* spores in risky industrial processes—such as tanning hides and processing wool or bone—where spores are generated in an enclosed, poorly-ventilated area. Anthrax associated with the handling of animal hides outside of an industrial processing plant is rare, and is most often of the cutaneous form. Cases of both cutaneous and inhalation anthrax have been reported among drum makers.

Examples of laboratory-acquired infection exist, and an extensive outbreak with numerous deaths in both humans and animals occurred in the former USSR in 1979 as the result of an accidental release from a military research institute. Anthrax may also occur through deliberate release of spores. In 2001, spores deliberately released through the postal system in the USA resulted in 11 cutaneous and 11 inhalation cases, including 5 deaths. The distal proximity of some of the cases to original source suggests exposure to low concentrations of spores. The risk of inhalation anthrax is determined not only by bacillary virulence factors, but also by infectious aerosol production and removal rates, and by host factors.

The disease spreads among grazing animals through contaminated soil and feed, and probably by biting flies; in some endemic regions, non-biting flies, such as blowflies, are important in the spread of disease among omnivorous browsers (e.g. goats and various wild animal species), through depositing the organism on the leaves of shrubbery after feeding on the tissue or fluids of the anthrax carcass. Omnivorous and carnivorous animals acquire anthrax through contaminated meat, bone meal or other feeds derived from infected carcasses.

6. Incubation period—From 1 to 7 days, although incubation periods of up to 60 days are possible. In the 1979 USSR outbreak, incubation periods extended to 43 days.

7. Period of communicability—Person-to-person transmission is very rare. It has not been reported for inhalation or gastrointestinal forms of anthrax, and has only been rarely reported for cutaneous anthrax, where it requires direct contact with skin lesions. Articles and soil contaminated with spores may remain infective for several years.

8. Susceptibility—Circumstantial evidence indicates humans are moderately resistant to anthrax infection. There is some evidence of inapparent infection, including by the ingestion and inhalation routes, among people in frequent contact with the infectious agent; second attacks can occur, but reports are rare.

9. Methods of control—

    A. Preventive measures:

       1) Immunize high-risk persons with a cell-free vaccine prepared from a culture filtrate containing the protective antigen (in the USA, marketed under the trade name Biothrax). This vaccine is effective in preventing cutaneous and inhalational anthrax: it is recommended for laboratory workers who routinely work with *B. anthracis*, and workers who handle potentially contaminated industrial raw materials and engage in activities with high potential for production of or exposure to *B. anthracis* spore-containing aerosols. It may also be used to protect military personnel against exposure to anthrax used as a biological warfare agent. Vaccination may be indicated for veterinarians and other persons handling potentially infected animals in areas with high incidence of epizootic anthrax. Annual booster injections are recommended if the risk of exposure continues. Vaccines for administration to humans

are only produced in the USA and UK (protein-based non-living vaccines) and China and Russia (live spore vaccines analogous to livestock vaccines). They are restricted in availability outside these countries, and are essentially for administration to persons known to be in at-risk occupations as detailed above. The protein-based vaccines, requiring several doses over several weeks, are not really suitable for "after-the-event" response in incidents of naturally-acquired anthrax, but they could be administered together with prolonged antibiotic therapy after a substantial deliberate release exposure (see F[v] below).

i) Prevention of naturally-acquired human anthrax begins with prevention in animals. Effective control centers around vaccination of livestock in endemic regions, and appropriate procedures in the event of incidents of livestock anthrax—correct disposal of carcasses; decontamination of carcass sites and items in contact with the carcasses or sites; vaccination of unvaccinated animals in the affected herd; treatment of symptomatic animals in such herds with penicillin or other suitable antibiotic; and quarantine. (Note: since the vaccine is a live vaccine, antibiotics and the vaccine should not be administered simultaneously).

(ii) Educate employees who handle potentially contaminated articles about modes of anthrax transmission, care of skin abrasions, and personal cleanliness.

iii) Control dust and properly ventilate work areas in hazardous industries, especially those handling raw animal materials. Maintain continued medical supervision of employees, and provide prompt medical care for all suspicious skin lesions. Workers must wear protective clothing (gloves, boots, impermeable gowns, etc); adequate facilities must be provided for washing and changing clothes after work. Where possible, workers in at-risk occupations should be vaccinated. Locate eating facilities away from places of work. Vaporized formaldehyde has been used for disinfection of workplaces contaminated with *B. anthracis*.

iv) Thoroughly wash, disinfect or sterilize hair, wool and bone meal—or other feed of animal origin—prior to processing, using disinfecting protocols demonstrated effective against *B anthracis* spores, such as the duckering process of irradiation.

(v) Do not sell the hides of animals exposed to anthrax, or use their carcasses as food or feed supplements (bone or blood meal).

(vi) If anthrax is suspected in an animal, do not necropsy the animal; instead, aseptically collect a blood sample for smear and/or culture. Avoid contamination of the area. If a necropsy is inadvertently performed, autoclave, incinerate or chemically disinfect/fumigate all instruments or materials used.

Because anthrax spores may survive for years in the soil if carcasses are buried (there are many instances on record of outbreaks following disturbance of old burial sites), preferred disposal techniques are incineration at the site of death or removal to an incinerator or rendering plant, ensuring that no contamination occurs en route to the plant. Should these methods prove impossible, bury carcasses at the site of death as deeply as possible, without digging below the local water table level. Laboratory studies of close relatives of *B. anthracis* in the Bacillus genus have shown that exposure to elevated levels of calcium cations can extend the viable lifespan of spores. The same phenomenon could occur with *B. anthracis* spores, and so the addition of lye or quicklime to a carcass on burial (originally applied in the hope of speeding up putrefaction and discouraging scavengers) is now no longer recommended, as it is thought Ca^{++} ions may actually assist in the survival of anthrax spores.

(vii) Control effluents and wastes from rendering plants that handle potentially infected animals, and from factories that manufacture products from hair, wool, bones or hides likely to be contaminated. If appropriate, decontaminate.

viii) Promptly immunize, and annually re-immunize, all domestic animals at risk. Treat symptomatic animals with penicillin or tetracyclines; immunize them after cessation of treatment. These animals should not be used for food until a few months have passed. Treatment in lieu of immunization may be used for animals exposed to a discrete source of infection, such as contaminated commercial feed

(ix) The affected herd or flock should be quarantined for at least 14 days, preferably 20 days, after the last case.

B. Control of patient, contacts and the immediate environment:

1) Report to local health authority: Case report obligatory in most countries, Class 2 (see *Reporting*). Also report to the appropriate livestock or agriculture authority. Even a single case of human anthrax, especially of the inhalation variety, is

so unusual in industrialized countries and centers that it warrants immediate reporting to public health and law enforcement authorities for consideration of deliberate use.

2) Isolation: Anthrax is essentially non-contagious. Standard hygienic precautions (wearing disposable gloves; changing dressings; disinfecting clothing and bedding soiled with lesion fluid; washing hands after any of these procedures) for the duration of the lesion or illness in the living patient.

3) Concurrent disinfection: Of discharges from lesions and articles soiled therewith. Hypochlorite is sporicidal, and good when organic matter is not overwhelming and the item is not corrodable; to ensure adequacy of disinfection, free chlorine concentrations should be verified. Hydrogen peroxide, peracetic acid or glutaraldehyde may be alternatives; formaldehyde, ethylene oxide and cobalt irradiation have been used. Spores require steam sterilization, autoclaving or burning to ensure complete destruction. Fumigation and chemical disinfection may be used for valuable equipment.

In the event of death, the body fluids of the deceased person should be assumed to have very high concentrations of *B. anthracis* (although antibiotic treatment before death will probably have greatly reduced this) and suitable overclothing as well as gloves should be worn to place the body in a body bag. Bedding is probably best bagged and incinerated rather than simply disinfected. Whether the room should be fumigated depends on the perceived level of contamination beyond bedding.

4) Quarantine: Not applicable.

5) Immunization of contacts: Not applicable.

6) Investigation of contacts and source of infection: Search for history of exposure to infected animals or animal products and trace to place of origin. In a manufacturing plant, inspect for adequacy of preventive measures as outlined in 9A. As mentioned in 9B, there may be reason to consider deliberate use for all human cases of anthrax, but particularly those with no obvious occupational source of infection, or in other unusual circumstances.

7) Specific treatment: Ciprofloxacin is the recommended first-line treatment. Alternatives are doxycycline and amoxicillin (if isolate is susceptible). In inhalation anthrax, use of one or two additional antimicrobial agents, such as rifampicin, linezolid, macrolides, aminoglycosides, vancomycin, chloramphenicol, penicillin or ampicillin, clindamycin, and clarithromycin is recommended. Initial intravenous therapy with two or more antimicrobial agents effective against B anthracis is recommended for treatment of all forms of anthrax except localized cutaneous anthrax. Localized cutaneous

anthrax can be treated with oral doxycycline or ciprofloxa-cin monotherapy, except in young children (<8 years), for whom initial therapy of cutaneous anthrax should be IV, and therapy with two or more additional antimicrobials should be considered. Cephalosporins and trimethoprim-sulfame-thoxazole should not be used to treat anthrax.

In life-threatening cases, a combination of antibiotics, with at least one having good penetration to the CNS, may be appropriate, reverting to one drug when progression of symptoms ceases, and with overall duration 10–14 days. Supportive symptomatic (intensive care) treatment is also important.

C. *Epidemic measures:* Outbreaks in livestock may be an occu-pational hazard of animal husbandry, with consequent risk to humans. Occasional epidemics in industrialized countries have been local industrial outbreaks among employees working with animal products, especially goat hair. These appear to be very rare in industrialized countries, although complacency is not advised. Outbreaks related to handling and consuming meat from infected cattle have occurred in Africa, Asia, and Russia.

D. *Disaster implications:* None, except in case of floods in previously infected areas, which may raise the risk of new cases occurring in livestock.

E. *International measures:* In line with The Terrestrial Animal Health Code (Organisation Mondiale de La Santé Animale (OIE), Paris, France, 2007), imported animals or animal products should be accompanied by international veterinary certificates that the animals involved were free from anthrax and were not on premises quarantined for anthrax at the time of harvesting. Imported bone meal should be sterilized if used as animal feed. Disinfect wool, hair hides, etc. when indicated and feasible.

F. *Measures in case of deliberate use:* The general procedures for dealing with deliberate civilian release occurrences include the following:

(i) Anyone who receives a threat about dissemination of anthrax organisms, or who receives a suspicious package or enve-lope, should immediately notify the relevant local criminal investigative authorities with responsibility for the investiga-tion of such biological threats, including local police.

(ii) Other agencies must cooperate and provide assistance as requested.

(iii) Where appropriate, local and state health departments should also be notified, and should be ready to provide public health management and follow-up as needed.

(iv) Quarantine is not appropriate (see Quarantine, above).

(v) If the threat of exposure to aerosolized anthrax is credible or confirmed, persons at risk should begin post-exposure prophylaxis (PEP) with both an appropriate antibiotic (Ciprofloxacin is the drug of choice; doxycycline is an alternative). If one of the non-living vaccines is available, because of uncertainty as to when or if inhaled spores may germinate or be cleared by the alveolar immune system, PEP consists of 3 doses of cell free vaccine at 0, 2, and 4 weeks in combination with 60 days of antimicrobials. The vaccine has not been evaluated for safety and efficacy in children under 18 or in adults aged 60 or older. Where it is known that the patient has had a substantial exposure to aerosolized anthrax spores, antibiotic treatment must be continued for about 6 weeks to allow development of adequate vaccine-induced immunity.

vi) Responders should use an approved, pressure-demand self-contained breathing apparatus (SCBA) in conjunction with a Level A protective suit in responding to a suspected biological incident where any of the following information is unknown or the event is uncontrolled: the type(s) of airborne agent(s); the dissemination method; if aerosol dissemination is still occurring or it has stopped but there is no information on the duration of dissemination; or what the exposure concentration might be.

vii) Responders may use a Level B protective suit with an exposed or enclosed, approved pressure-demand SCBA in a situation in which the suspected biological aerosol is no longer being generated, or in which other conditions may present a splash hazard.

viii) Responders may use a full face piece respirator with a P100 filter or powered air-purifying respirator (PAPR) with high efficiency particulate air (HEPA) filters when it can be determined that: an aerosol-generating device was not used to create high airborne concentration; or dissemination was by a letter or package that can be easily bagged.

ix) Persons who may have been exposed and may be contaminated should be decontaminated with soap and copious amounts of water in a shower. Bleach solutions are usually not required; a 1:10 dilution of household bleach (final hypochlorite concentration 0.5%) should be used only if there is gross contamination with the agent and it is impossible to remove the materials through soap and water decontamination. The bleach solution, to be used only after soap and water decontamination, must be rinsed off after 10 to 15 minutes.

x) All persons who are to be decontaminated should remove clothing and personal effects and place all items in plastic bags, which should be labeled clearly with the owner's name, contact telephone number, and inventory of contents. Personal items may be kept as evidence in a criminal trial or returned to the owner if the threat is unsubstantiated.

xi) If the suspect item associated with an anthrax threat remains sealed (unopened), first responders should not take any action other than notifying the relevant authority and packaging the evidence. Quarantine, evacuation, decontamination and chemoprophylaxis will be dictated by subsequent epidemiologic and environmental investigation.

For more information on the deliberate use of infectious agents to cause harm, see the section on *Deliberate use*.

ARENAVIRAL HEMORRHAGIC FEVERS IN THE WESTERN HEMISPHERE	ICD-9 078.7; ICD-10 A96
JUNÍN (ARGENTINIAN) HEMORRHAGIC FEVER	ICD-10 A96.0
MACHUPO (BOLIVIAN) HEMORRHAGIC FEVER	ICD-10 A96.1
GUANARITO (VENEZUELAN) HEMORRHAGIC FEVER	ICD-10 A96.8
SABIÁ (BRAZILIAN) HEMORRHAGIC FEVER	ICD-10 A96.8

[CCDM19: P. Rollin]
[CCDM18: K. Leitmeyer]

1. Identification—Acute febrile viral illnesses; duration is 7–15 days. Onset is gradual, with malaise, headache, retro-orbital pain, conjunctival injection, sustained fever and sweats, followed by prostration. There may be petechiae and ecchymoses, accompanied by erythema of the face, neck and upper thorax. An enanthem with petechiae on the soft palate is frequent. Severe infections result in epistaxis, hematemesis, melena, hematuria and gingival hemorrhage. Encephalopathies, intention tremors and depressed deep tendon reflexes are frequent. Bradycardia and hypotension with clinical shock are common findings, and leukopenia and thrombocytopenia are characteristic. Moderate albuminuria is present, with cellular and granular casts and vacuolated epithelial cells in the urine. Case-fatality rates range from 15% to 30% in untreated individuals.

Diagnosis is made through virus isolation or antigen detection in blood or organs; by PCR, or serologically by IgM capture ELISA; or through the detection of neutralizing antibody or rises in titer thereof by ELISA or IFA. Laboratory studies for virus isolation and neutralizing antibody tests require BSL-4.

2. Infectious agents—Among the 18 known New World arenaviruses belonging to the Tacaribe complex, 4 have been associated with hemorrhagic fever in humans: Junín for the Argentine disease; the closely related Machupo virus for the Bolivian; Guanarito virus for the Venezuelan; and the Sabiá virus for the Brazilian. These viruses are related to the Old World arenaviruses that include the agents of Lassa fever and lymphocytic choriomeningitis. A further virus, Whitewater Arroyo Virus, has been found in rodents in North America.

3. Occurrence—Argentine hemorrhagic fever was first described among corn harvesters in Argentina in 1955. Since then, the number of cases reported from the endemic areas of the Argentine pampas has ranged from 100 to 4 000 per year, with an estimated cumulative total of 30 000 symptomatic cases. The region at risk has been expanding northwards, and now potentially affects a population of 5 million. Disease occurs seasonally from late February to October, predominantly in males, and 63% of cases are in the age group 20–49.

A similar disease, Bolivian hemorrhagic fever, caused by the related virus, occurs sporadically or in epidemics in small villages of rural northeastern Bolivia. In July–September 1994, there were 9 cases with 7 deaths.

In 1989, an outbreak of severe hemorrhagic illness occurred in the municipality of Guanarito, Venezuela; 104 cases with 26 deaths occurred between May 1990 and March 1991 among rural residents in Guanarito and neighboring areas. To date, about 200 confirmed cases have been reported. Although the virus continued to circulate in the rodent population, there was an unexplained drop in human cases between 1992 and 2002 (one outbreak with 18 cases).

Sabiá virus caused a fatal illness with hemorrhage and jaundice in Brazil in 1990, a laboratory infection in Brazil in 1992, and a laboratory infection treated with ribavirin in the USA in 1994.

4. Reservoir—In Argentina, wild rodents of the pampas (*Calomys musculinus* and *Calomys laucha*) are the hosts for Junín virus. In Bolivia, *Calomys callosus* is the reservoir animal. Cane rats (*Zygodontomys brevicauda*) were shown to be the main reservoir of Guanarito virus. The reservoir of Sabiá virus is not known, although a rodent host is presumed. Arenaviruses persist in nature by chronically infecting rodents with a one-virus-one rodent species relationship. Rodent infections result in long term virus excretion and lifelong viremia; vertical infection is also common.

5. Mode of transmission—Transmission to humans occurs primarily by inhalation of small particle aerosols from rodent excreta containing virus, from saliva, or from rodents disrupted by mechanical harvesters. Viruses deposited in the environment may also be infective when secondary aerosols are generated by farming and grain processing, when ingested, or by contact with cuts or abrasions. While uncommon, person-to-person transmission of Machupo virus has been documented in health care and family settings. Fatal scalpel accidents during necropsy as and laboratory infections without further person-to-person transmission have been described.

6. Incubation period—Usually 7–14 days (in extreme cases 5–21 days).

7. Period of communicability—Rarely transmitted directly from person to person, although this has occurred in both Argentine and Bolivian diseases.

8. Susceptibility—All ages appear to be susceptible, but protective immunity of unknown duration follows infection. Subclinical infections occur.

9. Methods of control—

   A. *Preventive measures:* Specific rodent control in houses has been successful in Bolivia. In Argentina, human contact most commonly occurs in the fields, and rodent dispersion makes control more difficult. An effective live attenuated Junín vaccine has been administered to more than 150 000 persons in Argentina. In experimental animals, this vaccine is effective against Machupo but not Guanarito virus; it is still not known whether it provides effective cross-protection in humans.

   B. *Control of patient, contacts and the immediate environment:*

      1) Report to local health authority: In selected endemic areas; in most countries not a reportable disease, Class 3 (see *Reporting*); category A pathogen list as defined by the CDC.
      2) Isolation: Strict isolation during the acute febrile period. Respiratory protection may be desirable along with other barrier methods.
      3) Concurrent disinfection: Of sputum and respiratory secretions, and blood-contaminated materials.
      4) Quarantine: Not applicable
      5) Immunization of contacts: Not applicable.

6) Investigation of contacts and source of infection: Monitoring and, where feasible, control of rodents.

7) Specific treatment: Convalescent serum given within 8 days of onset reduced the case fatality rate in Argentine disease to less than 1%. Ribavirin is likely to be useful in all 4 diseases. Other compounds (inosine-5 monophosphate dehydrogenate inhibitors, phenothiazines and myristic acid analog s) were recently shown to inhibit arenavirus replication in cell culture and animals.

C. Epidemic measures: Rodent control; consider immunization.

D. Disaster implications: None.

E. International measures: None.

ARTHROPOD-BORNE VIRAL DISEASES
(Arboviral Diseases)
[CCDM19: E. Hayes, J. Mackenzie, R. Shope]
[CCDM19: J. Mackenzie, R. Shope]

Introduction

Many arboviruses produce clinical and sub-clinical infection in humans. There are 4 main clinical syndromes:

1. Acute central nervous system (CNS) illness ranging in severity from mild aseptic meningitis to encephalitis or flaccid paralysis
2. Acute self-limited fevers, with or without exanthem, and often accompanied by headache; some may give rise to more serious illness with CNS involvement or hemorrhages
3. Hemorrhagic fevers, often associated with capillary leakage, shock and high case-fatality rates (these may be accompanied by liver damage with jaundice, particularly in cases of yellow fever)
4. Polyarthritis and rash, with or without fever and of variable duration, self-limited or with arthralgic sequelae lasting several weeks to years.

Many of the arboviruses are transmitted primarily in zoonotic cycles. With these zoonotic viruses, such as West Nile virus, Japanese encephalitis virus, and LaCrosse virus, humans are incidentally infected and are usually not important in maintaining transmission cycles. With other arboviruses, such as dengue, yellow fever and chikungunya viruses, humans are often the principal source of virus amplification and vector infection. Most arboviruses are transmitted by mosquitoes, but some are transmitted by

DISEASES IN HUMANS CAUSED BY ARTHROPOD-BORNE VIRUSES

Virus family, genus, group	Name of virus	Vector	Disease in humans	Where found
TOGAVIRIDAE				
Alphavirus	Barmah Forest	Mosquito	Fever, arthralgia, rash	Australia
	Chikungunya	Mosquito	Fever, arthralgia, rash (hemorrhage rare)	Africa, SE Asia, Philippines
	Eastern equine encephalomyelitis	Mosquito	Encephalitis	Americas
	Mayaro (Uruma)	Mosquito	Fever, arthralgia, rash	S America
	O'nyong-nyong	Mosquito	Fever, arthralgia, rash	Africa
	Ross River	Mosquito	Fever, arthralgia, rash	Australia, S Pacific
	Semliki Forest	Mosquito	Encephalitis	Africa
	Sindbis (Ockelbo, Babanki)	Mosquito	Fever, arthralgia, rash	Africa, India, SE Asia, Europe, Philippines, Australia, Russia
	Venezuelan equine encephalomyelitis	Mosquito	Fever, encephalitis	Americas
	Western equine encephalomyelitis	Mosquito	Fever, encephalitis	Americas
FLAVIVIRIDAE				
Flavivirus	Alkurma	Tick	Fever Encephalitis	Saudi Arabia
	Banzi	Mosquito	Fever	Africa
	Bussuquara	Mosquito	Fever, arthralgia	S America
	Dengue 1, 2, 3 and 4	Mosquito	Fever, hemorrhage, rash	Throughout tropics
	Edge Hill	Mosquito	Fever, arthralgia	Australia
	Ilhéus	Mosquito	Fever, encephalitis	Central & S America
	Japanese encephalitis	Mosquito	Encephalitis, fever	Asia, Pacific islands, Torres Strait of Australia, Papua New Guinea
	Kokobera	Mosquito	Fever, arthralgia	Australia
	Koutango	Mosquito	Fever, rash	Africa
	Kunjin (West Nile subtype)	Mosquito	Fever, encephalitis	Australia, Sarawak
	Kyasanur Forest disease	Tick	Hemorrhage, fever, meningoencephalitis	India

DISEASES IN HUMANS CAUSED BY ARTHROPOD-BORNE VIRUSES

Virus family, genus, group	Name of virus	Vector	Disease in humans	Where found
FLAVIVIRIDAE *Flavivirus (cont).*	Louping ill	Tick	Encephalitis	United Kingdom, western Europe
	Murray Valley encephalitis	Mosquito	Encephalitis	Australia, N. Guinea
	Negishi	Unknown	Encephalitis	Japan
	Omsk hemorrhagic fever	Tick	Hemorrhage, fever	Russia
	Powassan	Tick	Encephalitis	Canada, Russia, USA
	Rocio	Mosquito	Encephalitis	Brazil
	Sepik	Mosquito	Fever	Papua New Guinea
	Spondweni	Mosquito	Fever	Africa
	St. Louis encephalitis	Mosquito	Encephalitis, fever	Americas
	Tick-borne encephalitis	Tick	Encephalitis, paralysis, fever	Europe, Asia
	Usutu	Mosquito	Fever, rash	Africa, Europe
	Wesselsbron	Mosquito	Fever	Africa, SE Asia
	West Nile	Mosquito	Fever, encephalitis, paralysis, fever, rash	Africa, North America, Caribbean, S & Central America, India, Australia (Kunjin) subcontinent, Middle East, Russia, Europe, SE Asia
	Yellow fever	Mosquito	Hemorrhagic fever	Africa, S & Central America
	Zika	Mosquito	Fever	Africa, SE Asia
BUNYAVIRIDAE *Bunyavirus* Group C	Apeu	Mosquito	Fever	S America
	Caraparu	Mosquito	Fever	S and Central America

BUNYAVIRIDAE

Bunyavirus (cont.)

Itaqui	Mosquito	Fever	S America
Madrid	Mosquito	Fever	Panama
Marituba	Mosquito	Fever	S America
Murutucu	Mosquito	Fever	S America
Nepuyo	Mosquito	Fever	S and Central America
Oriboca	Mosquito	Fever	S America
Ossa	Mosquito	Fever	Panama
Restan	Mosquito	Fever	Trinidad, Suriname
Bunyamwera group			
Bunyamwera	Mosquito	Fever, rash	Africa
Germiston	Mosquito	Fever, rash	Africa
Ilesha	Unknown	Fever, rash, hemorrhage	Africa
Tensaw	Mosquito	Encephalitis	N America
Bwamba group			
Bwamba	Mosquito	Fever, rash	Africa
California group			
California encephalitis	Mosquito	Encephalitis	USA
Guaroa	Mosquito	Fever	S America, Panama
Jamestown Canyon	Mosquito	Encephalitis	USA, Canada
LaCrosse	Mosquito	Encephalitis	USA
Snowshoe hare	Mosquito	Encephalitis	Canada, China, Russia, USA
Tahyna (Lumbo)	Mosquito	Fever	Africa, Asia, Europe
Trivittatus	Mosquito	Fever	N America
Guama group			
Catu	Mosquito	Fever	S America
Guama	Mosquito	Fever	S America
Simbu group			
Oropouche	Midges (*Culicoides*)	Fever, meningitis	S America, Panama
Phlebovirus **(Sandfly fever group)**			
Candiru	Unknown	Fever	S. America
Chagres	Phlebotomine	Fever	Central America
Sandfly Naples type	Phlebotomine	Fever	Africa, Asia, Europe
Punta Toro	Phlebotomine	Fever	Panama

DISEASES IN HUMANS CAUSED BY ARTHROPOD-BORNE VIRUSES

Virus family, genus, group	Name of virus	Vector	Disease in humans	Where found
	Rift Valley fever	Mosquito	Fever, hemorrhage, encephalitis, retinitis	Africa, Arabia
	Sandfly Sicilian type	Phlebotomine	Fever	Africa, Asia, Europe
	Toscana	Phlebotomine	Aseptic meningitis	Italy, Portugal
BUNYAVIRIDAE				
Nairovirus	Nairobi sheep disease	Tick	Fever	Africa, India
	Dugbe	Tick	Fever	Africa
	Crimean-Congo hemorrhagic fever	Tick	Hemorrhagic fever	Africa, central Asia, Europe, Middle East
Unclassified	Bhanja	Tick	Fever	Africa, Asia, Europe
	Tataguine	Mosquito	Fever, rash	Africa
REOVIRIDAE				
Orbivirus				
Changuinola group	Changuinola	Phlebotomine	Fever	Central America
Kemerovo group	Kemerovo	Tick	Fever	Russia
Colorado tick fever	Colorado tick fever	Tick	Fever	Canada, USA
RHABDOVIRIDAE				
Ungrouped	Orungo	Mosquito	Fever	Africa
Vesicular stomatitis group	Vesicular stomatitis, Indiana & New Jersey	Phlebotomine	Fever, encephalitis	Americas
	Vesicular stomatitis, Alagoas	Phlebotomine	Fever	S America
	Chandipura	Mosquito	Fever	Africa, India
ORTHOMYXOVIRIDAE	Thogoto	Tick	Meningitis	Africa, Europe
NOT CLASSIFIED	Quaranfil	Tick	Fever	Africa, Arabia

ticks, sandflies or biting midges. Direct person-to-person transmission does not generally occur, except through blood transfusion and in some instances from mother to child. Laboratory infections may occur, including aerosol infections.

The main viruses thought to be associated with human disease are listed in the accompanying table with type of vector, predominant character of recognized disease, and geographical distribution. In some instances, observed cases of disease due to particular viruses are too few to be certain of the usual clinical course. Some viruses capable of causing disease have only been recognized through laboratory exposure. Viruses in which evidence of human infection is based solely on serological surveys are not included. Those viruses that are believed to be the most prominent causes of human disease are covered in more detail in subsequent chapters.

Over 100 viruses currently classified as arboviruses produce disease in humans. Most of these are further classified by antigenic relationships, morphology and replicative mechanisms into families and genera, of which *Togaviridae* (Alphavirus), *Flaviviridae* (Flavivirus) and *Bunyaviridae* (Bunyavirus, Phlebovirus, Nairovirus) are the best known. Alphaviruses and bunyaviruses are usually mosquito-borne; flaviviruses are usually either mosquito- or tick-borne; phleboviruses are generally transmitted by sandflies—apart from Rift Valley fever virus, which is transmitted by mosquitoes. Other viruses of the family *Bunyaviridae* and of several other groups mainly produce febrile diseases or hemorrhagic fevers, and may be transmitted by mosquitoes, ticks, sandflies or midges.

ARTHROPOD-BORNE VIRAL
ARTHRITIS AND RASH   ICD-9 066.3; ICD-10 B33.1
(Polyarthritis and rash, Ross River fever, Epidemic polyarthritis)

CHIKUNGUNYA VIRUS DISEASE	ICD-10 A92.0
MAYARO VIRUS DISEASE	ICD-10 A92.8
(Mayaro fever, Uruma fever)	
O'NYONG-NYONG FEVER	ICD-10 A92.1
SINDBIS (OCKELBO) VIRUS	
DISEASE AND OTHERS	ICD-10 A92.8

(Pogosta disease, Karelian fever)
[CCDM19: J. Mackenzie, D. Smith]
[CCDM18: J. Mackenzie, R. Shope]

1. Identification—A self-limiting viral disease characterized by arthralgia or arthritis, primarily in the wrist, knee, ankle and small joints of the extremities, lasting days to months. In many patients, onset of arthritis is followed after 1–10 days by a maculopapular rash, usually non-pruritic, affecting mainly the trunk and limbs. Buccal and palatal enanthema may occur. The rash resolves within 7–10 days, and is followed by a fine desquamation. Myalgia, fatigue, fever and lymphadenopathy are common. Paresthesias and tenderness of palms and soles occur in a small percentage of cases. Persistence of joint pains, arthritis, myalgia and/or fatigue occurs in 10–50% of cases.

Chikungunya causes a more severe illness, with high fever, prominent lymphadenopathy and leukopenia, and a prolonged convalescence. Mild hemorrhagic disease can occur with Mayaro virus disease and with chikungunya virus disease (see *Dengue hemorrhagic fever*). Rare deaths and occasional severe congenital infections occur due to chikungunya virus infection.

Serological tests show IgM in acute serum samples, and a rise in titers to alphaviruses between acute and convalescent samples. IgM commonly persists for weeks or months. Diagnosis may be made by RT-PCR on blood, particularly for chikungunya. Virus may be isolated from blood in the first few days of illness, using newborn mice, mosquito inoculation, or cell culture.

2. Infectious agents—Ross River, Barmah Forest viruses, Sindbis (in Africa and Europe), Mayaro, chikungunya and o'nyong-nyong viruses cause similar illnesses. Ockelbo, Pogosta and Karelian fever are due to Sindbis virus.

3. Occurrence—Outbreaks of disease occur during warm and wet conditions that favor proliferation of the mosquito vectors. Ross River virus disease occurs annually in Australia, occurring in December to March in temperate regions, and in the wet season from December to June in tropical areas. Infections may also occur in normally arid regions following irregular heavy rain with flooding. Sporadic cases occur in the colder regions of southern Australia and in Papua New Guinea. In 1979, an outbreak in Fiji spread to other Pacific islands, including American Samoa, the Cook Islands, and Tonga. Barmah Forest virus infection occurs in the same regions as Ross River virus infections, but is less common. Chikungunya virus occurs in Africa, southeastern Asia, India, Sri Lanka, and the Philippines, and has caused a major epidemic throughout the Indian Ocean region since 2004. Sindbis virus disease occurs in Africa and northern Europe, but is rare in Asia and Australia. Outbreaks occur in summer and autumn in Europe and South Africa. Pogosta disease in Finland has a seven-year cycle. O'nyong-nyong virus is known only from Africa; epidemics in 1959–1963 and 1996–1997 involved millions of cases throughout eastern Africa. Mayaro virus occurs in Central America, northern South America and Trinidad. Sporadic cases and occasional outbreaks occur in endemic areas.

4. Reservoir—Marsupials, especially kangaroos and wallabies for Ross River virus and Barmah Forest virus; primates for chikungunya; birds for

Sindbis; unknown for Mayaro virus and o'nyong-nyong virus. Trans-ovarial transmission of Ross River virus has been demonstrated in *Aedes vigilax*.

5. Mode of transmission—Ross River virus and Barmah Forest virus are transmitted by *Culex annulirostris*, *Ae. vigilax*, and other *Aedes* spp.; chikungunya virus by *Ae. aegypti* and *Ae. albopictus* in Asia, other *Ae.* Spp in Africa and Australia; o'nyong-nyong virus by *Anopheles* spp.; Sindbis virus by various *Culex* spp., Ae. spp. and *Culex* spp.; Mayaro virus by *Haemagogus* spp.

6. Incubation period—From 3 to 12 days, usually 7 to 9 days.

7. Period of communicability—No evidence of direct person-to-person transmission. Humans are infectious to mosquitoes for the first few days after onset of illness. Infected individuals can introduce virus into receptive areas, e.g. chikungunya virus and Ross River virus.

8. Susceptibility—Recovery is universal, though some take several months, and followed by lasting homologous immunity; second attacks are unknown. Unapparent infections are common, especially in children, among whom the overt disease is rare.

9. Methods of control—

    A. Preventive measures: General measures applicable to mosqui-to-borne viral encephalitides (see *Arthropod-borne viral encephalitides*, I9A, 1–5 and 8).

    B. Control of patient, contacts and the immediate environment:

        1) Report to local health authority: In selected endemic areas; in many countries, not a reportable disease, Class 3 (see *Reporting*).

        2) Isolation: To avoid further transmission, advise patients not to travel to areas with vector mosquito species for the first few days after onset of symptoms, and provide advice about mosquito protection.

        3) Concurrent disinfection: Not applicable.

        4) Quarantine: Not applicable.

        5) Immunization of contacts: Not applicable.

        6) Investigation of contacts and source of infection: Search for unreported or undiagnosed cases wherever the patient lived during the 2 weeks prior to onset; check all family members serologically.

        7) Specific treatment: None.

    C. Epidemic measures: Same as for arthropod-borne viral fevers (see *Dengue fever*, 9C).

    D. Disaster implications: None.

E. International measures: WHO Collaborating Centres provide support as required. More information can be found at: <http://www.who.int/collaboratingcentres/database/en/>

ARTHROPOD-BORNE VIRAL ENCEPHALITIDES
[CCDM19: J. Mackenzie, D. Smith]
[CCDM18: J. Mackenzie, R. Shope]

I. MOSQUITO-BORNE VIRAL ENCEPHALITIDES	ICD-9 062
JAPANESE ENCEPHALITIS	ICD-10 A83.0
WESTERN EQUINE ENCEPHALITIS	ICD-10 A83.1
EASTERN EQUINE ENCEPHALITIS	ICD-10 A83.2
ST. LOUIS ENCEPHALITIS	ICD-10 A83.3
MURRAY VALLEY ENCEPHALITIS	ICD-10 A83.4
KUNJIN ENCEPHALITIS (NOTE: KUNV IS A STRAIN OF WEST NILE VIRUS)	ICD-10 A83.4
LACROSSE ENCEPHALITIS	ICD-10 A83.5
CALIFORNIA ENCEPHALITIS	ICD-10 A83.5
ROCIO ENCEPHALITIS (INCLUDING ENCEPHALITIS DUE TO ILHÉUS VIRUS)	ICD-10 A83.6
JAMESTOWN CANYON ENCEPHALITIS	ICD-10 A83.8

The following are classified as ARTHROPOD-BORNE VIRAL FEVERS AND HEMORRHAGIC FEVERS under the ICD codes, but are included here as encephalitis is the most important clinical manifestation:

VENEZUELAN EQUINE ENCEPHALITIS	ICD-10 A92.2
WEST NILE ENCEPHALITIS	ICD-10 A92.3

1. Identification—A group of acute inflammatory viral diseases of short duration involving parts of the brain, spinal cord and meninges. Signs and symptoms of these diseases are similar, but vary in severity and rate of progress. Most infections are asymptomatic; mild cases often occur as fever with headache, or as aseptic meningitis. Severe infections are usually marked by acute onset of headache, high fever, meningeal signs, altered mental state, tremors, occasionally convulsions (especially in young children), and rarely acute flaccid paralysis. Case-fatality rates for encephalitis range from 0.3% to 60%; rates for encephalitis due to Japanese encephalitis virus (JEV), Murray Valley encephalitis virus (MVEV), West Nile virus (WNV) and eastern equine encephalitis virus (EEEV) are among the highest, with an overall mortality of about 25%. Neurological sequelae varying from mild peripheral or cranial nerve palsies to spastic quadraparesis occur in up to 50% of survivors, particularly infants and older patients. Late onset Parkinsonism and neuropsychiatries illness can occur.

The CSF usually shows a mild leukocytosis, predominantly lymphocytes, ranging from 50 to 500 × 106/L, and may be 1000 × 106/L or greater in some cases. During acute illness, CT scans are usually normal or nonspecific, while MRI scans may show thalamic, brain stem, cervical cord and/or temporal lobe abnormalities. CT or MRI scan lesions in the thalamus and brain stem may appear late in the course of illness.

These diseases require differentiation from other infectious and noninfectious causes of acute neurological disease. Infectious causes include other insect-borne encephalitides (see below); herpes encephalitis; aseptic meningitis due to enteroviruses; encephalitic and non-paralytic poliomyelitis; rabies; meningoencephalitis due to mumps or measles; post-vaccination or post-infectious encephalitides; and bacterial, mycoplasmal, protozoal, leptospiral and mycotic meningitides or encephalitides.

Within the first few days after onset of illness, virus may be detected in the CSF or serum using RT-PCR. Virus may occasionally be isolated from the brain tissue of fatal cases, or rarely from blood or CSF, by inoculation of suckling mice or by cell culture. However, diagnosis is usually based on serological testing. Detection of IgM in acute serum (by EIA or IFA) accompanied by a rise in IgG between acute and convalescent serum (by HI, IFA or CFT) indicates recent infection. Neutralization titers or epitope-blocking EIA assays are needed to confirm the specific infecting virus, especially with the flaviviruses. Detection of IgM in CSF confirms encephalitis and is usually only reactive against the infecting virus, but is not present in all patients. Serum IgM persists for months after acute infection. Histopathological changes are not specific for individual viruses.

2. **Infectious agents**—Each disease is caused by a specific virus in one of 3 genera: EEEV, WEEV, VEEV, Semliki Forest virus and Me Tri virus for the alphaviruses (Togaviridae, *Alphavirus*); JEV, WNV (including KUNV), MVEV, SLEV, Ilhéus virus, Rocio virus and Wesselsbron virus in the flaviviruses (Flaviviridae, *Flavivirus*); and LaCrosse, California, encephalitis, Jamestown Canyon and snowshoe hare viruses in the California group of bunyaviruses (Bunyaviridae, *Bunyavirus*) and Toscana virus in the phleboviruses (Bunyaviridae, *Phlebovirus*).

3. Occurrence—EEE occurs in eastern, Gulf, and north central USA and adjacent Canada, in scattered areas of Central and South America and in the Caribbean islands; WEE in western and central USA, Canada and parts of South America; VEE (including Everglades, Mucambo and Tocate encephalitis) in Central America, northern South America, southern North America and Trinidad; JE in western Pacific islands from the Republic of Korea to the Philippines and to Pakistan, through southern and southeastern Asia, extending to far North Queensland. Kunjin virus (KUNV) encephalitis and MVE occur in parts of Australia and Papua New Guinea; SLE in most of the USA, in Canada and in Central America and Brazil; Ilhéus and Rocio encephalitis in Brazil; LaCrosse encephalitis in the USA from Minnesota and Texas to New York and Georgia; snowshoe hare encephalitis in Canada, China and Russia. Other arboviruses are rare causes of encephalitis, including Semliki Forest virus in Africa and Asia; Me Tri virus in Vietnam; Wesselsbron virus in Africa; snowshoe hare virus in Canada, Alaska, and northern Eurasia; and Toscana virus in southern Europe. Cases due to these viruses occur during warm, wet conditions that favor an increase in mosquito numbers, which is usually summer and early autumn in temperate latitudes, and during the wet season in tropical and subtropical areas. A similar seasonality is seen with the viruses transmitted by biting midges or sandflies.

4. Reservoir—California group viruses and WNV overwinter in *Aedes and Culex* spp., respectively, though the true reservoir or means of winter carryover for arboviruses is not established. MVEV can survive in desiccation-resistant eggs during dry seasons. LaCrosse virus is trans-ovarially and venereally transmitted in *Ae. triseriatus* mosquitoes. The mechanisms probably differ for each virus. A range of bird and mammalian species act as amplifying hosts and maintain the viruses in animal-mosquito cycles. The hosts include pigs for JEV, and birds for EEEV, WEEV, JEV, WNV, MVE and SLEV.

5. Mode of transmission to humans—Bite of infected mosquitoes, midges or sandflies. The most important mosquito vectors are as follows:

- EEEV in the USA and Canada: probably *Culiseta melanura* from bird to bird, and one or more *Aedes* or *Coquillettidia* spp. from birds or other animals to humans.
- WEEV in western USA and Canada: *Cx. tarsalis*.
- JEV: *Cx. tritaeniorhynchus*, *Cx. vishnui* complex, and in the tropics, *Cx. gelidus*
- WNV in the USA: *Cx. tarsalis*, the *Cx. pipiens pipiens*, *Cx. quinquefasciatus*, and *Cx. tarsalis*; in Africa and the Middle East: *Cx. univittatus*.
- MVEV in Australia: *Cx. annulirostris*
- SLEV in the USA: *Cx. tarsalis*, the *Cx. pipiens-quinquefasciatus* complex, and *Cx. nigripalpus*.
- LaCrosse virus: *Ae. triseriatus*.

Human-to-human transmission occurs only in special circumstances. For example, rare cases of transplacental transmission, and transmission by organ transplant and blood transfusion, have occurred with WNV in the USA.

6. Incubation period—Usually 5–15 days.

7. Period of communicability—Humans are not infectious to other humans, other than in the special situations mentioned above; nor do they play a major role in the spread of these viruses. The virus is not usually detectable in human blood after onset of disease. Horses develop active disease with the two equine viruses, with WNV and with JEV, but viremia is rarely present in high titer or for long periods and, like humans, they are unlikely sources of mosquito infection. Viremia in birds usually lasts several days. Mosquitoes remain infective for life.

8. Susceptibility—Susceptibility to clinical disease is usually highest in infancy and old age; unapparent or undiagnosed infection is more common at other ages. Susceptibility varies with virus, e.g. LaCrosse encephalitis is usually a disease of children, while severity of SLE and WNV increases with age. Infection results in homologous immunity, but little is known about heterologous protection in humans. In highly endemic areas, adults are largely immune to local strains by reason of mild and inapparent infection, and illness occurs mainly in children, visitors or people new to the area.

9. Methods of control—

    A. Preventive measures:

        1) Educate the public about modes of spread and control.
        2) Destroy larvae and eliminate breeding places of known and suspected vector mosquitoes.
        3) Kill mosquitoes through space and residual spraying of human habitations (see *Malaria*, 9A1-5).
        4) Screen sleeping and living quarters; use bed nets, preferably insecticide-treated mosquito nets (ITNs) or long-lasting insecticidal nets (LLINs) pre-treated with pyrethroid insecticides during manufacture.
        5) Avoid exposure to mosquitoes during hours of biting, or use repellents (see *Malaria*, 9A2-4).
        6) In endemic areas, immunize domestic animals or house them away from living quarters (e.g. pigs in JE endemic areas). An equine vaccine for EEV is available.
        7) Mouse-brain inactivated vaccine against JEV infection is used most widely. It is commercially available and is recommended for those traveling to endemic areas for extended visits to rural areas, and for laboratory staff working with live JEV. Mass vaccination of children is carried out in some

endemic areas. Live attenuated and formalin-inactivated primary hamster kidney cell vaccines are licensed and widely used in China.

8) Protect accidentally exposed laboratory workers passively with human immune serum if available.

B. Control of patient, contacts and the immediate environment:

1) Report to local health authority: Case report obligatory in several countries, Class 2 (see *Reporting*). Report under appropriate disease; or as "encephalitis, other forms"; or as "aseptic meningitis." Specify cause or clinical type when known.

2) Isolation: Not applicable. Virus is not usually found in blood, secretions or discharges during clinical disease. Standard blood and body substance precautions are sufficient. Patients in the first few days after onset of illness should avoid mosquito exposure, especially if they are in areas that are receptive to introduction of arboviruses.

3) Concurrent disinfection: Not applicable.

4) Quarantine: Not applicable.

5) Immunization of contacts: Not applicable.

6) Investigation of contacts and source of infection: Search for missed cases and the presence of vector mosquitoes, and consider testing symptomatic close contacts. Primarily a community vector control problem (see 9C).

7) Specific treatment: None established.

C. Epidemic measures:

1) Identification of infection among horses or birds and recognition of human cases in the community have epidemiological value by indicating frequency of infection and areas involved. Immunization of horses probably does not limit spread of the virus in the community; immunization of pigs against JE should have a significant effect.

2) Fogging or spraying from aircraft with suitable insecticides has shown promise for aborting urban epidemics of SLE.

3) Identify and control breeding areas for insect vector species.

D. Disaster implications: None.

E. International measures: Spray with insecticide those aircraft arriving from recognized areas of prevalence. WHO Collaborating Centres provide support as required. More information can be found at:
<http://www.who.int/collaboratingcentres/database/en/>

II. TICKBORNE VIRAL
ENCEPHALITIDES   ICD-9 063; ICD-10 A84

FAR EASTERN TICK-BORNE
ENCEPHALITIS   ICD-10 A84.0

(Russian spring-summer encephalitis)

CENTRAL EUROPEAN TICK-
BORNE ENCEPHALITIS   ICD-10 A84.1

SIBERIAN TICK-BORNE
ENCEPHALITIS   ICD-10 A84.8

LOUPING ILL   ICD-10 A84.8

POWASSAN VIRUS
ENCEPHALITIS   ICD-10 A84.8

1. Identification—A group of viral diseases clinically resembling the mosquito-borne encephalitides, caused by tick-borne encephalitis virus (TBEV), louping ill virus (LIV), and Powassan encephalitis virus (POWV). There are three subtypes of TBEV: Far Eastern, Central European and Siberian. The Far Eastern subtype causes the most severe disease, with up to 50% of cases developing neurological disease, and 20% mortality; the others cause an uncommon and milder neurological illness, with 1-3% mortality for the Siberian subtype and 1-2% for the Central European subtype. Central European TBEV typically causes a diphasic illness with a week of influenza-like illness, followed by an asymptomatic period of a few days, then neurological illness in one-third of cases. Powassan encephalitis (PE) has a similar clinical course, with a 10% case-fatality rate and neurological sequelae among 50% of survivors. LIV is closely related to Central European TBEV and causes a similar illness. All may cause a polio-like flaccid paralysis.

Specific identification is made through demonstration of specific IgM or nucleic acid in acute phase serum or CSF, serological tests of paired sera, virus isolation from blood during acute illness, or from brain postmortem (inoculation of suckling mice or cell culture). Common serological tests distinguish the group from most other similar diseases, but differentiating within this group requires characterization of the viral RNA.

2. Infectious agents—A complex within the flaviviruses; minor antigenic differences exist, more with Powassan than others, but viruses causing these diseases are closely related.

3. Occurrence—Disease of the CNS caused by this complex is distributed spottily over much of Russia, other parts of eastern and central Europe, Scandinavia, and the UK. Far Eastern TBEV is in northeast Russia, China, and northern Japan; Central European TBEV is found in an area extending from Scandinavia down to the Adriatic region, and east to the Urals; and the Siberian TBEV is found in Siberia and the Baltic region.

Ixodes persulcatus is the major vector of the Far Eastern and Siberian subtypes, and *Ix. ricinus* for the central European subtype. LIV is found in the UK and Ireland and southwestern Europe, and is transmitted by *Ix. ricinus*. Powassan virus is present in Canada, the USA, and Russia, and is transmitted by *Ix. cookei* in North America and by *Ix. persulcatus* and *Haemaphysalis longicornis* in Russia. Seasonal incidence depends on density of the tick vectors: activity peaks in spring and early summer in eastern Asia; early summer and early autumn in Europe; and June to September in Canada and the USA.

Areas of highest incidence are those where humans have intimate association with large numbers of infected ticks, generally in rural or forested areas but also in urban populations. Local epidemics of Central European TBEV disease have occurred among people consuming unpasteurized milk and dairy products from goats and sheep, hence the name "diphasic milk fever." The age pattern varies in different regions and is influenced by opportunity for exposure to ticks, consumption of milk from infected animals, and previously acquired immunity. Laboratory infections are common, some with serious sequelae, including death.

4. Reservoir—The tick, or ticks and mammals in combination, appear to be the true reservoir; trans-ovarian tick passage of some tick-borne encephalitis viruses has been demonstrated. Sheep and deer are the primary vertebrate hosts for LIV, while rodents and other small mammals and birds serve as sources of tick infections with TBEV and POWV.

5. Mode of transmission—Bites of infective ticks or consumption of milk from certain infected animals. Larval ticks ingest virus by feeding on infected vertebrates, including rodents, other mammals or birds. Central European TBEV may be acquired through consumption of infected raw milk.

6. Incubation period—Usually 7–14 days.

7. Period of communicability—No direct person-to-person transmission. A tick infected at any stage remains infective for life. Viremia may last for days in vertebrates; in humans, up to 7–10 days.

8. Susceptibility—Men and women of all ages are susceptible. Infection, whether unapparent or overt, leads to immunity.

9. Methods of control—

> **A. Preventive measures:**
>
> 1) See *Lyme Disease*, 9A, for measures against ticks.
> 2) Inactivated virus vaccines have been used extensively in Europe and the Russian Federation, with reported safety and effectiveness.
> 3) Boil or pasteurize milk of susceptible animals in areas where Central European TBEV occurs.

B. Control of patient, contacts and the immediate environment:

1) Report to local health authority: In selected endemic areas; in most countries not a reportable disease, Class 3 (see *Reporting*).
2) Isolation: None, after tick removal.
3) Concurrent disinfection: Not applicable.
4) Quarantine: Not applicable.
5) Immunization of contacts: Not applicable.
6) Investigation of contacts and source of infection: Search for missed cases, presence of tick vectors, and animals excreting virus in milk.
7) Specific treatment: None.

C. Epidemic measures: See *Lyme disease*, 9C.

D. Disaster implications: None.

E. International measures: WHO Collaborating Centres provide support as required. More information can be found at: <http://www.who.int/collaboratingcentres/database/en/>

ARTHROPOD-BORNE VIRAL FEVERS
[CCDM19: E. Hayes, J. Mackenzie]
[CCDM18: J. Mackenzie, R. Shope]

I. MOSQUITO-BORNE AND CULICOIDES-BORNE VIRAL FEVERS:
(Yellow fever and dengue are presented separately)

I. A. VENEZUELAN EQUINE ENCEPHALOMYELITIS VIRUS DISEASE   ICD-9 066.2; ICD-10 A92.2
(Venezuelan equine encephalitis, Venezuelan equine fever)

1. Identification—Infection with Venezuelan equine encephalomyelitis (VEE) virus causes abrupt onset of severe headache, chills, fever, myalgia, retro-orbital pain, nausea and vomiting. Conjunctival and pharyngeal congestion as well as pneumonia may occur. Most infections are relatively mild, with symptoms lasting 3–5 days. Some cases may have a diphasic fever course; after a few days of fever, particularly in children,

CNS involvement may range from somnolence to frank encephalitis with disorientation, convulsions, paralysis, coma and death.

Presumptive diagnosis is based on clinical and epidemiological grounds (such as exposure in an area where an equine epizootic is in progress), and is confirmed by virus isolation, rise in VEE-specific antibody, or detection of VEE RNA. Virus can be isolated in cell culture or in newborn mice, from specimens including blood, throat swabs, or nasopharyngeal washings during the first 72 hours of symptoms; acute and convalescent sera drawn 10 days apart may show rising antibody titers. Laboratory infections may occur in the absence of proper containment facilities.

2. Infectious agent—VEE virus, an alphavirus (Togaviridae, *Alphavirus*), with enzootic subtypes and epizootic varieties of subtype 1.

3. Occurrence—Endemic in northern South America, Trinidad and Central America. The disease appears as epizootics, mainly in northern and western South America. In 1971, VEE spread temporarily into the southern part of the USA.

4. Reservoir—Enzootic subtypes of VEE are maintained in a rodent-mosquito cycle. Epizootic varieties of subtype 1 are believed to arise periodically from enzootic VEE 1D viruses in northern South America. During outbreaks, epizootic VEE virus is transmitted in a cycle involving horses, which serve as the major source of virus, to mosquitoes, which in turn infect humans. Humans also develop sufficient viremia to serve as hosts in a human-mosquito-human transmission cycle.

5. Mode of transmission—Bite of an infected mosquito. VEE viruses have been isolated from *Culex* (*Melanoconion*), *Aedes*, *Mansonia*, *Psorophora*, *Haemagogus*, *Sabethes*, *Deinocerites* and *Anopheles* mosquitoes, *Simulium*, and possibly ceratopogonid gnats. Infection by aerosol transmission is common, primarily in laboratories; there is no evidence of direct horse-to-human transmission.

6. Incubation period—Usually 2-6 days; can be as short as 1 day.

7. Period of communicability—Infected humans and horses are infectious for mosquitoes for up to 72 hours; infected mosquitoes probably transmit virus throughout life.

8. Susceptibility—General. Mild infections and subsequent immunity occur frequently in endemic areas. Children are at greatest risk for CNS infection.

9. **Methods of control —**

   A. *Preventive measures:*

   1) Use general mosquito control procedures.
   2) Avoid forested endemic areas, especially at night.
   3) Live attenuated virus (TC-83) and inactivated vaccines for VEE have been used to protect laboratory workers and other adults at high risk. Vaccine for use in horses is commercially available.

   B. *Control of patient, contacts and the immediate environment:*

   1) Report to local health authority: In selected endemic areas; in most countries, not a reportable disease, Class 3 (see *Reporting*).
   2) Isolation: Blood and body fluid precautions. Patients should be treated in a screened room or in quarters treated with a residual insecticide for at least 5 days after onset, or until afebrile.
   3) Concurrent disinfection: Not applicable.
   4) Quarantine: Not applicable.
   5) Immunization of contacts: Not applicable.
   6) Investigation of contacts and source of infection: Search for unreported or undiagnosed cases.
   7) Specific treatment: None.

   C. *Epidemic measures:*

   1) Determine extent of the infected areas; immunize horses and/or restrict their movement from the affected area.
   2) Use approved mosquito repellents for those exposed.
   3) Conduct a community survey to determine density of vector mosquitoes, their breeding places, and effective control measures.
   4) Identify infected horses, prevent mosquitoes from feeding on them, and intensify mosquito control efforts in the affected area.

   D. *Disaster implications:* None.

   E. *International measures:* Immunize animals and restrict their movement from epizootic areas to areas free of the disease.

I. B. OTHER MOSQUITO-BORNE AND CULICOIDES-BORNE

FEVERS	ICD-9 066.3
BUNYAMWERA VIRAL FEVER	ICD-10 A92.8
BWAMBA VIRUS DISEASE	ICD-10 A92.8
RIFT VALLEY FEVER	ICD-10 A92.4
WEST NILE FEVER (INCLUDING KUNJIN VIRAL FEVER)	ICD-10 A92.3
GROUP C VIRUS DISEASE	ICD-10 A92.8
OROPOUCHE VIRUS DISEASE	ICD-10 A93.0
ZIKA VIRUS DISEASE	ICD-10 A93

1. Identification—A group of viruses that cause febrile illnesses usually lasting a week or less, many of which are dengue-like. Initial symptoms include fever, headache, malaise, arthralgia or myalgia, and occasionally nausea and vomiting; generally, there is some conjunctivitis and photophobia. Fever may or may not be diphasic. Rash can occur.

Encephalitis occurs with West Nile (including Kunjin virus subtype of West Nile) and Oropouche virus infections. It has been recognized since 1999 in the USA, and later in Canada, as a prominent complication of West Nile virus infection, especially among the elderly. Persons with Rift Valley fever (RVF) may develop retinitis, encephalitis or hepatitis associated with hemorrhages that may be fatal. Several group C viruses are reported to produce weakness in the lower limbs; they are not fatal. Epidemics of RVF, West Nile virus disease, and Oropouche fever may involve thousands of patients. An outbreak of Zika virus disease recently struck on Yap Island in the Federated States of Micronesia.

Serological tests may show a rise in virus-specific antibody. Viral nucleic acid can be detected in blood and cerebrospinal fluid. Virus can be isolated by inoculation into cell culture or suckling mice, from blood drawn early during the febrile period. Laboratory infections may occur with many of these viruses.

2. Infectious agents—Each disease is caused by a distinct virus with the same name as the disease. West Nile, Banzi, Kunjin, Spondweni and Zika viruses are flaviviruses; the group C bunyaviruses are Apeu, Caraparu, Itaqui, Madrid, Marituba, Murutucu, Nepuyo, Oriboca, Ossa and Restan. Oropouche is a bunyavirus of the Simbu group. RVF is a phlebovirus.

3. Occurrence—West Nile virus is widespread in Africa, North America, Europe, the Middle East, India, southeast Asia, and Australasia (in Australasia it is called Kunjin virus, a subtype of West Nile); and has spread into the Caribbean and Central and South America. It has caused outbreaks in Canada, the Czech Republic, Egypt, France, Italy, India, Israel, Romania, Russia and the USA. Bwamba and Bunyamwera fevers have been identified only in Africa. West Nile virus also causes equine encephalitis and a fatal encephalitis in some birds, especially the American crow. The first epidemic of Rift Valley fever outside Africa occurred in 2000 in the Arabian peninsula (probable vector *Ae. vexans arabiensis*). Group C virus fevers occur in tropical South America, Panama and Trinidad; Oropouche fever occurs in Brazil, Panama, Peru and Trinidad; Kunjin virus occurs in Australia. Seasonal incidence depends on vector density. Occurrence is primarily rural, although occasionally Oropouche, RVF, and West Nile have been involved in explosive urban and suburban outbreaks.

4. **Reservoir**—Some of these viruses are maintained in a continuous vertebrate-mosquito cycle. Oropouche virus may be transmitted by *Culicoides*. Birds are a source of mosquito infection for West Nile virus; rodents serve as reservoirs for group C viruses.

5. **Mode of transmission**—In most instances, bite of an infective mosquito:

- West Nile: *Culex univittatus* in southern Africa, *C. modestus* in France, *C. pipiens molestus* in Israel; *C. pipiens/restuans*, *C. quinquefasciatus*, *C. tarsalis* and *Ae. albopictus* in North America; *C. annulirostris* in Australasia. Virus also isolated from *Aedes* and *Mansonia*, and from ticks.
- Bunyamwera: *Aedes* spp.
- Group C viruses: *Aedes* and *Culex* (*Melanoconion*)
- Rift Valley (in sheep and other animals): potential vectors include *Aedes* mosquitoes; *Ae. mcintoshi* may be infected trans-ovarially and may account for maintenance of RVF virus in enzootic foci. *C. pipiens* was implicated in a 1977 epidemic of RVF in Egypt with at least 600 deaths. Mechanical transmission by hematophagous flies and transmission by aerosols or contact with highly infective blood may contribute to RVF outbreaks. Many human infections of RVF are associated with the handling of animal tissues during necropsy or butchering. Other arthropods may be vectors, such as *Culicoides paraensis* for the Oropouche virus.

6. **Incubation period**—Usually 2–14 days.

7. **Period of communicability**—No direct person-to-person transmission except for some viruses through blood transfusion, and possibly from mother to child. Infected mosquitoes probably transmit virus throughout life.

Viremia, essential for vector infection, often occurs during early clinical illness in humans.

8. **Susceptibility**—Susceptibility appears to be general in both sexes at all ages. Unapparent infections and mild disease are common. Since infection leads to immunity, susceptibles in endemic areas are mainly young children.

9. **Methods of control—**

   A. *Preventive measures:*

   1) Follow measures applicable to mosquito-borne viral encephalitides (see 9A). For RVF, precautions in care and handling of infected animals and their products, as well as human acute phase blood, are important.
   2) An inactivated cell culture RVF vaccine is available for humans as an investigational new drug; live and inactivated vaccines are available for sheep, goats and cattle.

   B. *Control of patient, contacts and the immediate environment:*

   1) Report to local health authority: In selected endemic areas; in most countries, not a reportable disease, Class 3 (see *Reporting*). For RVF, notify WHO, FAO and the International Office of Epizootics in Paris.
   2) Isolation: Blood and body fluid precautions. Keep patient in screened room, or in quarters treated with an insecticide, for at least 5 days after onset or until afebrile. Blood of RVF patients may be infectious. Screen blood for West Nile nucleic acid in North America before transfusion.
   3) Concurrent disinfection: Not applicable.
   4) Quarantine: Not applicable.
   5) Immunization of contacts: Not applicable.
   6) Investigation of contacts and source of infection: Determine patient's place of residence during fortnight before onset. Search for unreported or undiagnosed cases.
   7) Specific treatment: None.

   C. *Epidemic measures:*

   1) Use approved mosquito repellents for people exposed to bites of vectors.
   2) Do not slaughter sick or dying domestic animals suspected of being infected with RVF.
   3) Determine density of vector mosquitoes; identify and treat their breeding places with larvicides. Consider strategies to reduce abundance of adult mosquitoes, such as aerial spraying of insecticide.
   4) Immunize sheep, goats and cattle against RVF.

   D. *Disaster implications:* None.

   E. *International measures:* For RVF, immunize animals and restrict their movement from enzootic areas to clean areas; do not butcher sick animals; for others, none except enforcement of international agreements designed to prevent transfer of

mosquitoes and infected vertebrates by ships, airplanes and land transport. WHO Collaborating Centres provide support as required. More information can be found at:
<http://www.who.int/collaboratingcentres/database/en/>

II. TICK-BORNE VIRAL FEVERS ICD-9 066.1
COLORADO TICK FEVER ICD-10 A93.2
OTHER TICK-BORNE FEVERS ICD-10 A93.8

1. Identification—Colorado tick fever (CTF) is an acute febrile (often diphasic) viral disease with infrequent rash. After initial onset, a brief remission is usual, followed by a second bout of fever lasting 2–3 days; neutropenia and thrombocytopenia almost always occur on the 4th to 5th day of fever. Characteristically, CTF is a moderately severe disease, with occasional encephalitis, myocarditis or tendency to bleed. Deaths are rare. Bhanja virus can cause severe neurological disease and death; CNS infections also occur with Kemerovo and Thogoto viruses (the latter may cause hepatitis).

Laboratory confirmation of CTF is made by isolation of virus from blood inoculated into suckling mice or cell cultures, by demonstration of antigen in erythrocytes by IF, or by detection of viral RNA by PCR (CTF virus may persist in erythrocytes for up to 120 days). IFA and neutralization assays detect serum antibodies as early as 10 days after onset of illness, but in contrast to most arboviral infections, IgM antibodies do not usually appear until 14 to 21 days after onset of illness. Diagnostic methods for confirming other tick-borne viral fevers vary only slightly, except that serum is used for virus isolation instead of erythrocytes.

2. Infectious agents—Colorado tick fever, Nairobi sheep disease (Ganjam), Kemerovo, Lipovnik, Quaranfil, Bhanja, Thogoto and Dugbe viruses.

3. Occurrence—Colorado tick fever is endemic in mountainous regions above 1 500 meters (5 000 feet) in Canada and the western USA. Virus has been isolated from *Dermacentor andersoni* ticks in Alberta and British Columbia (Canada). CTF occurs most frequently in those with recreational or occupational exposure (hiking, fishing) in enzootic loci; seasonal incidence parallels the period of greatest tick activity (April–June in the Rocky Mountains of the USA). Geographic distribution of other viruses is shown in the introductory table.

4. Reservoir—Reservoirs for CTF include small mammals such as ground squirrels, porcupines, chipmunks and *Peromyscus* spp.; also ticks, principally *D. andersoni*.

5. Mode of transmission—By bite of an infective tick. Immature ticks (*D. andersoni*) acquire CTF virus by feeding on viremic animals; they pass the virus trans-stadially and transmit virus to humans during subsequent feeding.

6. Incubation period—Usually 3-4 days.

7. Period of communicability—Not directly transmitted from person to person except by transfusion. The wildlife cycle is maintained by ticks, which remain infective throughout life. Virus is present in blood during the febrile stage and in CTF, in erythrocytes from 2 to 16 weeks or more after onset.

8. Susceptibility—Susceptibility apparently universal. Second attacks are rare.

9. Methods of control—

A. *Preventive measures:* Personal protective measures to avoid tick bites; control of ticks and rodent hosts (see *Lyme disease*, 9A).

B. *Control of patient, contacts and the immediate environment:*

1) Report to local health authority: In endemic areas; in most states and countries, not a reportable disease, Class 3 (see *Reporting*).
2) Isolation: Blood and body fluid precautions. No blood donations for 4 months.
3) Concurrent disinfection: Remove ticks from patients.
4) Quarantine: Not applicable.
5) Immunization of contacts: Not applicable.
6) Investigation of contacts and source of infection: Identification of tick-infested areas.
7) Specific treatment: None.

C. *Epidemic measures:* Not applicable.

D. *Disaster implications:* None.

E. *International measures:* WHO Collaborating Centres provide support as required. More information can be found at: <http://www.who.int/collaboratingcentres/database/en/>

III. PHLEBOTOMINE-BORNE VIRAL FEVERS

SANDFLY FEVER   ICD-9 066.0; ICD-10 A93.1
(Phlebotomus fever, Papatasi fever)

CHANGUINOLA VIRUS DISEASE   ICD-9 066.0; ICD-10 A93.8
(Changuinola fever)

VESICULAR STOMATITIS VIRUS DISEASE   ICD-9 066.8; ICD-10 A93.8
(Vesicular stomatitis fever)

1. Identification—A group of arboviral diseases that cause headache, fever, retrobulbar pain on motion of the eyes, injected sclerae, malaise, nausea, and pain in the limbs and back. Pharyngitis, oral mucosal vesicular lesions and cervical adenopathy are characteristic of vesicular stomatitis virus (VSV) infections. Leukopenia is usual on the 4th to 5th day after onset of fever. Symptoms may be alarming, but death is very rare. Complete recovery may be preceded by prolonged mental depression. Encephalitis may occur following Toscana and Chandipura virus infections.

A presumptive diagnosis is based on the clinical picture and the occurrence of multiple similar cases. Diagnoses may be confirmed serologically by detection of specific IgM antibodies or by antibody titer rise, or by isolation of virus from blood inoculated into newborn mice or cell culture; for VSV infections, from throat swabs and vesicular fluid.

2. Infectious agents—The sandfly fever group of viruses (Bunyaviridae, *Phlebovirus*); several related immunological types have been isolated from humans and differentiated. In addition, Changuinola virus (an orbivirus) and VSV of the Indiana type (a rhabdovirus), both of which produce febrile disease in humans, have been isolated from *Lutzomyia* spp. sandflies. Chandipura virus is also a rhabdovirus.

3. Occurrence—A disease of subtropical and tropical areas: areas in Europe with long periods of hot, dry weather; Asia, distributed in a belt extending around the Mediterranean and eastward into China; Africa; and tropical rain forests in Central and South America and Myanmar. The disease is seasonal in temperate zones north of the equator, occurring between April and October, and is prone to affect military personnel and travelers from non-endemic areas.

4. Reservoir—The main reservoir is the sandfly, in which the virus is maintained trans-ovarially. Arboreal rodents and nonhuman primates may harbor VSV. Rodents (gerbils) have been implicated as a reservoir for Eastern Hemisphere sandfly viruses.

5. Mode of transmission—Bite of an infective sandfly. The vector of the classic virus is a small, hairy, blood-sucking midge (*Phlebotomus papatasi*, the common sandfly), which bites at night and has a limited flight range. Sandflies of the genus *Sergentomyia* have also been found to be infected and may be vectors. Members of the genus *Lutzomyia* are involved in Central and South America.

6. Incubation period—Up to 6 days, usually 3-4 days, rarely less.

7. Period of communicability—Virus is present in the blood of an infected person at least 24 hours before and 24 hours after onset of fever. Phlebotomines become infective about 7 days after biting an infected person, and remain so for their normal life span of about 1 month.

8. Susceptibility—Susceptibility is universal; homologous acquired immunity is probably lasting. Relative resistance of native populations in sandfly areas is probably attributable to infection early in life.

9. Methods of control—

   A. *Preventive measures:* Personal protective measures to prevent sandfly feeding; control of sandflies is the principal objective (see *Leishmaniasis*, cutaneous and mucosal, 9A2).

   B. *Control of patient, contacts and the immediate environment:*

   1) Report to local health authority: In selected endemic areas; in most countries, not a reportable disease, Class 3 (see *Reporting*).
   2) Isolation: None; consider preventing access of sandflies to infected individuals for the first few days of illness, by using very fine screening or mosquito bed nets (10-12 mesh/cm or 25-30 mesh/inch, aperture size not more than 0.085 cm or 0.035 inch), and by spraying quarters with insecticide.
   3) Concurrent disinfection: Destroy sandflies in residences.
   4) Quarantine: Not applicable.
   5) Immunization of contacts: Not currently available.
   6) Investigation of contacts and source of infection: In the Eastern Hemisphere, search for breeding areas of sandflies around dwellings, especially in rubble heaps, in masonry cracks, and under stones.
   7) Specific treatment: None.

   C. *Epidemic measures:*

   1) Educate the public about conditions leading to infection and the importance of preventing sandfly bites by use of repellents, particularly after sundown.
   2) Use insecticides to control sandflies in and about human habitations, community-wide.

D. Disaster implications: None.

E. International measures: WHO Collaborating Centres provide support as required. More information can be found at: <http://www.who.int/collaboratingcentres/database/en/>

ARTHROPOD-BORNE VIRAL HEMORRHAGIC FEVERS
[CCDM19: J. Mackenzie, D. Smith]
[CCDM18: P. Formenty, J. Mackenzie, R. Shope]

I. MOSQUITO-BORNE DISEASES
(Dengue hemorrhagic fever and yellow fever are presented separately)
II. TICK-BORNE DISEASES
II.A. CRIMEAN-CONGO HEMORRHAGIC FEVER   ICD-9 065.0; ICD-10 A98.0
(Central Asian hemorrhagic fever)

1. Identification—A viral disease with sudden onset of fever, malaise, weakness, irritability, headache, severe pain in limbs and loins, and marked anorexia. Vomiting, abdominal pain and diarrhea occur occasionally. Flush on face and chest and conjunctival injection develop early. Hemorrhagic enanthem of soft palate, uvula and pharynx, and a fine petechial rash spreading from the chest and abdomen to the rest of the body, sometimes with large purpuric areas, are generally associated with the disease.

There may be bleeding from the gums, nose, lungs, uterus and intestine, but only in serious or fatal cases does this occur in large amounts, when it is often associated with severe liver damage. Hematuria and albuminuria are common but usually not massive. Fever is constantly elevated for 5–12 days or may be biphasic; it falls rapidly by lysis. Convalescence is prolonged. Other findings are leukopenia, with lymphopenia more marked than neutropenia. Thrombocytopenia is common. The reported case-fatality rate ranges from 2% to 50%, with most fatalities occurring 5–14 days after onset. In Russia, it is estimated that five infections occur for each hemorrhagic case.

Diagnosis is through isolation of virus from blood (inoculation of cell cultures or suckling mice), by PCR, or by antigen detection. Serological diagnosis is by ELISA, reverse passive HI, IFA, CF, immunodiffusion, or plaque-reduction neutralization test. Specific IgM may be present during the acute phase; convalescent sera often have low neutralization antibody titers. Due to the high risk of transmission to health care personnel and laboratory workers, handling of specimens requires high-level precautions.

2. Infectious agent—The Crimean-Congo hemorrhagic fever virus (Bunyaviridae, *Nairovirus*).

3. Occurrence—Observed in the steppes of western Crimea and in the Rostov and Astrakhan regions of Russia, as well as in Afghanistan, Albania, Bosnia and Herzegovina, Bulgaria, western China, northern Greece, the Islamic Republic of Iran, Iraq, Kazakhstan, Pakistan, South Africa, Turkey, Uzbekistan, the Arabian Peninsula, and throughout sub-Saharan Africa. Most patients have close contact with animals or are health care personnel. Seasonal occurrence in Russia is from June to September, the period of vector activity.

4. Reservoir—Maintained in host tick species, especially *Hyalomma* spp., as well as *Boophilus* and *Rhipicephalus* ticks. Domestic animals (sheep, cattle, ostriches, and goats), wild herbivores, hedgehogs and hares act as amplifying hosts.

5. Mode of transmission—Bite of infective adult ticks, or by crushing those ticks on removal. Immature ticks are believed to acquire infection from the animal hosts and by trans-ovarial transmission. Nosocomial infection of medical workers, occurring after exposure to blood and secretions from patients, has been important in recent outbreaks; tertiary cases have occurred in family members of medical workers. Infection is also associated with butchering or other contact with infected animal blood.

6. Incubation period—Usually 3 to 7 days, with a range of 1–12 days.

7. Period of communicability—Highly infectious in the hospital setting. Nosocomial infections are common after exposure to blood and secretions.

8. Susceptibility—Immunity after infection probably lifelong.

9. Methods of control—

    A. Preventive measures: See *Lyme disease*, 9A, for preventive measures against ticks. An inactivated mouse brain vaccine has been used in eastern Europe and Russia (not available in the USA).

    B. Control of patient, contacts and the immediate environment:

        1) Report to local health authority: In selected epidemic areas; in most countries, not a reportable disease, Class 3 (see *Reporting*).

2) Isolation: Patient isolated in a single room, under negative pressure if available. Strict blood and body fluid precautions.
3) Concurrent disinfection: Bloody discharges are infective; decontaminate with heat or chlorine disinfectants. Careful disposal or disinfection of all blood-contaminated instruments, equipment, linen, clothing and other objects.
4) Quarantine: Not applicable.
5) Immunization: Not applicable, except in eastern Europe.
6) Investigation of contacts and source of infection: Search for missed cases and the presence of infective animals and possible vectors.
7) Specific treatment: Intravenous ribavirin, and convalescent plasma with a high neutralizing antibody titer, are regarded as useful.

C. Epidemic measures: See *Lyme disease*, 9C.

D. Disaster implications: None.

E. International measures: WHO Collaborating Centres provide support as required. More information can be found at: <http://www.who.int/collaboratingcentres/database/en/>

ARTHROPOD-BORNE VIRAL HEMORRHAGIC FEVERS
II.B. OMSK HEMORRHAGIC FEVER   ICD-9 065.1; ICD-10 A98.1
KYASANUR FOREST DISEASE   ICD-9 065.2; ICD-10 A98.2

1. Identification—These two viral diseases have marked similarities. Onset is sudden, with chills, headache, fever, pain in lower back and limbs, and severe prostration, often associated with conjunctivitis, diarrhea and vomiting by the third or fourth day. A papulovesicular eruption on the soft palate, cervical lymphadenopathy and conjunctival suffusion are usually present. Severe cases are associated with hemorrhages but with no cutaneous rash. Bleeding occurs from gums, nose, GI tract, uterus and lungs (rarely from the kidneys), sometimes for many days. When severe, this results in shock and death; shock may also occur without manifest hemorrhage. Leukopenia and thrombocytopenia are marked. The febrile period ranges from 5 days to 2 weeks. Sometimes there is a biphasic course of illness with an afebrile period of 1–2 weeks, after which a small proportion of patients develop meningoencephalitis.

Convalescence tends to be slow and prolonged, but most recover without sequelae. Estimated case-fatality rate is from 1% to 3% for Omsk hemorrhagic fever (OHF) and 3 to 5% for Kyasanur Forest disease (KFD).

Diagnosis is made by isolation of virus from blood in suckling mice or cell cultures (virus may be present up to 12 days following onset); or through EIA, IF, HI, CF or neutralizing antibody titers.

2. Infectious agents—The OHF and KFD viruses are closely related; they belong to the tick-borne encephalitis/louping ill complex of flaviviruses, and are antigenically similar to the other viruses in the complex.

3. Occurrence—In the Kyasanur Forest of the Shimoga and Kanara districts of Karnataka, India, principally in young adult males exposed in the forest during the dry season, from November to June. In 1983, there were 1 155 cases with 150 deaths, the largest epidemic of KFD ever reported. OHF occurs in the forest steppe regions of western Siberia, within the Omsk, Novosibirsk, Kurgan and Tjumen regions. The Novosibirsk district reported 2 to 41 cases per year between 1989 and 1998, mostly in muskrat trappers. Seasonal occurrence in each area coincides with vector activity. Laboratory infections are common with both viruses.

4. Reservoir—In KFD, probably rodents, shrews, and monkeys in combination with ticks; in OHF, rodents, muskrats and ticks.

5. Mode of transmission—Bite of infective (especially nymphal) ticks, probably *Haemaphysalis spinigera* in KFD. In OHF, infective ticks are possibly *Dermacentor reticulatus (pictus)* and *D. marginatus*; direct transmission from muskrats to humans does occur, with disease in the families of muskrat trappers.

6. Incubation period—Usually 3–8 days.

7. Period of communicability—Not directly transmitted from person to person. Infected ticks remain so for life.

8. Susceptibility and resistance—Men and women of all ages are probably susceptible; previous infection leads to immunity.

9. Methods of control—See *Tick-borne viral encephalitides* and *Lyme disease*, 9A. Formalin-inactivated mouse-brain virus vaccine has been used for OHF; tick-borne encephalitis vaccine has also been used to protect against OHF, without proof of efficacy. A formalin-inactivated cell-culture vaccine is used to prevent KFD in endemic areas of India.

ASCARIASIS   ICD-9 127.0; ICD-10 B77
(Roundworm infection, Ascaridiasis)
[CCDM19: M. Eberhard, A. Gabrielli, L. Savioli]
[CCDM18: L. Savioli]

1. Identification—A helminthic infection of the small intestine generally associated with few or no overt clinical symptoms. Live worms, passed in stools or occasionally from the mouth, anus, or nose, are often the first recognized sign of infection. Some patients have pulmonary manifestations (pneumonitis, Löffler syndrome) caused by larval migration (mainly during re-infections) and characterized by wheezing, cough, fever, eosinophilia and pulmonary infiltration. Heavy parasite burdens may aggravate nutritional deficiency and, if chronic, may affect work and school performance. Serious complications, sometimes fatal, include bowel obstruction by a bolus of worms, particularly in children; or obstruction of bile duct, pancreatic duct or appendix by one or more adult worms. Reports of ascaris pancreatitis are increasing.

Diagnosis is made by identifying eggs in feces, or adult worms passed from the anus, mouth or nose. Intestinal worms may be visualized by radiological and sonographic techniques; more rarely, pulmonary involvement may be confirmed by identifying ascarid larvae in sputum or gastric washings.

2. Infectious agent—*Ascaris lumbricoides*, the large intestinal roundworm of humans. *A. suum*, a similar parasite of pigs, rarely, if ever, develops to maturity in humans, although it may cause larva migrans.

3. Occurrence—Common and worldwide, with greatest frequency in moist tropical countries where prevalence often exceeds 50%. Prevalence and intensity of infection are usually highest in children between 3 and 8 years.

4. Reservoir—Humans; ascarid eggs in soil.

5. Mode of transmission—Ingestion of infective eggs from soil contaminated with human feces or from uncooked produce contaminated with soil containing infective eggs, but not directly from person to person or from fresh feces. Transmission occurs mainly in the vicinity of the home, where children, in the absence of sanitary facilities, fecally pollute the area; heavy infections in children are frequently the result of ingesting soil (pica). Contaminated soil may be carried long distances on feet or footwear into houses and conveyances; transmission of infection by dust is also possible.

Eggs reach the soil in the feces, and then undergo development (embryonation); at summer temperatures they become infective after 2–3 weeks, and may remain infective for several months or years in favorable soil. Ingested embryonated eggs hatch in the intestinal lumen; the larvae penetrate the gut wall and reach the lungs via the circulatory system. Larvae grow and develop in the lungs, pass into the alveoli 9-10 days after infection, ascend the trachea, and are swallowed, reaching the small intestine 14-20 days after infection, where they grow to maturity, mate and begin laying eggs 45-60 days after initial ingestion of the embryonated eggs. Eggs passed by gravid females are discharged in feces.

6. **Incubation period**—The life cycle requires 4-8 weeks to for completion.

7. **Period of communicability**—As long as mature, fertilized female worms continue to live in the intestine. Usual life span of adult worms is 12 months; maximum lifespan may reach 24 months. The female worm can produce more than 200 000 eggs a day. Under favorable conditions, embryonated eggs can remain viable in soil for years.

8. **Susceptibility**—Susceptibility is general.

9. **Methods of control**—

   A. *Preventive measures:*

   1) Educate the public in the use of proper toilet facilities and—especially for children—the need to avoid direct contact with contaminated soils.
   2) Provide adequate facilities for proper disposal of feces, and prevent soil contamination in areas immediately adjacent to houses, particularly children's play areas.
   3) In rural areas, construct latrines that prevent dissemination of ascarid eggs through overflow, drainage, or otherwise. Treating human feces by composting for later use as fertilizer may not kill all eggs.
   4) Encourage satisfactory hygienic habits in children; in particular, train them to wash hands before eating and handling food.
   5) In endemic areas, protect food from dirt. Food that has been dropped on the floor should not be eaten unless washed or reheated.
   6) WHO recommends a "preventive chemotherapy" strategy focused on treatment of high-risk groups at regular intervals, for the control of morbidity due to soil-transmitted helminth (STH) infections, including ascariasis, trichuriasis and hookworm disease. Recommended drugs and dosages are: single-dose mebendazole (500 mg) or albendazole (400 mg, half dose for children 12-24 months). Action to be taken is differentiated according to prevalence of any STH (soil transmitted helminths) infection (infection with at least one STH) among children aged 6-15 years.

Recommended treatment strategy for STH in preventive chemotherapy[a]

Category	Prevalence of infection among school-aged children	Action to be taken	
High-risk community	≥50%	Treat all school-age children (enrolled and not enrolled) twice each year[b].	Also treat with the same frequency:
			• Preschool children (aged 1–5)
			• Women of childbearing age, including women in the 2nd and 3rd trimesters and lactating women
			• Adults at high risk in certain occupations (e.g. tea pickers and miners).
Low-risk community	≥20% and <50%	Treat all school-age children (enrolled and not enrolled) once each year.	Also treat with the same frequency:
			• Preschool children (aged 1–5)
			• Women of childbearing age, including women in the 2nd and 3rd trimesters and lactating women
			• Adults at high risk in certain occupations (e.g. tea pickers and miners).

[a]When prevalence of any STH infection is less than 20%, large-scale intermittent chemotherapy interventions are not recommended. Affected individuals should be treated on a case-by-case basis.

[b]If resources are available, a third drug distribution intervention might be added. In this case, the appropriate frequency of treatment would be every 4 months.

Extensive monitoring has shown no significant ill effects of administration of antihelminthics to pregnant women, but as a precautionary measure, women in the 1st trimester of pregnancy should not be treated. Administration to very young children (1–2 years old) is safe, but key recommendations should be followed in order to avoid choking: (1) children should never be forced to swallow tablets; (2) tablets should be crushed and mixed with water; (3) treatment should be supervised by trained personnel.

B. Control of patient, contacts and the immediate environment:

1) Report to local health authority: Official report not ordinarily justifiable, Class 5 (see *Reporting*).
2) Isolation: Not applicable.
3) Concurrent disinfection: Sanitary disposal of feces.
4) Quarantine: Not applicable.
5) Immunization of contacts: Not applicable.
6) Investigate contacts and source of infection: Determine others who should be treated. Environmental sources of infection should be sought, particularly on premises of affected families.
7) Specific treatment: Single-dose oral mebendazole (500 mg) or albendazole (400 mg, half dose for children 12–24 months); on theoretical grounds, both are contraindicated during the first trimester of pregnancy unless there are specific medical or public health indications. Erratic migration of ascarid worms has been reported following mebendazole therapy; this may also occur with other medications, or spontaneously in heavy infections. Single-dose ivermectin 200 micrograms/kg single-dose is also highly effective against ascaris. Single-dose pyrantel pamoate (10 mg/kg) or levamisole (2.5 mg/kg) are also effective (and also effective against hookworm, but not against *T. trichiura*).

C. Epidemic measures: Survey for prevalence in highly endemic areas and educate the community in environmental sanitation and in personal hygiene. Provide treatment facilities and community treatment for high-risk groups— especially children— or for the whole population.

D. Disaster implications: None.

E. International measures: None.

ASPERGILLOSIS
ICD-9 117.3; ICD-10 B44

[CCDM19: M. Brandt]
[CCDM18: D. Denning]

1. Identification—A fungal disease that may present with a variety of clinical syndromes produced by several of the *Aspergillus* species. Allergic bronchopulmonary aspergillosis (ABPA), with symptoms similar to those of asthma, is an allergy to the spores of *Aspergillus* molds. Up to 5% of adult asthmatics may develop it at some time during their lives; it is also common in cystic fibrosis patients reaching adolescence and adulthood. Some patients have central bronchiectasis.

In the long term, ABPA can lead to permanent lung damage (fibrosis) if untreated. Increasing evidence suggests that fungal allergy is associated with increasing severity of asthma. The diagnosis of ABPA in patients with asthma is based on a combination of radiographic, clinical and laboratory findings, including central bronchiectasis on chest computed tomography

(CAT) scans, infiltrates on chest radiographs, positive *Aspergillus* skin-prick testing, elevated total serum IgE (1 000 ng/mL), elevated serum IgE and/or IgG antibodies to *Aspergillus fumigatus*, peripheral blood eosinophilia, and positive *Aspergillus* precipitins. In patients with cystic fibrosis, the diagnosis of ABPA is challenging, and consensus criteria have been developed.

There are several subacute-to-chronic forms of pulmonary aspergillosis, including chronic necrotizing pulmonary aspergillosis, chronic cavitary pulmonary aspergillosis, chronic fibrosing pulmonary aspergillosis, and aspergilloma. Aspergilloma is a non-invasive form of aspergillosis in which the fungus grows inside a cavity, typically in a previously damaged area of the lung (such as those damaged by tuberculosis, sarcoidosis, or other cavity-causing lung diseases); the conidia penetrate the cavity and germinate therein, forming a fungal ball. Aspergillomas may be asymptomatic, or may lead to hemoptysis. In the other forms of chronic aspergillosis, symptoms such as weight loss, chronic cough, and fatigue may be slowly progressive over months to years. Hemoptysis may also occur. Diagnosis is made by X-rays, lung scans, and *Aspergillus* precipitins testing.

Acute *Aspergillus* sinusitis (a form of invasive aspergillosis) may occur in cases of neutropenia or following a hematopoietic stem cell transplant. Symptoms include fever, facial pain, nasal discharge, and headaches. Diagnosis is made by finding the fungus in sinus fluid or tissue, and with scans. Invasive aspergillosis usually occurs in persons with significant immunosuppression (e.g. due to hematopoietic stem cell transplant, neutropenia, HIV/AIDS, therapy with corticosteroids and/or other immunosuppressive medications, and solid organ transplantation). A rare inherited condition, chronic granulomatous disease, puts affected people at moderate risk. Symptoms usually include fever, cough, chest pain and/or breathlessness that do not respond to standard antibiotics. X-rays and CT scans are abnormal. Bronchoscopy may confirm the diagnosis, together with microscopy and culture. Sputum cultures have low sensitivity and specificity. Newer tests, such as the galactomannan antigen assay, may help confirm diagnosis.

In up to 40% of infected people with poor immune systems, hematogenous dissemination occurs to the brain or to other organs—including the eye, heart, kidneys and skin—with worsening of the prognosis. In some cases, however, skin infection allows earlier diagnosis and treatment. *Aspergillus* spp. may cause keratitis after minor injury to the cornea, often leading to unilateral blindness. The organisms may infect the implantation site of a cardiac prosthetic valve or other surgical sites.

2. Infectious agents—Of the 180-odd species of *Aspergillus*, about 40 have been reported to cause disease in humans. The species that most commonly cause invasive infection in humans are *A. flavus*, *A. fumigatus*, *A. nidulans*, *A. niger*, and *A. terreus*. Common allergenic species include *A. fumigatus*, *A. clavatus* and *A. versicolor*. *A. fumigatus* causes most cases of fungus ball; *A. niger* is the commonest fungal cause of external otitis.

3. Occurrence—Worldwide; uncommon and sporadic; occasional outbreaks recognized in healthcare settings; no distinctive differences in incidence by race or gender. On certain foods, many isolates of *A. flavus* and *A. parasiticus* (occasionally other species) will produce aflatoxins or other mycotoxins that cause disease in animals and fish and are highly carcinogenic for experimental animals. An association between high aflatoxin levels in foods and hepatocellular cancer has been noted in Africa and southeastern Asia. Outbreaks of acute aflatoxicosis (liver necrosis with ascites) have been described in humans in India and Kenya, and in animals.

4. Reservoir—*Aspergillus* species are ubiquitous in nature, particularly in decaying vegetation, such as in piles of leaves or compost piles. Conidia are commonly present in the air, both outdoors and indoors, and during all seasons of the year. Water and foods may also be contaminated.

5. Mode of transmission—Inhalation of airborne conidia.

6. Incubation period—Probably between 2 days and 3 months.

7. Period of communicability—No person-to-person transmission.

8. Susceptibility—The ubiquity of *Aspergillus* species and the usual occurrence of the disease as an opportunistic infection suggest that most people are naturally immune and do not develop disease caused by *Aspergillus*. Immunosuppressive or cytotoxic therapy increase susceptibility, and invasive disease is seen primarily in those with prolonged neutropenia or corticosteroid treatment. Transplant recipients, patients with HIV infection and persons with chronic granulomatous disease are also susceptible.

9. Methods of control—

 A. *Preventive measures:* High efficiency particulate air (HEPA) filtration and other air quality improvement measures may decrease the incidence of invasive aspergillosis in hospitalized patients with profound and prolonged neutropenia.

 B. *Control of patient, contacts and the immediate environment:*

   1) Report to local health authority: Official report not ordinarily justifiable, Class 5 (see *Reporting*).
   2) Isolation: Not applicable.
   3) Concurrent disinfection: Ordinary cleanliness. Terminal cleaning.
   4) Quarantine: Not applicable.
   5) Immunization of contacts: Not applicable.
   6) Investigation of contacts: Not ordinarily indicated.

7) Specific treatment: ABPA is treated with steroids by aerosol or by mouth, especially during attacks, and treatment is usually prolonged. Itraconazole is useful in reducing the amount of steroids needed. The role of newer azoles, such as voriconazole, in the treatment of ABPA remains to be determined. Surgical resection, if possible, is the treatment of choice for patients with aspergilloma who cough blood, but it is best reserved for single cavities. Asymptomatic patients may require no treatment; oral itraconazole (400 mg/day) or the newer voriconazole may help symptoms, but do not kill the fungi within the cavity. Voriconazole (IV or orally) is the treatment of choice in tissue-invasive forms. Alternatives are itraconazole (IV or orally), amphotericin B formulations (IV only), and other echinocandins such as caspofungin (IV only). Immunosuppressive therapy should be discontinued or reduced as much as possible. Endobronchial colonization should be treated by measures to improve bronchopulmonary drainage. In sinusitis, surgery may help in eradicating the fungus. Treatment with amphotericin B, caspofungin, voriconazole or itraconazole is usually effective, although relapse is common.

C. *Epidemic measures:* Not generally applicable; a sporadic disease. Outbreaks have been reported in healthcare settings, particularly during periods of construction.

D. *Disaster implications:* None. Aflatoxin is one possible substance that could be used deliberately to cause harm, through adding to water and/or food.

For more information on the deliberate use of infectious agents to cause harm, see the section on *Deliberate use.*

E. *International measures:* None.

BABESIOSIS   ICD-9 088.8; ICD-10 B60.0
[CCDM19: B. Herwaldt]
[CCDM18: F. Meslin, K. Western]

1. Identification—A zoonotic infection caused by intraerythrocytic protozoan parasites of the *Babesia* genus. The clinical spectrum ranges from asymptomatic to life threatening, in part dependent on host and parasite factors. If clinically manifest, *Babesia* infection is typified by the presence of fever, nonspecific flu-like symptoms, and hemolytic anemia. Common findings include fever, chills, myalgia, fatigue and jaundice secondary to a hemolytic anemia that may last from several days to a few months. Seroprevalence studies indicate that most infections are asymptomatic. Even persons with asymptomatic infection may have low-level (sub-patent) parasitemia for months, sometimes for longer than a year, making transmission via blood transfusion an issue. Dual infection with *Borrelia burgdorferi*, causal agent of Lyme disease, may increase the severity of both diseases.

Diagnosis of acute cases with parasitemia is through light-microscopic identification of intraerythrocytic *Babesia* parasites on Wright- or Giemsa-stained blood smears. In some circumstances, distinguishing *Babesia* species from *Plasmodium falciparum* can be difficult. Some *Babesia* species (e.g. *B. Microti* and *B. duncani*) are also morphologically indistinguishable from one another. Confirmation of the diagnosis/species by a reference laboratory—through blood-smear examination and other means (e.g., serologic testing, molecular analyses, animal inoculation)—should be considered.

2. Infectious agents—Several species have been established to cause disease in humans, some of which have only recently been identified or characterized. In the USA, these include, predominantly, *Babesia microti* (see *Occurrence*); also *B. duncani* (formerly, the WA1-type parasite) and related organisms (in several western states), as well as *B. divergens*-like parasites. In Europe, these include: *B. divergens*, EU1, and *B. microti*. In other regions, these include various *Babesia* species and strains.

3. Occurrence—Worldwide, scattered. Overall, most of the documented zoonotic cases have occurred in the United States, some in Europe, and a few in other areas. However, with increased awareness of new *Babesia* species, patterns of documented cases may change. In the United States, most cases have been attributed to *B. microti* and acquired in the Northeast (particularly, but not exclusively, in parts of Connecticut, Massachusetts, New Jersey, New York, and Rhode Island), and to a lesser extent in the upper Midwest (Wisconsin and Minnesota). In Europe, human infections caused by *B. divergens* have been reported from France, Germany, Ireland, Russia, Serbia and Montenegro (formerly the Federal Republic of Yugoslavia), Spain, Sweden and the United Kingdom (Scotland). Human infections with less well-characterized species have been reported from China (including Taiwan), Egypt, Japan, Spain (Canary Islands), and South Africa.

4. Reservoir—Deer mice (*Peromyscus leucopus*) and other small mammals for *B. microti* in the United States; cattle for *B. divergens* in Europe; not definitively established for other zoonotic *Babesia* species.

5. Mode of transmission—Tickborne in nature, although the tick bite typically is not noticed, and the tick vector has not been identified for some *Babesia* species. The vectors include *Ixodes scapularis* for *B. microti* in the United States (typically, the nymphal stage, from late spring through early fall) and *I. ricinus* for *B. divergens* in Europe. Nymphal Ixodes ticks have typically fed on infected deer mice (*Peromyscus leucopus*) and other small mammals (e.g. voles, *Microtus pennsylvanicus*). The adult tick is normally found on deer (which are not infected by the parasite) but may also feed on other mammalian and avian hosts.

Babesia species are also transmissible by blood transfusion (documented for *B. microti* and *B. duncani*); bloodborne transmission is not inherently restricted by geographic region or season. There are rare cases of congenital/perinatal transmission.

6. Incubation period—Variable, in part dependent on host, parasite, and epidemiologic factors. Around 1-3 weeks or longer for tickborne transmission, and from weeks to months for bloodborne transmission. Symptoms may appear or recrudesce many months (even >1 year) after initial exposure, particularly in the context of immunosuppression.

7. Period of communicability—No person-to-person transmission other than through blood transfusion, which may occur months to >1 year after the donor is infected; asymptomatic, undiagnosed parasitemia may be protracted.

8. Susceptibility—Susceptibility to *B. microti* is assumed to be universal. Persons who are asplenic, immunocompromised, elderly, or otherwise debilitated are at increased risk for clinically manifest infection, which can be severe.

9. Methods of control—

  A. Preventive measures:

  1) Tickborne transmission (in babesiosis-endemic areas): Educate the public about personal protective measures to reduce the risk for tick exposures. Control rodents around human habitation and use tick repellents. See *Lyme disease*, 9A, and *Tick-borne rickettsioses*, 9A.
  2) Bloodborne transmission: Tests for screening blood donations for evidence of *Babesia* infection are not available.

  B. Control of patient, contacts and the immediate environment:

  1) Report to local health authority: Reporting of newly suspected cases in some countries, particularly in areas not previously known to be endemic, Class 3 (see *Reporting*).
  2) Isolation: Blood and body fluid precautions.
  3) Concurrent disinfection: Not applicable.
  4) Quarantine: Not applicable.
  5) Protection of contacts: If indicated by the epidemiologic and clinical context (see #6 below), evaluate other persons who

might have become infected in the same setting as the patient.

6) Investigation of contacts and source of infection: Cases occurring in a new area deserve careful study (e.g., to identify/characterize the *Babesia* species, tick vector, and reservoir hosts). Investigations of blood-transfusion-acquired cases require medical and public health attention: the implicated blood donor must be investigated promptly and refrain from future donations, and the recipients of cellular blood products from all potentially relevant donations must be promptly evaluated.

7) Specific treatment: Combination therapy with clindamycin and quinine is the standard of care for severe *B. microti* infection. In a controlled clinical trial restricted to adults with non–life-threatening infection, combination therapy with atovaquone plus azithromycin had comparable efficacy to clindamycin plus quinine, and was better tolerated. Isolated case reports describe success with other drug combinations (e.g., atovaquone plus quinine). Adjunctive exchange transfusion should be considered for critically ill patients, particularly, but not exclusively, for patients with a high proportion of parasitized red blood cells (e.g., ≥10%). Some patients require dialysis and mechanical ventilation. If indicated by the epidemiologic and clinical context, consider the possibility of co-infection with *Borrelia burgdorferi* (Lyme disease) or *Anaplasma phagocytophilum* (human granulocytic anaplasmosis). Dialysis may be necessary for patients with renal failure.

C. Epidemic measures: None.

D. Disaster implications: None.

E. International measures: None.

BALANTIDIASIS   ICD-9 007.0; ICD-10 A07.0
(Balantidiosis, Balantidial dysentery)
[CCDM19: A. Gabrielli, L. Savioli]
[CCDM18: L. Savioli]

1. Identification—A protozoan infection of the colon characteristically producing diarrhea or dysentery, accompanied by abdominal colic, tenesmus, nausea, and vomiting. Occasionally the dysentery resembles that due to amebiasis, with stools containing much blood and mucus, but relatively little pus. Peritoneal or urogenital invasion is rare.

Diagnosis is made by identifying the trophozoites or cysts of *Balantidium coli* in fresh feces, or trophozoites in material obtained by sigmoidoscopy.

2. Infectious agent—*Balantidium coli*, a large ciliated protozoan.

3. Occurrence—Worldwide; the incidence of human disease is low. Waterborne epidemics occasionally occur in areas of poor environmental sanitation. Environmental contamination with swine feces may result in higher incidence. Laboratory pigs may carry this parasite. Epidemics have rarely been identified.

4. Reservoir—Swine, and possibly other animals, such as rats and nonhuman primates.

5. Mode of transmission—Ingestion of contaminated food or water containing cysts from feces of infected hosts; in epidemics, mainly through fecally contaminated water. Sporadic transmission is by transfer of feces to mouth, via hands or contaminated water or food.

6. Incubation period—Unknown; may be only a few days.

7. Period of communicability—As long as the infection persists.

8. Susceptibility—Humans appear to have a high natural resistance. In individuals debilitated by other diseases, the infection may be serious, and even fatal.

9. Methods of control—

    A. *Preventive measures:*

        1) Educate the general public in personal hygiene.
        2) Educate and supervise food handlers through health agencies.
        3) Dispose of feces in a sanitary manner.
        4) Minimize contact with swine feces.
        5) Protect public water supplies against contamination with swine feces. Diatomaceous earth and sand filters remove all cysts, but ordinary water chlorination does not destroy cysts. Small quantities of water are best treated by boiling.

    B. *Control of patient, contacts and the immediate environment:*

        1) Report to local health authority: Official report not ordinarily justifiable, Class 5 (see *Reporting*).
        2) Isolation: Not applicable.
        3) Concurrent disinfection: Sanitary disposal of feces.
        4) Quarantine: Not applicable.
        5) Immunization of contacts: Not applicable.

6) Investigation of contacts and source of infection: Microscopic examination of feces of household members and suspected contacts. Also investigate contact with swine; consider treating infected pigs with tetracycline.

7) Specific treatment: Tetracycline 500 mg four times daily for 10 days eliminates infection (though tetracycline cannot be used in children less than eight years of age); ampicillin, bacitracin, iodoquinol, metronidazole and paramomycin are also effective.

C. Epidemic measures: Any grouping of several cases in an area or institution requires prompt epidemiological investigation, especially of environmental sanitation.

D. Disaster implications: None.

E. International measures: None.

BARTONELLA INFECTIONS ICD9 088.0 Bartonellosis; ICD10 A44.8

Other forms of bartonellosis; A44.9 Bartonellosis, unspecified
[CCDM19: W. Nicholson]
[CCDM18: D. Raoult]

A number of species and subspecies of the genus *Bartonella* have been described and found to be associated with human disease, including acute febrile illness, ocular manifestations, and endocarditis. These are as follows:

- *Bartonella clarridgeiae*
- *Bartonella elizabethae*
- *Bartonella grahamii*
- *Bartonella koehlerae*
- *Bartonella vinsonii* subsp. *arupensis*
- *Bartonella vinsonii* subsp. *berkhoffii*
- *Bartonella rochalimae* sp. nov.
- *"Bartonella washoensis"* (distinct recognized species, but name not formally introduced).

These agents are generally associated with pet dogs and cats, wild carnivores, or wild rodents (including mice, rats, and squirrels). The arthropod vectors for the pathogens among reservoir species are suspected to be fleas or ticks, although the specific arthropods associated with transmission to humans are yet to be determined. These pathogens are listed here for completeness, and their treatment and clinical management are similar to those for *Bartonella henselae*. It is of note that diagnostic methods targeting *B. henselae*, *B. quintana*, or *B. bacilliformis* may not perform well with all *Bartonella* species, so specific requests at reference centers may be needed to confirm these infections.

Please note that **Cat-scratch disease** and **Trench fever** are dealt with in separate chapters.

BARTONELLOSIS ICD-9 088.0; ICD-10 A44 [A44.0 Systemic bartonellosis; A44.1 verruga peruana, cutaneous and mucocutaneous bartonellosis]
(Oroya fever, Verruga peruana, Carrion disease)

1. Identification—A bacterial infection with two clinical forms: a febrile anemia (Oroya fever, ICD-10 A44.0) and a benign dermal eruption (verruga peruana, ICD-10 A44.1). Asymptomatic infection and a carrier state may both occur. Oroya fever is characterized by irregular fever, headache, myalgia, arthralgia, pallor, severe hemolytic anemia (macro- or normocytic, usually hypochromic), and generalized non-tender lymphadenopathy. Verruga peruana has a pre-eruptive stage characterized by shifting pains in muscles, bones and joints; the pain, often severe, lasts minutes to several days at any one site. The dermal eruption may be miliary with widely disseminated small hemangioma-like nodules, or nodular with fewer – but larger – deep-seated lesions, most prominent on the extensor surfaces of the limbs. Individual nodules, particularly near joints, may develop into tumor-like masses with an ulcerated surface. Atypical cases with milder manifestations (prolonged splenomegaly and mild anemia) may occur.

Verruga peruana may be preceded by Oroya fever or by an asymptomatic infection, with an interval of weeks to months between the stages. The case-fatality rate of untreated Oroya fever ranges from 10% to 90%; death is often associated with protozoal and bacterial superinfections, including salmonella septicemia. Verruga peruana has a prolonged course, but seldom results in death.

Laboratory diagnosis depends upon: Giemsa detection of the agent adherent to or within RBCs during the acute stage; immunohistochemical or silver staining of antigen or agent respectively in sections of skin lesions during the eruptive stage; or, most commonly, culture isolation of the agent during either stage. Serology and, increasingly, PCR may also be used to establish the diagnosis.

2. Infectious agent—*Bartonella bacilliformis*.

3. Occurrence— Historically limited to mountain valleys of southwestern Colombia, of Ecuador, and of Peru, at altitudes between 600 and 2 800 meters (2 000 to 9 200 ft), where the sand fly vector is present; no predilection for age, race, or gender. During the past two decades, Peruvian outbreaks have been documented at lower altitudes between highlands and jungle, while coastal lowlands in Ecuador have become endemic.

4. Reservoir—Humans with the agent present in the blood. In endemic areas, the asymptomatic carrier rate may reach 5%. There is no known animal reservoir.

5. Mode of transmission—Through the bite of sand flies of the genus *Lutzomyia* (Family *Phlebotomidae*). Species are not identified for all areas; *Lutzomyia verrucarum* is important in Peru. These insects feed only from dusk to dawn. Blood transfusion, particularly during the Oroya fever stage, may transmit infection.

6. Incubation period—Usually 16–22 days, occasionally 3–4 months.

7. Period of communicability—No direct person-to-person transmission other than via transfused blood. Humans are infectious for the sand fly for a long period; the agent may be present in blood for weeks before, and up to several years after, clinical illness. Duration of infectivity of the sand fly is unknown.

8. Susceptibility—Susceptibility is general; the disease is milder in children than in adults. Unapparent infections and carriers are known. Recovery from untreated Oroya fever almost invariably gives permanent immunity to this form; the verruga stage may recur.

9. Methods of control—

   A. Preventive measures:

     1) Control sand flies (see *Leishmaniasis*, cutaneous, 9A).

     2) Avoid known endemic areas after sundown; apply insect repellent (e.g. DEET) to exposed parts of the body; and use fine-mesh bednets, preferably insecticide-treated. For more information on insecticide-treated mosquito nets (ITNs), see *Malaria*, (9AI1). Further information on WHO-recommended nets can be found at:
       <http:// www.who.int/whopes/en/>

     3) Blood from residents of endemic areas should not be used for transfusions until it has tested negative.

   B. Control of patient, contacts and the immediate environment:

     1) Report to local health authority: In selected endemic areas; in most countries not a reportable disease, Class 3 (see *Reporting*).

     2) Isolation: Blood and body fluid precautions. The infected individual should be protected from sand fly bites (see 9A).

     3) Concurrent disinfection: Not applicable.

4) Quarantine: Not applicable.

5) Immunization of contacts: Not applicable.

6) Investigation of contacts and source of infection: Identification of sand flies, particularly in localities where the infected person was exposed after sundown during the preceding 3–8 weeks.

7) Specific treatment: Penicillin, streptomycin, chloramphenicol, and tetracyclines are all effective in reducing fever and bacteremia in the acute stages, though tetracycline and doxycycline cannot be used in children less than eight years of age. Recent treatment protocols use ciprofloxacin for 10–14 days. Ampicillin and chloramphenicol are also effective against the frequent secondary complication, salmonellosis. They do not prevent evolution to verruga peruana, which must be treated by streptomycin or rifampicin. Laboratory evidence suggests that doxycycline in association with gentamicin may be the preferred regimen for acute and eruptive stages, but clinical trials are needed.

C. *Epidemic measures:* Intensify case-finding and systematically spray houses with a residual insecticide.

D. *Disaster implications:* Only if refugee centers are established in an endemic locus.

E. *International measures:* None.

BLASTOMYCOSIS   ICD-9 116.0; ICD-10 B40
(North American blastomycosis, Gilchrist disease)
[CCDM19: M. Brandt]
[CCDM18: L. Severo]

1. **Identification**—A granulomatous systemic mycosis that primary affects the lungs, and is often subclinical. Hematogenous dissemination may occur, and in the majority of cases involves skin, bones and genitourinary tract. Pulmonary blastomycosis may be acute or chronic. Acute infection is rarely recognized, but presents with the sudden onset of fever, cough, and a pulmonary infiltrate on chest X-ray. The acute disease resolves spontaneously after 1–3 weeks of illness. Some patients exhibit extrapulmonary infection during or after the resolution of pneumonia. More commonly, there is an indolent onset that evolves into chronic disease.

Cough and chest ache may be mild or absent so that patients may present with infection already spread to other sites, particularly the skin, and less often to bone, prostate or epididymis. Cutaneous lesions begin as erythematous papules that become verrucous, crusted or ulcerated, and which spread slowly. Most commonly, cutaneous lesions are located on the face and distal extremities. Weight loss, weakness and low-grade fever are often present; pulmonary lesions may cavitate. Untreated disseminated or chronic pulmonary blastomycosis eventually progresses to death.

Clinical diagnosis is confirmed by culture, DNA probe, or by visualizing the fungus through direct microscopic examination of unstained smears of sputum and lesional material, which shows characteristic "broad-based" budding forms of the fungus, often dumbbell-shaped. Serological tests have some limitations, as sensitivity and specificity vary with the test employed. The immunodiffusion test is more sensitive and specific than the CF test, and antibodies against A antigen have been reported in 52% to 80% of patients with blastomycosis.

2. Infectious agent—*Blastomyces dermatitidis* (teleomorph *Ajellomyces dermatitidis*), a dimorphic fungus that grows as a yeast in tissue and in enriched culture media at 37°C (98.6°F), and as a mold at room temperature (25°C/77°F).

3. Occurrence—Uncommon. Endemic areas in North America include the southeastern and southern states, especially those bordering the Mississippi and Ohio river basins, the Midwestern states and Canadian provinces that border the great Lakes, and a small area in New York and Canada along the St. Lawrence River. Outside North America, well-documented autochthonous cases have been reported in Africa, and occasional cases have been reported in Central America, South America, India, and the Middle East. There is no commercially available skin test for blastomycosis.

Rare in children; males are more frequently affected than females. Disease is common in dogs, and has also been reported in cats, a horse, a captive African lion, and a sea lion.

4. Reservoir—Moist soil, particularly in wooded areas along waterways, and in undisturbed places, such as under porches or sheds.

5. Mode of transmission—Inhalation of conidia in spore-laden dust, typically of the mold or saprophytic growth forms.

6. Incubation period—Indefinite; probably weeks to months. For symptomatic infections, median is 45 days.

7. Period of communicability—No direct person-to-person or animal-to-person transmission.

8. Susceptibility—Unknown. Inapparent pulmonary infections are probable but of unknown frequency. Cell-mediated immunity plays a role in controlling lung infection. The rarity of the natural disease and of laboratory-acquired infections suggests humans are relatively resistant.

9. **Methods of control—**

A. *Preventive measures:* Unknown.

B. *Control of patient, contacts and the immediate environment:*

1) Report to local health authority: Official report not ordinarily justifiable, Class 5 (see *Reporting*).
2) Isolation: Not applicable.
3) Concurrent disinfection: Sputum, discharges and all contaminated articles. Terminal cleaning.
4) Quarantine: Not applicable.
5) Immunization of contacts: Not applicable.
6) Investigation of contacts and source of infection: Not beneficial unless clusters of disease occur.
7) Specific treatment: Itraconazole is the drug of choice; amphotericin B is indicated in severely ill patients or those with brain lesions, followed by itraconazole after the patient's condition has stabilized.

C. *Epidemic measures:* Not applicable, a sporadic disease.

D. *Disaster implications:* None.

E. *International measures:* None.

BOTULISM

INTESTINAL BOTULISM
FORMERLY INFANT
BOTULISM   ICD-9 005.1; ICD-10 A05.1
[CCDM19: E. Barzilay, J. Schlundt]
[CCDM18: H. Toyofuku]

1. **Identification**—There are four naturally occurring forms of botulism:
   i) Foodborne, caused by the ingestion of foods contaminated with a clostridial neurotoxin
   ii) Wound botulism, caused by contamination of a wound by *C. botulinum* spores that germinate and produce toxin
   iii) Infant botulism, caused by intestinal colonization of the infant gastrointestinal tract
   iv) Adult intestinal toxemia botulism.

In addition, two forms of botulism are recognized which do not occur naturally:

   i) Inhalational botulism, which can result from inhalation of aerosolized botulism neurotoxin

   ii) Iatrogenic botulism, which can result from accidental injection of the botulism neurotoxin into the systemic circulation instead of the intended therapeutic locus.

The site of toxin production differs for each form, but all share the stereotypical flaccid paralysis that results from the action of *botulinum* neurotoxin on the neuromuscular junction.

Foodborne botulism is a severe intoxication resulting from ingestion of preformed toxin present in contaminated food. The symptoms, which may begin as early as a few hours to as late as several days after ingestion of the contaminated food, follow a classic pattern of flaccid, symmetric, descending paralysis. Early symptoms are often marked fatigue, weakness and vertigo, usually followed by blurred vision, dry mouth, and difficulty in swallowing and speaking as the toxin affects the cranial nerves. Neurological symptoms always descend through the body: shoulders are first affected, then the upper arms, lower arms, thighs, calves, and so on. Paralysis of breathing muscles can cause loss of breathing and death, unless assistance with breathing (mechanical ventilation) is provided. There is no fever and no loss of consciousness. Gastrointestinal symptoms, including nausea, vomiting, constipation and abdominal swelling and— less commonly— diarrhea, may occur. Similar symptoms usually appear in individuals who shared the same food. Most cases recover, if diagnosed and treated promptly, including early administration of antitoxin and intensive respiratory care. The case-fatality rate in the USA is 5%–10%. Recovery may take months.

Infant botulism is the most common form of botulism. It affects children under 12 months of age, with the majority of cases occurring in infants aged between 6 weeks and 6 months. Ingested spores germinate in the infant intestine, where they produce bacteria that reproduce in the gut and release toxin. Colonization is believed to occur because normal bowel florae that could compete with *C. botulinum* have not been fully established. Clinical symptoms in infants start with constipation, and may include loss of appetite, weakness, poor suck, an altered cry, and a striking loss of head control.

Infant botulism ranges from a mild illness with gradual onset that never requires hospitalization, to sudden infant death; progression is more severe in infants younger than 2 months. Some studies suggest that infant botulism may cause an estimated 5% of cases of sudden infant death syndrome (SIDS). The case fatality rate of hospitalized cases is less than 1%; it is much higher without access to hospitals with pediatric intensive care units.

Wound botulism occurs when spores get into an open wound and reproduce in an anaerobic environment, and is normally associated with severe trauma. Symptoms are similar to the foodborne form, but may take up to 2 weeks to appear.

Adult intestinal toxemia botulism, similar to infant botulism, is relatively rare. It occurs in immunocompromised adults, those using antimicrobials, or those with some anatomical or functional bowel abnormality, when ingested spores germinate in their intestine and produce bacteria that reproduce in the gut and release toxin.

Diagnosis of foodborne botulism is made by demonstration of *botulinum* toxin in serum, stool, gastric aspirate and/or incriminated food, or through culture of *C. botulinum* from gastric aspirate or stool in a clinical case. Identification of organisms in suspected food is helpful but not diagnostic because *botulinum* spores are ubiquitous; the presence of toxin in a suspect food source is highly significant. The diagnosis may be accepted in a person with the clinical syndrome who had consumed a food item incriminated in a laboratory-confirmed case. Toxin in serum or positive wound culture confirms the diagnosis of wound botulism. Electromyographic diagnostics can corroborate the clinical diagnosis for all forms of botulism.

Identification of *C. botulinum* and/or toxin in patient's feces or in autopsy specimens helps establish the diagnosis of intestinal botulism. Toxin is rarely detected in the sera of patients.

2. Infectious agent—Human botulism is a serious but relatively rare neuroparalytic progressive disorder caused by potent toxins produced by *Clostridium botulinum*. Of the 7 recognized subtypes of clostridial neurotoxins (*botulinum* types A, B, C, D, E, and, rarely, F and G), only types A, B, E, and rarely type F cause human illness. The botulism neurotoxin (BoNT) is thought to be one of the most lethal substances known; the medial lethal dose (LD_{50}) is 1 nanogram of toxin per kilogram of body mass.

Most human outbreaks are due to types A, B, E and rarely F; type G has been isolated from soil and autopsy specimens, but a causal role in botulism is not established. Type E outbreaks are usually related to *Clostridium botulinum* in fish, seafood and meat from marine mammals. Proteolytic (A, some B and F) and nonproteolytic (E, some B and F) groups differ in water activity, temperature, pH and salt requirements for growth. Currently, the mouse bioassay is the standard method for quantification of botulism toxin.

Toxin is produced in improperly processed, canned, low-salt, low-acid or alkaline foods, and in pasteurized and lightly cured foods held without refrigeration, especially in airtight packaging. More recently, some outbreaks have been linked to minimally heated, chilled food that has been kept at too high a temperature (temperature abuse). Toxin is destroyed by boiling (e.g. 85°C/185°F for 5 minutes or longer); inactivation of spores requires much higher temperatures (120°C/248°F for 10 minutes or longer). Type E toxin can be produced slowly at temperatures as low as 3°C (37.4°F), lower than that of ordinary refrigeration.

3. Occurrence—Worldwide. Sporadic cases, family and general outbreaks occur where food is prepared or preserved by methods that do not destroy spores and which permit toxin formation. Cases rarely result from commercially processed products, although in 2007 mistakes in the retort canning process led to two outbreaks of foodborne botulism in commercially canned products in the US; outbreaks have also occurred from contamination via cans damaged after processing. Cases of infant botulism have been reported from the Americas, Asia, Australia and Europe. Actual incidence and distribution of infant botulism are likely to be underreported, because symptoms may be mild, and physician awareness and diagnostic testing remain limited. The vast majority of recent global cases were reported by the USA, with close to half of those reported in California. Internationally, a number of cases have been detected in Argentina, Australia, Japan, Canada and in Europe (mostly Italy and the United Kingdom), with scattered further reports from Chile, China, Egypt, the Islamic Republic of Iran, Israel, and Yemen.

4. Reservoir—Spores, ubiquitous in soil worldwide. Spores are frequently recovered from agricultural products, including honey, and are also found in marine sediments and in the intestinal tract of animals, including fish.

5. Mode of transmission—Foodborne botulism occurs when *C. botulinum* is allowed to grow and produce toxin in food that is then eaten without sufficient heating or post-production cooking to inactivate the toxin. Growth of this anaerobic bacteria and formation of toxin tend to occur in products with low acidity and oxygen content, and in the right combination of storage temperature and preservative parameters (low salt and sugar content). These conditions are most often present in lightly preserved foods (such as fermented, salted or smoked fish and meat products) and in inadequately processed, home-canned or home-bottled, low-acid, low-salt and low-sugar foods. The food implicated reflect local eating habits and food-preservation procedures. Occasionally, commercially prepared foods are involved.

Poisonings are often due to home-canned vegetables and fruits; meat is less frequently implicated. Several outbreaks have occurred following consumption of uneviscerated fish, baked potatoes, improperly handled commercial potpies, sautéed onions, minced garlic in oil, and so on. Some recent outbreaks originated in restaurants. Garden foods such as tomatoes, formerly considered too acidic to support growth of *C. botulinum*, may no longer be considered low-hazard foods for home canning.

In the arctic, outbreaks have been associated with seal meat, fermented whale blubber, smoked salmon, fermented salmon eggs, and other traditional foods which are fermented and consumed without cooking; these outbreaks are almost exclusively caused by toxin type E. In Europe, most cases are due to sausages and smoked or preserved meats; in Japan, to seafood. The biggest outbreak to date occurred in Thailand on 14 March

2006 and affected 209 people, of whom 42 developed respiratory failure, with no deaths. The outbreak was caused by home-prepared bamboo shoots. Treatment of severe cases relied on imported anti-toxin from four countries.

Inhalation botulism, following inhalation of the toxin (aerosol), has only been reported in laboratory workers. In these cases, neurological symptoms were the same as in foodborne botulism, but the incubation period was longer. All affected persons recovered within two weeks, following antitoxin treatment. Studies suggest that following inhalational botulism exposure, there would be an irritant upper airway prodrome with the initial contact, followed by variable onset of different degrees of paralysis in exposed victims.

Waterborne botulism could theoretically also result from the ingestion of the preformed toxin, which is stable in fluids. Although botulinum toxin has been shown to retain much of its activity for up to 70 days in untreated water and beverages, the risk of inadvertent waterborne botulism is considered low, since water treatment processes inactivate the toxin.

Wound botulism often results from contamination of wounds by soil or gravel or from improperly treated open fractures. Since the 1990s, there has been an alarming and continuing emergence of wound botulism among chronic drug abusers in some parts of Europe and North America, primarily in dermal abscesses from subcutaneous or intramuscular injection (skin or muscle "popping") of pure "black-tar" heroin, but also from sinusitis in cocaine "sniffers." Use of adulterants or acidulants (such as citric acid), often used to solubilize heroin for injection, increase the risk of wound botulism by causing more extensive tissue damage upon injection.

Intestinal botulism (infant or adult intestinal toxemia) arises from ingestion of *C. botulinum* spores that germinate in the colon, rather than through ingestion of preformed toxin. Possible sources of spores for infants include foods and dust. In several studies, infant botulism been associated with ingestion of honey contaminated with botulism spores, and mothers are warned not to feed raw honey to their infants before the age of one year.

Adult intestinal toxemia botulism usually occurs in adults who have altered intestinal flora because of antimicrobial use, or because of anatomical or functional bowel abnormalities.

6. Incubation period—Neurological symptoms of foodborne botulism usually appear within 12–36 hours, but sometimes occur several days after eating contaminated food. The shorter the incubation period, the more severe the disease and the higher the case-fatality rate. The incubation period of intestinal botulism in infants is unknown, since the precise time of ingestion often cannot be determined. In the case of inhalational botulism, the incubation period is thought to be longer, ranging from 12 to 80 hours after exposure.

7. **Period of communicability**—Despite excretion of *C. botulinum* toxin and organisms at high levels (about 10^6 organisms/gram) in the feces of intestinal botulism patients for weeks to months after onset of illness, no instance of secondary person-to-person transmission has ever been documented. Foodborne botulism patients typically excrete the toxin for shorter periods.

8. **Susceptibility**—Susceptibility is general. Almost all patients hospitalized with infant botulism are between 2 weeks and 1 year old; 95% are aged less than 6 months; the median age at onset is 7.6 weeks for formula-fed infants and 13.7 weeks for breast-fed infants. Adults with special bowel problems leading to unusual GI flora (or with a flora unintentionally altered by antibiotic treatment for other purposes) may be susceptible to intestinal botulism.

9. **Methods of control**—

   A. *Preventive measures:* Good practices in food preparation (particularly preservation) and hygiene; inactivation of bacterial spores in heat-sterilized or canned products and inhibition of growth in all other products. Commercial heat pasteurization (e.g. in vacuum-packed pasteurized and hot smoked products) may not suffice to kill all spores, and the safety of these products must be predicated on preventing growth and toxin production. Refrigeration combined with control of salt content, sugar content, and/or acidity will prevent the growth or formation of toxin. If exposure to the toxin via an aerosol is suspected, the patient's clothing must be removed and stored in plastic bags until it can be washed with soap and water. The patient must shower thoroughly.

   Food and water samples associated with suspect cases must be obtained immediately, stored in sealed containers and sent to reference laboratories.

   B. *Control of patient, contacts and the immediate environment:*

   1) Report to local health authority: Case report of suspected and confirmed cases obligatory in most countries, Class 2 (see *Reporting*); immediate telephone report indicated.
   2) Isolation: Not required; handwashing indicated after handling soiled material, including diapers.
   3) Concurrent disinfection: Detoxify implicated food(s) by boiling before discarding, or break the containers and bury them deeply in soil to prevent ingestion by animals. Sterilize contaminated utensils by boiling or by chlorine disinfection, to inactivate any remaining toxin. Usual sanitary disposal of feces from infant cases. Terminal cleaning.
   4) Quarantine: Not applicable.

5) Management of contacts: None for simple direct contacts; naturally occurring botulism is not transmissible among humans. Those known to have eaten incriminated food should be kept under close medical observation. The decision to provide presumptive treatment with polyvalent (equine type AB or ABE) antitoxin to asymptomatic exposed individuals should be weighed carefully, balancing the potential protection of antitoxin administered early (within 1–2 days after ingestion) against the risk of adverse reactions and sensitization to horse serum.

6) Investigation of contacts and source of toxin: Study recent food history of those who are ill, and recover all suspected foods for appropriate testing and disposal. Search for other cases of botulism to rule out foodborne botulism.

7) Specific treatment: Intravenous administration of 1 vial of polyvalent (AB or ABE) *botulinum* antitoxin as soon as possible (obtained from national or international sources) is part of routine treatment. In the USA, consultation and antitoxin is available from the Centers for Disease Control and Prevention, by calling +1-770-488-7100. Serum (10 mL), vomitus or gastric secretions, and stool (25 gr) should be collected to identify the specific toxin before antitoxin is administered, but antitoxin should not be withheld pending test results. Procedures for collecting, storing and shipping samples from patients with suspected botulism can be found at the American Society for Microbiology website: http://www.asm.org/Policy/index.asp?bid=6342. It should be noted that inadequate stocking of antitoxin is a worldwide problem, especially in developing countries. The possibility of maintaining internationally-available stockpiles is presently under investigation. Immediate access to an intensive care unit is essential, so that respiratory failure—the usual cause of death —can be anticipated and managed promptly. For wound botulism, in addition to antitoxin the wound should be debrided and/or drainage should be established, with appropriate antibiotics (e.g. penicillin).

In infant botulism, meticulous supportive care is essential. Human-derived botulism immune globulin (BabyBIG®) is used for the treatment of infant botulism caused by *C. botulinum* type A or type B. Clinical consultations and BabyBIG®, made and distributed by the California Department of Public Health, are available on a 24-hour basis by calling the Infant Botulism Treatment and Prevention Program (1-510-231-7600, http://www.infantbotulism.org). Equine-derived antitoxin is not used for infant botulism. Such treatment is reported to result in significant reduction in hospital stay, and in the length of time for which mechanical ventilation and tube feeding are necessary. Antibiotics do not improve the course of the disease, and aminoglycoside antibiotics in particular may worsen it, by causing a synergistic neuromuscular blockade. Antibiotics should be used only to treat secondary infections. Assisted respiration may be required.

There is a vaccine against botulism, but its effectiveness and side-effects have not been fully evaluated.

C. **Epidemic measures:** Suspicion of a single case of botulism should immediately raise the question of a group outbreak involving a family or others who have shared food. Home-preserved foods are the prime suspect until ruled out, although restaurant foods or widely-distributed commercially-preserved foods are occasionally identified as the source of intoxication, and pose a greater public health threat.

Recent outbreaks have implicated unusual food items, and even unlikely foods should be considered. Any food implicated by epidemiological or laboratory findings requires immediate recall. An immediate search is necessary for people sharing the suspect food, and for any remaining food from the same source, which may be similarly contaminated; if found, it should be submitted for laboratory examination. Sera, gastric aspirates and stool from patients and (when indicated) others exposed but not ill should be collected and forwarded immediately to a reference laboratory, before administration of antitoxin.

D. **Disaster implications:** None, with the exception of large-scale deliberate use (see F).

E. **International measures:** Commercial products may have been distributed widely; international efforts may be required to recover and test implicated foods. International common source outbreaks have occurred.

F. **Measures in case of deliberate use:** There have been attempts to use *botulinum* toxin as a bioweapon. Although the greatest threat may be aerosol use, the more common threat may be intentional foodborne or waterborne contamination. Two or more seemingly unrelated cases in the same time frame raise the possibility of deliberate use of botulism toxin. All such cases must be reported immediately so that appropriate investigations can be initiated without delay. Because outbreaks of botulism are often associated with home-canned food, outbreaks associated with commercial food products should be investigated with the possibility of intentional contamination in mind.

Sensible precautions, coupled with strong surveillance and response capacity, constitute the most efficient and effective way of countering all such potential assaults, including food terrorism. The WHO document entitled *Terrorist threats to food: guidance for establishing and strengthening prevention and response systems* (<http://whqlibdoc.who.int/publications/2002/9241545844.pdf>) provides guidance on integrating consideration of deliberate food sabotage into existing programs for controlling the production of safe food. It also provides guidance on strengthening communicable disease control systems to ensure that surveillance, preparedness and response systems are sufficiently sensitive. Such systems and programs will increase the capacity to reduce the burden of foodborne illness and to address the threat of food terrorism.

BRUCELLOSIS   ICD-9 023; ICD-10 A23
Undulant fever, Malta fever, Mediterranean fever)
[CCDM19: K. Glynn]
[CCDM18: D. Dragon]

1. Identification—A systemic bacterial disease of acute or insidious onset, with continued, intermittent or irregular fever of variable duration; headache; weakness; profuse sweating; chills; arthralgia; depression; weight loss; and generalized aching. Localized suppurative infections of organs, including liver and spleen, may occur, as well as chronic localized infections; sub-clinical disease has been reported. The disease may last days, months or occasionally a year or more, if not adequately treated.

Osteoarticular complications occur in 20%–60% of cases; sacroiliitis is the most frequent joint manifestation. Genitourinary involvement is seen in 2%–20% of cases, with orchitis and epididymitis as common manifestations. Recovery is usual but disability is often pronounced. Neurobrucellosis is a less common but more severe manifestation, which occurs in 3–7% of cases. The case-fatality rate of untreated brucellosis is 2% or less, and usually results from endocarditis caused by *B. melitensis* infection. Part or all of the original syndrome may reappear as relapses. A neurotic symptom complex is sometimes misdiagnosed as chronic brucellosis.

Laboratory diagnosis is through appropriate isolation of the infectious agent from blood, bone marrow or other tissues, or discharges. Current serological tests allow precise diagnosis in over 95% of cases, but it is necessary to combine a test (Rose Bengal and seroagglutination) detecting agglutinating antibodies (IgM, IgG and IgA) with others detecting non-agglutinating antibodies (Coombs–IgG or ELISA-IgG) developing in later stages. These methods do not apply for *B. canis*, where diagnosis requires tests detecting antibodies to rough-lipopolysaccharide antigens.

2. Infectious agents—*Brucella abortus*, biovars 1-6 and 9; *B. melitensis*, biovars 1-3; *B. suis*, biovars 1-5; and *B. canis*; *B. ceti* and *B. pinnepedialis* (nov. sp.).

3. Occurrence—Worldwide, especially in Mediterranean countries (Europe and Africa), the Middle East, Africa, central Asia, central and South America, India, and Mexico. Sources of infection and responsible organism vary according to geographic area. Cases are increasingly documented in non-endemic regions subsequent to international travel. Brucellosis is predominantly an occupational disease of those working with infected animals or their tissues, especially farm workers, veterinarians and abattoir workers; hence it is more frequent among males. Another major risk factor for cases and outbreaks is consumption of raw milk and milk products (especially unpasteurized soft cheese) from infected cows, sheep and goats. Isolated cases of infection with *B. canis* occur in animal handlers from contact with dogs, and with *B. suis* in hunters from contact with feral swine. The disease is often unrecognized and unreported. Rare cases of infection with newly-described marine-associated *Brucella* spp. have been reported. Brucellosis remains among the most common laboratory-acquired bacterial infections.

4. Reservoir—Cattle, swine, goats and sheep. Infection may occur in camels, bison, elk, equids, caribou and some species of deer. *B. canis* is an occasional problem in laboratory dog colonies and kennels; a small percentage of pet dogs and a higher proportion of stray dogs have positive *B. canis* antibody titers. Coyotes have been found to be infected. Marine mammals can be infected with *B. ceti* (whales, porpoises, dolphins) and *B. pinnepedialis* (seals, sea lions, walruses).

5. Mode of transmission—Contact through breaks in the skin with animal tissues, blood, urine, vaginal discharges, aborted fetuses and especially placentas; ingestion of raw milk and dairy products (unpasteurized cheese) from infected animals. Airborne infection occurs in pens and stables for animals, and for humans in laboratories and abattoirs. A small number of cases have resulted from accidental self-inoculation of strain 19 Brucella animal vaccine; the same risk is present when Rev-1 vaccine is handled. Rare infections have resulted from accidental inoculation with the attenuated RB51 *Brucella* cattle vaccine.

6. Incubation period—Variable and difficult to ascertain; usually 5-60 days. 1-2 months is commonplace; occasionally several months.

7. Period of communicability—Rare person-to-person communicability. Risk may exist for medical personnel in endemic regions participating in activities characterized by gross exposure to contaminated fomites or tissues or massive bleeding, such as certain obstetric procedures.

8. Susceptibility—Severity and duration of clinical illness vary. Duration of acquired immunity uncertain.

9. Methods of control—The control of human brucellosis rests on the elimination of the disease among domestic animals.

A. Preventive measures:

1) Educate the public (especially tourists) regarding the risks associated with drinking untreated milk or eating products made from unpasteurized or otherwise untreated milk.

2) Educate farmers and workers in slaughterhouses, meat processing plants and butcher shops about the nature of the disease and the risk in handling carcasses and products from potentially infected animals—particularly products of parturition—together with proper operation of abattoirs to reduce exposure. Give emphasis to the importance of appropriate ventilation.

3) Educate hunters to use protective outfits (gloves, clothing) when handling feral swine or other potentially infected wildlife such as elk; to practice good hygiene such as hand washing when possible; to avoid eating meat from animals that appear sick; and to bury animal remains.

4) Search for infection among livestock by serological testing and by ELISA or testing of cows' milk ("ring test"); eliminate infected animals (segregation and/or slaughtering). Infection among swine usually requires slaughter of the herd. In high-prevalence areas, immunize young goats and sheep with live attenuated Rev-1 strain of *B. melitensis*, and immunize calves and sometimes adult animals with strain 19, *B. abortus*. Since 1996, strain RB51 of *B. abortus* has largely replaced strain 19 for immunization of cattle against *B. abortus*. RB51 vaccine was designed to be less virulent for humans than strain 19 when accidentally injected.

5) Rev 1 is resistant to streptomycin, and RB51 to rifampicin. This must be taken into account when treating human cases of animal vaccine infections, which are otherwise to be treated like other human cases of brucellosis.

6) Pasteurize milk and dairy products from cows, sheep and goats. Boiling milk is effective when pasteurization is impossible. Do not eat meat from animals that appear ill.

7) Exercise care in handling and disposal of placenta, discharges and fetuses. Disinfect contaminated areas.

B. Control of patient, contacts and the immediate environment:

1) Report to local health authority: Case report obligatory in most countries, Class 2 (see *Reporting*).

2) Isolation: Draining and secretion precautions if there are draining lesions; otherwise none.

3) Concurrent disinfection: Of purulent discharges.

4) Quarantine: Not applicable.
5) Immunization of contacts: Not applicable.
6) Investigation of contacts and source of infection: Trace infection to the common or individual source, usually infected domestic goats, swine or cattle, or raw milk or dairy products from cows and goats. Test suspected animals, and remove reactors.
7) Specific treatment: The treatment of choice is a combination of doxycycline (200 mg daily) and rifampicin (600-900 mg daily) or streptomycin (1 gram daily) for at least 6 weeks, though doxycyline cannot be used in children less than eight years of age. The streptomycin-containing regimen is generally associated with a lower rate of relapse, although may be less effective in treating neurobrucellosis, due to low penetration into cerebrospinal fluid and potential for neurotoxicity. Doxycycline (as above) in combination with gentamicin (5 mg/kg daily) for 7 days may be an acceptable alternative. In severely ill toxic patients, corticosteroids may be helpful. Trimethoprim-sufamethoxazole-containing regimens can be effective, but relapses occur in up to 30% of cases. Relapses also occur in about 5-15% of patients with uncomplicated infections treated with doxycycline and rifampicin, and are due to sequestered rather than resistant organisms; patients should be treated again with the original regimen. Monotherapy should be avoided, as relapse rates can be as high as 50%. Arthritis may occur in recurrent cases.

C. **Epidemic measures:** Search for common vehicle of infection, usually raw milk or milk products—especially cheese—from an infected herd. Recall incriminated products; stop production and distribution unless pasteurization is instituted.

D. **Disaster implications:** None.

E. **International measures:** Control of domestic animals and animal products in international trade and transport. WHO Collaborating Centres provide support as required. More information can be found at:

http://www.who.int/collaboratingcentres/database/en/

F. **Measures in the case of deliberate use:** Their potential to infect humans and animals through aerosol exposure, combined with a low infectious dose of 10-100 organisms, is such that *Brucella* species may be used as potent biological weapons.

For more information on the deliberate use of infectious agents to cause harm, see the section on *Deliberate use*.

BURULI ULCER ICD-9 031.1; ICD-10 A31.1
[CCDM19: K. Glynn]
[CCDM18: K. Asiedu]

1. **Identification**—A bacterial infection caused by a mycobacterium. Classically presents as a chronic, essentially painless, skin ulcer, with undermined edges and a necrotic white or yellow base ("cotton wool" appearance). Most lesions are located on the extremities and occur among children living near wetlands in rural tropical environments. Buruli ulcer often starts as a painless nodule or a papule, which eventually ulcerates; other presentations, such as plaques and indurated edematous lesions, represent a rapidly disseminated form that does not pass through a nodular stage. Bones and joints may be affected by direct spread from an overlying cutaneous lesion of Buruli ulcer or through the bloodstream; osteomyelitis due to *Mycobacterium ulcerans* is being reported with increasing frequency. Long-neglected or poorly-managed patients usually present with scars that are sometimes hypertrophic or keloid, with partially healed areas or disabling contractures, especially for lesions that cross joints. Marjolin ulcers (squamous cell carcinoma) may develop in unstable or chronic nonpigmented scars.

If diagnosed by an experienced clinician, and in endemic areas, diagnosis can usually be made on clinical grounds. Smears and biopsy specimens can be sent to the laboratory for confirmation by the Ziehl-Neelsen stain for acid-fast bacilli, culture, PCR, and histopathology.

Histopathologically, active lesions have contiguous coagulation necrosis of subcutaneous fat and acid-fast bacilli present. The differential diagnosis of *M. ulcerans* disease includes the following, by dermatologic manifestation:

1) Minor infections: insect bites and a variety of dermatological conditions
2) Nodules: cysts; lipomas, boils, onchocercomas, lymphadenitis, mycoses
3) Plaques: leprosy, cellulites, mycoses, psoriasis
5) Edematous forms: cellulites, elephantiasis, actinomycosis
6) Ulcers: tropical phagedenic ulcer, leishmaniasis, neurogenic ulcer, yaws, squamous cell carcinoma, pyoderma gangrenosum, noma.

2. **Infectious agent**—The infectious agent, *M. ulcerans*, is an acid-fast bacillus, a slow-growing environmental mycobacterium. It can be identified through culture (in 6 weeks) and genetic sequence analysis using PCR. *M. ulcerans* secretes mycolactone, a virulence factor that destroys tissues and locally suppresses immune activity. Molecular analysis defines 4 strains of *M. ulcerans*: African, American, Asian, and Australian. Mycolactone production varies with the different groups, and is maximal in the African strain.

3. **Occurrence**—*M. ulcerans* infection has been reported in over 30 countries worldwide, mostly tropical. The global burden of the disease is yet to be determined. Africa is the continent most affected. Numbers of reported cases have been increasing over the last 25 years, most strikingly in western Africa, where M. *ulcerans* disease is second only to tuberculosis in terms of mycobacterial disease prevalence (in some endemic districts and communities, it is the most prevalent mycobacterial disease).

4. **Reservoir**—Evidence points to the fauna, flora and other ecological aspects of the wetlands. Insects, snails and fish are naturally infected and may serve as natural hosts for *M. ulcerans*. In Australia, it has been described not only in humans but also in native animals including the koala (*Phascolarctos cinereus*), the brushtail and ringtail possums (family Phalangeridae), and the long-footed potoroo (*Potorous longipes*). There has been a case reported in a domesticated alpaca (*Lama pacos*); all of these except for those in the potoroo occurred in the focal areas where human cases occurred.

5. **Mode of transmission**—In most studies a significant number of patients had antecedent trauma at the site of the lesion. Circumstances suggest that trauma introduces the causal agent into the skin. Recent evidence suggests that insects may be natural reservoirs and their bite may transmit the disease to humans. Snails belonging to the families of *Ampullariidae* and *Planorbidae* could be contaminated after feeding on aquatic plants covered by a biofilm of *M. ulcerans*. Aerosols arising from stagnant waters may disseminate *M. ulcerans*.

Environmental changes that promote flooding, such as deforestation, dam construction and irrigation systems, are often associated with outbreaks of Buruli ulcer. Population increases in rural wetlands place populations at risk during manual farming activities. Lack of protected water supplies contributes to dependence on pond water for domestic use, and potential exposure.

6. **Incubation period**—Incubation period is about 2–3 months; anecdotal observations suggest that *M. ulcerans* infections may have long periods of latency. Similarly to tuberculosis, it is believed that only a small proportion of infected people develop disease.

7. **Period of communicability**—Interhuman transmission of Buruli ulcer in the field is exceptional; rare cases have developed in caretakers of Buruli ulcer patients.

8. **Susceptibility**—Probably all persons can be infected. Most are believed to abort the disease in a preclinical stage and others show only small lesions that are rapidly self-healing. Residence or travel to the permanent wetlands of endemic areas, regular contact with the contaminated aquatic environment, and local trauma to the skin are known risk factors. Factors that probably determine the type of disease are dose of

agent, depth of inoculation of the agent, and host immunological response. BCG neonatal vaccination, for example, appears to protect against *M. ulcerans* osteomyelitis in patients with skin lesions. HIV infection is not a risk factor, but may exacerbate the clinical course of the disease.

9. **Methods of control—**

A. *Preventive measures:*

1) Avoidance of insect bites, including wearing clothing that covers the extremities, and use of bednets.
2) Provision of a protected water supply.
3) Health education on the disease for populations at risk.
4) BCG neonatal vaccination may provide short-term prophylaxis.
5) Prompt cleansing of abrasions or wounds antiseptically.
6) Early detection and early treatment of suspicious skin lesions helps avoid complications and deformities.

B. *Control of patients, contacts and immediate environment:*

1) Report to local health authority: Although neither a notifiable nor a contagious disease, it is recommended that cases be reported to local health authorities so that its distribution can be clearly defined.
2) Isolation: Not applicable.
3) Concurrent disinfection: Not applicable.
4) Quarantine: Not applicable.
5) Immunization of contacts: Not applicable.
6) Investigation of contacts and source of infection: Investigation of possible places where the patient has been over the last 3 months or longer.
7) Specific treatment: Surgical excision and primary suturing or skin graft, depending on the severity of the disease. Antimicrobial therapy with rifampicin and an aminoglycoside (streptomycin or amikacin) for at least 4 weeks and not more than 12 weeks. Antimicrobial therapy should be started 1 or 2 days before the initial surgery to minimize *M. ulcerans* bacteremia. Clinical improvements will dictate continuation of antimicrobial therapy or further surgical intervention.

C. *Epidemic measures.* Epidemics are very uncommon and call for education, cleanliness, early reporting, and the provision of wound care materials.

D. *Disaster implications:* During wars and other conflicts, diagnosis and treatment of patients is neglected because the health care infrastructure needed to treat patients is disrupted or destroyed. This may lead to severe superinfection of lesions.

E. International measures: Endemic countries should coordinate efforts across borders. Health workers in non-endemic areas must be aware of the disease and its management because of international travel. Further information is available at http://www.who.int/gtb-buruli or from WHO Collaborating Centres, which provide support as required. More information on WHO Collaborating Centres can be found at: <http://www.who.int/collaboratingcentres/database/en/>

CAMPYLOBACTER ENTERITIS   ICD-9 008.4; ICD-10 A04.5

(Vibrionic enteritis)
[CCDM19: M. Patrick, J. Schlundt]
[CCDM18: H. P. Braam]

1. Identification—An acute zoonotic bacterial enteric disease of variable severity characterized by diarrhea (frequently with bloody stools), abdominal pain, malaise, fever, nausea and/or vomiting. In 50% of patients, diarrhea is preceded by a febrile period. Symptoms usually occur 2–5 days after exposure and may persist for one to two weeks. Prolonged illness and/or relapses may occur in adults. Gross or occult blood with mucus and WBCs is often present in liquid stools. Less common forms include a typhoid-like syndrome, febrile convulsions, or a meningeal syndrome; rarely, post-infectious complications include reactive arthritis (approx. 1% of cases), urticaria, erythema nodosum, febrile convulsions or Guillain-Barré syndrome (approx. 0.1% of cases). Cases may mimic acute appendicitis or inflammatory bowel disease. Many infections are asymptomatic, and occasionally self-limited. The number of campylobacteriosis cases is comparable to or higher than cases of non-typhoid salmonellosis in most countries. Patients with fluoroquinolone-resistant Campylobacter may have a 6-fold increased risk of invasive disease or death. While most cases will recover, there are still a significant number of deaths caused by *Campylobacter*— comparable in the USA to the number of deaths caused by enterohemorrhagic *E. coli* (approx. 100 per year in the US).

Diagnosis is based on isolation of the organisms from stools using selective media, reduced oxygen tension, and incubation at 43°C (109.4°F). Bacteremia is detected in <1% of patients. Visualization of motile and curved, spiral or S-shaped rods similar to those of *Vibrio cholerae* by stool phase contrast or darkfield microscopy can provide rapid presumptive evidence for *Campylobacter* enteritis. Antibody-based and PCR detection methods have also been developed for early diagnosis.

2. Infectious agents—*Campylobacter jejuni* and, less commonly, *C. coli* are the usual causes of *Campylobacter* diarrhea in humans. There is substantial phenotypic and genotypic diversity within these two species and at least 20 biotypes and serotypes occur; their identification may be helpful for epidemiological purposes. Other *Campylobacter* organisms, including *C. lari, C. fetus* subsp. *fetus* and *C. upsaliensis*, have been associated with diarrhea in normal hosts; standard culture methods may not detect all strains of *C. fetus* and *C. upsaliensis*.

3. Occurrence—*Campylobacter* is an important cause of diarrheal illness in all age groups, causing 5%–14% of diarrhea worldwide. In the United States, campylobacteriosis is estimated to affect 2.4 million persons every year, or 0.8% of the population. It is an important cause of travelers' diarrhea; 12% of cases in the United States can be attributed to international travel. In industrialized countries, children under five and young adults and males have the highest incidence of illness. In developing countries, illness is confined largely to children under two, especially infants. Persons who are immunocompromised show an increased risk for infection and recurrences, more severe symptoms, and a greater likelihood of being chronic carriers. Decreased stomach acidity has been reported as a risk for infection. Since campylobacter is commonly isolated with other intestinal pathogens, case incidence might be significantly underestimated. Common-source outbreaks are rare but have occurred, most often associated with foods, especially undercooked poultry, unpasteurized milk and non-chlorinated water. The largest numbers of sporadic cases in temperate areas occur in the warmer months.

4. Reservoir—Animals, most frequently poultry and cattle. Puppies, kittens, other pets, swine, sheep, rodents and birds may also be sources of human infection. In many countries, raw poultry meat is commonly contaminated with *C. jejuni*.

5. Mode of transmission—Ingestion of the organisms in under-cooked meat—particularly poultry—other contaminated food and water, or raw milk; and from contact with infected pets (especially puppies and kittens), farm animals or infected infants. Water is an important vehicle, and highly resistant 'viable but not culturable' forms of Campylobacter can be found in water sources contaminated with animal feces. In general, Campylobacter may be more robust to physical conditions than other foodborne pathogens, and might therefore present a more difficult food safety problem. Contamination of milk usually occurs from intestinal carrier cattle; people and food can be infected through ingestion of raw or undercooked poultry, or from common cutting boards contaminated when raw poultry is cut on them. The infective dose is often low, typically fewer than 500 organisms. Person-to-person transmission with *C. jejuni* appears uncommon. Newer risk assessment modeling has enabled the preparation of dose-response curves, reflecting the fact that the infection process should be viewed as a probability of infection related to the dose ingested. These models seem to suggest a 5–50% probability for infection with a dose of 100 organisms, and a 50–80% probability for infection at 10 000 organisms.

6. Incubation period—Usually 2 to 5 days, with a range of 1–10 days, depending on dose ingested.

7. Period of communicability—Throughout the course of infection; usually several days to several weeks. Individuals not treated with antibiotics may excrete organisms for 2–7 weeks. The temporary carrier state is probably of little epidemiological importance, except for infants and others who are incontinent of stool. Chronic infection of poultry and other animals constitutes the primary source of infection.

8. Susceptibility—Immune mechanisms are not well understood, but lasting immunity to serologically related strains follows infection. In developing countries, most people develop immunity in the first 2 years of life.

9. Methods of control—

    A. Preventive measures:

        1) Control and prevention measures at all stages of the food chain, from agricultural production on the farm to processing, manufacturing and preparation of foods in both commercial establishments and the domestic environment.

        2) Pasteurize all milk and chlorinate or boil water supplies. Thoroughly cook all animal foodstuffs, especially poultry, which should meet a minimum internal temperature of 165° F. Avoid using common cutting boards for raw and cooked products. Avoid recontamination from uncooked foods within the kitchen after cooking is completed.

        3) Reduce incidence of *Campylobacter* on farms through specific interventions. Institute comprehensive control programs and hygienic measures to prevent spread of organisms in poultry and animal farms (e.g. changes of boots and clothes, and thorough cleaning and disinfection). Vaccines as well as competitive exclusion (intestinal) are being investigated as control measures. Good slaughtering and handling practices will reduce contamination of carcasses and meat products. Further reduction of contamination can be achieved through freezing, chemical carcass decontamination, or irradiation.

        4) Recognize, prevent and control *Campylobacter* infections among domestic animals and pets. Puppies and kittens with diarrhea are possible sources of infection; erythromycin may be used to treat their infections, reducing risk of transmission to children. Keep pets out of kitchens. Stress handwashing after animal contact.

5) Minimize contact with poultry and their feces. Stress handwashing after animal contact when this cannot be avoided.

B. *Control of patient, contacts and the immediate environment:*

1) Report to local health authority: Obligatory case report in several countries, Class 2 (see *Reporting*).

2) Isolation: Enteric precautions for hospitalized patients. Exclude symptomatic individuals from food handling or care of people in hospitals, custodial institutions and day care centers; exclude asymptomatic convalescent stool-positive individuals only for those with questionable handwashing habits. Stress proper handwashing.

3) Concurrent disinfection: Cleaning of areas and articles soiled with stools. In communities with an adequate sewage disposal system, feces can be discharged directly into sewers without preliminary disinfection. Terminal cleaning required.

4) Quarantine: Not applicable.

5) Immunization of contacts: Not applicable.

6) Investigation of contacts and source of infection: Useful only to detect outbreaks; investigate outbreaks to identify implicated food, water or raw milk to which others may have been exposed. Note that most cases of campylobacteriosis are sporadic.

7) Specific treatment: None generally indicated except rehydration and electrolyte replacement (see *Cholera*, 9B7). *C. jejuni* or *C. coli* organisms are susceptible in vitro to many antimicrobial agents, including erythromycin, tetracyclines and quinolones, but these are of value only to eliminate the carrier state, or in invasive cases only early in the illness and when the identity of the infecting organism is known. Worldwide incidence of fluoroquinolone resistance has increased markedly in the last twenty years, which may be related to veterinary use of fluoroquinolones; although methods for susceptibility testing vary, resistance rates greater than 30% have been reported in Europe, and 50% in the Middle East. Health professionals should have a higher degree of suspicion of resistance in travelers returning from abroad, or in those with precedent use of fluoroquinolones. Longer durations of illness and increased likelihood of hospitalization have been reported in those with resistant disease, although these findings have been controversial. In many areas, quinolone resistance of *Campylobacter* is increasing (documented in USA, Europe, and Asia).

C. Epidemic measures: Report groups of cases (e.g. in a classroom) to the local health authority, with search for vehicle and mode of spread.

D. Disaster implications: A risk when mass feeding and poor sanitation coexist.

E. International measures: WHO Collaborating Centres provide support as required. More information can be found at:

http://www.who.int/collaboratingcentres/database/en/

See also *Joint FAO/WHO Expert Committee on Risk Assessment of [. . .] Campylobacter spp. in broiler chickens*, 2001, available at:

<http://www.who.int/foodsafety/micro/jemra/assessment/campy/en/>

- and the website of the Pan-American Health Organization:

<http://www.paho.org/english/hcp/hct/eer/campylobacter.htm>

CANDIDIASIS   ICD-9 112; ICD-10 B37
(Moniliasis, Thrush, Candidosis)
[CCDM19: M. Brandt, F. Ndowa]
[CCDM18: F. Ndowa]

1. Identification—A mycosis usually confined to the superficial layers of skin or mucous membranes, presenting clinically as oral thrush, intertrigo, vulvovaginitis, paronychia or onychomycosis. Ulcers or pseudomembranes may form in the esophagus, stomach or intestine. Invasive candidiasis, including candidemia, usually occurs in patients with specific risk factors for infection, such as central venous catheters, immunosuppression, antibiotic therapy, surgery, or critical illness. Candidemia may be uncomplicated, or may disseminate and cause deep-seated infection in many organs, including the eyes, kidneys, liver, spleen, and heart and central nervous system.

Diagnosis requires both laboratory and clinical evidence of candidiasis. The single most valuable laboratory test is microscopic demonstration of pseudohyphae and/or yeast cells in infected tissue or normally sterile body fluids. Culture confirmation is important, but isolation from sputum, bronchial washings, stools, urine, mucosal surfaces, skin or wounds is not proof of a causal relationship to the disease. Severe or recurrent oropharyngeal infection in an adult with no obvious underlying cause should suggest the possibility of HIV infection.

2. Infectious agents—*Candida albicans*, *Candida* (formerly *Torulopsis) glabrata*, *C. parapsilosis*, *C. tropicalis*, and *C. krusei* are most common. Numerous less common species, such as *C. dubliniensis*, have also been reported to cause disease.

3. Occurrence—Worldwide. *Candida* species are often part of the normal flora.

4. Reservoir—Humans.

5. Mode of transmission—Contact with secretions or excretions of mouth, skin, vagina and feces, from patients or carriers; by passage from mother to neonate during childbirth; and by endogenous spread. The role of spread by the sexual route is limited, although some studies have demonstrated significant asymptomatic male genital colonization with species of candida, more commonly in male sexual partners of infected women.

6. Incubation period—Variable, 2–5 days for thrush in infants.

7. Period of communicability—Presumably while lesions are present.

8. Susceptibility—The frequent isolation of *Candida* species from sputum, throat, feces and urine in the absence of clinical evidence of infection suggests a low level of pathogenicity or widespread immunity. Oral thrush is a common, usually benign condition during the first few weeks of life. Clinical disease occurs when host defenses are low. Local factors contributing to superficial candidiasis include interdigital intertrigo and paronychia on hands with excessive water exposure (e.g. cannery and laundry workers), and intertrigo in moist skinfolds of obese individuals. Repeated clinical skin or mucosal eruptions are common.

Prominent among systemic factors predisposing to superficial candidiasis are diabetes mellitus, HIV infection, and treatment with broad-spectrum antibiotics or supraphysiological doses of adrenal corticosteroids. Women in the third trimester of pregnancy are prone to vulvovaginal candidiasis. Factors predisposing to invasive candidiasis include immunosuppression, indwelling intravenous catheters, neutropenia, hematological malignancies, burns, postoperative complications, and very low birth weight in neonates. Urinary tract candidiasis usually arises as a complication of prolonged catheterization of the bladder or renal pelvis. Most adults and older children have a delayed dermal hypersensitivity to the fungus and possess humoral antibodies.

9. **Methods of control—**

A. *Preventive measures:* To prevent systemic spread, early detection and local treatment of any infection in the mouth, esophagus or urinary bladder, of those with predisposing systemic factors (see *Susceptibility*). Fluconazole chemoprophylaxis decreases the incidence of invasive candidiasis following hematopoietic stem cell transplantation in some studies of high-risk intensive care unit patients and liver transplant recipients, and in very low birth weight neonates. Micafungin has also been effective in preventing *Candida* infections in hematopoietic stem cell transplant recipients. Posaconazole is effective in preventing invasive candidiasis in hematopoietic stem cell transplant recipients with graft-versus-host disease, and patients with prolonged, chemotherapy-induced neutropenia.

B. *Control of patient, contacts and the immediate environment:*

1) Report to local health authority: Official report not ordinarily justifiable, Class 5 (see *Reporting*).
2) Isolation: Not applicable.
3) Concurrent disinfection: Of secretions and contaminated articles.
4) Quarantine: Not applicable.
5) Immunization of contacts: Not applicable.
6) Investigation of contacts and source of infection: Not beneficial in sporadic cases.
7) Specific treatment: Ameliorating the underlying causes of candidiasis, e.g. removal of indwelling central venous catheters, may facilitate cure. Topical nystatin or an azole (miconazole, clotrimazole, ketoconazole, fluconazole) is useful in many forms of superficial candidiasis. Oral clotrimazole troches or nystatin suspension are effective for treatment of oral thrush. Itraconazole suspension or fluconazole are effective in oral and esophageal candidiasis. A number of newer antifungals, such as voriconazole, posaconazole and the echinocandins (caspofungin, micafungin, and anidulafungin) are also effective in oropharyngeal and esophageal candidiasis, but their use should generally be reserved for patients with disease refractory to standard therapy. Vaginal infection may be treated with oral fluconazole or topical clotrimazole, miconazole, butoconazole, terconazole, tioconazole or nystatin. Initial treatment for invasive candidiasis in a critically ill patient should consist of an echinocandin or an amphotericin B formulation. Fluconazole is an acceptable choice for initial treatment of candidemia in a stable patient who is unlikely to be infected by an organism with reduced suscep-

tibility to fluconazole. Treatment may be adjusted once the infecting species is known.

C. Epidemic measures: Outbreaks are most frequently due to contaminated intravenous solutions and thrush in nurseries for newborns. Outbreaks of *Candida parapsilosis* fungemia in neonatal intensive care units have been linked to transmission from healthcare workers. Concurrent disinfection and terminal cleaning comparable to that used for epidemic diarrhea in hospital nurseries (see *Diarrhea*, section IV, 9A).

D. Disaster implications: None.

E. International measures: None.

CAPILLARIASIS

Three types of nematodes of the superfamily Trichuroidea, genus *Capillaria*, produce disease in humans.
[CCDM19: Editorial Board]
[CCDM18: D. Engels]

I. CAPILLARIASIS DUE TO CAPILLARIA PHILIPPINENSIS   ICD-9 127.5; ICD-10 B81.1
(Intestinal capillariasis)

1. Identification—First described in Luzon, Philippines, in the early 1960s, the disease is clinically an enteropathy with massive protein loss and a malabsorption syndrome leading to progressive weight loss and emaciation. Fatal cases are characterized by the presence of great numbers of parasites in the small intestine together with ascites and pleural transudate. Case-fatality rates of 10% have been reported. Subclinical cases also occur, but usually become symptomatic over time.

Diagnosis is based on clinical findings plus the identification of eggs or larval or adult parasites in the stool. The eggs resemble those of *Trichuris trichuria*. Jejunal biopsy may show worms in the mucosa.

2. Infectious agent—*Capillaria philippinensis*.

3. Occurrence—Intestinal capillariasis is endemic in the Philippines and in Thailand; cases have been reported from Egypt, Japan, the Republic of Korea and Taiwan (China). Isolated cases have also been reported from Colombia, India, Indonesia, and the Islamic Republic of Iran. In

Luzon (Philippines), more than 1 800 cases have been seen since 1967. Males between the ages of 20 and 45 appear to be particularly at risk.

4. Reservoir—Unknown; possibly aquatic birds. Fish are considered intermediate hosts.

5. Mode of transmission—Patients usually have a history of ingestion of raw or inadequately cooked small fish, eaten whole. Experimentally, infective larvae develop in the intestines of freshwater fish that ingest eggs; these fish are then eaten by monkeys, Mongolian gerbils and some birds, which become infected. The parasite then matures within their intestines.

6. Incubation period—Unknown in humans; in animal studies, about a month or more.

7. Period of communicability—Not transmitted directly from person to person.

8. Susceptibility—Susceptibility appears to be general in those geographic areas in which the parasite is prevalent. Attack rates are often high.

9. Methods of control—

   A. Preventive measures:

   1) Avoid eating uncooked fish or other aquatic animal life in known endemic areas.
   2) Provide adequate facilities for the disposal of feces.

   B. Control of patient, contacts and the immediate environment:

   1) Report to local health authority: Case report by most practicable means, Class 3 (see *Reporting*).
   2) Isolation: Not applicable.
   3) Concurrent disinfection: Sanitary disposal of feces.
   4) Quarantine: Not applicable.
   5) Immunization of contacts: Not applicable.
   6) Investigation of contacts and source of infection: Stool examination for all members of family groups and others with common exposure to raw or undercooked fish, with treatment of infected individuals.
   7) Specific treatment: Mebendazole or albendazole as drugs of choice.

   C. Epidemic measures: Prompt investigation of cases and contacts; treatment of cases as indicated. Education on the need to cook all fish prior to eating.

   D. Disaster implications: None.

   E. International measures: None.

II. CAPILLARIASIS DUE TO
CAPILLARIA HEPATICA   ICD-9 128.8; ICD-10 B83.8
(Hepatic capillariasis)

1. Identification—An uncommon and occasionally fatal disease in humans due to the presence of adult *Capillaria hepatica* in the liver. The picture is that of an acute or subacute hepatitis with marked eosinophilia resembling that of visceral larva migrans; the organism can disseminate to the lungs and other viscera.

Diagnosis is made by demonstrating eggs or the parasite in a liver biopsy or at necropsy.

2. Infectious agent—*Capillaria hepatica* (*Hepaticola hepatica*).

3. Occurrence—Since identification as a human disease in 1924, about 30 cases have been reported from Africa, North and South America, Asia, Europe and the Pacific area.

4. Reservoir—Primarily rats (as many as 86% infected in some reports) and other rodents, but also a large variety of domestic and wild mammals. The adult worms live and produce eggs in the liver.

5. Mode of transmission—The adult worms produce fertilized eggs that remain in the liver until the death of the host animal. When infected liver is eaten, the eggs are freed by digestion, reach the soil in the feces and develop to the infective stage in 2-4 weeks. When ingested by a suitable host, embryonated eggs hatch in the intestine; larvae migrate through the wall of the gut and are transported via the portal system to the liver, where they mature and produce eggs. Spurious infection in humans may be detected when eggs are found in stools after consumption of infected liver, raw or cooked; since these eggs are not embryonated, infection cannot be established.

6. Incubation period—From 3 to 4 weeks.

7. Period of communicability—Not directly transmitted from person to person.

8. Susceptibility—Susceptibility is universal; malnourished children appear more often infected.

9. Methods of control—

   A. Preventive measures:

   1) Avoid ingestion of dirt, whether directly (pica), in contaminated food or water, or on hands.
   2) Protect water supplies and food from soil contamination.

B. *Control of patient, contacts and the immediate environment:*

1) Report to local health authority: Official report not ordinarily justifiable, Class 5 (see *Reporting*).
2) Isolation: Not applicable.
3) Concurrent disinfection: Not applicable.
4) Quarantine: Not applicable.
5) Immunization of contacts: Not applicable.
6) Investigation of contacts and source of infection: Not applicable.
7) Specific treatment: Thiabendazole and albendazole effectively kill the worms in the liver.

C. *Epidemic measures:* Not applicable.

D. *Disaster implications:* None.

E. *International measures:* None.

III. PULMONARY CAPILLARIASIS   ICD-9 128.8; ICD-10 B 83.8

A pulmonary disease manifested by fever, cough and asthmatic breathing, caused by *Capillaria aerophila* (*Thominx aerophila*), a nematode parasite of cats, dogs and other carnivorous mammals. Pneumonitis may be severe; heavy infections may be fatal. The worms live in tunnels in the epithelial lining of the trachea, bronchi and bronchioles; fertilized eggs are sloughed into the air passages, coughed up, swallowed and discharged from the body in the feces. In the soil, larvae develop in the eggs and remain infective for a year or longer. Infection is acquired mainly by children, through ingestion of infective eggs in soil or in soil-contaminated food or water. Eggs may appear in the sputum in 4 weeks; symptoms may appear earlier or later. Human cases have been recorded from the Islamic Republic of Iran, Morocco and Russia; animal infection has been reported in North and South America, Europe, Asia and Australia.

CAT-SCRATCH DISEASE   ICD-9 078.3; ICD-10 A28.1
(Cat-scratch fever, Benign lymphoreticulosis)
[CCDM19: W. Nicholson]
[CCDM18: D. Raoult]

1. Identification—A sub-acute, usually self-limited bacterial disease characterized by malaise, granulomatous lymphadenitis, and variable patterns of fever. Often preceded by a cat scratch, lick or bite that produces a red papular lesion with involvement of a regional lymph node, usually within 2 weeks; may progress to suppuration. The papule at the inoculation site can be found in 50%–90% of cases. Parinaud oculoglandular syndrome (granulomatous conjunctivitis with pretragal adenopathy) can occur after direct or indirect conjunctival inoculation; neurological complications such as encephalopathy and optic neuritis can also occur. Prolonged high fever may be accompanied by osteolytic lesions and/or hepatic and splenic granulomata. Bacteremia, hepatic extravasation of blood (peliosis hepatis) and bacillary angiomatosis due to this infection may occur among young children and among immunocompromised persons, particularly those with HIV infection.

Cat-scratch disease can be clinically confused with other diseases that cause regional lymphadenopathies (e.g. tularemia, brucellosis, tuberculosis, plague, pasteurellosis, and lymphoma).

Diagnosis is based on a consistent clinical picture combined with serological evidence of antibody to *Bartonella henselae*. A titer of 1/64 or greater by IFA assay is considered positive.

Histopathological examination of affected lymph nodes may show consistent characteristics, but is not diagnostic. Pus obtained from lymph nodes is usually bacteriologically sterile by conventional techniques. Immunodetection and PCR are highly efficient in detecting *Bartonella* in biopsies or aspirates of lymph nodes. *Bartonella* has been grown from blood and from lymph node aspirates after prolonged incubation on rabbit blood agar in 5% CO_2 at 36°C (96.8°F), and in other cell culture systems.

2. Infectious agent—*Bartonella* (formerly *Rochalimaea*) *henselae* has been implicated epidemiologically, bacteriologically and serologically as the causal agent of most cat-scratch disease. Related bartonellae, such as *B. quintana* and *B. clarridgeiae*, may also produce illnesses among immunocompromised hosts.

3. Occurrence—Worldwide, but uncommon; affects men and women equally; more common in children and young adults. Familial clustering rarely occurs. Most cases are seen during the late summer, autumn, and winter months.

4. Reservoir—Domestic cats are the main vectors and reservoirs for *B. henselae*; no evidence of clinical illness in cats even when chronic bacteremia has been demonstrated. Cat fleas and ticks may be infected, but their role in transmission is not well defined.

5. Mode of transmission—Over 90% of patients give a history of scratch, bite, lick or other exposure to a healthy, usually young, cat or kitten. Dog scratch or bite, monkey bite, and contact with rabbits, chickens or horses have also been reported prior to the syndrome, but cat involvement was not excluded in all cases. Cat fleas (*Ctenocephalides felis*) transmit *B. henselae* among cats, but play no clear role in direct transmission to humans.

6. Incubation period—Variable, usually 3–14 days from inoculation to primary lesion and 5–50 days from inoculation to lymphadenopathy.

7. Period of communicability—Not directly transmitted from person to person.

8. Susceptibility—Unknown.

9. Methods of control—

A. *Preventive measures:* Thorough cleaning of cat scratches and bites may help. Flea control is very important to prevent continuing infection of cats.

B. *Control of patient, contacts and the immediate environment:*

1) Report to local health authority: Official report not ordinarily justifiable, Class 5 (see *Reporting*).
2) Isolation: Not applicable.
3) Concurrent disinfection: Of discharges from purulent lesions.
4) Quarantine: Not applicable.
5) Immunization of contacts: Not applicable.
6) Investigation of contacts and source of infection: Not applicable.
7) Specific treatment: Treatment of uncomplicated disease in immunocompetent patients is not indicated, but all immunocompromised patients must be treated for 1–3 months. Prolonged administration (at least 1 month) of antibiotics such as erythromycin, rifampicin, ciprofloxacin or gentamicin is effective in the disseminated forms seen in persons with HIV infection. Needle aspiration of suppurative lymphadenitis may be required for relief of pain, but incisional biopsy of lymph nodes may be avoided.

C. *Epidemic measures:* Not applicable.

D. *Disaster implications:* None.

E. *International measures:* None.

CHANCROID ICD-9 099.0; ICD-10 A57
(Ulcus molle, Soft chancre)
[CCDM19: R. Ballard, F. Ndowa, Ye Tun]
[CCDM18: F. Ndowa]

1. Identification—An acute, sexually transmitted bacterial infection usually localized in the genital area and characterized clinically by a single or multiple painful, necrotic ulcers that bleed on contact. Chancroid ulcers are more frequently found in uncircumcised men, on the foreskin or in the coronal sulcus, and may cause a phimosis. These primary lesions are frequently accompanied by painful, swollen and suppurating regional lymph nodes. In women, asymptomatic carriage is rare, but minimally symptomatic or painless lesions may occur on the vaginal wall or cervix. Extragenital lesions have been reported. Chancroid ulcers, like other genital ulcers, are associated with an increased risk of HIV infection. Culture and polymerase chain reaction (PCR) tests are the preferred tests for a definitive diagnosis, but PCR is not commonly available and requires training and stringent quality control. Diagnosis is by isolation of the organism from lesion exudates on a selective medium incorporating vancomycin into chocolated horse blood agar enriched with fetal calf serum IsoVitaleX and activated charcoal. PCR and direct immunofluorescence have also been used successfully to detect organisms in ulcer exudates, on a research basis.

2. Infectious agent—*Haemophilus ducreyi*, a Gram-negative coccobacillus, or Ducrey's bacillus.

3. Occurrence—Most prevalent in tropical and subtropical regions, where incidence may be higher than that of syphilis, and approaching that of gonorrhea in men. With an exclusively human reservoir—and more often diagnosed in men, especially clients of sex workers— chancroid has disappeared from many regions with increased access to condoms and provision of appropriate antimicrobial chemotherapy, often as a component of syndromic case management of genital ulcer disease. The disease is much less common in temperate zones, where it may occur in small outbreaks. In the USA and other industrialized countries, outbreaks and some endemic transmission have occurred, but principally among migrant workers and poor inner city residents who are clients of sex workers, and among persons with risk factors such as drugs or crack cocaine use.

4. Reservoir—Humans.

5. Mode of transmission—Direct sexual contact with discharges from open lesions and pus from buboes. Auto-inoculation to non-genital sites may occur in infected persons. Beyond the neonatal period, sexual abuse must be considered when chancroid is found in children.

6. **Incubation period**—From 3 to 5 days, up to 14 days.

7. **Period of communicability**—Until healing of the primary lesions, and as long as infectious agent persists in the original lesion or discharging regional lymph nodes— up to several weeks or months without effective antibiotic chemotherapy. Initiation of appropriate antibiotic treatment results in the elimination of *H. ducreyi*, and lesions heal in 1–2 weeks.

8. **Susceptibility**—Susceptibility is general; the uncircumcised are at higher risk than the circumcised. There is no evidence of natural immunity.

9. **Methods of control**—

   A. *Preventive measures:*

   1) See Syphilis, 9A.
   2) Perform serological follow-up for syphilis and HIV in all patients with no herpetic genital ulcerations.

   B. *Control of patient, contacts and the immediate environment:*

   1) Report to local health authority: Case report obligatory in many countries, Class 2 (see *Reporting*).
   2) Isolation: Avoid sexual contact until all lesions are healed.
   3) Concurrent disinfection: Not applicable.
   4) Quarantine: Not applicable.
   5) Immunization of contacts: Not applicable.
   6) Investigation of contacts and source of infection: Examine and treat all sexual contacts within the 10 days preceding onset of symptoms. Women without external signs of infection may have small, inapparent intravaginal lesions. Sexual contacts even without obvious signs of disease should receive prophylactic treatment.
   7) Specific treatment: Ceftriaxone, erythromycin, azithromycin, ceftriaxone, or, for adults only, ciprofloxacin. Alternatives include amoxicillin with clavulanic acid. Fluctuant inguinal nodes must be aspirated through intact skin to prevent spontaneous rupture, even after initiation of effective therapy.

   C. *Epidemic measures:* Persistent occurrence or increased incidence is an indication for stricter application of measures outlined in 9A and 9B above. When compliance with treatment is a problem, consideration should be given to single dose therapy with azithromycin or ceftriaxone. Empirical therapy to high-risk groups with or without lesions, including sex workers; to clinic patients reporting contact with sex workers; and to clinic patients with genital ulcers and a negative syphilis diagnosis may be required to control an outbreak. Interventions providing periodic presumptive treatment to sex workers and their clients have an impact on the prevalence of chancroid and provide valuable information for strategies to eliminate the disease in areas of high prevalence.

D. Disaster implications: None.

E. International measures: See *Syphilis*, 9E.

CHICKENPOX/HERPES ZOSTER   ICD-9 052-053;
ICD-10 B01-B02

(Varicella/Shingles)
[CCDM19: A. Jumaan, D. Lavanchy]
[CCDM18: D. Lavanchy]

1. Identification—The varicella-zoster virus (VZV) causes two distinct diseases, varicella (chickenpox) as the primary infection, and later, when VZV reactivates, herpes zoster (shingles). Varicella is an acute illness characterized by fever and generalized, pruritic, vesicular rash typically consisting of 250 to 500 lesions in varying stages of development and resolution. The rash is maculopapular for a few hours, vesicular for 3 to 4 days, then crusts, leaving granular scabs. The vesicles are unilocular and collapse on puncture, in contrast to the multilocular, non-collapsing vesicles of smallpox. Lesions commonly occur in successive crops, with several stages of maturity present at the same time; they tend to have central distribution, and are more abundant on covered than on exposed parts of the body. Lesions may appear on the scalp, high in the axilla, on mucous membranes of the mouth and upper respiratory tract, and on the conjunctivae; they tend to occur in areas of irritation, such as sunburn or diaper rash. They may be so few as to escape observation.

Mild, atypical and inapparent infections occur, especially among vaccinated individuals (breakthrough varicella). Breakthrough varicella is defined as varicella developing more than 42 days after vaccination; most breakthrough disease is mild, without fever, and with skin rash of <50 lesions that are atypical, with papules that do not progress to vesicles, and which may be so few in numbers as to escape observation.

Occasionally, especially in adults and in persons with cellular immune deficiencies such as malignancies and HIV/AIDS, fever and constitutional manifestations may be severe. Although varicella is usually a benign childhood disease, and is rarely rated as an important public health problem, varicella zoster virus may induce pneumonia or encephalitis, sometimes with persistent sequelae or death. Secondary bacterial infections of the vesicles may leave disfiguring scars, or result in necrotizing fasciitis or septicemia.

The case-fatality rate is lower for children (1:100 000 infected in the 5-9 age group) than for adults (1:5 000). Serious complications include pneumonia (viral and bacterial), secondary bacterial infections, hemorrhagic complications and encephalitis. Children with acute leukemia, including those in remission after chemotherapy, are at increased risk of disseminated disease, which is fatal in 5%-10% of cases. Neonates who develop varicella between ages 5 and 10 days are at increased risk of developing severe generalized varicella. Among neonates whose mothers develop the disease 5 days prior to or within 2 days after delivery and who do not receive VZIG (see below) or antiviral therapy, the case-fatality rate can reach 30%. Infection early in pregnancy, at 0-12 weeks, may be associated with fetal death or congenital varicella syndrome in 1% of cases, and at 13-20 weeks gestation with a 2% risk. Cases consistent with congenital varicella syndrome have been reported post 20 weeks gestation. Clinical varicella was a frequent antecedent of Reye syndrome, before the association of Reye syndrome with aspirin use for viral infections was identified.

Herpes zoster (shingles), which occurs in about 10-20% of the population, is a local manifestation of reactivation of latent varicella infection in the dorsal root ganglia. Vesicles with an erythematous base are restricted to skin areas supplied by sensory nerves of a single or associated group of dorsal root ganglia. Rash is typically unilateral, and most commonly affects thoracic, cervical, and ophthalmic dermatomes. Small numbers of lesions may appear outside the primary dermatome. Lesions are histologically identical to those of varicella, deeper seated, and more closely aggregated. The rash lasts about 7-10 days, and heals within 2-4 weeks. Complications develop in about 30% of herpes zoster cases; the most common is chronic severe pain or post-herpetic neuralgia (PHN). Although the definition of PHN has been inconsistent, PHN is defined as pain that persists after the rash heals, ranging from any duration to 30-90 days after rash resolution; it can, however, last for months, or even years. Herpes zoster may result in permanent neurological damage such as cranial nerve palsy and contralateral hemiplegia, or visual impairment following herpes zoster ophthalmia. The incidence of both herpes zoster and post-herpetic neuralgia increase with age; persons with malignant neoplasm and those infected with HIV also have a high risk of herpes zoster, with higher rates among children. Herpes zoster is more common following hematopoietic stem cell and solid organ transplants, especially in the first year. In the immunosuppressed and those with malignancies, but sometimes in otherwise healthy individuals with fewer lesions, extensive chickenpox-like lesions may appear outside the dermatome. Intrauterine infection is associated with herpes zoster in children. Occasionally, a varicelliform eruption follows shortly after herpes zoster, and rarely there is a secondary eruption of zoster after chickenpox.

Laboratory tests—such as visualization of virus by electron micrograph (EM); virus isolation in cell cultures; demonstration of viral antigen in smears using direct fluorescent antibody (DFA) of viral DNA by PCR, or of a rise in serum antibodies—are not routinely required for diagnosis, but are useful in complicated cases and in epidemiological studies. In the vaccine era, viral strain identification may be needed (e.g. to document whether herpes zoster in a vaccine recipient is due to vaccine or wild virus). Several antibody assays are now commercially available, but they are not sensitive enough to be used for post-immunization testing of immunity. Multinucleated giant cells may be detected in Giemsa-stained (Tzanck smear) scrapings from the base of a lesion; these are not found in vaccinia lesions, but do occur in herpes simplex lesions. They are not specific for varicella infections, and the availability of rapid direct fluorescent antibody testing has limited their value for clinical testing.

2. Infectious agent—Human (alpha) herpesvirus 3 (varicella-zoster virus, VZV), a member of the *Herpesvirus* group.

3. Occurrence—Worldwide. Infection with human (alpha) herpesvirus 3 is nearly universal. In temperate climates, at least 90% of the population has had chickenpox by age 15, and at least 95% by young adulthood. In temperate zones, chickenpox occurs most frequently in winter and early spring. The epidemiology of varicella in tropical countries differs from temperate climates, with a higher proportion of cases occurring among adults. Herpes zoster occurrence has been described most commonly in developed countries where Zoster occurs more commonly in older people 50 years of age.

4. Reservoir—Humans.

5. Mode of transmission—Person-to-person by direct contact, droplet or airborne spread of vesicle fluid, or secretions of the respiratory tract of chickenpox cases, or of vesicle fluid of patients with herpes zoster; indirectly through articles freshly soiled by discharges from vesicles and mucous membranes of infected people. In contrast to vaccinia and variola, scabs from varicella lesions are not infective. Varicella in unvaccinated persons is one of the most readily communicable of diseases, especially in the early stages of the eruption; secondary attack rates in susceptible household contacts range from 61% to 100%. Herpes zoster has a lower rate of transmission: data from a household study showed that 20% of those who are varicella seronegative develop varicella when they are in contact with persons who have herpes zoster.

6. Incubation period—10–21 days; commonly 14–16 days; may be prolonged as long as 28 days after passive immunization against varicella (see 9A2), and may be shortened in the immunodeficient.

7. Period of communicability—As long as 5 days, but usually 1–2 days before onset of rash, and continuing until all lesions are crusted (usually about 5 days). Contagiousness may be prolonged in patients with altered immunity. The secondary attack rate among susceptible siblings is 60%–100%. Patients with herpes zoster may be infectious for a week after the appearance of vesiculopustular lesions. Susceptible individuals should be considered infectious for 10–21 days following exposure.

8. **Susceptibility**—Susceptibility to varicella is universal among those not previously infected or vaccinated; ordinarily a more severe disease of adults than of children. Infection usually confers long immunity; second attacks are rare in immunocompetent persons but have been documented; subclinical reinfection is common. Viral infection remains latent; disease may recur years later as herpes zoster. Herpes zoster occurs in about 15% of older adults, and rarely in children.

Neonates whose mothers are not immune and patients with leukemia may suffer severe, prolonged or fatal chickenpox. Adults with cancer—especially of lymphoid tissue, with or without steroid therapy—immuno-deficient patients and those on immunosuppressive therapy may have an increased frequency of severe herpes zoster, both localized and disseminated.

9. **Methods of control**—

   A. *Preventive measures:*

      1) Live attenuated varicella virus vaccines are licensed through-out the world. A quadrivalent vaccine (MMRV) has been licensed for use in healthy children aged 12 months to 12 years. In industrialized countries, a first dose is recommended for routine immunization of children aged 12 to 18 months and a second dose is routinely recommended at 4–6 years of age for children up to 12 years who have not had varicella. The second dose may be given at early as 3 months after the first. One dose of the vaccine has a cumulative preventive efficacy estimated at 70%–90% in children followed for up to 10 years. A second dose catch-up vaccination is recommended for persons who previously received only one dose. If an immunized person does get "break-through varicella," it is usually a mild case with fewer lesions (up to 50, frequently not vesicular), mild or no fever, and of shorter duration. If administered within 3 days of exposure, varicella vaccine is likely to prevent or at least modify disease in a case contact. The protection against herpes zoster induced by varicella vaccine, administered either in childhood or in adult populations, is not yet sufficiently documented in the general population; however, postlicensure data, mostly among immunocompromised children, indicate that children immunized with varicella vaccine seem to have a lower risk and milder herpes zoster than children who had natural varicella

infection. Large scale vaccination of children and older adults may have an important impact on the incidence of herpes zoster and post herpetic neuralgia.

For persons ≥13 years of age, two doses of varicella vaccine 4-8 weeks apart are also recommended for susceptible persons without evidence of immunity. The criteria for evidence of VZV immunity were revised in 2006. People born after 1980 with a history of a typical disease are considered immune and exempt from varicella vaccination, if their history is verified by a health care provider; however, for those with a history of atypical disease, a physician or a designee assessment is recommended in addition to evidence of a typical or a lab-confirmed varicella case.

Vaccination is offered without confirmation of seronegativity. Priority groups for adult immunization include close contacts of persons at high risk for serious complications; persons who live or work in environments where transmission of varicella is likely (e.g. teachers of young children, day care employees, residents and staff in institutional settings) or can occur (e.g. college students, inmates and staff members of correctional institutions and military personnel); nonpregnant women of childbearing age; adolescents and adults in households with children; and international travelers.

In immunocompromised persons, including persons with advanced HIV infection, varicella vaccination is currently contraindicated. However, varicella vaccine should be considered for HIV-infected children with CD4+ T-lymphocyte counts ≥200 cells/μL (≥15%). Varicella vaccine may also be considered for HIV-infected adolescents and adults with CD4+ counts ≥200 cells/μL. Other contraindications for varicella vaccination include a history of anaphylactic reactions to any component of the vaccine (including neomycin), pregnancy (theoretical risk to the fetus—pregnancy should be avoided for 4 weeks following vaccination), ongoing severe illness, and advanced immune disorders.

Except for patients with acute lymphatic leukemia in stable remission, ongoing treatment with systemic steroids (adults 20 mg/day, children 1 mg/kg/day) is considered a contraindication for varicella vaccination. However, persons who have discontinued corticosteroid therapy for at least a month can be vaccinated. Varicella vaccine may be administered to people on inhaled, nasal, and topical steroids. A history of congenital immune disorders in close family members is a relative contraindication. Routine childhood immunization against varicella may be considered in countries where the disease is a public health and socioeconomic problem, where immunization is affordable, and where sustained high vaccine coverage (85%–90%) can be achieved. Persons over 13 years of age require 2 doses of vaccine 4–8 weeks apart.

A mild varicella-like rash at the site of vaccine injection or at distant sites has been observed in 2%–4% of children and about 5% of adults. Rare occasions of mild herpes zoster following vaccination show that the currently used vaccine strains may induce latency, with the subsequent risk of reactivation, although the rate seems to be lower than after natural disease. Duration of immunity after one dose is unknown, but antibodies have persisted for at least 10 years; persistence of antibody has occurred in the presence of circulating wild virus. At time of writing in early 2008, one study has found that incidence and severity of breakthrough varicella increased with time since vaccination, while another study did not find a loss of vaccine effectiveness over time.

2) Protect high-risk individuals who cannot be immunized— e.g. non-immune neonates and the immunodeficient—from exposure, by immunizing household or other close contacts.

3) Varicella-zoster immune globulin (VZIG or VariZIG), prepared from the plasma of normal blood donors with high VZV antibody titer, effectively modifies or prevents disease if given within 96 hours after exposure (see 9B5).

A herpes zoster vaccine for older adults has been approved and recommended for use in the USA for healthy persons aged 60 years or older.

B. *Control of patient, contacts and the immediate environment:*

1) Report to local health authority: In many countries, not a reportable disease; varicella-related deaths became nationally notifiable in the USA on January 1, 1999 and cases became nationally notifiable on January 2005; Class 3 (see *Reporting*).

2) Isolation: Exclude children from school, medical offices, emergency rooms or public places until vesicles become dry and crusted, usually after 5 days in non-immunized children and 1–4 days with breakthrough varicella in immunized children; exclude infected adults from workplace and avoid contact with susceptibles. In hospital, observe strict isolation, because of the risk of varicella in susceptible immuno-compromised patients.

3) Concurrent disinfection: Articles soiled by discharges from the nose and throat.

4) Quarantine: Usually none. However, in places where susceptible children with known recent exposure must remain for

medical reasons, the risk of spread to steroid-treated or immunodeficient patients may justify quarantine of known contacts for at least 10–21 days after exposure (up to 28 days if VZIG was given).

5) Protection of contacts: Varicella vaccine is effective in preventing illness or modifying severity if used within 3 days, and possibly up to 5 days, of exposure; it is recommended for susceptible persons following exposure to varicella.

VZIG within 96 hours of exposure may prevent or modify disease in susceptible close contacts of cases. It is available in several countries for high-risk persons exposed to chickenpox, and indicated for newborns of mothers who develop chickenpox within 5 days prior to or 2 days after delivery. There is no assurance that administering VZIG to a pregnant woman will prevent congenital malformations in the fetus, but it may modify varicella severity in the pregnant woman.

Antiviral drugs such as acyclovir appear useful in preventing or modifying varicella in exposed individuals if given within a week of exposure. Most studies have been carried out in immunocompromised children, with few data available for healthy children. A dose of 80 mg/kg/day in 4 divided doses has been used, but no regimen is as yet generally recommended for this purpose.

6) Investigation of contacts and source of infection: The source of infection may be a case of varicella or herpes zoster. All contacts, especially if ineligible for post-exposure immunization, should be evaluated promptly for administration of VZIG. Infectious patients should be isolated until all lesions are crusted; exposed susceptibles eligible for immunization should receive vaccine immediately to control or prevent an outbreak.

7) Specific treatment: Antiviral therapy is moderately effective in treating varicella and herpes zoster infections: acyclovir, valacyclovir or famcyclovir are considered the agents of choice for treatment of varicella. These drugs, as well as brivudin, have been shown to help shorten the duration of the infection and possibly post-herpetic neuralgia in herpes zoster; they may shorten the duration of symptoms and reduce acute and chronic pain, especially if administered within 48–72 hours of rash onset. In case of resistance, foscarnet is considered the second line drug. For the treatment of post-herpetic neuralgia, amptryptilin, gabapentin, pregabalin or carbamazepine are recommended.

C. **Epidemic measures:** Outbreaks of varicella are common in schools and other institutional settings; they may be protracted, disruptive and associated with complications. Infectious cases should be isolated, and susceptible contacts immunized promptly (or referred to their health care provider for immunization). Persons ineligible for immunization, such as susceptible pregnant females and those at high risk for severe disease (as above), should be evaluated immediately for administration of VZIG.

D. Disaster implications: Outbreaks of chickenpox may occur among children crowded together in emergency housing situations.

E. International measures: See C.

CHLAMYDIAL INFECTIONS
[CCDM19: R. Johnson, F. Ndowa]
[CCDM18: F. Ndowa]

As laboratory techniques improve, chlamydial organisms are increasingly implicated as causes of human disease. Chlamydiae are obligate intracellular bacteria that differ from viruses and rickettsiae but, like the latter, are sensitive to broad-spectrum antimicrobials. Those that cause human disease are classified into 3 species:

1) *Chlamydia psittaci*, a common pathogen of avian species and domestic animals, but also the etiologic agent of psittacosis (q.v.) in humans.

2) *C. trachomatis*, including serotypes that cause trachoma (q.v.), genital infections (see below), chlamydial conjunctivitis (q.v.), and infant pneumonia (q.v.); and other serotypes that cause lymphogranuloma venereum (q.v.).

3) *C. pneumoniae*, the cause of respiratory disease including pneumonia (q.v.), and implicated in coronary artery disease.

Chlamydiae are increasingly recognized as important pathogens responsible for several sexually transmitted infections, with infant eye and lung infections consequent to maternal genital infection.

GENITAL INFECTIONS, CHLAMYDIAL   ICD-9 099.8; ICD-10 A56

1. Identification—Sexually transmitted genital infection is manifested in males primarily as a urethritis, and in females as a cervical infection. Clinical manifestations of urethritis are often difficult to distinguish from gonorrhea and include moderate or scanty mucopurulent discharges, urethral itching, and burning on urination. Although most men develop symptoms following infection, the majority of men identified through screening or population surveys report no or only mild symptoms. Asymptomatic infection may be found in 1%–25% of sexually active men. Possible complications or sequelae of male urethral infections include epididymitis, infertility, and Reiter syndrome. In homosexual men, receptive anorectal intercourse may result in chlamydial proctitis.

In the female, clinical manifestations may be similar to those of gonorrhea and may present as a mucopurulent endocervical discharge, with edema, erythema and easily induced endocervical bleeding caused by inflammation of the endocervical columnar epithelium. Up to 70% of sexually active women with chlamydial infections are asymptomatic. Complications and sequelae include salpingitis with subsequent risk of infertility, ectopic pregnancy, or chronic pelvic pain. Asymptomatic chronic infections of endometrium and fallopian tubes may lead to the same outcome. Less frequent manifestations include Bartholinitis, urethral syndrome with dysuria and pyuria, perihepatitis (Fitz-Hugh-Curtis syndrome), and proctitis. Infection during pregnancy may result in premature rupture of membranes and preterm delivery, and conjunctival and pneumonic infection of the newborn. Endocervical chlamydial infection has been associated with increased risk of acquiring HIV infection. Chlamydial infections may be acquired concurrently with *N. gonorrhoeae*, and may persist after gonorrhea has been successfully treated. Because gonococcal and chlamydial cervicitis are often difficult to distinguish clinically, and because dual infection is common, treatment for both organisms is recommended when one is suspected.

Diagnosis of chlamydial infections has undergone considerable transformation in recent years, following the advent of molecular tests. Culture is technically difficult and not as sensitive as molecular assays. Antigen detection using enzyme-linked immunoassay (EIA) has been shown not to be as sensitive as the molecular assays, though it is still widely used. Nucleic acid amplification tests (NAATs), including polymerase chain reaction (PCR), transcription mediated amplification (e.g. Gen-Probe) and strand displacement amplification, offer excellent sensitivity (usually well above 90%) and high specificity. NAATs can be used with urine specimens. The choice of diagnostic test, however, is determined by cost and ease of performance. Amplification tests are expensive and require stringent quality control. Less sensitive tests will continue to be used, especially in resource-constrained settings, until new technologies become more affordable or easy to perform. For other agents, see *Urethritis, nongonococcal* (below).

2. Infectious agent—*Chlamydia trachomatis* immunotypes D through K are responsible for sexually-acquired genital infections in the adult and perinatally transmitted infections of the neonate and infant. Other immunotypes are responsible for trachoma and lymphogranuloma venereum.

3. Occurrence—Common worldwide; recognition has increased steadily in the last two decades.

4. Reservoir—Humans.

5. Mode of transmission—Sexual intercourse. Neonatal infection results from exposure to the mother's infected cervix.

6. Incubation period—Poorly defined, probably 7–14 days or longer.

7. Period of communicability—Unknown—infected individuals are presumed to be infectious. Without treatment, infection can persist for months. Relapses are probably common.

8. Susceptibility—Susceptibility is general. Reinfection is common; immunity induced by chlamydial infections is not well understood. Cellular immunity is immunotype-specific.

9. Methods of control—

    A. Preventive measures:

        1) Health and sex education, same as for syphilis (see *Syphilis*, 9A), with emphasis on use of a condom when engaging in sexual intercourse.

        2) Screening of women for *C. trachomatis* has been shown to reduce the risk of pelvic inflammatory disease. Annual screening of sexually active adolescent girls should be routine. Screening of adult women should also be considered if they are under 25 or are at increased risk, (e.g. have multiple or new sex partners, and/or use barrier contraceptives inconsistently). Newer tests for *C. trachomatis* infection, which also enable screening of adolescent and young adult males, may be used on urine specimens.

    B. Control of patient, contacts and the immediate environment:

        1) Report to local health authority: Case report is required in many industrialized countries, Class 2 (see *Reporting*).

        2) Isolation: Universal precautions, as appropriate for hospitalized patients. Appropriate antibiotherapy renders discharges noninfectious; patients should refrain from sexual intercourse until treatment of index patient and current sexual partners is completed.

        3) Concurrent disinfection: Care in disposal of articles contaminated with urethral and vaginal discharges.

        4) Quarantine: Not applicable.

        5) Immunization of contacts: Not applicable.

        6) Investigation of contacts and source of infection: Presumptive treatment of sexual partners is recommended. As a

minimum, concurrent treatment of regular sex partners is a practical approach to management. The mothers of infants who have chlamydial infection and the sex partners of these women should be evaluated and treated. If neonates born to infected mothers have not received systemic treatment, chest X-rays at 3 weeks of age and again after 12–18 weeks may be considered to exclude subclinical chlamydial pneumonia.

7) Specific treatment: Doxycycline (PO), 100 mg twice daily for 7 days; or azithromycin (PO), 1 gram in a single dose. Tetracycline (PO), 500 mg 4 times daily for 7 days, is an alternative, but is cumbersome in terms of frequency and the need to avoid food and milk products before ingestion, thus negatively affecting patient compliance. In addition, tetracycline and doxycycline cannot be used in children less than eight years of age. Erythromycin is the recommended drug of choice for infants, and azithromycin is recommended for women with a known or suspected pregnancy.

C. *Epidemic measures:* None.

D. *Disaster implications:* None.

E. *International measures:* None.

URETHRITIS, NONGONOCOCCAL AND NONSPECIFIC (NGU, NSU) ICD-9 099.4; ICD-10 N34.1

While chlamydiae are the most frequently isolated causal agents in cases of non-gonococcal urethritis, other agents are involved in a significant number of cases. *Ureaplasma urealyticum* is considered the causal agent in approximately 10%–20% of NGU cases, and *Mycoplasma genitalium* has been implicated in some studies. Herpesvirus simplex type 2 is rarely implicated; *Trichomonas vaginalis*, though rarely implicated, has been shown to be a significant cause of urethritis in some high prevalence settings. If laboratory facilities for demonstration of chlamydia are not available, all cases of NGU (together with their sexual partners) are best managed as though their infections were due to chlamydia, especially since many chlamydia-negative cases also respond to antibiotherapy.

CHOLERA AND OTHER
VIBRIOSES   ICD-9 001; ICD-10 A00

I. *VIBRIO CHOLERAE*
SEROGROUPS O1 AND O139
[CCDM19: A. Boore, M. Iwamoto, E. Mintz, P. Yu]
[CCDM18: C. Chaignat]

1. Identification—An acute bacterial enteric disease characterized in its severe form by sudden onset, profuse painless watery stools (rice-water stool) provoked by an enterotoxin that affects the small intestine; nausea; and profuse vomiting early in the course of illness. In untreated cases, rapid dehydration, acidosis, circulatory collapse, hypoglycemia in children, and renal failure can rapidly lead to death. In most cases infection is asymptomatic or causes mild diarrhea, especially with organisms of the El Tor biotype; asymptomatic carriers can transmit the infection. In severe dehydrated cases (cholera gravis), death may occur within a few hours, and the case-fatality rate may exceed 50%. With proper and timely rehydration, this can be less than 1%.

Diagnosis is confirmed by isolating *Vibrio cholerae* of the serogroup O1 or O139 from feces. Ideally, in cases of sporadic infection, clinical isolates of *V. cholerae* O1 and O139 should be tested for the presence of the cholera toxin gene. Strains of *V. cholerae* O1 or O139 that do not possess cholera toxin can cause acute watery diarrhea, but do not cause cholera or epidemic disease. *V. cholerae* grows well on standard culture media, but the use of selective media, such as thiosulfate citrate bile-salts (TCBS) agar, is recommended. The strains are further characterized by O1 and O139 specific antisera. Strains that agglutinate in O1 antisera are further characterized for serotype. If laboratory facilities are not nearby or immediately available, Cary Blair transport medium can be used to transport or store a fecal or rectal swab. For clinical purposes, a quick presumptive diagnosis can be made by darkfield or phase microscopic visualization of the vibrios moving like "shooting stars," inhibited by preservative-free, serotype-specific antiserum. For epidemiological purposes, a presumptive diagnosis can be based on the demonstration of a significant rise in titer of anti-cholera toxin or vibriocidal antibodies. In nonendemic areas, organisms isolated from initial suspected cases should be confirmed in a reference laboratory through appropriate biochemical and serological reactions, and by testing the organisms for cholera toxin production or for the presence of cholera toxin genes. One-step dipstick tests for rapid detection of *V. cholerae* O1 and O139 are available on the market, and have shown promise in initial field evaluations; however, these tests do not yield isolates for subtyping or antimicrobial resistance testing that may be useful for epidemiologic and treatment decisions. In epidemics, once laboratory confirmation and antibiotic sensitivity have been established, it is unnecessary to confirm all subsequent cases. Shift should be made to primary use of proposed WHO clinical case definitions, as follows:

- Disease unknown in area: severe dehydration or death from acute watery diarrhea in a patient aged 5 or more
- Endemic cholera: acute watery diarrhea with or without vomiting in a patient aged 5 or more
- Epidemic cholera: acute watery diarrhea with or without vomiting in any patient.

However, monitoring an epidemic should include laboratory confirmation and antimicrobial sensitivity testing of a small proportion of cases on a regular basis.

2. Infectious agent—Only *Vibrio cholerae* serogroups O1 and O139 are associated with the epidemiological characteristics of cholera. Serogroup O1 occurs as two biotypes—classical and El Tor—each of which occurs as three serotypes (Inaba, Ogawa and, rarely, Hikojima). The clinical illness caused by *V. cholerae* O1 of either biotype and by *V. cholerae* O139 is similar because these organisms elaborate an almost identical enterotoxin. In any single epidemic, one particular serogroup and biotype tends to be dominant, but serogroup switching is common. The current seventh pandemic is characterized by the O1 serogroup El Tor biotype, *V. cholerae* O1. The classical biotype has not been diagnosed outside of south Asia in many years, and *V. cholerae* O139 remains confined to South East Asia.

Before 1992, non-O1 strains were recognized as causing sporadic cases and rare outbreaks of diarrheal disease, but were not associated with large epidemics. However, in 1992–1993, large-scale epidemics of cholera-like disease were reported in India and Bangladesh, caused by a new organism, *V. cholerae* serogroup O139. This organism elaborates the same cholera toxin but differs from O1 strains in lipopolysaccharide (LPS) structure and in the production of capsular antigen. The clinical and epidemiological picture of illness it causes is typical of cholera, and cases should be reported as such. The epidemic O139 strain, which possesses the virulence factors of *V. cholerae* O1 El Tor, was apparently derived by a deletion in the genes that encode the O1 lipopolysaccharide antigen of an El Tor strain, followed by the acquisition of a large fragment of new DNA encoding the enzymes that allow synthesis of O139 lipopolysaccharide and capsule.

The reporting as cholera of illness due to non-O1 or non-O139 serogroups of *V. cholerae* is inaccurate and leads to confusion, even if these strains do possess the cholera toxin gene.

3. Occurrence—Cholera is one of the oldest and best-understood epidemic diseases. Epidemics and pandemics are strongly linked to the consumption of unsafe water and food, poor hygiene, poor sanitation and crowded living conditions. Conditions leading to epidemics exist in many developing countries where cholera is either endemic or a recurring problem in a large number of areas. Typical settings for cholera are peri-urban slums where basic urban infrastructure is missing. Outbreaks of cholera can also occur on a seasonal basis in endemic areas of Asia and Africa. In 2000–2001, for example, KwaZulu-Natal, South Africa experienced an outbreak that resulted in more than 125 000 cases with a low case fatality rate of less than 0.5%—a low rate that had never previously been observed in an outbreak of that magnitude.

Man-made or natural disasters such as complex emergencies and floods resulting in population movements and overcrowded refugee camps are potentially fertile ground for explosive outbreaks with high case fatality rates. In July 1994, an outbreak of *V. cholerae* El Tor among Rwandan refugees in Goma, Democratic Republic of Congo (DRC), resulted in more than 50 000 cases and 24 000 deaths over the course of little more than one month.

In 2006, 52 countries reported 236 896 cases of cholera and 6 311 deaths to WHO—an overall case fatality rate of 2.7%. These numbers represent a 76% increase in reported cases compared to 2005, and were the highest numbers reported since the late 1990s. Approximately 99% of all reported cases and all but a very few deaths were in sub-Saharan Africa. Reported case fatality rates by country ranged from 0 to 9%. Globally, actual numbers of cholera cases and deaths are likely to be much higher because of underreporting and poor surveillance.

During the 19th century, cholera spread repeatedly, through 6 pandemic waves, from the Gulf of Bengal to most of the world. During the first half of the 20th century, the disease was confined largely to Asia, except for a severe epidemic in Egypt in 1947. During the latter half of the 20th century, the epidemiology of cholera has been marked by: (1) the global spread of the seventh pandemic of cholera caused by *V. cholerae* O1 El Tor; (2) the recognition of environmental reservoirs of cholera, such as on the shore of the Gulf of Bengal and along the US coast of the Gulf of Mexico; and (3) the appearance for the first time of large explosive epidemics of cholera caused by *V. cholerae* organisms of a serogroup other than O1 (*V. cholerae* O139).

During the current (seventh) pandemic, which started in 1961, *V. cholerae* of the El Tor biotype spread worldwide from Indonesia, reaching the Asian mainland in 1963, and Africa in 1970, where it has remained endemic in many countries. Cholera reached Latin America in 1991 after nearly a century of absence, causing explosive epidemics along the Pacific coast of Peru and in many countries— by 1994, approximately one million cholera cases had been recorded in Latin America. Although the clinical disease was as severe as in other regions of the world, the overall case fatality rate in Latin America was low, at 1%, except in highly rural areas in the Andes and Amazon region where patients were often far from medical care.

In late 1992, the new serogroup of *V. cholerae* designated O139 Bengal emerged in Southern India and Bangladesh and spread rapidly throughout the region over the next few months, infecting several hundred thousand persons. During this epidemic period, *V. cholerae* O139 almost completely replaced *V. cholerae* O1 strains in hospitalized cholera patients and in samples of surface water. The epidemic continued to spread through 1994, with cases of O139 cholera reported from 11 countries in Asia. This new strain was soon introduced to other continents by infected travelers, but secondary spread outside of Asia has not been reported and *V. cholerae* O139 remains confined at time of writing to the southeastern areas of the Asian continent. It is not known whether this new strain has the potential to generate a new pandemic; however, the earlier explosive spread through Asia suggests that continued international surveillance is warranted.

Cases of cholera are regularly imported into industrialized countries. Several prospective studies using optimized bacteriological methods (TCBS medium) have shown that the incidence of traveler's cholera in travelers from industrialized countries is considerably higher than previously estimated. However, safe water and adequate sanitation limit the potential for outbreaks, and secondary transmission in developed countries is exceedingly rare.

Since 1973, the occurrence of laboratory and sporadic cases in the Gulf coast area of the USA, all due to a single indigenous strain, has led to the identification of an environmental reservoir of *V. cholerae* O1 El Tor Inaba in the Gulf of Mexico.

4. Reservoir—The main reservoir is humans. Observations in Australia, Bangladesh and the USA have shown that environmental reservoirs exist, apparently in association with copepods or other zooplankton in brackish water or estuaries.

5. Mode of transmission—Cholera is acquired through ingestion of an infective dose of contaminated food or water and can be transmitted through many mechanisms. Water is usually contaminated by feces of infected individuals and can itself contaminate, directly or through the contamination of food. Contamination of drinking water usually occurs at source, during transportation, or during storage at home. Food may also be contaminated by soiled hands, during preparation, or while eating. In funeral ceremonies transmission may occur through consumption of food and beverages prepared by family members after they handled the corpse for burial. *V. cholerae* O1 and O139 can persist in water for long periods and multiply in moist leftover food.

Beverages prepared with contaminated water and sold by street vendors, ice and even commercial bottled water have been incriminated as vehicles in cholera transmission, as have cooked vegetables and fruit "freshened" with untreated wastewater have also served as vehicles of transmission. Outbreaks or epidemics as well as sporadic cases are often attributed to raw or undercooked seafood. In other instances, sporadic cases of cholera follow the ingestion of raw or inadequately cooked seafood from non-polluted waters. Cases have been traced to eating shellfish from coastal and estuarine waters where a natural reservoir of

V. cholerae O1, serotype Inaba, exists in an estuarine environment not characterized by sewage contamination. Clinical cholera in endemic areas is usually confined to the lowest socioeconomic groups.

6. Incubation period—From a few hours to 5 days, usually 2–3 days.

7. Period of communicability—As long as stools are positive, usually only a few days after recovery. Occasionally the carrier state may persist for several months. Antibiotics known to be effective against the infecting strains (e.g. tetracycline or doxycycline) shorten the period of communicability, but are recommended only for treatment of severely ill patients. Rarely, chronic biliary infection lasting for years, associated with intermittent shedding of vibrios in the stool, has been observed in adults.

8. Susceptibility—Variable; gastric achlorhydria increases the risk of illness, and breastfed infants are protected. Severe cholera occurs significantly more often among persons with blood group O. Infection with either *V. cholerae* O1 or O139 results in a rise in agglutinating and antitoxic antibodies, and increased resistance to reinfection. Serum vibriocidal antibodies, which are readily detected following O1 infection, are the best immunological correlate of protection against O1 cholera, but comparably specific, sensitive and reliable assays are not available for O139 infection. Field studies show that an initial clinical infection by *V. cholerae* O1 of the classical biotype confers protection against either classical or El Tor biotypes; in contrast an initial clinical infection caused by biotype El Tor results in only a modest level of long-term protection that is limited to El Tor infections. In endemic areas, most people acquire antibodies by early adulthood. However, infection with O1 strains affords no protection against O139 infection, and vice-versa. In experimental challenge studies in volunteers, an initial clinical infection due to *V. cholerae* O139 conferred significant protection against diarrhea upon re-challenge with *V. cholerae* O139.

9. Methods of control—

   A. Preventive measures:

   1) See Typhoid fever, 9A, 1–10.
   2) Traditional injectable cholera vaccines based on killed whole cell microorganisms provide only partial protection (50% efficacy) of short duration (3–6 months), do not prevent asymptomatic infection, and are associated with adverse effects. Their use has never been recommended by WHO, and they are no longer available in most countries.

   Two oral cholera vaccines (OCV) that are safe and which provide significant protection for several months against cholera caused by O1 strains have been licensed in many countries. OCVs are mainly used by travelers from industrialized countries. The first is a single-dose live vaccine (strain

CVD 103-HgR) which, although licensed, is not currently available, as the manufacturer ceased production in 2004. The second is a killed vaccine consisting of inactivated vibrios plus B-subunit of the cholera toxin, given on a 2-dose regimen. As of mid-2008, these vaccines were not licensed in the USA. A third killed whole-cell oral cholera vaccine containing no B-subunit has been produced via technology-transfer to Vietnam, though this vaccine is currently only licensed for use in that country.

A 2003–2004 mass vaccination trial in Mozambique showed that OCVs are effective in preventing cholera in the short-term in African populations with a high prevalence of HIV infection, and that large-scale vaccination campaigns are feasible. Additional questions, such as the duration of protection and cost-effectiveness, remain to be answered before widespread vaccination can be widely recommended. It has been suggested that herd immunity can be achieved with a 50–70% OCV coverage rate, a finding that—if supported by future observations in the field—would further support a scaling up of OCV use in endemic areas.

3) Measures that inhibit or otherwise compromise the movement of people, foods or other goods are not epidemiologically justified and have never proved effective to control cholera.

B. Control of patient, contacts and the immediate environment:

1) Report to local health authority: Case report is no longer routinely required by the International Health Regulations [2005] (see sections on *Reporting* and on the *IHR (2005)*); but the Regulations do make obligatory the reporting of outbreaks that have public health impact, are unusual or unexpected, or which pose a threat of international spread or trade or travel restrictions.

2) Isolation: Hospitalization with enteric precautions is desirable for severely ill patients; strict isolation is not necessary. Less severe cases can be managed on an outpatient basis with oral rehydration. An appropriate antimicrobial agent can be administered to decrease the likelihood of further spread, but antimicrobials are clinically indicated for severe cases only as their injudicious use fosters the development of antimicrobial resistant strains. Cholera wards can be operated even when crowded without hazard to staff and visitors, provided standard procedures are observed for hand washing and cleanliness and for the circulation of staff and visitors. Fly control should be practiced.

3) Concurrent disinfection: Of feces and vomit and of linens and articles used by patients, using heat, carbolic acid or other

disinfectant. In communities with a modern and adequate sewage disposal system, feces can be discharged directly into the sewers without preliminary disinfection.

4) Quarantine: Not applicable. WHO does not advise routine screening or quarantine of travelers coming from cholera affected areas. For more information, please see the WHO statement relating to international travel and trade to and from countries experiencing outbreaks of cholera, which can be found at:

<http://www.who.int/cholera/choleratravelandtradeadvice 161107.pdf>

5) Management of contacts: Surveillance of persons who shared food and drink with a cholera patient for 5 days from last exposure. Chemoprophylaxis is rarely advisable—often by the time it can be delivered to contacts of an individual case, the targeted individuals have either already acquired the infection, or have little chance of acquiring it from the case in question. However, chemoprophylaxis of institutionalized populations, such as those in jail, which are rapidly accessible following the identification of an index case, has been successfully accomplished. The same antimicrobials used for treatment can be used for chemoprophylaxis, with attention to the resistance patterns of circulating strains. Mass chemoprophylaxis of whole communities is never indicated, as it is a waste of resources and can quickly lead to antibiotic resistance.

6) Investigation of contacts and source of infection: Investigate possibilities of infection from polluted drinking water and contaminated food. Meal companions for the 5 days prior to onset should be interviewed. A search by stool culture for unreported cases is recommended only among household members or those exposed to a possible common source in a previously uninfected area.

7) Specific treatment: The cornerstone of cholera treatment is timely and adequate rehydration. Patients presenting mild dehydration can be treated successfully by oral rehydration solutions (ORS) therapy. Only severely dehydrated patients need rehydration through intravenous routes to repair fluid and electrolyte loss through diarrhea. As rehydration therapy becomes increasingly effective, patients who survive hypovolemic shock and severe dehydration may manifest certain complications, such as hypoglycemia, that must be recognized and treated promptly.

Most patients with mild or moderate fluid loss can be treated entirely with oral rehydration solutions that contain:

glucose 75 mmol/L; NaCl 75 mmol/L; KCl 20 mmol/L; and trisodium citrate dihydrate 10 mmol/L. This new formula of ORS was approved by a WHO expert committee in June 2002; it has a total osmolarity of 245 mOsm/L and is particularly effective for treatment of children with acute non-cholera diarrhea in both developing and industrialized areas. Mild and moderate volume depletion should be corrected with oral solutions, replacing over 4–6 hours a volume matching the estimated fluid loss (approximately 5% of body weight for mild dehydration and 7% for moderate dehydration). Continuing losses are replaced by giving, over 4 hours, a volume of oral solution equal to 1.5 times the stool volume lost in the previous 4 hours. In children, daily supplementation with 30mg elemental zinc during illness has been shown to reduce both duration and severity of cholera.

Severely dehydrated patients or patients in shock should be given rapid IV rehydration with a balanced multi-electrolyte solution containing approximately 130 mEq/L of Na+, 25 48 mEq/L of bicarbonate, acetate or lactate ions, and 10 15 mEq/L of K+. Useful solutions include Ringer lactate (4 grams NaCl, 1 gram KCl, 6.5 grams sodium acetate and 8 grams glucose/L), and "Dacca solution" (5 grams NaCl, 4 grams NaHCO3 and 1 gram KCl/L), which can be prepared locally in an emergency. The initial fluid replacement should be 30 mL/kg in the first hour for infants and in the first 30 minutes for persons over 1 year, after which the patient should be reassessed. After circulatory collapse has been effectively reversed, most patients can continue on oral rehydration to complete the 10% initial fluid deficit replacement and to match continuing fluid loss.

In severe cases, appropriate antimicrobial agents can shorten the duration of diarrhea, reduce the volume of rehydration solutions required, and shorten the duration of vibrio excretion. Adults are given a single 300 mg dose of doxycycline, or tetracycline 500 mg 4 times a day for 3 days. Children may be given 12.5 mg/kg of tetracycline 4 times daily, for 3 days (there is little risk of dental staining with short course tetracycline treatment). Where tetracycline-resistant strains of *V. cholerae* are prevalent, alternative antimicrobial regimens include furazolidone (100 mg 4 times daily for adults and 1.25 mg/kg 4 times daily for children, for 3 days); or erythromycin (250 mg 4 times daily for adults and 30 mg/kg 4 times daily for children, for 3 days). Ciprofloxacin, 250 mg once daily for 3 days, is also a useful regimen for adults. *V. cholerae* O1 and O139 strains are often resistant to cotrimoxazole or trimethoprim-sulfamet. Since individual strains of *V. cholerae* O1 or O139 may be resistant to any of these antimicrobials, knowledge of the sensitivity of local strains to these agents, if available, should always be used to guide the choice of antimicrobial therapy.

C. Epidemic measures:

1) Educate the population at risk concerning the need to seek appropriate treatment without delay.
2) Provide effective treatment facilities.
3) Adopt emergency measures to ensure a safe water supply. Chlorinate public water supplies, even if the source water appears uncontaminated. Chlorinate or boil water used for drinking, cooking and washing dishes and food containers, unless the water supply is adequately chlorinated and subsequently protected from contamination. Households that store drinking water should ensure that protective storage containers are used to prevent recontamination of treated water by hands or objects during storage.
4) Ensure careful preparation and supervision of food and drinks. After cooking or boiling, protect against contamination by flies and unsanitary handling; leftover foods should be thoroughly reheated (70°C/158°F for at least 15 minutes) before ingestion. Persons with diarrhea should not prepare food or haul water for others. Food served at funerals of cholera victims may be particularly hazardous if the body has been prepared for burial by the participants without stringent precautions; this practice should be discouraged during epidemics.
5) Initiate a thorough investigation designed to find the predominant vehicle(s) of infection and circumstances (time, place, and person) of transmission, and plan control measures accordingly.
6) Provide appropriate safe facilities for sewage disposal.
7) Parenteral whole cell vaccine is not recommended.
8) Oral cholera vaccines can be used as an additional public health tool, but should not replace other recommended control measures, or detract from surveillance or clinical management of cases. The use of the currently available OCV is not recommended in populations currently experiencing an outbreak, due to the time required to administer—and receive full immunologic benefits from—the 2-dose regimen, and the heavy financial and logistical requirements.

D. Disaster implications:

Outbreak risks are high in endemic areas if large groups of people are crowded together without sufficient quantities of safe water, adequate food handling, or sanitary facilities.

E. International measures:

1) Governments are required to report cholera cases due to *V. cholerae* O1 and O139, and outbreaks or epidemics of acute watery diarrhea, to WHO when they are unusual or unexpected, or when they present significant risk of international spread or of international travel or trade restrictions (International Health regulations 2005).

2) Measures applicable to ships, aircraft and land transport arriving from cholera areas are to be applied within the framework of the revised *International Health Regulations* (2005).

3) International travelers: No country is authorized under the International Health Regulations 2005 to require proof of cholera vaccination as a condition of entry, and the International Certificate of Vaccination no longer provides a specific space for the recording of cholera vaccination. Immunization with either of the new oral vaccines can be recommended for individuals from industrialized countries traveling to areas of endemic or epidemic cholera. As of mid-2008, no cholera vaccines are licensed and available in the United States. In countries where the new oral vaccines are already licensed, immunization may be particularly recommended for travelers with known risk factors such as hypochlorhydria (consequent to partial gastrectomy or medication) or cardiac disease (e.g. arrhythmia), and for the elderly or individuals of blood group O.

4) Further information can be found at:
   <http://www.who.int/csr/disease/cholera>
   In addition, WHO Collaborating Centres provide support as required. More information can be found at:
   <http://www.who.int/collaboratingcentres/database/en/>

II. VIBRIO CHOLERAE SEROGROUPS OTHER THAN O1 AND O139   ICD-9 005.8; ICD-10 A05.8

1. Identification—Of the more than 200 *V. cholerae* serogroups that exist, only O1 and O139 are associated with the clinical syndrome of cholera and can cause large epidemics. Organisms of *V. cholerae* serogroups other than O1 and O139 have been associated with sporadic cases of gastroenteritis, but have not spread in epidemic form. They have been associated with wound infection and also, rarely, isolated from patients (usually immunocompromised hosts) with septicemic disease.

2. Infectious agent—*V. cholerae* pathogens of serogroups other than O1 and O139. Serogroups of *V. cholerae* have been defined on the basis of their surface antigen (lipopolysaccharide O antigen). *Vibrio*s formerly known as non-agglutinable vibrios [NAGs] or non-cholera vibrios [NCVs] are now included in the species *V. cholerae*. Some strains elaborate cholera enterotoxin, but most do not.

As with all *V. cholerae*, growth is enhanced in an environment of 1% NaCl. Rarely do non-O1/non-O139 *V. cholerae* strains elaborate cholera toxin or harbor the colonization factors of O1 and O139 epidemic strains. Some non-O1/non-O139 strains produce a heat-stable enterotoxin (so-called NAG-ST). Epidemiological and volunteer challenge studies have documented the pathogenicity of strains producing NAG-ST. The non-O1/non-O139 strains isolated from blood of septicemic patients have been heavily encapsulated.

The reporting of non-toxinogenic *V. cholerae* O1, or of non-O1/non-O139 *V. cholerae* infections, as cholera is inaccurate and leads to confusion.

3. Occurrence—Non-O1/non-O139 *V. cholerae* strains are associated with 2%–3% of cases (including travelers) of diarrheal illness in tropical developing countries. Isolation rates are higher in coastal areas. Most non-O1 non-O139 *V. cholerae* are of little public health importance.

4. Reservoir—Non-O1/non-O139 *V. cholerae* are found in aquatic environments worldwide, particularly in mildly brackish waters, where they constitute indigenous flora. Although halophilic, they can also proliferate in fresh water (e.g. lakes). *Vibrio* counts vary according to the season, and peak in warm seasons. In brackish waters they are found adherent to chitinous zooplankton and shellfish. Isolates of *V. cholerae* other than O1 and O139 are able to survive and multiply in a variety of foodstuffs.

5. Mode of transmission—Cases of non-O1/non-O139 gastroenteritis are usually linked to consumption of raw or undercooked seafood, particularly shellfish. In tropical endemic areas, some infections may be due to ingestion of surface waters. Wound infections arise from environmental exposure, usually to brackish water, or from occupational accidents among professions such as fishermen and shellfish harvesters. In high-risk hosts, septicemia may result from a wound infection or from ingestion of contaminated seafood.

6. Incubation period—Short, 12–24 hours with an average of 10 hours in experimental challenge of volunteers (range 5.5–96 hours).

7. Period of communicability—It is not known whether in nature these infections can be transmitted from person to person or by humans contaminating vehicles such as food. If the latter does occur, the period of potential communicability is likely to be limited to the period of vibrio excretion, usually several days.

8. **Susceptibility**—All humans are believed to be susceptible to gastroenteritis if they ingest a sufficient number of non-O1/non-O139 *V. cholerae* in an appropriate food vehicle, or to developing a wound infection if the wound is exposed to vibrio-containing water or shellfish. Septicemia develops most commonly in hosts who are immunocompromised, have chronic liver disease or severe malnutrition.

9. **Methods of control**—

   A. *Preventive measures:*

   1) Educate consumers about the risks associated with eating seafood unless it has been irradiated or cooked for 15 minutes at 70°C/158°F.
   2) Educate seafood handlers and processors on the following preventive measures:

      a) Ensure that cooked seafood reaches temperatures adequate to kill the organism by heating for 15 minutes at 70°C/158°F (organisms may survive at 60°C/140°F for up to 15 minutes and at 80°C/176°F for several minutes).
      b) Handle cooked seafood in a manner that precludes contamination from raw seafood or contaminated seawater.
      c) Keep all seafood, raw and cooked, adequately refrigerated before eating.
      d) Avoid use of seawater in food handling areas, e.g. on cruise ships.

   B., C. and D. *Control of patient, contacts and immediate environment; Epidemic measures* and *Disaster implications:* See Staphylococcal food intoxication (section I, 9B except for B2, 9C and 9D).

   Isolation: Enteric precautions. Report to local health authority. Reporting mandatory in some areas. Recognition and report of outbreaks associated with common seafood are of particular importance.

   Patients with liver disease or who are immunosuppressed (because of treatment or underlying disease) and alcoholics should be warned not to eat raw seafood. When disease occurs in these individuals, a history of eating seafood and—especially—the presence of bullous skin lesions justify early institution of antibiotic therapy, with a combination of oral minocycline (100 mg every 12 h) and intravenous cefotaxime (2 grams every 8 h) as the treatment regimen of choice. Tetracyclines and ciprofloxacin are also effective.

III. *VIBRIO PARAHAEMOLYTICUS*
ENTERITIS   ICD-9 005.4; ICD-10 A05.3
(*Vibrio parahaemolyticus* infection)

1. Identification—An intestinal disorder characterized by watery diarrhea and abdominal cramps in nearly all cases, usually with nausea, vomiting, fever and headache. About one quarter of patients experience a dysentery-like illness with bloody or mucoid stools, high fever, and high WBC count. Typically, it is a disease of moderate severity lasting 1–7 days; systemic infection and death rarely occur.

Diagnosis is confirmed by isolating *Vibrio parahaemolyticus* from the patient's stool on appropriate media (typically TCBS media).

2. Infectious agent—*Vibrio parahaemolyticus*, a halophilic vibrio. More than a dozen different O antigen groups and approximately 60 different K antigen types have been identified. Clinical isolates from humans are generally (but not always) capable of producing a characteristic hemolytic reaction (the "Kanagawa phenomenon"). Newer methods use DNA gene probes for a thermostable direct hemolysin (TDH) and thermostable direct related hemolysin (TRH) in order to determine virulence.

3. Occurrence—Sporadic cases and common-source outbreaks have been reported in many parts of the world, particularly Japan, southeastern Asia and the USA. Several large foodborne outbreaks have occurred in the USA in which undercooked seafood was the food vehicle; consumption of raw or undercooked clams or oysters is often implicated in individual cases. Cases occur primarily in warm months.

4. Reservoir—Marine coastal environs are the natural habitat. During the cold season, organisms are found in marine silt; during the warm season, they are found free in coastal waters and in fish and shellfish.

5. Mode of transmission—Ingestion of raw or inadequately cooked seafood, or any food contaminated by handling raw seafood, or by rinsing with contaminated water.

6. Incubation period—Usually between 12 and 24 hours, but can range from 4 to 96 hours.

7. Period of communicability—Not normally communicable from person to person (except fecal-oral transmission).

8. Susceptibility—Most people are probably susceptible, especially those with liver disease, decreased gastric acidity, diabetes, peptic ulcers, or immunosuppression.

9. **Methods of control—**

    A. ***Preventive measures:*** See *non toxigenic V. cholerae* infections; monitor shellfish and coastal waters for pathogenic *V. parahaemolyticus*.

    B., C. and D. ***Control of patient, contacts and immediate environment; Epidemic measures*** and ***Disaster implications:*** See Staphylococcal food intoxication (section I, 9C and 9D).

    Isolation: Enteric precautions. Report to local health authority. Obligatory case report, class 2B. Recognition and reporting of cases associated with recent shellfish consumption is especially important for trace back investigations.

    1) Specific treatment: Rehydration as appropriate. If septicemia occurs, effective antimicrobials (aminoglycosides, third-generation cephalosporins, fluoroquinolones, tetracycline).

IV. INFECTION WITH *VIBRIO VULNIFICUS*   ICD-9 005.8; ICD-10 A05.8

1. **Identification**—Infection with *Vibrio vulnificus* produces septicemia in persons with chronic liver disease, chronic alcoholism or hemochromatosis, or those who are immunosuppressed. The disease appears 12 hours to 3 days after eating raw or undercooked seafood, especially oysters. One-third of patients are in shock when they present for care or develop hypotension within 12 hours of hospital admission. Three-quarters of patients have distinctive bullous skin lesions; thrombocytopenia is common and there is often evidence of disseminated intravascular coagulation. Over 50% of patients with primary septicemia die; case-fatality rate exceeds 90% among those who become hypotensive. *V. vulnificus* can also infect wounds sustained in coastal or estuarine waters; wounds range from mild, self-limited lesions to rapidly progressive cellulitis and myositis that can mimic clostridial myonecrosis in rapidity of spread and destructiveness.

2. **Infectious agent**—A halophilic, usually lactose-positive (85% of isolates) marine *Vibrio* that is biochemically quite similar to *V. parahaemolyticus*. Confirmation of species identity sometimes requires use of DNA probes or numerical taxonomy in a reference laboratory. *V. vulnificus* expresses a polysaccharide capsule, of which there are multiple antigenic types on its surface.

3. **Occurrence**—*V. vulnificus* infection has been reported in many areas of the world—e.g. Israel, Japan, the Republic of Korea, Spain, Taiwan (China) and Turkey—and is the most common agent of serious infections caused by *Vibrio* species in north America. The annual inci-

dence of *V. vulnificus* in the USA is about 0.5 cases per 100 000 population, with the areas surrounding the Gulf of Mexico having the highest rates at about 1.0 cases per 100 000. Approximately two-thirds of cases in these Gulf state areas are primary septicemia.

4. Reservoir—*V. vulnificus* is a free-living autochthonous element of flora of estuarine environments. It is recovered from estuarine waters and from shellfish, particularly oysters. During warm summer months it can be isolated routinely from most cultured oysters.

5. Mode of transmission—Infection is acquired through ingestion of raw or undercooked seafood, after exposure of wounds to estuarine water (e.g. in boating accidents), or from occupational wounds (in oyster shuckers, fishermen, and so on).

6. Incubation period—Usually 12 to 72 hours after eating raw or undercooked seafood.

7. Period of communicability—This is not considered to be an infection that is transmitted directly from person to person.

8. Susceptibility—Persons with cirrhosis, hemochromatosis and other chronic liver disease, and immunocompromised hosts (from either underlying disease or medication), are at increased risk for the septicemic form of disease. For the period 1981–1992 the annual incidence of *V. vulnificus* illness among adults with liver disease in Florida, USA who ate raw oysters was 7.2 per 100 000, versus 0.09 for adults without known liver disease.

9. Methods of control—

    A. Preventive measures: The same as those for prevention of non-O1/non-O139 *V. cholerae* infections.

V. INFECTION WITH OTHER VIBRIOS   ICD-9 005.8; ICD-10 A05.8

Infection with certain other *Vibrio* species has been associated with sporadic cases of diarrheal disease and rarely with outbreaks. These include *V. cholerae* of serogroups other than O1 and O139, *V. mimicus* (some strains elaborate an enterotoxin indistinguishable from that produced by *V. cholerae* O1 and O139), *V. fluvialis*, *V. furnissii*, and *V. hollisae*. Septicemic disease in hosts with underlying liver disease, severe malnutrition or immunocompetence has, rarely, been associated with *V. hollisae*. *V. alginolyticus* and *V. damsela* have been associated with wound infections.

CHROMOBLASTOMYCOSIS

CHROMOMYCOSIS   ICD-9 117.2; ICD-10 B43
(Dermatitis verrucosa)
[CCDM19: M. Brandt, A. Gabrielli, L. Savioli]
[CCDM18: L. Savioli]

1. **Identification**—A chronic spreading mycosis of the skin and subcutaneous tissues, usually of the lower extremities, although other areas can be involved. The initial lesion appears as a papule or a nodule. Progression to contiguous tissues is slow, over a period of years, with eventual large, nodular, verrucous or even cauliflower-like masses. Invasion to muscle or bone can occur, although disseminated disease is rare. Rarely is a cause of death.

Microscopic examination of scrapings or biopsies from lesions shows characteristic muriform cells—large, brown, thick-walled rounded cells that divide by fission in two planes. Confirmation of diagnosis should be made by biopsy and attempted cultures of the fungus.

2. **Infectious agents**—*Fonsecaea* (*Phialophora*) *pedrosoi, Phialophora verrucosa, Cladosporium carrionii, Rhinocladiella aquaspersa, Botryomyces caespitatus, Exophiala spinifera* and *E. jeanselmei.*

3. **Occurrence**—Worldwide; sporadic cases in widely scattered areas, but mainly southern USA, central America, Latin America, Caribbean islands, South Pacific islands, Africa (including Madagascar), Australia, and Japan. Primarily a disease of barefoot rural agricultural workers in tropical regions, probably due to frequent traumatic inoculation. The disease is most common among men aged 30–50 years.

4. **Reservoir**—Wood, soil and decaying vegetation.

5. **Mode of transmission**—Minor penetrating trauma, usually a sliver of contaminated wood or other material.

6. **Incubation period**—Unknown; probably months.

7. **Period of communicability**—Not transmitted from person to person.

8. **Susceptibility**—Unknown; rarity of disease and absence of laboratory-acquired infections suggest that humans are relatively resistant.

9. **Methods of control**—

    A. ***Preventive measures:*** Protect against small puncture wounds by wearing shoes or protective clothing.

B. Control of patient, contacts and the immediate environment:

1) Report to local health authority: Official report not ordinarily justifiable, Class 5 (see *Reporting*).
2) Isolation: Not applicable.
3) Concurrent disinfection: Of discharges from lesions and articles soiled therewith.
4) Quarantine: Not applicable.
5) Immunization of contacts: Not applicable.
6) Investigation of contacts and source of infection: Not indicated.
7) Specific treatment: No guidelines exist; chromomycosis is not easy to cure medically, and multiple long-term treatment approaches are often used. Itraconazole is currently the most effective antifungal agent, but its effectiveness appears to depend on the etiologic agent. Terbinafine or terbinafine plus itraconazole have also been used in some patients. Oral flucytosine has been shown to benefit some patients, but relapse and development of resistance have been common. Oral 5-fluorocytosine or itraconazole benefit some patients. Large lesions may respond better when flucytosine is combined with amphotericin B IV. Voriconazole has also shown some efficacy. Small lesions are sometimes cured by surgical excision or cryotherapy.

C. Epidemic measures: Not applicable; a sporadic disease.

D. Disaster implications: None.

E. International measures: None.

CLONORCHIASIS   ICD-9 121.1; ICD-10 B66.1
(Chinese or oriental liver fluke disease)
[CDDM19: Editorial Board]
[CCDM18: D. Engels]

1. Identification—A trematode disease of the bile ducts. Clinical complaints may be slight or absent in light infections; symptoms result from local irritation of bile ducts by the flukes. Loss of appetite, diarrhea and a sensation of abdominal pressure are common early symptoms. Rarely, bile duct obstruction producing jaundice may be followed by cirrhosis, enlargement and tenderness of the liver, with progressive ascites and edema. Clonorchiasis is a chronic disease, sometimes of 30 years duration or longer, but rarely a direct or contributing cause of death, and it is often completely asymptomatic. However, it is a significant risk factor for development of cholangiocarcinoma.

Diagnosis is made by finding the characteristic eggs in feces or duodenal drainage fluid, to be differentiated from those of other flukes. Serological diagnosis by ELISA can be performed, but is not always specific. "Antigenic cocktails" for serodiagnosis are under development at time of writing.

2. Infectious agent—*Clonorchis sinensis*, the Chinese liver fluke.

3. Occurrence—Present throughout China (including Taiwan), except in northwestern areas, and highly endemic in southeastern China; occurs in Japan (rarely), the Republic of Korea, Viet Nam and probably in Cambodia and Lao Democratic Republic, principally in the Mekong River delta. In other parts of the world, imported cases may be recognized in immigrants from Asia. In most endemic areas, highest prevalence is among adults over the age of 30.

4. Reservoir—Humans, cats, dogs, swine, rats and other animals.

5. Mode of transmission—People are infected by eating raw or undercooked freshwater fish containing encysted larvae. During digestion, larvae are freed from cysts and migrate via the common bile duct to biliary radicles. Eggs deposited in the bile passages are evacuated in feces. Eggs in feces contain fully developed miracidia; when ingested by a susceptible operculate snail (e.g. *Parafossarulus*), they hatch in its intestine, penetrate the tissues, and asexually generate larvae (cercariae) that emerge into the water. On contact with a second intermediate host (about 110 species of freshwater fish belonging mostly to the family Cyprinidae), cercariae penetrate the host fish and encyst, usually in muscle, occasionally on the underside of scales. The complete life cycle, from person to snail to fish to person, requires at least 3 months.

6. Incubation period—Unpredictable, as it varies with the number of worms present; flukes reach maturity within 1 month after encysted larvae are ingested.

7. Period of communicability—Infected individuals may pass viable eggs for as long as 30 years; infection is not directly transmitted from person to person.

8. Susceptibility and resistance—Susceptibility is universal.

9. Methods of control—

    A. Preventive measures:

        1) Thoroughly cook or irradiate all freshwater fish, or freeze at −10°C (14°F) for at least 5 days. Storage of fish for several weeks in a saturated salt solution has been recommended, but effectiveness remains unproven.

2) In endemic areas, educate the public to the dangers of eating raw or improperly treated fish, and the necessity of sanitary disposal of feces to avoid contaminating sources of food fish. Prohibit disposal of night soil and animal waste (excreta) in fishponds.

B. Control of patient, contacts and the immediate environment:

1) Report to local health authority: Official report not ordinarily justifiable, Class 5 (see *Reporting*).
2) Isolation: Not applicable.
3) Concurrent disinfection: Sanitary disposal of feces.
4) Quarantine: Not applicable.
5) Immunization of contacts: Not applicable.
6) Investigation of contacts and source of infection: Of the individual case, not usually indicated. A community problem (see C).
7) Specific treatment: The drug of choice is praziquantel. Albendazole is under investigation.

C. Epidemic measures: Locate source of infected fish. Shipments of dried or pickled fish are the likely source in nonendemic areas, as are fresh or chilled freshwater fish brought from endemic areas.

D. Disaster implications: None.

E. International measures: Control of fish or fish products imported from endemic areas.

OPISTHORCHIASIS   ICD-9 121.0; ICD-10 B66.0

Opisthorchiasis is caused by small liver flukes of cats and some other fish-eating mammals. *Opisthorchis felineus* occurs in Europe and Asia, and has infected over 2 million people in Russia; *O. viverrini* is endemic in southeastern Asia, especially Thailand, where approximately 8 million infections have been reported. These worms are the leading cause of cholangiocarcinoma throughout the world; in northern Thailand, rates for the latter are as high as 85/10 000 population. The biology of these flatworms, the characteristics of the disease and methods of control are essentially the same as those for clonorchiasis. Eggs cannot be easily distinguished from those of *Clonorchis*.

COCCIDIOIDOMYCOSIS ICD-9 114; ICD-10 B38
(Valley fever, San Joaquin fever, Desert fever, Desert
rheumatism, Coccidioidal granuloma)
[CCDM19: M. Brandt]
[CCDM18: L. Severo]

1. **Identification**—The primary infection may be entirely asymptomatic or may resemble an acute influenza-like illness with fever, chills, cough, rash and (rarely) pleuritic pain. About 1 in 5 clinically recognized cases (an estimated 5% of all primary infections) develop erythema nodosum. Primary infection may heal completely without detectable sequelae; may leave fibrosis, a pulmonary nodule that may or may not have calcified areas; may leave a persistent thin-walled cavity; or, most rarely, may progress to the disseminated form of the disease.

Less than 1% of symptomatic coccidioidomycosis becomes disseminated. Disseminated coccidioidomycosis is a progressive, severe granulomatous disease characterized by lesions in nearly any part of the body, especially in subcutaneous tissues, skin, bone and meninges. Coccidioidal meningitis is a form of disseminated infection that can resemble tuberculous meningitis, but which runs a more chronic course. Disseminated infection is uniformly fatal without treatment.

Diagnosis is made through demonstration of characteristic coccidioidal spherules on microscopic examination, or through culture of sputum, pus, urine, CSF or biopsies of skin lesions or organs. Handling cultures of the agent is extremely hazardous and must be carried out in a class II biological safety cabinet under BSL-3 containment. Clinical specimens should be handled under BSL-2 containment. Precipitin and CF tests are usually positive within the first 3 months of clinical disease. The precipitin test detects IgM antibody, which appears 1–2 weeks after symptoms appear and persists for 3–4 months. Complement fixation tests detect mostly IgG antibody, which appears 1–2 months after clinical symptoms start and persists for 6–8 months. Serial serological tests may be helpful in monitoring response to therapy; serological tests may be negative in the immunocompromised.

2. **Infectious agent**—*Coccidioides immitis* and *posadasii*, dimorphic fungi. *Coccidioides* grow in soil and culture media as a saprophytic mold that reproduces by arthroconidia; in tissues and under special conditions, the parasitic form grows as spherical cells (spherules) that reproduce by formation of endospores.

3. **Occurrence**—Primary infections are common only in arid and semi-arid areas of the Western Hemisphere: in the USA, from central/southern California to southern Texas; northern Argentina; northeastern Brazil; Colombia; Mexico; Paraguay; Venezuela; and Central America. Dusty fomites from endemic areas can transmit infection. Disease has occurred in people who have merely traveled through endemic areas.

Infection is seasonal, and most frequent following rainy seasons during hot and dry periods, especially after wind and dust storms. Coccidioidomycosis is an important disease among persons with potential occupational exposure and those who are visiting or have moved into endemic areas. Since 1998, a marked increase of coccidioidomycosis has been reported in the largest endemic US states, California and Arizona.

The disease affects all ages and all races, although men and the elderly are most frequently affected. Persons at highest risk for disseminated infection include pregnant women in the third trimester, persons of African or Filipino race/ethnicity, and immunocompromised persons, especially those with HIV or an organ transplant.

4. Reservoir—Soil; especially in and around rodent burrows, in regions with appropriate temperature, moisture and soil requirements; infects humans, cattle, cats, dogs, horses, burros, sheep, swine, wild desert rodents, coyotes, chinchillas, llamas, and other animal species.

5. Mode of transmission—Inhalation of infective arthroconidia from soil and in laboratory accidents from cultures. While the parasitic form is normally not infective, accidental inoculation of infected pus or culture suspension into the skin or bone can result in granuloma formation.

6. Incubation period—In primary infection, 1 to 4 weeks. Dissemination may develop insidiously years after the primary infection, sometimes without recognized symptoms of primary pulmonary infection.

7. Period of communicability—No direct person-to-person or animal- to-human transmission. *Coccidioides* spp. from skin abscesses or fistulas may change, rarely, from the parasitic to the infective saprophytic form.

8. Susceptibility—*Coccidioides* is highly infectious; disease may occur after inhalation of only a few arthroconidia. High frequency of subclinical infection has been indicated by the high prevalence of positive skin tests in endemic areas. Recovery is generally followed by solid, lifelong immunity. Reactivation can occur in those who become immunosuppressed therapeutically or through HIV infection.

9. Methods of control—

A. Preventive measures:

1) In endemic areas: Planting grass, paving airfields, and other dust control measures (including facemasks, air-conditioned cabs and wetted soil).
2) Individuals from nonendemic areas, or those who are immunocompromised or otherwise at risk, should be evaluated

before recruitment to dusty occupations such as road building.

B. **Control of patient, contacts and the immediate environment:**

1) Report to local health authority: Case report of all recognized cases, especially outbreaks, in selected endemic areas; in many countries, not a reportable disease, Class 3 (see *Reporting*). Isolates of *Coccidioides* are classified as select agents in the United States, and reporting to CDC or USDA is required [APHIS/CDC Form 4: "Report of Isolation of a Select Agent or Toxin in a Clinical or Diagnostic Laboratory"].
2) Isolation: Not applicable.
3) Concurrent disinfection: Discharges and soiled articles must be disinfected. Terminal cleaning.
4) Quarantine: Not applicable.
5) Immunization of contacts: Not applicable.
6) Investigation of contacts and source of infection: Not recommended except in cases appearing in nonendemic areas, where residence, work exposure and travel history should be obtained.
7) Specific treatment: Primary coccidioidomycosis usually resolves spontaneously without therapy, and the benefit of treating primary pulmonary disease is controversial. Amphotericin B IV is used in severe pulmonary infections. Fluconazole is currently the agent of choice for meningeal infection. Fluconazole, itraconazole, and ketoconazole have been useful in chronic, non-meningeal coccidioidomycosis. Posaconazole, a newer antifungal agent, has been shown to be of benefit in salvage studies of severe and disseminated infection.

C. **Epidemic measures:** Outbreaks occur when groups of susceptible persons are infected by airborne arthroconidia. Institute dust control measures where feasible (see 9A1).

D. **Disaster implications:** Possible hazard if large groups of susceptible persons are forced to move through or live in dusty conditions in areas where the fungus is prevalent.

E. **International measures:** None.

F. **Measures in case of deliberate use:** Coccidioides arthroconidia have low potential use as a weapon. See Anthrax, section F, for general measures to be taken when confronted with a threat such as that posed by *Coccidioides* arthroconidia.

For more information on the deliberate use of infectious agents to cause harm, see the section on *Deliberate use*.

CONJUNCTIVITIS/KERATITIS   ICD-9 372.0-372.3, 370; ICD-10 H10, H16

[CCDM18 & 19: S. Resnikoff]

I. ACUTE BACTERIAL CONJUNCTIVITIS   ICD-9 372.0; ICD-10 H10.0-H10.3
(Pinkeye, "Sticky eye," Brazilian purpuric fever [ICD-10 A48.4])

1. Identification—A clinical syndrome beginning with lacrimation, irritation and hyperemia of the palpebral and bulbar conjunctivae of one or both eyes, followed by edema of eyelids and mucopurulent discharge. In severe cases, ecchymoses of the bulbar conjunctiva and marginal infiltration of the cornea with mild photophobia may occur. Non-fatal (except as noted below), the disease may last from 2 days to 2–3 weeks; many patients have no more than hyperemia of the conjunctivae and slight exudate for a few days.

Confirmation of clinical diagnosis through microscopic examination of a stained smear or culture of the discharge is required to differentiate bacterial from viral or allergic conjunctivitis, or adenovirus/enterovirus infection. Inclusion conjunctivitis (see below), trachoma and gonococcal conjunctivitis are described separately.

2. Infectious agents—*Haemophilus influenzae* biogroup *aegyptius* (Koch-Weeks bacillus) and *Streptococcus pneumoniae* appear to be the most important; *H. influenzae* type b, *Moraxella* and *Branhamella* spp., *Neisseria meningitidis* and *Corynebacterium diphtheriae* may also produce the disease. *H. influenzae* biogroup *aegyptius*, gonococci (see Gonococcal infections), *S. pneumoniae*, *S. viridans*, various Gram-negative enteric bacilli and, rarely, *Pseudomonas aeruginosa* may produce the disease in newborn infants.

3. Occurrence—Widespread and common worldwide, particularly in warmer climates; frequently epidemic. In North America, infection with *H. influenzae* biogroup *aegyptius* occurs primarily during summer and early autumn; in North Africa and the Middle East, infections occur as seasonal epidemics. Infection due to other organisms occurs throughout the world, often associated with acute viral respiratory disease during cold seasons. Occasional cases of systemic disease have occurred among children in several communities in Brazil, 1–3 weeks after conjunctivitis due to a unique invasive clone of *Haemophilus influenzae* biogroup *aegyptius*. This severe Brazilian purpuric fever (BPF) had a 70% case-fatality rate among more than 100 cases recognized over a wide area of Brazil covering four states. The causal agent has been isolated from conjunctival, pharyngeal and blood cultures. The disease has been restricted essentially to Brazil; two cases in Australia were similar clinically, but the organism differed from the Brazilian strain.

4. Reservoir—Humans. Carriers of *H. influenzae* biogroup *aegyptius* and *S. pneumoniae* are common in many areas during inter-epidemic periods.

5. Mode of transmission—Contact with discharges from conjunctivae or upper respiratory tracts of infected people; contaminated fingers, clothing and other articles, including shared eye makeup applicators, multiple dose eye medications and inadequately sterilized instruments such as tonometers. Eye gnats or flies may transmit the organisms mechanically in some areas, but their importance as vectors is undetermined, and probably differs from area to area.

6. Incubation period—Usually 24-72 hours.

7. Period of communicability—During the course of active infection.

8. Susceptibility—Children aged less than five are most often affected; incidence decreases with age. The very young, the debilitated and the aged are particularly susceptible to staphylococcal infections. Immunity after attack is low grade, and varies with the infectious agent.

9. Methods of control—

   A. *Preventive measures:* Personal hygiene, hygienic care and treatment of affected eyes.

   B. *Control of patient, contacts and the immediate environment:*

      1) Report to local health authority: Obligatory report of epidemics; no case report for classic disease, Class 4; for systemic disease, Class 2 (see *Reporting*).
      2) Isolation: Drainage and secretion precautions. Children should not attend school during the acute stage.
      3) Concurrent disinfection: Of discharges and soiled articles. Terminal cleaning.
      4) Quarantine: Not applicable.
      5) Immunization of contacts: Not applicable.
      6) Investigation of contacts and source of infection: Usually not beneficial for conjunctivitis, but must be undertaken for Brazilian purpuric fever.
      7) Specific treatment: Local application of an ointment or drops containing a sulfonamide such as sodium sulfacetamide, gentamicin or combination antibiotics such as polymyxin B with neomycin or trimethoprim is generally effective. For BPF, systemic treatment is required; isolates are sensitive to both ampicillin and chloramphenicol and resistant to trimethoprim-sufamethoxazole. Oral rifampicin (20 mg/kg/day for 2 days) may be more effective than local chloramphenicol in eradication of the causal clone, and may be useful in

prevention among children with Brazilian purpuric fever clone conjunctivitis (see *Gonococcal conjunctivitis*, 9B7.)

C. Epidemic measures:

1) Prompt and adequate treatment of patients and their close contacts.
2) In areas where insects are suspected of mechanically transmitting infection, measures to prevent access of eye gnats or flies to the eyes of sick and well people.
3) Insect control, according to the suspected vector.

D. Disaster implications: None.

E. International measures: None.

II. KERATOCONJUNCTIVITIS, ADENOVIRAL ICD-9 077.1; ICD-10 B30.0
(Epidemic keratoconjunctivitis [EKC], Shipyard conjunctivitis, Shipyard eye)

1. Identification—An acute viral disease of the eye, with unilateral or bilateral inflammation of conjunctivae and edema of the lids and periorbital tissue. Onset is sudden with pain, photophobia, and blurred vision, and occasionally low-grade fever, headache, malaise and tender preauricular lymphadenopathy. Approximately seven days after onset in about half the cases, the cornea exhibits several small, round sub-epithelial infiltrates; these may eventually form punctate erosions that stain with fluorescein. Duration of acute conjunctivitis is about 2 weeks; it may continue to evolve, leaving discrete sub-epithelial opacities that may interfere with vision for a few weeks. In severe cases, permanent scarring may result. Diagnosis is confirmed by recovery of virus from appropriate cell cultures inoculated with eye swabs or conjunctival scrapings; virus may be visualized through FA staining of scrapings or through IEM; viral antigen may be detected by ELISA testing. Serum neutralization or HAI tests may identify type-specific titer rises.

2. Infectious agents—Typically, adenovirus types 8, 19 and 37 are responsible, though other adenovirus types have been involved. Most severe disease has been found in infections caused by types 8, 5 and 19.

3. Occurrence—Presumably worldwide. Both sporadic cases and large outbreaks have been reported from Asia, Europe, the Pacific Islands and North America.

4. Reservoir—Humans.

5. Mode of transmission—Direct contact with eye secretions of an infected person and, indirectly, through contaminated surfaces, instruments or solutions. In industrial plants, epidemics are centered in first-aid stations and dispensaries where treatment is frequently administered for minor trauma to the eye; transmission occurs through fingers, instruments and other contaminated items. Similar outbreaks have originated in eye clinics and medical offices. Dispensary and clinic personnel acquiring the disease may act as sources of infection. Family spread is common, with children typically introducing the infection.

6. Incubation period—Between 5 and 12 days, but in many instances this duration is exceeded.

7. Period of communicability—From late in the incubation period to 14 days after onset. Prolonged viral shedding has been reported.

8. Susceptibility—There is usually complete type-specific immunity after adenoviral infections. Trauma, even minor, and eye manipulation increase the risk of infection.

9. Methods of control—

    A. Preventive measures:

        1) Educate patients about personal cleanliness and the risk associated with use of common towels and toilet articles. Educate patients to minimize hand-to-eye contact.

        2) Avoid shared use of eyedroppers, medicines, eye makeup, instruments or towels.

        3) During ophthalmologic procedures in dispensaries, clinics and offices, asepsis should include vigorous handwashing before examining each patient, and systematic sterilization of instruments after use; high-level disinfection is recommended for instruments that will be in contact with the conjunctivae or eyelids. Clean gloves should be worn for examining eyes of patients with possible or confirmed epidemic keratoconjunctivitis. Any ophthalmic medicines or droppers that have come in contact with eyelids or conjunctivae must be discarded. Medical personnel with overt conjunctivitis should not have physical contact with patients.

        4) With persistent outbreaks, patients with epidemic keratoconjunctivitis should be seen in physically separate facilities.

        5) Use safety measures such as goggles in industrial plants.

    B. Control of patient, contacts and the immediate environment:

        1) Report to local health authority: Obligatory report of epidemics in some countries; no individual case report, Class 4 (see *Reporting*).

        2) Isolation: Drainage and secretion precautions; patients must use separate towels and linens during the acute stage.

Infected medical personnel or patients should not come in contact with uninfected patients.

3) Concurrent disinfection: Of conjunctival and nasal discharges and articles soiled therewith. Terminal cleaning.
4) Quarantine: Not applicable.
5) Immunization of contacts: Not applicable.
6) Investigation of contacts and source of infection: In outbreaks, the source of infection should be identified, and precautions taken to prevent further transmission.
7) Specific treatment: None during the acute phase. If residual opacities interfere with the patient's ability to work, topical corticosteroids may be administered by a qualified ophthalmologist.

C. Epidemic measures:

1) Strictly apply recommendations in 9A.
2) Organize convenient facilities for prompt diagnosis, with no or minimal contact between infected and uninfected individuals.

D. Disaster implications: None.

E. International measures: WHO Collaborating Centres provide support as required. More information can be found at: <http://www.who.int/collaboratingcentres/database/en/>

III. ADENOVIRAL HEMORRHAGIC CONJUNCTIVITIS   ICD-9 077.2; ICD-10 B30.1
(Pharyngoconjunctival fever)
ENTEROVIRAL HEMORRHAGIC CONJUNCTIVITIS   ICD-9 077.4; ICD-10 B30.3
(Apollo 11 disease, Acute hemorrhagic conjunctivitis)

1. Identification—In adenoviral conjunctivitis, lymphoid follicles usually develop, the conjunctivitis lasts 7-15 days, and there are frequently small sub-conjunctival hemorrhages. In one adenoviral syndrome, pharyngoconjunctival fever, there is upper respiratory disease and fever with minor degrees of corneal epithelial inflammation (epithelial keratitis). In enteroviral acute hemorrhagic conjunctivitis (AHC), onset is sudden, with redness, swelling and pain often in both eyes; the course of the inflammatory disease is 4-6 days, during which sub-conjunctival hemorrhages appear on the bulbar conjunctiva as petechiae that enlarge to form confluent sub-conjunctival hemorrhages. Large hemorrhages gradually resolve over 7-12 days. In major outbreaks of enteroviral origin, there has been a low incidence of a polio-like paralysis, including cranial nerve palsies, lumbosacral radiculomyelitis and lower motor neuron paralysis.

Neurological complications start a few days to a month after conjunctivitis, and often leave residual weakness.

Laboratory confirmation of adenovirus infections is through isolation of the virus from conjunctival swabs in cell culture, rising antibody titers, detection of viral antigens through IF, or identification of viral nucleic acid with a DNA probe. Enterovirus infection is diagnosed by isolation of the agent, immuno-fluorescence, demonstration of a rising antibody titer, or PCR.

2. Infectious agents—Adenoviruses and picornaviruses. Most adenoviruses can cause PCF, but types 3, 4 and 7 are the most common causes. The most prevalent picornavirus type has been designated as enterovirus 70; this and a variant of coxsackievirus A24 have caused large outbreaks of AHC.

3. Occurrence—PCF occurs during outbreaks of adenovirus-associated respiratory disease, or as summer epidemics in temperate climates, associated with swimming pools. Adenoviral hemorrhagic conjuctivitis was first recognized in Ghana in 1969 and Indonesia in 1970, during major epidemics that spread throughout Africa and the Pacific Islands; numerous epidemics have occurred since then in tropical areas of Asia, Africa, Central and South America, the Caribbean, the Pacific Islands and parts of North America and Mexico. An outbreak in American Samoa in 1986 due to coxsackievirus A24 variant affected an estimated 48% of the population. Smaller outbreaks have occurred in Europe, usually associated with eye clinics.

4. Reservoir—Humans.

5. Mode of transmission—Direct or indirect contact with discharge from infected eyes. Person-to-person transmission is most noticeable in families, where high attack rates often occur. Adenovirus can be transmitted in poorly chlorinated swimming pools, and has been reported as "swimming pool conjunctivitis"; it is also transmitted through respiratory droplets. Large AHC epidemics are often associated with overcrowding and low hygienic standards. Schoolchildren have been implicated in the rapid dissemination of AHC throughout communities.

6. Incubation period—For adenovirus infection, 4–12 days, with an average of 8 days. For picornavirus infection, 12 hours to 3 days.

7. Period of communicability—Adenovirus infections may be communicable up to 14 days after onset, picornavirus at least 4 days after onset.

8. Susceptibility—Infection can occur at all ages. Re-infections and/or relapses have been reported. The role and duration of the immune response are not yet clear.

9. Methods of control—

    A. Preventive measures: No effective treatment; prevention is critical. Personal hygiene should be emphasized, including use of non-shared towels and avoidance of overcrowding. Maintain strict asepsis in eye clinics; wash hands before examining each patient. Eye clinics must ensure high-level disinfection of potentially contaminated equipment. Adequate chlorination of swimming pools. Closing schools may be necessary.

B. Control of patient, contacts and the immediate environment:

1) Report to local health authority: Obligatory report of epidemics; no case report, Class 4 (see *Reporting*).
2) Isolation: Drainage and secretion precautions; restrict contact with cases while disease is active (e.g. children should not attend school).
3) Concurrent disinfection: Of conjunctival discharges and articles and equipment soiled therewith. Terminal cleaning.
4) Quarantine: Not applicable.
5) Immunization of contacts: Not applicable.
6) Investigation of contacts and source of infection: Locate other cases to determine whether a common source of infection is involved.
7) Specific treatment: None.

C. Epidemic measures:

1) Organize adequate facilities for the diagnosis and symptomatic treatment of cases.
2) Improve standards of hygiene and limit overcrowding wherever possible.

D. Disaster implications: None.

E. International measures: WHO Collaborating Centres provide support as required. More information can be found at: <http://www.who.int/collaboratingcentres/database/en/>

IV. CHLAMYDIAL CONJUNCTIVITIS ICD-9 077.0; ICD-10 A74.0
(Inclusion conjunctivitis, Paratrachoma, Neonatal inclusion blennorrhea, "Sticky eye") (See separate chapter for *Trachoma*)

1. **Identification**—In the newborn, an acute conjunctivitis with purulent discharge, usually recognized within 5–12 days after birth. The acute stage usually subsides spontaneously in a few weeks; inflammation of the eye may persist for more than a year if untreated, with mild scarring of the conjunctivae and infiltration of the cornea (micropannus). Chlamydial pneumonia (see *Pneumonia, chlamydial*) occurs in some infants with concurrent nasopharyngeal infection. Gonococcal infection must be ruled out. In children and adults, an acute follicular conjunctivitis is seen typically with preauricular lymphadenopathy on the involved side, hyperemia, infiltration,

and a slight mucopurulent discharge, often with superficial corneal involvement. In adults, there may be a chronic phase with scant discharge and symptoms that sometimes persist for more than a year if untreated. The agent may cause symptomatic infection of the urethral epithelium in men and women and the cervix in women, with or without associated conjunctivitis.

Laboratory methods to assist diagnosis include isolation in cell culture, antigen detection using IF staining of direct smears, EIA methods, and DNA probe.

2. **Infectious agents**—*Chlamydia trachomatis* of serovars D through K. Feline strains of *C. psittaci* have also caused acute follicular keratoconjunctivitis in humans.

3. **Occurrence**—Sporadic cases of conjunctivitis are reported worldwide among sexually active adults. Neonatal conjunctivitis due to *C. trachomatis* is common and occurs in 15%–35% of newborns exposed to maternal infection. Among adults with genital chlamydial infection, 1 in 300 develops chlamydial eye disease.

4. **Reservoir**—Humans for *C. trachomatis*; cats for *C. psittaci*.

5. **Mode of transmission**—Generally transmitted in adults during sexual intercourse; the genital discharges of infected people are infectious. In the newborn, conjunctivitis is usually acquired by direct contact with infectious secretions during transit through the birth canal. *In utero* infection may also occur. The eyes of adults become infected by the transmission of genital secretions to the eye, usually by the fingers. Children may acquire conjunctivitis from infected newborns or other household members; cases in children should be assessed for sexual abuse as appropriate. Outbreaks reported among swimmers in non-chlorinated pools have not been confirmed by culture, and may be due to adenoviruses or other known causes of "swimming pool conjunctivitis."

6. **Incubation period**—In newborns, 5–12 days, ranging from 3 days to 6 weeks; in adults, 6–19 days.

7. **Period of communicability**—While genital or ocular infection persists; carriage on mucous membranes has been observed for as long as two years after birth.

8. **Susceptibility**—There is no evidence of resistance to re-infection, although the severity of the disease may be decreased in succeeding infections.

9. **Methods of control**—

   A. *Preventive measures:*

   1) Correct and consistent use of condoms to prevent sexual transmission; prompt treatment of persons with chlamydial urethritis and cervicitis, including pregnant women.

2) General preventive measures as for other STIs (see *Syphilis*, 9A).

3) Identification of infection in high-risk pregnant women, by culture or antigen detection. Treatment of cervical infection in pregnant women will prevent subsequent transmission to the infant. Erythromycin base, 500 mg 4 times daily for 7 days, is usually effective, but frequent GI side effects interfere with compliance, and treatment must be observed to ensure completion. If compliance is a problem, consideration may be given to the use of other macrolides, based on the most recent medical literature. Evaluation and treatment of sexual partners should also be undertaken.

4) Routine prophylaxis for gonococcal ophthalmia neonatorum is effective against chlamydial infection, and should be practiced. The method of choice is a single application into the eyes of the newborn, within 1 hour after delivery, of one of the following: povidone-iodine (2.5% solution); tetracycline 1% eye ointment; erythromycin 0.5% eye ointment; or silver nitrate eye drops (1%). All methods give comparable results in preventing gonococcal conjunctivitis; in field studies povidone-iodine was significantly more effective in preventing neonatal eye infections. Ocular prophylaxis does not prevent nasopharyngeal colonization and risk of subsequent chlamydial pneumonia. Penicillin is ineffective against chlamydiae.

B. Control of patient, contacts and the immediate environment:

1) Report to local health authority: Case report of neonatal cases obligatory in many countries, Class 2 (see *Reporting*).

2) Isolation: Drainage and secretion precautions for the first 96 hours after starting treatment.

3) Concurrent disinfection: Aseptic techniques and handwashing by personnel appear to be adequate to prevent nursery transmission.

4) Quarantine: Not applicable.

5) Immunization of contacts: Not applicable.

6) Investigation of contacts and source of infection: All sexual contacts of adult cases, and mothers and fathers of neonatally infected infants, should be examined and treated. Infected adults should be investigated for evidence of ongoing infection with gonorrhea or syphilis.

7) Specific treatment: For ocular and genital infections of adults, tetracycline, erythromycin or ofloxacin is effective when given by mouth for up to 2 weeks (tetracycline cannot be used in children less than eight years of age). Azithromycin is an effective single-dose therapy.

Oral treatment of neonatal ocular infections with erythromycin for 2 weeks is recommended to eliminate the risk of chlamydial pneumonia as well; the dose is 10 mg/kg, given every 12 hours during the first week of life, and every 8 hours thereafter.

C. Epidemic measures: Sanitary control of swimming pools; ordinary chlorination suffices.

D. Disaster implications: None.

E. International measures: WHO Collaborating Centres provide support as required. More information can be found at:
<http://www.who.int/collaboratingcentres/database/en/>

COXSACKIEVIRUS DISEASES   ICD-9 074; ICD-10 B34.1
[CCDM18 & 19: D. Lavanchy]

The coxsackieviruses, members of the enterovirus group of the family Picornaviridae, are the causal agents of a group of diseases discussed in this chapter, as well as epidemic myalgia, enteroviral hemorrhagic conjunctivitis and meningitis (see under individual disease listings), pancreatitis, uveitis and coxsackievirus carditis (see below). They cause disseminated disease in newborns; there is evidence suggesting their involvement in the etiology of juvenile onset insulin-dependent diabetes.

I.A. ENTEROVIRAL VESICULAR PHARYNGITIS   ICD-9 074.0; ICD-10 B08.5
(Herpangina, Aphthous pharyngitis)
I.B. ENTEROVIRAL VESICULAR STOMATITIS WITH EXANTHEM   ICD-9 074.3; ICD-10 B08.4
(Hand, foot and mouth disease)
I.C. ENTEROVIRAL LYMPHONODULAR PHARYNGITIS   ICD-9 074.8; ICD-10 B08.8
(Acute lymphonodular pharyngitis, Vesicular pharyngitis)

1. Identification—Vesicular pharyngitis (herpangina) is an acute, self-limited, viral disease characterized by sudden onset, fever, sore throat and small (1–2 mm), discrete, grayish papulovesicular pharyngeal lesions on an erythematous base, gradually progressing to slightly larger ulcers. These lesions usually occur on the anterior pillars of the tonsillar fauces, soft palate, uvula and tonsils, and may persist 4–6 days after the onset of illness. No fatalities have been reported. In one series, febrile convulsions occurred in 5% of cases.

Vesicular stomatitis with exanthem (hand, foot and mouth disease) differs from vesicular pharyngitis in that oral lesions are more diffuse and may occur on the buccal surfaces of the cheeks and gums and on the sides of the tongue. Papulovesicular lesions, which may persist from 7 to 10 days, also occur commonly as an exanthem, especially on the palms, fingers and soles; maculopapular lesions occasionally appear on the buttocks. Although the disease is usually self-limited, rare cases have been fatal in infants.

Acute lymphonodular pharyngitis also differs from vesicular pharyngitis in that the lesions are firm, raised, discrete, whitish to yellowish nodules, surrounded by a 3–6 mm zone of erythema. They occur predominantly on the uvula, anterior tonsillar pillars and posterior pharynx, with no exanthem.

Stomatitis due to herpes simplex virus requires differentiation; it has larger, deeper, more painful ulcerative lesions, commonly located in the front part of the mouth. These diseases are not to be confused with vesicular stomatitis caused by the vesicular stomatitis virus, normally of cattle and horses, which in humans usually occurs among dairy workers, animal husbandrymen, and veterinarians. Foot-and-mouth disease of cattle, sheep and swine rarely affects laboratory workers handling the virus; however, humans can be a mechanical carrier of the virus and the source of animal outbreaks. A virus not serologically differentiable from coxsackievirus B-5 causes vesicular disease in swine, which may be transmitted to humans.

Differentiation of the related but distinct coxsackievirus syndromes is facilitated during epidemics. Virus may be isolated from lesions and nasopharyngeal and stool specimens through cell cultures and/or inoculation to suckling mice. Since many serotypes may produce the same syndrome and common antigens are lacking, serological diagnostic procedures are not routinely available unless the virus is isolated for use in the serological tests.

2. **Infectious agents**—For vesicular pharyngitis, coxsackievirus group A, types 1–10, 16 and 22. For vesicular stomatitis with or without exanthem (hand, foot and mouth disease), coxsackievirus group A, type A16 predominantly and types 4, 5, 9 and 10; group B, types 2 and 5; and (less often) enterovirus 71. For acute lymphonodular pharyngitis, coxsackievirus group A, type 10. Other enteroviruses have occasionally been associated with these diseases.

3. **Occurrence**—Probably worldwide for vesicular pharyngitis and vesicular stomatitis, both sporadically and in epidemics; maximal incidence in summer and early autumn; mainly in children under 10, but adult cases (especially young adults) are not unusual. Isolated outbreaks of acute

lymphonodular pharyngitis, predominantly in children, may occur in summer and early autumn. These diseases frequently occur in outbreaks among groups of children (e.g. in nursery schools, childcare centers).

4. Reservoir—Humans.

5. Mode of transmission—Direct contact with nose and throat discharges and feces of infected persons (who may be asymptomatic) and by aerosol droplet spread; no reliable evidence of spread by insects, water, food or sewage.

6. Incubation period—Usually 3–5 days for vesicular pharyngitis and vesicular stomatitis; 5 days for acute lymphonodular pharyngitis.

7. Period of communicability—During the acute stage of illness and perhaps longer, since viruses persist in stool for several weeks.

8. Susceptibility—Susceptibility to infection is universal. Immunity to the specific virus is probably acquired through clinical or unapparent infection; duration unknown. Second attacks may occur with group A coxsackievirus of a different serological type.

9. Methods of control—

  A. *Preventive measures:* Limit person-to-person contact, where practicable, by measures such as crowd reduction and ventilation. Promote handwashing and other hygienic measures in the home.

  B. *Control of patient, contacts and the immediate environment:*

  1) Report to local health authority: Obligatory report of epidemics in some countries; no case report, Class 4 (see *Reporting*).
  2) Isolation: Enteric precautions.
  3) Concurrent disinfection: Of nose and throat discharges. Wash or discard articles soiled therewith. Give careful attention to prompt handwashing when handling discharges, feces and articles soiled therewith.
  4) Quarantine: Not applicable.
  5) Immunization of contacts: Not applicable.
  6) Investigation of contacts and source of infection: Of no practical value except to detect other cases in groups of preschool children.
  7) Specific treatment: None.

  C. *Epidemic measures:* Give general notice to physicians of increased incidence of the disease, together with a description of onset and clinical characteristics. Isolate diagnosed cases and all children with fever, pending diagnosis, with special attention to respiratory secretions and feces.

D. Disaster implications: None.

E. International measures: WHO Collaborating Centres provide support as required. More information can be found at:

http://www.who.int/collaboratingcentres/database/en/

II. COXSACKIEVIRUS CARDITIS ICD-9 074.2; ICD-10 B33.2

(Viral carditis, Enteroviral carditis)

1. Identification—An acute or sub-acute viral myocarditis or pericarditis occurring (occasionally with other manifestations) as a manifestation of infection with enteroviruses, especially group B coxsackievirus. The myocardium is affected, particularly in neonates, in whom fever and lethargy may be followed rapidly by heart failure with pallor, cyanosis, dyspnea, tachycardia and enlargement of heart and liver. Heart failure may be progressive and fatal, or recovery may take place over a few weeks; some cases run a relapsing course over months and may show residual heart damage. In young adults, pericarditis is the more common manifestation, with acute chest pain, disturbance of heart rate, and often dyspnea. It may mimic myocardial infarction but is frequently associated with pulmonary or pleural manifestations (pleurodynia). The disease may be associated with aseptic meningitis; hepatitis; orchitis; pancreatitis; pneumonia; hand, foot and mouth disease; rash; or epidemic myalgia (see *Myalgia, epidemic*).

Serological studies or virus isolation from feces usually help diagnosis, but such results are inconclusive; a significant rise in specific antibody titers is diagnostic. Virus is, rarely, isolated from pericardial fluid, myocardial biopsy or postmortem heart tissue; such isolation provides a definitive diagnosis.

2. Infectious agents—Group B coxsackievirus (types 1–5); occasionally group A coxsackievirus (types 1, 4, 9, 16, 23) and other enteroviruses.

3. Occurrence—An uncommon disease, mainly sporadic, but increased during epidemics of group B coxsackievirus infection. Institutional outbreaks, with high case-fatality rates in newborns, have been described in maternity units.

4., 5., 6., 7., 8. and 9. Reservoir—Mode of transmission, Incubation period, Period of communicability, Susceptibility and **Methods of control**—See *Myalgia, epidemic*.

CRYPTOCOCCOSIS
(Torula)
[CCDM19: M. Brandt]
[CCDM18: L. Severo]

ICD-9 117.5; ICD-10 B45

1. Identification—Disease attributable to infection with fungi of the genus *Cryptococcus spp*. Infection occurs after inhalation of the fungal spores, which are present in the environment. Immunocompetent persons more commonly present with primary pulmonary infection, but immuno-compromised persons (including those with HIV or AIDS) often present after hematogenous spread to the meninges, with subacute or chronic meningitis; other sites of disseminated infection include the kidneys, prostate, bone, and skin (pustules, papules, plaques, ulcers, or subcutane-ous masses). Untreated meningitis terminates fatally within weeks to months.

Diagnosis of cryptococcal meningitis is aided by the evidence of the characteristic capsular halo or budding forms on microscopic examination of CSF mixed with India ink. Tests for antigen in serum and CSF are highly sensitive and specific. Diagnosis is confirmed through histopathology or culture (media containing cycloheximide inhibit the agent and should not be used). *Cryptococcus* can be stained using gomori-methenamine silver or periodic acid-Schiff staining; mucicarmine helps differentiate it from other yeasts, especially *Blastomyces* and *Histoplasma*.

2. Infectious agents—*Cryptococcus neoformans* var. *neoformans* and var. *grubii*, and *C. neoformans* var. *gattii*. The latter are more frequent in tropical or subtropical regions such as Australia and Africa. Recent reports have described an emergence of *C. neoformans* var. *gattii* in British Columbia, Canada.

3. Occurrence—Cases occur worldwide and tend to follow the AIDS epidemic in a given country or region. Infection is more frequent in adults than in children, males slightly more frequently than females. Patients with advanced HIV infection are at increased risk for developing cryptococco-sis, usually *C. neoformans*. Infection also occurs in cats, dogs, horses, cows, monkeys and other animals.

4. Reservoir—Saprophytic growth in the external environment. *C. neo-formans* can be isolated consistently from old pigeon nests and pigeon droppings and from soil in many parts of the world. Foliage and bark of certain species of eucalyptus have yielded *C. gattii*.

5. Mode of transmission—Presumably by inhalation.

6. Incubation period—Unknown. Pulmonary disease may precede brain infection by months or years.

7. Period of communicability—No person-to-person or animal-to-person transmission.

8. Susceptibility—No evidence for racial or population differences; the high prevalence of *C. neoformans* in the external environment and the rarity of infection suggest that humans have appreciable resistance. Susceptibility is increased during corticosteroid or other immunosuppressive therapy and by immune deficiency disorders (especially HIV infection).

9. Methods of control—

A. *Preventive measures:* There are no data that demonstrate that specific measures to avoid exposure are of any benefit in preventing infection. Fluconazole antifungal prophylaxis for patients with HIV has been shown to reduce the incidence of infection, but not overall survival.

B. *Control of patient, contacts and the immediate environment:*

1) Report to local health authority: Official report required in some jurisdictions as a possible manifestation of AIDS, Class 2 (see *Reporting*).
2) Isolation: Not applicable.
3) Concurrent disinfection: Of discharges and contaminated dressings. Terminal cleaning.
4) Quarantine: Not applicable.
5) Immunization of contacts: Not applicable.
6) Investigation of contacts and source of infection: None.
7) Specific treatment: The combination of amphotericin B and 5-flucytosine is the therapy of choice for disseminated infection, including meningitis, but has some toxicity; lipid formulation of amphotericin B can help avoid nephrotoxicity. For meningitis, consolidation therapy follows induction and is often long-term; fluconazole is used after an initial course of amphotericin B and 5-flucytosine. Management of elevated intracranial pressure in patients with meningeal involvement, through manometry and periodic therapeutic lumbar punctures, is essential.

C. *Epidemic measures:* None.

D. *Disaster implications:* None.

E. *International measures:* None.

CRYPTOSPORIDIOSIS   ICD-9 136.8; ICD-10 A07.2
[CCDM19: M. Arrowood, M. Eberhard, A. Gabrielli, L. Savioli]
[CCDM18: L. Savioli]

1. Identification—A parasitic infection of medical and veterinary importance affecting epithelial cells of the human GI, biliary and respiratory tracts, as well as over 45 different vertebrate species including poultry and other birds, fish, reptiles, small mammals (rodents, cats, dogs), and large mammals (particularly cattle and sheep). Asymptomatic infections are common and constitute a source of infection for others. The major symptom in human patients is diarrhea, which may be profuse and watery, preceded by anorexia and vomiting in children. The diarrhea is associated with cramping abdominal pain. General malaise, fever, anorexia, nausea and vomiting occur less often. Symptoms often wax and wane but remit in less than 30 days in most immunologically healthy people. In immunodeficient persons, especially those infected with HIV, who may be unable to clear the parasite, the disease has a prolonged and fulminant clinical course contributing to death. Symptoms of cholecystitis may occur in biliary tract infections; the relationship between respiratory tract infections and clinical symptoms is unclear.

Diagnosis is generally through identification of oocysts in fecal smears or of life cycle stages of the parasites in intestinal biopsy sections. Oocysts are small (4–6 micrometers) and may be confused with yeast unless appropriately stained. Most commonly used stains include auraminerhodamine, a modified acid-fast stain, and safranin-methylene blue. More sensitive immunobased ELISA assays have recently become available. A fluorescein-tagged monoclonal antibody is useful for detecting oocysts in stool and in environmental samples. Infection with this organism is not easily detected unless looked for specifically. Serological assays may help in epidemiological studies.

2. Infectious agent—*Cryptosporidium hominis* and *C. parvum*, coccidian protozoa, are the two species most often associated with human infection.

3. Occurrence—Worldwide. *Cryptosporidium* oocysts have been identified in human fecal specimens from more than 50 countries. In industrialized countries, prevalence of infection is less than 1%–4.5% of individuals surveyed by stool examination. In developing regions, prevalence ranges from 3% to 20%. Children under two, animal handlers, travelers, men who have sex with men and close personal contacts of infected individuals (families, health care and day care workers) are particularly prone to infection. Outbreaks have been reported in day care centers around the world, and have also been associated with: drinking water (at least 3 major outbreaks involved public water supplies); recreational use of water including waterslides, swimming pools and lakes; and consumption of contaminated beverages.

4. Reservoir—Humans, cattle and other domesticated and feral animals.

5. Mode of transmission—Fecal-oral, which includes person-to-person, animal-to-person, waterborne and foodborne transmission. The parasite infects intestinal epithelial cells and multiplies initially by meiogany (schizogony), followed by a sexual cycle resulting in fecal oocysts that can survive under adverse environmental conditions for long periods of time. Oocysts are highly resistant to chemical disinfectants used to purify drinking water. One or more autoinfectious cycles may occur in humans.

6. Incubation period—Variable; 1–12 days is the likely range, with an average of about 7 days.

7. Period of communicability—Oocysts, the infectious stage, appear in the stool at the onset of symptoms and are infectious immediately upon excretion. Excretion continues in stools for several weeks after symptoms resolve; outside the body, oocysts may remain infective for 2–6 months or longer in a moist environment.

8. Susceptibility—Immunocompetent people may have asymptomatic or self-limited symptomatic infections; it is not clear whether reinfection and latent infection with reactivation can occur. Immunodeficient individuals generally clear their infections when factors of immunosuppression (including malnutrition or intercurrent viral infections such as measles) are removed. In those with HIV infection, the clinical course may vary, and asymptomatic periods may occur, but the infection usually persists throughout the illness unless HAART is successful; approximately 2% of AIDS patients reported to CDC in the USA were infected with cryptosporidia when AIDS was diagnosed; hospital experience indicates that 10%–20% of AIDS patients develop the infection at some time during their illness.

9. Methods of control—

    A. Preventive measures:

        1) Educate the public in personal hygiene.
        2) Dispose of feces in a sanitary manner; use care in handling animal or human excreta.
        3) Have those in contact with calves and other animals with diarrhea (scours) wash their hands carefully.
        4) Boil drinking water supplies for 1 minute; chemical disinfectants are not effective against oocysts in drinking water.
           Only filters capable of removing particles 0.1–1.0 micrometers in diameter should be considered.
        5) Remove infected persons from jobs that require handling food that will not be subsequently cooked until cure can be verified.

6) Exclude infected children from day care facilities until diarrhea stops.

B. Control of patient, contacts and the immediate environment:

1) Report to local health authority: Case report in some countries by most practicable means, Class 3 (see *Reporting*).

2) Isolation: For hospitalized patients, enteric precautions in the handling of feces, vomitus and contaminated clothing and bed linen; exclusion of symptomatic individuals from food handling and from direct care of hospitalized and institutionalized patients; release to return to work in sensitive occupations when asymptomatic. Stress proper handwashing.

3) Concurrent disinfection: Of feces and articles soiled therewith. In communities with modern and adequate sewage disposal systems, feces can be discharged directly into sewers without preliminary disinfection. Terminal cleaning. Heating to 45°C (113°F) for 20 minutes (or, more conservatively, 50°C–60°C for 30 min) or to 64.2°C (147.5°F) for 2 minutes is effective, as is chemical disinfection with 10% formalin or 5% ammonia solution is effective.

4) Quarantine: Not applicable.

5) Immunization of contacts: Not applicable.

6) Investigation of contacts and source of infection: Microscopic examination of feces in household members and other suspected contacts, especially if symptomatic. Contact with cattle or domestic animals warrants investigation. If waterborne transmission is suspected, large volume water sampling filters can be used to look for oocysts in the water.

7) Specific treatment: Rehydration, when indicated, has been proven effective. FDA has approved nitazoxanide for immunocompetent children and adults (children under 4 years: 100 mg twice daily; children over 4 years: 200 mg twice daily), but not for the immunosuppressed or persons with HIV. Fluid and electrolyte replacement with oral rehydration solutions or intravenous fluids is essential. If the individual is taking immunosuppressive drugs, these should be stopped or reduced wherever possible.

C. Epidemic measures: Epidemiological investigation of clustered cases in an area or institution to determine source of infection and mode of transmission; search for common vehicle, such as recreational water, drinking water, raw milk or other potentially contaminated food or drink; institution of applicable prevention or control measures. Control of person-to-person or animal-to-person transmission requires emphasis on personal cleanliness and safe disposal of feces.

D. Disaster implications: None.

E. International measures: None.

DIARRHEA CAUSED BY *CYCLOSPORA* ICD-10 A07.8

This diarrheal disease is caused by *Cyclospora cayetanensis*, a sporulating coccidian protozoon infecting the upper small bowel. The clinical syndrome consists of watery diarrhea, nausea, anorexia, abdominal cramps, fatigue, myalgia and weight loss; fever is rare. The median incubation period is about 1 week. Persistence of symptoms, with remittance and relapse episodes, is typical: if untreated, diarrhea in the immunocompetent usually lasts for 10 to 24 days, but is self-limited; mean duration of organism shedding was 23 days in Peruvian children. In the immunocompromised, diarrhea can last for months in some patients.

Cyclosporiasis is most common in tropical and subtropical countries, where asymptomatic infections are not infrequent. It has also been associated with diarrhea in travelers to Asia, the Caribbean, and Latin America.

Diagnosis is made by identification in the stools of the 8–10 micrometer size oocysts, about twice the size of *Cryptosporidium parvum*, in wet mount under phase contrast microscopy. A modified acid-fast stain or modified safranin technique can be used. Organisms autofluoresce under ultraviolet illumination.

Cyclospora is endemic in many developing countries. Transmission can be foodborne or waterborne and occurs either through drinking (or swimming in) contaminated water, or through consumption of contaminated fresh fruits and vegetables. *Cyclospora* oocysts in freshly excreted stool are not infectious; they require days to weeks outside the host to sporulate and become infectious. *C. cayetanensis* was responsible for multiple foodborne outbreaks in North America linked to various types of fresh produce imported from developing countries. Raspberries, basil and lettuce are among the incriminated vehicles.

Produce should be washed thoroughly before it is eaten, although this practice does not eliminate the risk of cyclosporiasis. *Cyclospora* is resistant to chlorination.

Cyclosporiasis can be treated with a 7–10 day course of oral trimethoprimsulfamethoxazole, shown to cure about 90% of cases (for adults, 160 mg trimethoprim plus 800 mg sulfamethoxazole twice daily; for children, 5 mg/kg trimethoprim plus 25 mg/kg sulfamethoxazole twice daily). Patients with HIV infection may require higher dosage and longer treatment. Ciprofloxacin is less effective than trimethoprimsulfamethoxazole, but is the treatment of choice for patients who cannot tolerate sulfa drugs. In all patients, fluid and electrolyte balance should be monitored and maintained. In patients who are not treated, illness can be protracted, with remitting and relapsing symptoms.

Health care providers should consider the diagnosis of *Cyclospora* infection in persons with prolonged diarrheal illness, and should request stool specimens so that specific tests for this parasite can be made. In jurisdictions where formal reporting mechanisms are not yet established, clinicians and laboratory workers who identify cases of cyclosporiasis are encouraged to inform the appropriate health departments.

❖

CYTOMEGALOVIRUS INFECTIONS

| CYTOMEGALOVIRUS DISEASE | ICD-9 078.5; ICD-10 B25 |
| CONGENITAL CYTOMEGALOVIRUS INFECTION | ICD-9 771.1; ICD-10 P35.1 |

[CCDM18 & 19: D. Lavanchy]

1. Identification—While infection with cytomegalovirus (CMV) is common, it often passes undiagnosed as a febrile illness without specific characteristics. Serious manifestations of infection vary depending on the age and immunocompetence of the individual at the time of infection. The most severe form of the disease develops in 5%–10% of infants infected in utero. These show signs and symptoms of severe generalized infection, especially involving the CNS and liver. Lethargy, convulsions, jaundice, petechiae, purpura, hepatosplenomegaly, chorioretinitis, intracerebral calcifications and pulmonary infiltrates may occur. Survivors show mental retardation, microcephaly, motor disabilities, hearing loss and evidence of chronic liver disease. Death may occur in utero; the neonatal case-fatality rate is high for severely affected infants. Neonatal CMV is the leading cause of congenital viral infection, with an incidence of 0.5-3% of live births worldwide; 90%-95% of these intrauterine infections are inapparent but 15%-25% of these infants eventually manifest some degree of neurosensory disability. Fetal infection may occur during either primary or reactivated maternal infections; primary infections carry a much higher risk for symptomatic disease and sequelae. Seronegative newborns who receive blood transfusions from seropositive donors may also develop severe disease.

Primary infection in an immunocompetent host acquired later in life is generally inapparent, but may cause a syndrome clinically and hematologically similar to Epstein-Barr virus mononucleosis and hepatitis, distinguishable by virological or serological tests and the absence of heterophile antibodies. CMV causes up to 10% of all cases of mononucleosis seen among university students and hospitalized adults aged 25–34. It is the most common cause of mononucleosis following transfusion to non-immune individuals; many post-transfusion infections are clinically inapparent. Disseminated infection, with pneumonitis, retinitis, GI tract disorders (gastritis, enteritis, colitis) and hepatitis, occurs in immunodeficient and immunosuppressed patients—a serious manifestation of AIDS.

CMV is also the most common cause of post-transplant infection, both for solid organ and bone marrow transplants; in the former, this is particularly so with a seronegative recipient and a seropositive (carrier) donor, whereas reactivation is a common cause of disease after bone marrow transplant. In both cases, serious disease occurs in about 1 of 4 cases.

Optimal diagnosis in the newborn is through virus isolation or PCR, usually from urine. Positive tests for IgM antibodies to CMV are also helpful. Diagnosis of CMV disease in the adult is made difficult by the high frequency of asymptomatic and relapsing infections. Multiple diagnostic modalities should be used if possible. Virus isolation, CMV antigen detection (which can be done within 24 hours) and CMV DNA detection by PCR or in situ hybridization can be used to demonstrate virus in organs, blood, respiratory secretions, or urine. Serological studies should be done to demonstrate the presence of CMV specific IgM antibody or a 4-fold rise in antibody titer. Interpretation of the results requires knowledge of the patient's clinical and epidemiological background.

2. **Infectious agent**—Human (beta) herpesvirus 5 (human CMV), a member of the subfamily Betaherpesvirus of the family Herpesviridae; includes 4 major genotypes and many strains, although there often is cross-antigenicity among genotypes and strains.

3. **Occurrence**—Worldwide. In North America, intrauterine infection occurs in 0.5%–1% of pregnancies, usually as the result of a primary infection. In Europe, intrauterine infection is slightly less common. In Australia, the average annual incidence of children aged 0–14 years admitted to hospital with congenital CMV was 0.4–1.4 per 100 000. The situation in developing countries is not well described, but infection generally occurs early in life and most intrauterine infections are due to reactivation or reinfection of maternal infection. Serum antibody prevalence in young adults varies from 30% in highly industrialized countries to almost 100% in some developing countries; it is higher in women than in men and is inversely related to socioeconomic status within the USA. In the United Kingdom, antibody prevalence is related to ethnic group rather than social class. In various population groups, 8%–60% of infants begin shedding virus in the urine during their first year of life, as a result of infection acquired from the mother's cervix or breastmilk.

4. **Reservoir**—Humans are the only known reservoir of human CMV; strains found in many animal species are not infectious for humans.

5. **Mode of transmission**—Intimate exposure through mucosal contact with infectious tissues, secretions and excretions. CMV is excreted in

urine, saliva, breastmilk, cervical secretions and semen during primary and reactivated infections. Persistent excretion may occur in infected newborns and immunosuppressed individuals. The fetus may be infected in utero from either a primary or reactivated maternal infection; serious fetal infection with manifest disease at birth occurs most commonly during a mother's primary infection, but infection (usually without disease) may develop even when maternal antibodies existed prior to conception. Postnatal infection occurs more commonly in infants born to mothers shedding CMV in cervical secretions at delivery; thus, transmission of the virus from the infected cervix at delivery is a common means of neonatal infection. Virus can be transmitted to infants through infected breastmilk, an important source of infection but not of disease, except when milk from a surrogate mother is given to seronegative infants. Viremia may be present in asymptomatic people, so the virus may be transmitted by blood transfusion, probably associated with leukocytes. Many children in day care centers excrete CMV; this may represent a community reservoir. Transmission through sexual intercourse is common and is reflected by the almost universal infection of men who have many male sexual partners.

6. Incubation period—Illness following a transplant or transfusion with infected blood begins within 3-8 weeks. Infection acquired during birth is first demonstrable 3-12 weeks after delivery.

7. Period of communicability—Virus is excreted in urine and saliva for many months and may persist or be episodic for several years following primary infection. After neonatal infection, virus may be excreted for 5-6 years. Adults appear to excrete virus for shorter periods, but the virus persists as a latent infection. Fewer than 3% of healthy adults are pharyngeal excreters. Excretion recurs with immunodeficiency and immunosuppression.

8. Susceptibility—Infection is ubiquitous. Fetuses, patients with debilitating diseases, those on immunosuppressive drugs and especially organ allograft recipients (kidney, heart, bone marrow) and patients with AIDS are more susceptible to overt and severe disease.

9. Methods of control—

  A. Preventive measures:

  1) Take care in handling diapers/nappies; wash hands after diaper changes and toilet care of newborns and infants.
  2) Women of childbearing age who work in hospitals (especially delivery and pediatric wards) should use "universal precautions". Workers in day care centers and preschools (especially those dealing with mentally retarded populations) should observe strict standards of hygiene, including handwashing.
  3) Avoid transfusing neonates of seronegative mothers with blood from CMV-seropositive donors.

4) Avoid transplanting organs from CMV-seropositive donors to seronegative recipients. If unavoidable, hyperimmune IG or prophylactic administration of antivirals may be helpful. Antivirals are also helpful in seropositive bone-marrow transplant recipients who carry latent CMV.

B. Control of patient, contacts and the immediate environment:

1) Report to local health authority: Official report not ordinarily justifiable, Class 5 (see *Reporting*).
2) Isolation: Secretion precautions may be applied while in hospital for patients known to excrete virus.
3) Concurrent disinfection: Discharges from hospitalized patients and articles soiled therewith.
4) Quarantine: Not applicable.
5) Immunization of contacts: Currently there is no vaccine available.
6) Investigation of contacts and source of infection: None, because of the high prevalence of asymptomatic shedders in the population.
7) Specific treatment: The drugs of choice for prophylaxis and treatment of CMV disease are ganciclovir IV or valganciclovir, administered orally. Alternatively, cidofovir IV (together with probenecid), foscarnet IV and fomivirsen have been approved for the treatment of CMV retinitis in immunocompromised persons. Ganciclovir, valganciclovir, cidofovir and foscarnet may also be helpful— especially when combined with anti-CMV immune globulin—for pneumonitis and possibly GI disease in immunocompromised persons; these drugs are licensed for use in CMV infections occurring after organ transplantation. Maribavir is an important candidate currently undergoing phase 3 clinical trials.

C. Epidemic measures: None.

D. Disaster implications: None.

E. International measures: None.

DENGUE FEVER ICD-9 061; ICD-10 A90
(Breakbone fever)
[CCDM19: W. Sun]

1. Identification—An acute febrile viral disease characterized by sudden onset, fever for 2-7 days (sometimes biphasic), intense headache, myalgia, arthralgia, retro-orbital pain, anorexia, nausea, vomiting and rash. Early generalized erythema occurs in some cases. A generalized maculopapular rash may appear about the time of defervescence. Rash is frequently not visible in dark-skinned patients. Minor bleeding phenomena, such as petechiae, epistaxis or gum bleeding, may occur at any time during the febrile phase. With underlying conditions, adults may have major bleeding phenomena, such as GI hemorrhage in peptic ulcer cases or menorrhagia. Dengue fever with unusual hemorrhage should be differentiated from DHF with increased vascular permeability, bleeding manifestations and involvement of specific organs. Recovery may be associated with prolonged fatigue and depression. Lymphadenopathy and leukopenia with relative lymphocytosis are usual; mild thrombocytopenia (less than 100×10^3 cells per mm^3; or 100 SI units $\times 10^9$ per L) and elevated transaminases occur less frequently. Epidemics are explosive, but fatalities, usually rare, can be minimized by timely medical intervention.

Differential diagnosis includes chikungunya and other epidemiologically relevant diseases listed under arthropod-borne viral fevers; influenza; measles; rubella; malaria; leptospirosis; typhoid; scrub typhus; and other systemic febrile illnesses, especially those accompanied by rash.

Laboratory confirmation of dengue infection is through detection either of virus in acute phase blood/serum within 5 days of onset of illness, or of specific antibodies in convalescent phase serum obtained 6 days or more after onset of illness. Virus identification in blood is by reverse transcriptase polymerase chain reaction (RT-PCR), culture in mosquito cell lines, or inoculation to mosquitoes then identified through immunofluorescence with serotype-specific monoclonal antibodies. These procedures provide a definitive diagnosis, but practical considerations limit their use in endemic countries. The IgM capture ELISA is the most commonly used serological procedure for diagnosis, and is particularly suitable for high-volume testing. IgM antibody, indicating current or recent infection, is usually detectable 6–7 days after onset of illness. A positive test result in a single serum indicates presumptive recent infection; a definitive diagnosis requires increased antibody levels in paired sera. New immunoassays that detect dengue non-structural protein-1 (NS1) show some promise in diagnosis early in the febrile phase, prior to IgM rise. RT-PCR amplification protocols using dengue oligonucleotide primers can also detect dengue virus RNA in tissue from fatal cases. PCR with specific primers can distinguish among the dengue virus serotypes; PCR with nucleotide sequencing can characterize dengue strains and genotypes. Since these genome-based assays are costly, demand meticulous technique, and are highly prone to false-positives through contamination, they are not yet applicable for wide use in all settings.

2. Infectious agent—The viruses of dengue fever are flaviviruses and include serotypes 1, 2, 3 and 4 (dengue-1, -2, -3, -4). The same viruses are responsible for dengue hemorrhagic fever (see below).

3. Occurrence—Dengue viruses of multiple types are endemic in most countries in the tropics. In Asia, 2-5 year dengue/DHF epidemic cycles are established in southern Cambodia, China, Indonesia, Lao Democratic Republic, Malaysia, Myanmar, the Philippines, Thailand, and Viet Nam, with increasing epidemic activity and geographic spread in Bangladesh, India, Maldives, Pakistan, and Sri Lanka, and lower endemicity in New Guinea, Singapore and Taiwan (China). Dengue viruses of several types have regularly been reintroduced into countries of the Pacific Rim, and into northern Queensland, Australia, since 1981.

Dengue-1, -2, -3 and -4 are endemic in Africa. In large areas of western Africa, dengue viruses are probably transmitted epizootically in monkeys; urban dengue involving humans is also common in this area. In recent years, outbreaks of dengue fever have occurred on the eastern coast of Africa from Ethiopia to Mozambique, and on offshore islands such as the Comoros and the Seychelles, with a small number of dengue and DHF-like cases reported from the Arabian Peninsula.

Successive introduction and circulation of all 4 serotypes in tropical and subtropical areas of the Americas has occurred since 1977; dengue entered Texas in 1980, 1986, 1995, 1997, and 2005. As of 2007, two or more dengue viruses are endemic or periodically epidemic in virtually all of the Caribbean and Latin America, including Brazil, Bolivia, Colombia, Ecuador, the Guyanas, Mexico, Paraguay, Peru, Suriname, Venezuela, and Central America. There are now areas, such as Puerto Rico, parts of Venezuela and Mexico, where all 4 serotypes are co-circulating. Dengue was introduced into Easter Island, Chile, in 2002, and reintroduced into Argentina at the northern border with Brazil. Epidemics may occur wherever vectors are present and virus is introduced, whether in urban or rural areas.

4. Reservoir—The viruses are maintained in a human/*Aedes aegypti* mosquito cycle in tropical urban centers; a monkey/mosquito cycle may serve as a reservoir in the forests of southeastern Asia and western Africa.

5. Mode of transmission—Bite of infective mosquitoes, principally *Aedes aegypti*. This is a day-biting species, with increased biting activity for 2 hours after sunrise and several hours before sunset. Dengue outbreaks have been attributed to *Ae. aegypti* and *Ae. albopictus*, an urban species abundant in Asia that has now spread to Latin America and the USA, the Caribbean, and the Pacific parts of southern Europe and Africa. *Ae. albopictus* is less anthropophilic than *Ae. aegypti* and hence a less efficient epidemic vector. In Polynesia, one of the *Ae. scutellaris* spp. complex serves as the vector. Mosquitoes of *Ae. niveaus* complex in Malaysia and *Ae. furcifer-taylori* complex in western Africa are involved in enzootic monkey/mosquito transmission.

6. Incubation period—From 3 to 14 days, commonly 4-7 days.

7. Period of communicability—No direct person-to-person transmission. Patients are infective for mosquitoes during the period of high viremia, from shortly before the febrile period to the end thereof, usually 3-5 days. The mosquito becomes infective 8-12 days after the viremic blood-meal, and remains so for life.

8. Susceptibility—Susceptibility in humans is universal, but children usually have a milder disease than adults. Asymptomatic infections can occur. Recovery from infection with one serotype provides lifelong homologous immunity, but only short-term protection against other serotypes, and may exacerbate disease upon subsequent infections—presumably through immune enhancement, though this is not well understood. Given a particular patient who presents with dengue, it may be difficult, especially at the early stages, to predict its eventual severity (see *Dengue hemorrhagic fever*).

9. Methods of control—

   A. Preventive measures:

     1) Educate the public and promote behaviors to remove, destroy or manage mosquito vector larval habitats, which for *Ae. aegypti* are usually artificial water-holding containers close to or inside human habitations (e.g. old tires, flowerpots, and discarded containers for food or water storage).

     2) Survey the community to determine the abundance of vector mosquitoes, identify the most productive larval habitats, and promote and implement plans for their elimination, management or treatment with appropriate larvicides.

     3) Personal protection against day-biting mosquitoes through repellents, screening and protective clothing (see *Malaria*, 9A3 and 9A4).

   B. Control of patient, contacts and the immediate environment:

     1) Report to local health authority: Obligatory report of epidemics; case reports, Class 4 (see *Reporting*).

     2) Isolation: Blood precautions. Until the fever subsides, prevent access of day-biting mosquitoes to patients by screening the sickroom or using a mosquito bed net, preferably insecticide-impregnated, for febrile patients; or by spraying quarters with a knockdown adulticide or residual insecticide.

     3) Concurrent disinfection: Not applicable.

     4) Quarantine: Not applicable.

     5) Immunization of contacts: Not applicable. If dengue occurs near possible jungle foci of yellow fever, immunize the population against yellow fever, because the urban vector for the two diseases is the same.

     6) Investigation of contacts and source of infection: Determine patient's place of residence during the 2 weeks before onset of illness, and search for unreported or undiagnosed cases.

7) Specific treatment: Supportive, including oral rehydration. Acetylsalicylic acid (aspirin) is contraindicated because of its hemorrhagic potential. Severe illness is usually secondary to capillary leak syndrome, and requires appropriate intravenous fluid resuscitation.

C. Epidemic measures:

1) Search for and destroy *Aedes* mosquitoes in sites of human habitation, and eliminate or apply larvicide to all potential *Ae. aegypti* larval habitats. Adulticide should target indoor mosquitoes where most of the transmission takes place.
2) Use mosquito repellents for people exposed to vector mosquitoes.

D. Disaster implications: Epidemics can be extensive and affect a high percentage of the population.

E. International measures: Enforce international agreements designed to prevent the spread of *Ae. aegypti* via ships, airplanes and land transport. Improve international surveillance and exchange of data between countries. WHO Collaborating Centres provide support as required. More information can be found at:

<http://www.who.int/collaboratingcentres/database/en/>
Further information can be found on the following websites:
<http://www.cdc.gov/ncidod/dvbid/dengue/>
<http://www.who.int/denguenet>
<http://www.who.int/health_topics/dengue/en>
<http://www.paho.org/english/ad/dpc/cd/Dengue.htm>
<http://www.searo.who.int/en/Section10/Section332/Section1026.htm>

DENGUE HEMORRHAGIC FEVER/DENGUE SHOCK SYNDROME (DHF/DSS)   ICD-9 065.4; ICD-10 A91
[CCDM19: Editorial Board]
[CCDM18: R. Dayal-Drager]

1. Identification—A severe mosquito-transmitted viral illness endemic in much of southern and southeastern Asia, the Pacific, sub-Saharan Africa and Latin America, characterized by acute febrile illness, hemorrhagic diathesis with abnormal blood clotting, and increased vascular permeability with a tendency to develop hypovolemic shock. It is recognized principally in children, but also occurs in adults. The WHO proposed clinical case definition (1997) for DHF is:

1) Fever or history of recent fever lasting 2–7 days.
2) At least 1 of the following hemorrhagic manifestations: positive tourniquet test; petechiae; ecchymoses; purpura; hematemesis; melena; other overt bleeding.
3) Thrombocytopenia; $100 \times 10^3/mm^3$ or less (SI units $100 \times 10^9/L$ or less).
4) Evidence of plasma leakage by at least 1 of the following: (20% rise in hematocrit or 20% drop in hematocrit following volume replacement, pleural effusion, ascites, hypoproteinemia).

Dengue shock syndrome (DSS) includes all above criteria plus signs of shock:

a) Rapid, weak pulse.
b) Narrow pulse pressure (less than 20 mm Hg).
c) Hypotension for age.
d) Cold, clammy skin and restlessness.

Early oral or prompt intravenous fluid therapy may reduce hematocrit rise and require alternate observations to document increased plasma leakage or bleeding.

Illness begins abruptly with fever and, in children, mild or no upper respiratory complaints, often anorexia, facial flush, and mild GI disturbances. The liver may be enlarged, with occasional tenderness. Coincident with defervescence and decreasing platelet count, the patient's condition suddenly worsens in severe cases, with marked weakness, restlessness, facial pallor and often diaphoresis, severe abdominal pain, cool extremities, and circumoral cyanosis. Warning signs include intense continuous abdominal pain with persistent vomiting, and oliguria.

Hemorrhagic phenomena occur frequently, mostly on skin during febrile illness (see earlier). GI hemorrhage is an ominous sign that usually follows a prolonged period of shock. Pathophysiologic findings include accumulation of fluids in serosal cavities, low serum albumin, elevated transaminases, a prolonged prothrombin time and low levels of C3 complement protein. DHF cases with severe liver damage (with or without encephalopathy) have been observed during large epidemics of dengue-3 in Indonesia and Thailand. Case-fatality rates in new outbreak areas where diagnosis is not made or where shock is mistreated have been as high as 40%–50%; with prompt and proper physiological fluid replacement therapy, rates should be 1%-2%.

Serological tests show a rise in antibody titer against dengue viruses. IgM antibody, indicating a current or recent flavivirus infection, is usually detectable by day 6-7 after onset of illness. Viruses can be isolated from blood during the acute febrile stage of illness, by inoculation to mosquitoes or cell cultures. Inoculation to mosquitoes improves the chances of isolating viruses from organs examined at autopsy; PCR may detect virus-specific nucleic acid sequences.

Infection with dengue viruses with or without hemorrhagic manifestations is covered above. The related yellow fever and other hemorrhagic fevers are presented separately.

2. Infectious agent—See *Dengue fever*. All 4 dengue serotypes can cause DHF/DSS (in descending order of frequency, types 2, 3, 4 and 1). There is evidence that serotypes 2 and 4 need to be secondary infection in order to cause DHF/DSS, while primary infection with serotype 1 and 3 can cause DHF/DSS.

3. Occurrence—Recent epidemics of DHF have occurred in Asia (Cambodia, China, India, Indonesia, Lao People's Democratic Republic, Malaysia, Maldives, Myanmar, New Caledonia, Pakistan, Philippines, Singapore, Sri Lanka, Tahiti, Thailand and Viet Nam) and in the Americas (Brazil, Colombia, Cuba, Ecuador, El Salvador, French Guiana, Guatemala, Honduras, Nicaragua, Puerto Rico, Suriname and Venezuela). In an unprecedented pandemic in 1998, 56 countries reported 1.2 million cases of dengue and DHF. In tropical Asia, DHF/DSS is observed primarily among children of the local population under 15. In outbreaks in the Americas, the disease is observed in all age groups although two-thirds of fatalities occur among children. Malaysia, the Philippines, and Thailand report an increase in the number of DHF adult cases. Occurrence is greatest during the rainy season and in areas of high *Ae. aegypti* prevalence. It is estimated that there are over 500 000 cases of DHF each year, the majority of which occur in persons under 15 years of age.

4., 5., 6., and 7. Reservoir, Mode of transmission, Incubation period and **Period of communicability**—See *Dengue fever*.

8. Susceptibility—The best-described risk factor is the circulation of heterologous dengue antibody, acquired passively in infants or actively from an earlier infection. Such antibodies may enhance infection of mononuclear phagocytes through the formation of infectious immune complexes. Geographic origin of dengue strain, age, gender and human genetic susceptibility may also be important risk factors. In the 1981

Cuban outbreak caused by a southeastern Asian dengue-2 virus, DHF/DSS was observed 5 times more often in white than in black patients. In Myanmar, Burmese and Indians were equally susceptible to DHF, while in Viet Nam evidence of an association with genetic variations in the vitamin D receptor has recently been hypothesized as a factor in susceptibility.

9. **Methods of control—**

   A. *Preventive measures:* See *Dengue fever.*

   B. *Control of patient, contacts and immediate environment:*

   1), 2), 3), 4), 5) and 6) Report to local health authority, Isolation, Concurrent disinfection, Quarantine, Immunization of contacts and Investigation of contacts and source of infection: See *Dengue fever.*

   7) Specific treatment: Hypovolemic shock (which occurs most commonly at defervescence) resulting from significant plasma leakage often responds to rapid replacement with fluid and electrolyte solution (acetated Ringer solution or physiological saline at 10–20 ml/kg/hour). In more severe cases of shock, additional plasma and/or plasma expanders should be used. The rate of fluid administration must be judged by estimates of loss, usually through serial microhematocrit, urine output and clinical monitoring. A continued rise in hematocrit value in the presence of vigorous IV fluid administration indicates a need for plasma or other colloid. Care must be taken to monitor IV fluid and adjust the volume rate accordingly to the rate of plasma leakage, to avoid over-hydration. Blood transfusions are indicated for massive bleeding or in cases with refractory shock with unstable signs or a true fall in hematocrit due to concealed bleeding. The use of heparin to manage clinically significant hemorrhage occurring in the presence of well-documented, disseminated intravascular coagulation is a high risk and of no proven benefit. Fresh plasma, fibrinogen and platelet concentrate may be used to treat severe hemorrhage. Aspirin is contraindicated because of its hemorrhagic potential, and the risk that it may precipitate Reye's syndrome.

   C., D. and E. *Epidemic measures, Disaster implications* and *International measures:* See *Dengue fever.*

DERMATOPHYTOSIS ICD-9 110; ICD-10 B35
(Tinea, Ringworm, Dermatomycosis, Epidermophytosis,
Trichophytosis, Microsporosis)
[CCDM19: M. Brandt]
[CCDM18: R. Hay]

Dermatophytosis and tinea are general terms, essentially synonymous, applied to fungal infection of keratinized areas of the body (hair, skin and nails). Various genera and species of fungi known collectively as the dermatophytes are causative agents. The dermatophytoses are subdivided according to the site of infection.

I. TINEA BARBAE AND
   TINEA CAPITIS ICD-9 110.0; ICD-10 B35.0
(Ringworm of the beard and scalp, Kerion, Favus)

1. Identification—A fungal disease that begins as a small area of erythema and/or scaling and spreads peripherally, leaving scaly patches of temporary baldness. Infected hairs become brittle and break off easily. Occasionally, boggy, raised suppurative lesions develop, called kerions. Favus of the scalp (ICD-9 110.0; ICD-10 B35.0) is a variety of tinea capitis caused by *Trichophyton schoenleinii*. It is characterized by a mousy smell and by the formation of small, yellowish, cuplike crusts (scutulae) that amalgamate to form a pale or yellow visible mat on the scalp surface. Affected hairs do not break off, but become grey and lusterless, eventually falling out and leaving baldness that may be permanent.

Tinea capitis is easily distinguished from black piedra, a fungus infection of the hair occurring in tropical areas of South America, southeastern Asia and Africa. Black piedra is characterized by black, hard "gritty" nodules on hair shafts, caused by *Piedraia hortai*. There is a white form in which *Trichosporon* species, particularly *T. ovoides* or *T. inkin*, produce white, soft, pasty nodules.

Examination of the scalp under UV light (Wood lamp) for yellow-green fluorescence is helpful in diagnosing tinea capitis caused by *Microsporum* species such as *M. canis* and *M. audouinii*; *Trichophyton* species do not fluoresce. In infections caused by *Microsporum* spp., microscopic examination of scales and hair in 10% potassium hydroxide or under UV microscopy of a calcofluor white preparation reveals characteristic nonpigmented ectothrix (outside the hair) arthrospores; many *Trichophyton* spp. present an endothrix (inside the hair) pattern of invasion; and *T. verrucosum*, the cause of cattle ringworm, produces large ectothrix spores. Confirmation of the diagnosis requires culture of the fungus. Genetic identification methods are a useful supplement to traditional morphology-based methods of identification.

2. Infectious agents—Various species of *Microsporum* and *Trichophyton*. Species and genus identification is important for epidemiological, prognostic and therapeutic reasons.

3. Occurrence—Tinea capitis caused by *Trichophyton tonsurans* has been epidemic in urban areas in Australia, Mexico, the United Kingdom, eastern USA and Puerto Rico, as well as in many developing countries. *M. canis* infections occur in rural and urban areas wherever infected cats and dogs are present. *M. audouinii* is endemic in western Africa and was formerly widespread in Europe and North America, particularly in urban areas; *T. verrucosum* and *T. mentagrophytes* var. *mentagrophytes* infections occur primarily in rural areas where the disease exists in cattle, horses, rodents and wild animals.

4. Reservoir—Humans for *T. tonsurans*, *T. schoenleinii* and *M. audouinii*; animals, especially dogs, cats and cattle, harbour the other organisms noted above.

5. Mode of transmission—Direct skin-to-skin or indirect contact, especially from the backs of seats, barber clippers, toilet articles (combs, hairbrushes), clothing and hats that are contaminated with hair from infected people or animals. Infected humans can generate considerable aerosols of infective arthrospores.

6. Incubation period—Usually 10 to 14 days.

7. Period of communicability—Viable fungus and infective arthrospores may persist on contaminated materials for long periods.

8. Susceptibility—Children below the age of puberty are highly susceptible to *M. canis*; all ages are subject to *Trichophyton* infections. Reinfections mainly occur for infections spread amongst humans.

9. Methods of control—

    A. Preventive measures:

        1) Educate the public, especially parents, to the danger of acquiring infection from infected individuals, as well as from dogs, cats and other animals.
        2) In the presence of epidemics or in hyperendemic areas where non-*Trichophyton* species are prevalent, survey heads of young children by UV light (Wood lamp) before school entry.

    B. Control of patient, contacts and the immediate environment:

        1) Report to local health authority: Obligatory report of epidemics in some countries; no individual case report, Class 4 (see

Reporting). Outbreaks in schools must be reported to school authorities.

2) Isolation: Not applicable.

3) Concurrent disinfection: In mild cases, daily washing of scalp removes loose hair. Selenium sulfide or ketoconazole shampoos help remove scale. In severe cases, wash scalp daily and cover hair with a cap, which should be boiled after use.

4) Quarantine: Not practical.

5) Immunization of contacts: Not applicable.

6) Investigation of contacts and source of infection: Study household contacts, pets and farm animals for evidence of infection; treat if infected. Some animals, especially cats, may be inapparent carriers. With some agents (e.g. *T. tonsurans*), children may have mild infections accompanied by hair invasion; careful clinical examination of contacts is required.

7) Specific treatment: Topical agents are ineffective in true infections. Oral griseofulvin for at least 4 weeks is effective. Terbinafine and itraconazole are also effective. Terbinafine is more active than griseofulvin against agents such as *T. tonsurans*, but higher doses of this drug should be used in *Microsporum* infections. Systemic antibacterial agents are useful if lesions become secondarily infected by bacteria; in the case of kerions, also use an antiseptic cream, and remove scaly crusts from the scalp by gentle soaking. Examine regularly and take cultures; when cultures become negative, complete recovery may be assumed.

C. *Epidemic measures:* In school or other institutional epidemics, educate children and parents as to mode of spread, prevention and personal hygiene. If more than 2 infected children are present in a class, examine the others. Enlist services of physicians and nurses for diagnosis; carry out follow-up surveys.

D. *Disaster implications:* None.

E. *International measures:* None.

II. TINEA CRURIS   ICD-9 110.3; ICD-10 B35.6
(Ringworm of groin and perianal region)
TINEA CORPORIS
(Ringworm of the body)

1. **Identification**—A fungal disease of the skin other than of the scalp, bearded areas and feet, characteristically appearing as flat, spreading, ring-shaped or circular lesion with a characteristic raised edge around all or part of the lesion. This periphery is usually reddish, vesicular or pustular, and may be dry and scaly or moist and crusted. As the lesion

progresses peripherally, the central area often clears, leaving apparently normal skin. Differentiation from inguinal candidiasis, often distinguished by the presence of "satellite" pustules outside the lesion margins, is necessary, because treatment differs.

Presumptive diagnosis is made by taking scrapings from the advancing lesion margins, clearing in 10% potassium hydroxide, and examining microscopically or under UV microscopy of calcofluor white preparations for segmented, branched non-pigmented fungal filaments. Final identification is through culture.

2. Infectious agents—Most species of *Microsporum* and *Trichophyton*; also *Epidermophyton floccosum*.

3. Occurrence—Worldwide and relatively frequent. Males are infected more often than females.

4. Reservoir—Humans, animals and soil.

5. Mode of transmission—Direct or indirect contact with skin and scalp lesions of infected people or lesions of animals, contaminated floors, shower stalls, benches, and similar articles.

6. Incubation period—Usually 4 to 10 days.

7. Period of communicability—As long as lesions are present and viable fungus persists on contaminated materials.

8. Susceptibility—Susceptibility is widespread, aggravated by friction and excessive perspiration in axillary and inguinal regions, and when environmental temperatures and humidity are high. All ages are susceptible.

9. Methods of control—

    A. Preventive measures: Launder towels and clothing with hot water and/or fungicidal agent; general cleanliness in public showers and dressing rooms (repeated washing of benches; frequent hosing and rapid draining of shower rooms). A fungicidal agent such as cresol should be used to disinfect benches and floors.

    B. Control of patient, contacts and the immediate environment:

       1) Report to local health authority: Obligatory report of epidemics in some countries; no individual case report, Class 4 (see *Reporting*). Report infections of schoolchildren to school authorities.

       2) Isolation: While under treatment, infected persons should be excluded from swimming pools and activities likely to lead to exposure of others.

3) Concurrent disinfection: Effective and frequent laundering of clothing.
4) Quarantine: Not applicable.
5) Immunization of contacts: Not applicable.
6) Investigation of contacts and source of infection: Examine school and household contacts, household pets and farm animals; treat infections as indicated.
7) Specific treatment: Thorough bathing with soap and water, removal of scabs and crusts, and application of an effective topical fungicide (miconazole, ketoconazole, clotrimazole, econazole, naftifine, terbinafine, tolnaftate or ciclopirox) may suffice. Oral griseofulvin is effective, as are oral itraconazole and oral terbinafine.

C. Epidemic measures: Educate children and parents about the infection, its mode of spread, and the need to maintain good personal hygiene. Outbreaks are common amongst military personnel.

D. Disaster implications: None.

E. International measures: None.

III. TINEA PEDIS   ICD-9 110.4; ICD-10 B35.3
(Ringworm of the foot, Athlete's foot)

1. Identification—This fungal disease presents with characteristic scaling or cracking of the skin, especially between the toes (interdigital), diffuse scaling over the sole of the foot (dry type), or blisters containing a thin watery fluid; commonly called athlete's foot. In severe cases, vesicular lesions appear on various parts of the body, especially the hands; these dermatophytids do not contain the fungus but are an allergic reaction to fungus products.

Presumptive diagnosis is verified by microscopic examination of potassium hydroxide- or calcofluor white-treated scrapings from lesions that reveal septate branching filaments. Clinical appearance is not diagnostic; final identification is through culture. Note that bacteria, including Gram-negative organisms and coryneforms as well as *Candida* and *Scytalidium* species, may produce similar lesions. Itching is often a clue that dermatophyte fungi are present. *Scytalidium* can also cause similar dry lesions on the sole.

2. Infectious agents—*Trichophyton rubrum*, *T. mentagrophytes* var. *interdigitale*, and *Epidermophyton floccosum*.

3. Occurrence—Common worldwide. Adults are more often affected than children, males more than females. Infections are more frequent and more severe in hot weather. They are also common in industrial workers, schoolchildren, athletes and military personnel who share shower or bathing facilities.

4. Reservoir—Humans.

5. Mode of transmission—Direct or indirect contact with skin lesions of infected people or with contaminated floors, shower stalls and other articles used by infected people.

6. Incubation period—Unknown.

7. Period of communicability—As long as lesions are present and viable spores persist on contaminated materials.

8. Susceptibility—Susceptibility is variable and infection may be inapparent. Repeated attacks and chronic infections are frequent.

9. Methods of control—

A. *Preventive measures:* See *Tinea corporis*. Educate the public to maintain strict personal hygiene; take special care in drying between toes after bathing; regularly use a dusting powder or cream containing an effective antifungal on the feet, and particularly between the toes. Occlusive shoes may predispose to infection and disease.

B. *Control of patient, contacts and the immediate environment:*

1) Report to local health authority: Obligatory report of epidemics in some countries; no individual case report, Class 4 (see *Reporting*). Report high incidence in schools to school authorities.
2) Isolation: Not applicable.
3) Concurrent disinfection: Launder socks of heavily infected individuals to prevent reinfection.
4) Quarantine: Not applicable.
5) Immunization of contacts: Not applicable.
6) Investigation of contacts and source of infection: Not applicable.
7) Specific treatment: Topical antifungals (miconazole, clotrimazole, ketoconazole, terbinafine, ciclopirox or tolnaftate). Expose feet to air by wearing sandals; use dusting powders. Oral terbinafine or itraconazole may be indicated in severe, extensive or protracted disease; griseofulvin, although less active, is an alternative.

C. *Epidemic measures:* Thoroughly clean and wash floors of showers and similar sources of infection; disinfect with a fungicidal agent such as cresol. Educate the public about the mode of spread.

    D. Disaster implications: None.

    E. International measures: None.

IV. ONYCHOMYCOSIS DUE TO DERMATOPHYTES   ICD-9 110.1; ICD-10 B35.1
(Tinea unguium, Ringworm of the nails, Onychomycosis)

1. Identification—A chronic fungal disease involving one or more nails of the hands or feet. The nail gradually becomes detached from the nail bed, thickens, and becomes discolored and brittle; an accumulation of soft keratinous material forms beneath the nail or the nail becomes chalky and disintegrates.

Diagnosis is made by microscopic examination of potassium hydroxide preparations of the nail and of detritus beneath the nail for hyaline fungal elements. Etiology should be confirmed by culture.

2. Infectious agents—Various species of *Trichophyton*; rarely, other dermatophytes. *Scytalidium dimidiatum* causes an almost identical disease (not strictly speaking a tinea infection), differentiated through culture on cycloheximide-free media.

3. Occurrence—Common.

4. Reservoir—Humans; rarely animals or soil.

5. Mode of transmission—Presumably through extension from skin infections acquired by direct contact with skin or nail lesions of infected people, or from indirect contact (contaminated floors and shower stalls). Low rate of transmission, even to close family associates.

6. Incubation period—Unknown.

7. Period of communicability—As long as an infected lesion is present.

8. Susceptibility—Susceptibility variable. Reinfection is frequent.

9. Methods of control—

    A. Preventive measures: Cleanliness and use of a fungicidal agent such as cresol for disinfecting floors in common use; frequent hosing and rapid draining of shower rooms.

    B. Control of patient, contacts and the immediate environment:

        1) Report to local health authority: Official report not ordinarily justifiable, Class 5 (see *Reporting*).

2), 3), 4), 5) and 6) Isolation, Concurrent disinfection, Quarantine, Immunization of contacts and Investigation of contacts and source of infection: Not practical.

7) Specific treatment: Oral itraconazole and terbinafine are the drugs of choice. Oral griseofulvin is less effective. Treatment to be given until nails grow out (about 3–6 months for fingernails, 12–18 months for toenails). At present there is no effective treatment for *Scytalidium* infections.

C, D, and *E. Epidemic measures, Disaster implications and International measures:* Not applicable.

DIARRHEA, ACUTE   ICD-9 001-009; ICD-10 A09

[CCDM19: O. Fontaine, P. Griffin, O. Henao, D. Lo Fo Wong, E. Mintz, R. Mody, C. O'Reilly, J. Schlundt]
[CCDM18: P. Braam]

Diarrhea is often accompanied by other clinical signs and symptoms, including vomiting, fever, dehydration and electrolyte disturbances. It can be a symptom of infection by many different bacterial, viral and parasitic enteric agents. Several of the more common gastrointestinal infections characterized by diarrhea—cholera, shigellosis, salmonellosis, *Campylobacter* enteritis, *Escherichia coli* infections, yersiniosis, giardiasis, cryptosporidiosis and viral gastroenteropathy—are described in detail under individual listings elsewhere in this book.

Diarrhea can also occur in association with other infectious diseases, such as malaria, measles, and avian influenza; and as a result of noninfectious processes, such as intoxication by chemical agents. Change in the enteric flora induced by antimicrobials may produce acute diarrhea by overgrowth and toxin production by *Klebsiella oxytoca* or *Clostridium difficile*.

Approximately 70%–80% of the vast number of sporadic diarrheal episodes in people visiting treatment facilities in less industrialized countries could be diagnosed etiologically if the complete battery of newer laboratory tests were available and used. From a practical clinical standpoint, diarrheal illnesses can be divided into 3 clinical presentations:

1) Acute watery diarrhea (including cholera), lasting several hours or days; the main danger is dehydration; weight loss occurs if feeding is not continued. For severe dehydration (one or more of the following—lethargic or unconscious; drinking poorly or not at all; eyes very sunken and dry; mouth very dry; very slow skin pinch—corresponding to a fluid deficit of 10% of body weight), the preferred treatment is rapid intravenous therapy followed by oral rehydration;

in other cases (no or some dehydration), give reduced osmolarity oral rehydration solution (ORS) (75 mEq/L sodium, 75 mmol/L glucose, total osmolarity of 245 mOsm/L) by mouth early in the illness. Immediately upon rehydration, an unrestricted regular diet (or breastfeeding, as applicable) should be started regardless of the severity of illness. In children under five years of age, zinc supplementation given during an episode of acute diarrhea reduces the duration and severity of the episode, and zinc supplementation given for 10 to 14 days lowers the incidence of diarrhea in the following 2 to 3 months. For these reasons, WHO and UNICEF now recommend 20 mg elemental zinc per day for 10 to 14 days to all children under 5 years of age with acute, presumed infectious diarrhea.

2) Acute bloody diarrhea or dysentery, caused by *Campylobacter, Salmonella, Shigella, E. coli* O157:H7, *E. histolytica,* and other organisms. The main dangers are intestinal damage, sepsis, and malnutrition; other complications, including dehydration, may occur. Use of antimicrobial agents should ideally be based on the results of stool cultures and, if amebiasis is suspected, microscopic stool examination. Empiric regimens may be considered in travelers with limited access to facilities offering microbiological diagnosis. Hydration treatment is the same as that for acute watery diarrhea. Frequent small portions of regular food should be administered throughout the illness; higher protein meals may improve recovery.

3) Persistent diarrhea, lasting 14 days or longer; the main danger is malnutrition and serious extraintestinal infection; dehydration may also occur. Zinc supplementation may both prevent persistent diarrhea and hasten recovery, especially among children in developing countries. Non-infectious causes should be considered, e.g. an initial presentation of inflammatory bowel disease.

SURVEILLANCE NETWORKS FOR DIARRHEA/HUMAN GASTROINTESTINAL INFECTIONS

The information in the following section is applicable to all the acute diarrheal diseases.

Since the early 1990s, specialized national and international surveillance networks have been developed to detect outbreaks that are dispersed over large geographical areas and that previously remained undetected. Two examples of well-established international surveillance networks are Enternet and PulseNet International.

Enter-net, which began in 1993 as Salm-Net, was the international surveillance network for human gastrointestinal infections due to Salmonella, verocytotoxin-producing Escherichia coli O157 (VTEC) and Campylobacter, including antimicrobial resistance, and involved all 27 countries of the European Union (EU), as well as Australia, Canada, Japan, South Africa, Switzerland and Norway. Since October 2007, Enter-Net has been subsumed into the food- and waterborne disease unit of the European

Centre for Disease Prevention and Control (ECDC) in Stockholm. More information can be found here:

<http://www.ecdc.europa.eu/Activities/surveillance/ENTER_NET/index.html>

PulseNet International is a network of networks dedicated to tracking food-borne pathogens and diseases worldwide through molecular subtyping of outbreak-related isolates and sharing of DNA-fingerprint patterns. Currently, PulseNet International consists of PulseNet USA, PulseNet Canada, PulseNet Latin America and the Caribbean, PulseNet Europe, PulseNet Middle East and PulseNet Asia Pacific. More information can be found here:

<http://www.cdc.gov/pulsenet/whatis.htm>

Through the efforts of international networks such as PulseNet International and Enter-net, food-borne outbreaks of international importance have been detected, reported and halted from spreading further.

DIARRHEA CAUSED BY
ESCHERICHIA COLI   ICD-9 008.0; ICD-10 A04.0–A04.4

Six major categories of *Escherichia coli* strains cause diarrhea:

1) Enterohemorrhagic
2) Enterotoxigenic
3) Enteroinvasive
4) Enteropathogenic
5) Enteroaggregative
6) Diffuse-adherence.

Each has a different pathogenesis, possesses distinct virulence properties, and comprises a separate set of O:H serotypes. Different clinical syndromes and epidemiological patterns may also be seen. Transmission is usually through contaminated food, water, or hands, or via direct contact with animals; airborne transmission can occur for some categories. Contamination from the environment can also play a role.

I. DIARRHEA CAUSED BY
ENTEROHEMORRHAGIC
STRAINS   ICD-9 008.0; ICD-10 A04.3
(EHEC, Shiga toxin-producing *E. coli* [STEC], Enterohemorrhagic *E. coli* [EHEC], *E. coli* O157:H7, Verotoxin-producing *E. coli* [VTEC])

1. Identification—This category of diarrhea-causing *E. coli* was recognized in 1982, when a USA outbreak of hemorrhagic colitis was shown to be due to a serotype, *E. coli* O157:H7, which had not previously been identified as an enteric pathogen.

E. coli O157:H7 and other strains of *E. coli* that produce Shiga toxins are collectively known as Shiga toxin-producing *E. coli* (STEC). The diarrhea may range from mild and non-bloody to stools that are virtually all blood. The most severe clinical manifestation of Shiga toxin-producing *E. coli* (STEC) infection is hemolytic uremic syndrome (HUS). With the recognition that STEC is the cause of diarrhea-associated HUS, the term HUS is now used to describe both children and adults with hemolytic anemia, thrombocytopenia, and acute renal dysfunction following STEC infection, whether or not they also have neurologic abnormalities and fever. *E. coli* O157:H7 has the strongest association with HUS worldwide. About 15% of children with *E. coli* O157:H7 diarrhea, and a much smaller proportion of adults, develop HUS. Fifty percent of patients require dialysis, and about 5% die. Rates vary for other STEC serotypes. STEC express potent cytotoxins called Shiga toxins (Stx) 1 and 2 (Stx1 and Stx2 are also called verocytotoxins or verotoxins, and were previously called Shiga-like toxins). Stx1 is identical to the toxin elaborated by *Shigella dysenteriae* 1; HUS is also a complication of *S. dysenteriae* 1 infection. The structural genes for the toxins are found on chromosomally encoded phages. Most STEC strains have a chromosomal pathogenicity island containing multiple virulence genes, including those encoding proteins that cause attaching and effacing lesions.

In North America most strains of the most common STEC serotype, O157:H7, can be identified in stool cultures on sorbitol-MacConkey media by their inability to ferment sorbitol. Because most other STEC strains ferment sorbitol, other techniques must be used, among which are demonstrating the ability to elaborate Shiga toxins (a commercial assay is available), or the use of DNA probes that identify the toxin genes. This most likely results in under-reporting of non-O157 STEC. All STEC strains should be sent to the state health department laboratory for serotyping to monitor the frequency of various serotypes and to help detect outbreaks. In addition, *E. coli* O157:H7 strains are subtyped by pulsed-field gel electrophoresis to help detect outbreaks.

2. Infectious agent—The main STEC serotype in North America is *E. coli* O157:H7; this serotype is thought to cause over 90% of cases of diarrhea-associated HUS. In Germany this figure is closer to 50%. The other most common serogroups in North America are O26, O111, O103, O45, and O121. In Europe the same serogroups are found, and O145 is also important.

3. Occurrence—These infections are an important problem in North America, Europe, Japan, the southern cone of South America, and southern Africa. Their importance in the rest of the world is less well established.

4. Reservoir—Cattle are the most important reservoir of STEC; humans may also serve as a reservoir for person-to-person transmission. Other ruminants, including sheep, goats and deer, may also carry STEC.

5. Mode of transmission—Transmission is mainly through ingestion of food contaminated with ruminant feces, and direct contact with animals or their environment. Serious outbreaks, including cases of hemorrhagic colitis, HUS, and some deaths, have occurred in the USA from beef (usually as inadequately cooked hamburgers); grocery produce (including melons, lettuce, fresh spinach, coleslaw, apple cider, alfalfa sprouts and spinach); and unpasteurized cows milk. Direct person-to-person transmission occurs in families, childcare centers, and custodial institutions. Waterborne transmission occurs both from contaminated drinking water and from recreational waters.

6. Incubation period—2–10 days, with a median of 3–4 days.

7. Period of communicability—The duration of excretion of the pathogen is typically 1 week or less in adults, but 3 weeks in one-third of children. Prolonged carriage is uncommon.

8. Susceptibility—The infectious dose is very low. Little is known about differences in susceptibility and immunity, but infections occur in persons of all ages. Children under 5 years old are most frequently diagnosed with infection and are at greatest risk of developing HUS. The elderly also appear to be at increased risk of complications.

9. Methods of control—

A. *Preventive measures:* The potential severity of this disease and the importance of infection in vulnerable groups such as children and the elderly calls for early involvement of local health authorities to identify the source and apply appropriate preventive measures. As soon as the diagnosis is suspected, it is of paramount importance to block person-to-person transmission by instructing family members about the need for frequent (especially post-defecatory) handwashing with soap and water, disposal of soiled diapers/nappies and human waste, and prevention of food and beverage contamination. Measures likely to reduce the incidence of illness include the following:

1) Investigate potential to limit the prevalence of carriers in cattle herds. Decrease the carriage and excretion of STEC in cattle on farms, through improved farm management practices, especially in the days just before slaughter.
2) Manage slaughterhouse operations to minimize contamination of meat by animal hides or intestinal contents.
3) Decrease contamination with animal feces of foods consumed with no or minimal cooking, including through limited use of animal waste for fertilization purposes.
4) Pasteurize milk and dairy products.
5) Wash fruits and vegetables carefully, particularly if eaten raw. They should preferably be peeled.

6) Wash hands thoroughly and frequently using soap, in particular after contact with farm animals or the farm environment.

7) Strengthen control measures for exhibits which allow direct animal contact in public settings, such as fairs, farm tours, and petting zoos, and educate populations at risk about the risks associated with attending such events.

8) Cook beef adequately, especially ground beef, to an internal temperature of 70°C (155°F). Reliance on cooking until all pink color is gone is not as reliable as using a meat thermometer.

9) Protect, purify and chlorinate public water supplies; chlorinate swimming pools. When the safety of drinking water is doubtful, boil it.

10) Ensure adequate hygiene in childcare centers, and encourage frequent handwashing, with soap.

B. Control of patient, contacts and the immediate environment:

1) Report to local health authority: Case report of STEC infection is obligatory in many countries, Class 2 (see *Reporting*). Recognition and reporting of outbreaks is especially important.

2) Isolation: During acute illness, enteric precautions. Because of the small infective dose, infected patients should not be employed to handle food or to provide child or patient care until 2 successive negative fecal samples or rectal swabs are obtained (collected 24 hours apart and not sooner than 48 hours after the last dose of antimicrobials).

3) Concurrent disinfection: Of feces and contaminated articles. In communities with an adequate sewage disposal system, feces can be discharged directly into sewers without preliminary disinfection. Terminal cleaning.

4) Quarantine: Not applicable.

5) Management of contacts: When feasible, contacts with diarrhea should be excluded from food handling and the care of children or patients until diarrhea ceases and 2 successive negative stool cultures are obtained. All contacts should be educated about thorough handwashing after defecation and before handling food or caring for children or patients.

6) Investigation of contacts and source of infection: Cultures of contacts should generally be confined to food handlers, attendants, and children in childcare centers and other situations where the spread of infection is particularly likely. Culture of suspected foods, livestock feces, or agricultural environmental samples has become more productive in recent years, particularly in outbreak settings, when laboratories use selective culture conditions, including selective broth enrichment, immunomagnetic separation methods,

and plating on selective media. If ground beef is suspected as the source of infection, laboratory testing of the leftover beef can be useful.

7) Specific treatment: Reasonable concern exists that some antimicrobial agents increase the risk of HUS, although proof is lacking. A meta-analysis failed to confirm an increased risk of HUS or to show a benefit from antimicrobial therapy. However, most experts would not use an antimicrobial agent to treat persons with *E. coli* O157:H7 infection, because no benefit has been proven, and harm is possible. Fluid replacement is the cornerstone of treatment for STEC diarrhea; some clinicians choose to hospitalize all patients with *E. coli* O157:H7 infection for hydration to prevent the development of hemolytic uremic syndrome.

C. *Epidemic measures:*

1) Report at once to the local health authority any group of persons with acute bloody diarrhea, HUS, or thrombotic thrombocytopenic purpura, even in the absence of specific identification of the causal agent.

2) Search intensively for the specific vehicle (food, water, animal contact, etc.) by which the infection was transmitted; evaluate potential for ongoing person-to-person transmission; and use the results of epidemiological investigations to guide specific control measures.

3) Collaborate with relevant regulatory agencies to trace the source of suspected food and recall any implicated product; in large common-source food-borne outbreaks, prompt recall may prevent many cases.

4) If a waterborne outbreak is suspected, issue an order to boil water and chlorinate suspected water supplies adequately under competent supervision, or do not use them.

5) If a swimming-associated outbreak is suspected, close pools or beaches until chlorinated or shown to be free of fecal contamination, and until adequate toilet facilities are provided to prevent further contamination of water by bathers.

6) If a milk-borne outbreak is suspected, pasteurize or boil the milk.

7) Prophylactic administration of antimicrobials is not recommended.

8) Publicize the importance of handwashing after defecation; provide equipment for proper handwashing with soap and individual paper towels in public venues.

D. *Disaster implications:* A potential problem where personal hygiene and environmental sanitation are deficient (see *Typhoid fever*, 9D).

E. *International measures:* WHO Collaborating Centres provide support as required. More information can be found at:
  <http://www.who.int/collaboratingcentres/database/en/>
  [NB Search for: WHO Collaborating Centre for Research on Enterotoxigenic Escherichia Coli (ETEC)]
  For further information, see also:
  WHO Guide on Hygiene in Food Service and Mass Catering Establishments
  <http://whqlibdoc.who.int/hq/1994/WHO_FNU_FOS_94.5.pdf>
  WHO Five Keys to Safer Food Manual (2007)
  <http://www.who.int/foodsafety/publications/consumer/manual_keys>

II. DIARRHEA CAUSED BY ENTEROTOXIGENIC STRAINS
(Enterotoxigenic *E. coli*, ETEC)

ICD-9 008.0; ICD-10 A04.1

1. **Identification**—Enterotoxigenic *E. coli* (ETEC) is a major cause of travelers' diarrhea in people from industrialized countries who visit developing countries. ETEC is also a major cause of dehydrating diarrhea in infants and children in developing countries, especially among children less than 2 years of age. It has been estimated (WHO) that globally ETEC causes as many as 380 000 deaths annually in children under five. ETEC produces one or both of two enterotoxins — heat-labile (LT) enterotoxin and heat-stable enterotoxin — and colonization factors that allow the organism readily to colonize the small intestine and thus cause diarrhea. The severity of illness can range from mild watery diarrhea to severe cholera-like purging, as the enterotoxigenic strains may behave like *Vibrio cholerae* in producing a profuse watery diarrhea without blood or mucus. Abdominal cramping, vomiting, acidosis, prostration and dehydration can occur; low grade fever may or may not be present; symptoms usually last less than 5 days, but may last longer in previously unexposed travelers.

ETEC can be identified through demonstration of enterotoxin production, immunoassays, bioassays, DNA probe techniques that identify LT and ST genes (for heat labile and heat stable toxins) in colony blots, or PCR methods. None of these assays are widely available in clinical laboratories, and therefore ETEC infections are under-diagnosed.

2. **Infectious agent**—ETEC elaborate a heat-labile enterotoxin (LT), a heat-stable toxin (ST) or both toxins (LT/ST). The most common O serogroups include O6, O8, O15, O20, O25, O27, O49, O63, O78, O128ac, O148, O153, O159, O167, and O169. Serotype O169: H41 has emerged as the most common cause of ETEC outbreaks in the USA.

3. Occurrence—An infection primarily of developing countries. During the first 3 years of life, children in developing countries experience multiple ETEC infections that lead to the acquisition of immunity; consequently, illness in older children and adults occurs less frequently.

Infection occurs among travelers from industrialized countries that visit developing countries. ETEC transmission on cruise ships has also been reported. The number of food-borne outbreaks in industrialized countries has increased in recent years. In an outbreak setting, ETEC testing should be considered if the clinical presentation is compatible and the results of bacterial cultures for routine enteric pathogens are negative.

4. Reservoir—Humans. Although ETEC infections occur in animals, people constitute the reservoir for strains causing diarrhea in humans.

5. Mode of transmission—Contaminated food and water. Transmission via contaminated weaning foods may be particularly important in infection of infants. Direct contact transmission through fecally contaminated hands is believed to be rare.

6. Incubation period—Incubations as short as 10–12 hours have been observed in outbreaks and in volunteer studies with certain LT-only and ST-only strains. The incubation period of LT/ST diarrhea in volunteer studies has usually been 24–72 hours.

7. Period of communicability—For the duration of excretion of the pathogenic ETEC, which may be prolonged.

8. Susceptibility—Epidemiological studies and rechallenge studies in volunteers demonstrate that ETEC infection is followed by serotype-specific immunity. Multiple infections with different serotypes are required to develop broad-spectrum immunity against ETEC. Pre-existing malnutrition, including micronutrient deficiency, can lead to more severe infections with ETEC.

9. Methods of control—

A. Preventive measures:

1) For general measures for prevention of fecal-oral spread of infection, see *Typhoid fever*, 9A.
2) For adult travelers going for short periods of time to high-risk areas where it is not easy to obtain safe food or water, the use of prophylactic bismuth subsalicylate (2 tablets 4 times a day) or antimicrobials (norfloxacin, 400 mg daily or rifaximin, 200 mg daily) may be considered; however each regimen is associated with health risks of its own. A much preferable approach is to initiate very early treatment, beginning with the onset of diarrhea, e.g. after the second or third loose stool (See section 9B7).

B. *Control of patient, contacts and the immediate environment:*

1) Report to local health authority: Obligatory report of epidemics; no individual case report, Class 4 (see *Reporting*).
2) Isolation: Enteric precautions for known and suspected cases.
3) Concurrent disinfection: Of all fecal discharges and soiled articles. In communities with an adequate sewage disposal system, feces can be discharged directly into sewers without preliminary disinfection.
4) Quarantine: Not applicable.
5) Immunization of contacts: Not applicable.
6) Investigation of contacts and source of infection: Not applicable.
7) Specific treatment: Electrolyte-fluid therapy to prevent or treat dehydration is the most important measure (see *Cholera*, section 9B7). Most cases do not require any other treatment. For severe travelers' diarrhea in adults, early treatment with an antibiotic such as a fluoroquinolone—ciprofloxacin (PO 500 mg twice daily) or norfloxacin (PO 400 mg daily) for 5 days. Fluoroquinolones are used as initial treatment because many ETEC strains worldwide are resistant to other antimicrobials.

   However, if local strains are known to be sensitive, trimethoprim-sulfoxazole (PO 160 mg–800 mg twice daily) or doxycycline (PO 100 mg once daily), for 5 days, are useful, though doxycyline cannot be used in children less than eight years of age. Feeding should be continued according to the patient's appetite.

C. *Epidemic measures:* Epidemiological investigation may be indicated to determine how transmission is occurring.

D. *Disaster implications:* None.

E. *International measures:* WHO Collaborating Centres provide support as required. More information can be found at:
   <http://www.who.int/collaboratingcentres/database/en/>

III. DIARRHEA CAUSED BY ENTEROINVASIVE STRAINS   ICD-9 008.0; ICD-10 A04.2
(Enteroinvasive *E. coli*, EIEC)

1. Identification—This inflammatory disease of the gut mucosa and submucosa caused by EIEC strains of *E. coli* closely resembles that produced by *Shigella*. The organisms possess the same plasmid-dependent ability to invade and multiply within epithelial cells. Clinically, the syndrome of watery diarrhea due to EIEC is much more common than dysentery. The O antigens of EIEC may cross-react with *Shigella* O antigens. Illness begins with severe abdominal cramps, malaise, watery stools, tenesmus and fever; in less than 10% of patients, it progresses to the passage of multiple, scanty, fluid stools containing blood and mucus. The presence of many fecal leukocytes visible in a stained smear of mucus, also seen in shigellosis, should raise the suspicion of EIEC. Tests available in reference laboratories include an immunoassay that detects the plasmid-encoded specific outer membrane proteins associated with epithelial cell invasiveness; a bioassay (guinea pig-keratoconjunctivitis test) detects epithelial cell invasiveness; DNA probes detect the enteroinvasiveness plasmid.

2. Infectious agent—Strains of *E. coli* shown to possess enteroinvasiveness dependent on the presence of a large virulence plasmid encoding invasion plasmid antigens. The main O serogroups in which EIEC fall include O28ac, O29, O112, O124, O136, O143, O144, O152, O164 and O167.

3. Occurrence—EIEC infections are endemic in developing countries, and cause about 1%–5% of diarrheal episodes among people visiting treatment centers. Rarely, infections and outbreaks of EIEC diarrhea have been reported in industrialized countries.

4. Reservoir—Humans.

5. Mode of transmission—The scant available evidence suggests that EIEC is transmitted by contaminated food.

6. Incubation period—Incubations as short as 10 and 18 hours have been observed in volunteer studies and outbreaks, respectively.

7. Period of communicability—Duration of excretion of EIEC strains.

8. Susceptibility—Little is known about susceptibility and immunity to EIEC.

9. Methods of control—Same as for ETEC, above. For the rare cases of severe diarrhea with enteroinvasive strains, as for shigellosis, treat using antimicrobials effective against local *Shigella* isolates.

IV. DIARRHEA CAUSED BY ENTEROPATHOGENIC STRAINS   ICD-9 008.0; ICD-10 A04.0
(Enteropathogenic *E. coli*, EPEC)

1. Identification—The oldest recognized category of diarrhea-producing *E. coli*, implicated in 1940s and 1950s studies in which certain O:H serotypes were found to be associated with infant summer diarrhea, outbreaks of diarrhea in infant nurseries, and community epidemics of infant diarrhea. Diarrheal disease in this category is virtually confined to children aged less than one year, in whom it causes watery diarrhea with mucus, fever and dehydration. The diarrhea in infants can be both severe and prolonged, and in developing countries may be associated with high case fatality.

EPEC is best identified by molecular methods that target EPEC-associated virulence markers. EPEC strains contain a pathogenicity island known as the locus of enterocyte effacement (LEE), which encodes proteins that enable strains to cause dissolution of the microvilli of enterocytes and initiate close attachment of the bacteria to enterocytes (attaching and effacing [A/E] lesions). In cell culture, these organisms exhibit localized adherence to HEp-2 cells, a property that correlates with the presence of a virulence plasmid called the EPEC adherence factor (EAF) plasmid. Commonly used markers to identify EPEC in PCR and nucleic acid hybridization assays include the LEE-associated gene encoding intimin (*eae*), a protein that enables the organism to adhere intimately to epithelial cells and cause A/E lesions; the EAF plasmid-associated gene encoding bundlin (*bfpA*), a structural protein forming the pilus structure that mediates the initial stages of attachment; or sequences of unknown function from the EAF plasmid. It is important to note that EPEC strains share some traits with STEC, notably the LEE pathogenicity island, but do not produce Shiga toxins. An advantage to employing molecular methods for detecting EPEC is that both classical (historically recognized) and newly recognized EPEC serotypes will be detected.

The classical serotypes of EPEC can be tentatively identified through agglutination with antisera that detect EPEC O serogroups, but confirmation requires both O and H typing with high-quality reagents. The importance of using high-quality reagents and following manufacturers' recommendations for the use of their products cannot be over-emphasized. Particular attention to the intended use of OK typing antisera is advised. Antibodies against capsular (K antigens) will be present in OK antisera, thereby necessitating the use of O-specific antisera for definitive O typing.

2. Infectious agent—Frequently encountered O:H serotypes of EPEC include O55:NM, O55:H6, O55:H7, O86:NM, O86:H34, O111:NM, O111:H2, O111:H12, O111:H21, O114:NM, O114:H2, O119:H6, O125:H21, O126:NM, O126:H27, O127:NM, O127:H6, O127:H9, O127:H21, O128:H2, O128:H7, O128:H12, O142:H6, and O157:H45. A molecular definition for EPEC based on the presence of certain EPEC-associated virulence markers and a lack of Shiga toxin production has been proposed, which has expanded the list of serotypes now classified as EPEC. A full list of classical and newly recognized serotypes of EPEC is maintained by the WHO Collaborating Centre for Reference and Research on *Escherichia* and *Klebsiella* in Copenhagen, Denmark.

3. Occurrence—Since the late 1960s, EPEC has largely disappeared as an important cause of infant diarrhea in North America and Europe. However, it remains a major agent of infant diarrhea in many developing areas, including South America, sub-Saharan Africa, and Asia.

4. Reservoir—Humans.

5. Mode of transmission—Through contaminated infant formula and weaning foods. In infant nurseries, transmission by fomites and by contaminated hands can occur if handwashing techniques are compromised. Outbreaks due to contaminated water and rice have been reported.

6. Incubation period—As short as 9-12 hours in adult volunteer studies. It is not known whether the same incubation applies to infants who acquire infection through natural transmission.

7. Period of communicability—Limited to the duration of excretion of EPEC, which may be prolonged.

8. Susceptibility and resistance—Although susceptibility to clinical infection appears to be confined to infants in nature, it is not known whether this is because of immunity or of age-related, nonspecific host factors. Since diarrhea can be induced experimentally in some adult volunteers, specific immunity may be important in determining susceptibility. EPEC infection is uncommon in breastfed infants.

9. Methods of control—

A. Preventive measures:

1) Encourage mothers to practice exclusive breastfeeding from birth to 4-6 months, and to continue breastfeeding until the infant reaches 24 months of age or more. Provide adequate support for breastfeeding. If a mother cannot or chooses not to breastfeed, the infant should be fed commercially sterile infant formula or pasteurized donor breast milk when possible. Infant formulas should be prepared according to WHO guidelines for safe preparation, storage and handling of powdered infant formula (2006), and should be held at room temperature only for short periods. Cup feeding is preferred to bottle-feeding as early as possible; feeding implements should be cleaned thoroughly before use.

2) Prevention of hospital outbreaks depends on washing hands between handling babies and maintaining high sanitary standards in the facilities in which babies are held. Provide individual equipment for each infant; include a thermometer, kept at the bassinet. No common bathing or dressing tables should be used, and no bassinet stands should be

used for holding or transporting more than one infant at a time.

3) Practice rooming-in for mothers and infants in maternity facilities, unless there is a firm medical indication for separation. If mother or infant has a GI or respiratory infection, keep the pair together but isolate them from healthy pairs. In special care facilities, separate infected infants from those who are premature or ill in other ways.

4) Train health professionals in safe preparation of infant and follow-up formula according to WHO guidelines for safe preparation, storage and handling of powdered infant formula (2006).

B. Control of patient, contacts and the immediate environment:

1) Report to local health authority: Obligatory report of epidemics; no individual case report, Class 4 (see *Reporting*). Two or more concurrent cases of diarrhea requiring treatment for these symptoms in a nursery or among those recently discharged are to be interpreted as an outbreak requiring investigation.

2) Isolation: Enteric precautions for known and suspected cases.

3) Concurrent disinfection: Of all fecal discharges and soiled articles. In communities with an adequate sewage disposal system, feces can be discharged directly into sewers without preliminary disinfection.

4) Quarantine: Use enteric precautions and cohort methods (see 9C).

5) Immunization of contacts: Not applicable.

6) Investigation of contacts and source of infection: Families of discharged babies should be followed up for diarrheal status of the baby (see 9C).

7) Specific treatment: Electrolyte-fluid replacement (oral or IV) is the most important measure (see *Cholera*, 9B7). In children less than five years of age, give 20 mg elemental zinc per day for 10 to 14 days. Most cases do not require any other treatment. For severe enteropathogenic infant diarrhea, oral trimethoprim-sufamethoxazole (10–50 mg/kg/day) has been shown to ameliorate the severity and duration of diarrheal illness; it should be administered in 3–4 divided doses for 5 days. Since many EPEC strains are resistant to a variety of antimicrobials, selection should be based on the sensitivity of local isolated strains. Feeding, including breastfeeding, must continue.

C. Epidemic measures: For nursery epidemics (see section 9B1) the following:

1) All babies with diarrhea should be placed in one nursery under enteric precautions. Admit no more babies to the contaminated nursery. Suspend maternity service unless a clean nursery is available with separate personnel and facilities; promptly discharge infected infants as soon as medically possible. For babies exposed in the contaminated nursery, provide separate medical and nursing personnel skilled in the care of infants with communicable diseases. Observe contacts for at least 2 weeks after the last case leaves the nursery; promptly remove each new infected case to the single nursery ward used for these infants. Maternity service may be resumed after discharge of all contact babies and mothers, and thorough cleaning and terminal disinfection. Put into practice the recommendations of 9A, insofar as feasible, in the emergency.

2) Carry out a thorough epidemiological investigation into the distribution of cases by time, place, person and exposure to risk factors, to determine how transmission is occurring.

D. Disaster implications: None.

E. International measures: WHO Collaborating Centres provide support as required. More information can be found at:
<http://www.who.int/collaboratingcentres/database/en/>
For further information, see:
WHO Guidelines for Safe Preparation, Storage and Handling of Powdered Infant Formula (2006)
<http://www.who.int/foodsafety/publications/micro/pif_guidelines.pdf>

V. DIARRHEA CAUSED BY ENTEROAGGREGATIVE E. COLI
ICD-9 008.0; ICD-10 A04.4
(Enteroaggregative *E. coli*, EAEC)

This category of diarrhea-producing *E. coli* is increasingly recognized as a cause of both acute and persistent diarrhea among children and adults in developing and developed countries. However, there is some debate about whether EAEC is a diarrheal pathogen, or whether only some strains are pathogens. Some studies have identified EAEC among healthy control subjects in similar proportions to patients with diarrhea. In animal models, these *E. coli* organisms evoke a characteristic histopathology in which EAEC adhere to enterocytes in a thick biofilm of aggregating bacteria and mucus. The most widely available method to identify EAEC is the HEp-2 assay, wherein these strains produce a characteristic "stacked brick" aggregative pattern as they attach to one another and to the HEp-2 cells; this is a plasmid-dependent characteristic mediated by novel fimbriae.

Most EAEC encode one or more cytotoxin/enterotoxins that are believed to be responsible for the watery diarrhea with mucus seen in infected persons. Other diagnostic tools include a DNA probe and PCR assays. A few studies suggest that there is an inflammatory component to EAEC infection that may help to distinguish it from ETEC or EPEC. The incubation period is estimated at 20–48 hours.

1. Identification—This category of diarrhea-producing *E. coli* was first associated with infant diarrhea in a study in Chile in the late 1980s. It was subsequently recognized in India as being associated with persistent diarrhea (continuing unabated for at least 14 days), an observation that has since been confirmed by reports from Bangladesh, Brazil and Mexico. More recently EAEC has been recognized as also being associated with acute diarrhea.

2. Infectious agent—EAEC harbor a virulence plasmid required for expression of the unique fimbriae that encode aggregative adherence and many strains express a cytotoxin/enterotoxin. Among the most common EAEC O:H serotypes are O3:H2 and O44:H18. Many EAggEC strains initially appear as rough strains lacking O antigens.

3. Occurrence—Reports associating EAEC with infant diarrhea, including persistent diarrhea, have come from countries in Latin America, Asia, and sub-Saharan Africa. Studies in Europe and the USA suggest that EAEC may be responsible for a proportion of diarrheal disease in developed countries. EAEC have also been associated with diarrhea in HIV-infected adults and international travelers to developing countries. A small number of outbreaks of EAEC have been reported. EAEC is an important cause of traveler's diarrhea, responsible for 10–20% of such cases.

VI. DIARRHEA CAUSED BY DIFFUSE-ADHERENCE *E. COLI* (DAEC)   ICD-9 008.0; ICD-10 A04.4

A sixth category of diarrhea-producing *E. coli* now recognized is diffuse-adherence *E. coli* (DAEC). The name derives from the characteristic pattern of adherence of these bacteria to HEp-2 cells in tissue culture. DAEC is the least well-defined category of diarrhea-causing *E. coli*. Data from several epidemiological field studies of child diarrhea in developing countries have found DAEC to be significantly more common in children with diarrhea than in matched controls; other studies have failed to find such a difference. Preliminary evidence suggests that DAEC may be more pathogenic in children of preschool age than in infants and toddlers. Two DAEC strains failed to cause diarrhea when fed to volunteers, and no outbreaks due to this category have yet been recognized. The presence of a gene coding for a heat stable enterotoxin has been described in DAEC strains. Recent studies suggest that DAEC in some regions could be the most prevalent fecal isolate among diarrheagenic *E. coli*. The ability to cause epithelial cells to secrete a high amount of chemokine IL-8 seems to be linked to disease for certain DAEC strains. In general, however, little is known at present about the reservoir, modes of transmission, host risk factors, or period of communicability of DAEC.

DIPHTHERIA
[CCDM19: T. Tiwari]
[CCDM18: J. Clements]

ICD-9 032; ICD-10 A36

1. Identification—An acute bacterial disease primarily involving the mucous membrane of the upper respiratory tract (nose, tonsils, pharynx, larynx), skin, or rarely other mucous membranes e.g. conjunctivae, vagina, or ear. Inapparent infections (colonization) outnumber clinical cases. The characteristic lesion, caused by reaction to a potent exotoxin, is an asymmetrical adherent greyish white membrane with surrounding inflammation. In moderate to severe cases of respiratory diphtheria, the throat may be moderately to severely sore with enlarged and tender cervical lymph nodes, and, together with marked swelling of the neck, can give rise to a "bull neck" appearance. Pharyngeal membranes may extend into the trachea or progress to cause airway obstruction. Nasal diphtheria can be mild and chronic with one-sided serosanguinous nasal discharge and excoriations. The lesions of cutaneous diphtheria are variable and may be indistinguishable from impetigo. Absorption of diphtheria toxin can lead to myocarditis, with heart block and progressive congestive failure beginning about 1 week after onset. Neurologic complications may occur about 2 weeks after onset of illness and include polyneuropathies that can mimic Guillain-Barré syndrome. The case-fatality rate is 5%–10% for respiratory diphtheria even with treatment, and has changed little in the past 50 years.

Respiratory diphtheria should be suspected in the differential diagnosis of membranous pharyngitis that includes streptococcal pharyngitis, Vincent angina, infectious mononucleosis, oral syphilis, oral candidiasis and adenoviruses.

Presumptive diagnosis is based on observation of an asymmetrical, adherent grayish membrane associated with tonsillitis, pharyngitis, or a serosanguinous nasal discharge. Bacteriological examination of lesions confirms the diagnosis. If respiratory diphtheria is strongly suspected, specific treatment with antitoxin and antibiotics should be initiated without awaiting laboratory confirmation by culture, and continued even if the laboratory report is negative. Delay in starting treatment is associated with increased risk for complications and death.

2. Infectious agent—Toxin-producing strains of *Corynebacterium diphtheriae*. There are four biotypes: gravis, mitis, intermedius, and belfanti. Toxin production results when bacteria are infected by coryne-bacteriophage containing the diphtheria toxin gene *tox*. Nontoxigenic strains may cause sore throat, but rarely produce membranous lesions; however, they are increasingly associated with infective endocarditis.

3. Occurrence—A disease of colder months in temperate zones, primarily involving nonimmunized or underimmunized children below 15 years of age, but which may be found among adult population groups with low vaccination coverage. In the tropics, seasonal trends are less distinct; inapparent, cutaneous and wound diphtheria cases are much more common.

Diphtheria epidemics can occur in susceptible populations. In 1990, for example, a massive outbreak began in the Russia and spread to all countries of the former Soviet Union and Mongolia. Contributing factors included increased susceptibility among adults due to waning of vaccine-induced immunity; and failure fully to immunize children because of unwarranted contraindications, antivaccine movements, and declining socioeconomic conditions. After peaking in 1995, the epidemic declined. It was responsible for more than 150 000 reported cases and 5 000 deaths between 1990 and 1997.

In Ecuador, an outbreak of about 200 cases occurred in 1993-94; about 50% cases occurred in persons aged 15 years or older. In both epidemics, control was achieved through mass immunization campaigns.

4. Reservoir—Humans.

5. Mode of transmission—Contact with a patient or carrier; more rarely, contact with articles soiled with discharges from lesions of infected people. Raw milk has served as a vehicle.

6. Incubation period—Usually 2-5 days, occasionally longer.

7. Period of communicability—Variable, until virulent bacilli have disappeared from discharges and lesions; usually 2 weeks or less, seldom more than 4 weeks for respiratory diphtheria. The rare chronic carrier may shed organisms for 6 months or more. Effective antibiotic therapy promptly terminates shedding.

8. Susceptibility—Infants born to immune mothers have passive protection, which is usually lost before the 6th month. Disease or inapparent infection may induce long-lasting or lifelong immunity, but does not always do so. Immunization with diphtheria toxoid produces prolonged but not lifelong immunity. Immunity wanes with increasing age. Serosurveys in the USA indicate that more than 40% of adults lack protective levels of circulating antibodies; decreasing antibody levels have also been found in Australia, Canada and several European countries. Older adults may have immunological memory and may be protected against disease after exposure. Immunity induced by diphtheria toxoid protects against toxin-mediated systemic disease but not against colonization in the nasopharynx.

9. **Methods of control—**

   A. *Preventive measures:*

   1) Educational measures are important: inform the public, particularly parents of young children, of the hazards of diphtheria and the need for active immunization.
   2) The only effective control is widespread active immunization with diphtheria toxoid. Immunization should be initiated in infancy with a formulation containing diphtheria toxoid, tetanus toxoid and either acellular pertussis antigens (DTaP, preferred in the USA) or whole cell pertussis vaccine (DTP). Some currently available formulations combine DTP or DTaP with one or more of the following: *Hemophilus influenzae* type B vaccine, inactivated poliomyelitis vaccine, or hepatitis B vaccine.
   3) The schedule recommended in developing countries is at least 3 primary doses IM at 6, 10 and 14 weeks of age; and a DTP booster at 18 months to 4 years.

   The following schedules are recommended for use in industrialized countries (some countries may recommend different ages or dosages):

   a) Recommended immunization schedule for persons aged 0–18 Years—

   Vaccination is recommended with a primary series of diphtheria toxoid combined with other antigens, such as DTaP, or DTP-Hib, DTaP-HepB-Inactivated Polio vaccine. The first 3 doses are given at 4- to 8-week intervals beginning when the infant is 6 to 8 weeks of age; a fourth dose is given 6–12 months after the third dose. This schedule should not entail restarting immunizations because of delays in administering scheduled doses. A fifth dose is given at 4–6 years, prior to school entry; this dose is not necessary if the fourth dose was given after the fourth birthday. If the pertussis component of DTP is contraindicated, diphtheria and tetanus toxoids for children (DT) should be substituted. A booster dose with an adult formulation, Tdap (or Td if Tdap is unavailable), is recommended at 11–18 years of age.

   b) Previously unvaccinated persons aged >7 years—

Because adverse reactions may increase with age, a preparation with a reduced concentration of diphtheria toxoid (adult Td) is usually given after the seventh birthday for booster doses. For a previously unimmunized person, a primary 3-dose series of adsorbed tetanus and diphtheria toxoids (Td) is advised. Two doses are given at 4- to 8-week intervals, and the third dose is given 6 months to 1 year after the second dose. If the person is aged 10 years or older, a dose of Tdap may be substituted for a single Td dose in the series. Limited data from Sweden suggest that the 3-dose Td regimen may not induce protective diphtheria antibody levels in most adults, and additional doses may be needed.

c) Active protection should be maintained by administering a dose of Td every 10 years thereafter. A one-time dose of Tdap may be substituted for the next Td dose in persons ages 19–64 years, for added protection against pertussis.

4) Special efforts should be made to ensure that those who are at higher risk of patient exposure, such as health workers, are fully immunized and receive a booster dose of Td every 10 years.

5) For those who are severely immunocompromised or infected with HIV, diphtheria immunization is indicated, with the same schedule and dose as for immunocompetent persons, even though immune response may be suboptimal.

B. Control of patient, contacts and the immediate environment:

1) Report to local health authority: Case report obligatory in most countries, Class 2 (see *Reporting*).

2) Isolation: Strict isolation for pharyngeal diphtheria and contact isolation for cutaneous diphtheria, until 2 cultures from both throat and nose (and skin lesions in cutaneous diphtheria), taken at least 24 hours apart and at least 24 hours after cessation of antibiotic therapy, fail to grow *C. diphtheriae*. Where culture is impractical, isolation may end after 14 days of appropriate antibiotic therapy (see 9B7).

3) Concurrent disinfection: Of all articles in contact with patient and all articles soiled by discharges of patient. Terminal cleaning.

4) Quarantine: Adult contacts whose occupations involve handling food (especially milk) or close association with nonimmunized children should be excluded from that work until treated as described below, and until bacteriological examination proves them not to be carriers.

5) Management of contacts: All close contacts should have swabs taken from nose and throat for culture of *C. diphthe-*

riae, and should be kept under surveillance for 7 days. A single dose of benzathine penicillin (IM), or a 7–10 day course of erythromycin (PO, 40 mg/kg/day for children and 1 gram/day for adults), is recommended for all persons with household exposure to diphtheria, regardless of immunization status (see 9.B.7 for dosing). Those who handle food or work with school children should be excluded from work or school until proven not to be carriers. Previously immunized contacts should receive a booster dose of diphtheria toxoid if more than 5 years have elapsed since their last dose, and in nonimmunized contacts, a primary series should be initiated; use Td, DT, DTP, DTaP or DTP-Hib, DTP-HepB-IPV, or Tdap combination vaccine, depending on the contact's age and indication for other components.

6) Investigation of contacts and source of infection: Searching for carriers by culture of nasal and throat specimens, other than among close contacts, is neither useful nor indicated if provisions of 9.B.5 are carried out.

7) Specific treatment: Diphtheria antitoxin is the specific treatment for respiratory diphtheria. Sensitivity testing (skin or eye testing) should be undertaken before giving antitoxin—only antitoxin of equine origin is available. After completion of tests to rule out hypersensitivity, if diphtheria is strongly suspected on the basis of clinical findings, a single dose of antitoxin (in the range of 20 000 units for anterior nasal diphtheria to 100 000 units for extensive disease of 3 days duration) should be given daily intramuscularly for 14 days immediately after bacteriological specimens are taken, without waiting for results (to obtain diphtheria antitoxin in the USA, contact Centers for Disease Control and Prevention, Tel: 1-770-488-7100). Antibiotics are not a substitute for antitoxin but will eliminate *C. diphtheriae* and halt toxin production, and reduce communicability. Procaine penicillin G (IM) (25 000 to 50 000 units/kg/day for children and 1.2 million units/kg/day for adults, in 2 divided doses) or parenteral erythromycin (40–50 mg/kg/day, with a maximum of 2 grams/day in divided doses), is recommended until the patient can swallow comfortably. Erythromycin PO in 4 divided doses or penicillin V PO (125–250 mg 4 times daily) may be substituted for a recommended total treatment period of 14 days. Erythromycin-resistant strains are uncommon and have not been a public health problem.

Prophylactic treatment of carriers: A single dose of benzathine penicillin G (IM) (600 000 units for persons under 6 years and 1.2 million units for persons 6 or older) or a 7–10 day course of erythromycin (PO, 40 mg/kg/day for children and 1 gram/day for adults) has been recommended. If culture is positive, treat as for patients.

C. Epidemic measures:

1) Immunize the largest possible proportion of the population group involved, especially infants and preschool children. In an epidemic involving adults, immunize groups that are most affected or at high risk. Repeat immunization procedures 1 month later to provide at least 2 doses to recipients.

2) Identify close contacts and define population groups at special risk. In areas with appropriate facilities, carry out a prompt field investigation of reported cases to verify the diagnosis and to determine the biotype and toxigenicity of *C. diphtheriae*.

D. Disaster implications: Outbreaks can occur when social or natural conditions lead to crowding of susceptible groups, especially infants and children. This frequently occurs when there are large-scale movements of susceptible populations.

E. International measures: People traveling to or through countries where either respiratory or cutaneous diphtheria is common should receive primary immunization if necessary, or a booster dose of Td for those previously immunized.

DIPHYLLOBOTHRIASIS   ICD-9 123.4; ICD-10 B70.0
(Dibothriocephaliasis, Broad or fish tapeworm infection)
[CCDM19: M. Eberhard, A. Gabrielli, L. Savioli]
[CCDM18: L. Savioli]

1. Identification—An intestinal tapeworm infection of long duration; symptoms are commonly trivial or absent; some patients, however, develop vitamin B12 deficiency anemia. Massive infections may be associated with diarrhea, obstruction of the bile duct or intestine, and toxic symptoms. Identification of eggs or segments (proglottids) of the worm in feces confirms the diagnosis.

2. Infectious agents—*Diphyllobothrium latum* (*Dibothriocephalus latus*), *D. pacificum*, *D. dendriticum*, *D. ursi*, *D. dalliae* and *D. klebanovskii*, all cestodes.

3. Occurrence—The disease occurs in lake regions in the northern hemisphere, and sub-arctic, temperate and tropical zones where eating raw or partly cooked freshwater fish is popular. Prevalence increases with age. In North America, endemic foci have been found among Eskimos in Alaska and Canada. Infections in the USA are sporadic and usually come from eating uncooked fish from Alaska or, less commonly, from midwestern or Canadian lakes. Japan and Peru report cases of *D. pacificum* infection among consumers of marine (but not freshwater) fish.

4. **Reservoir**—Primarily humans for *D. latum*; dogs, bears and other fish-eating mammals for the other *Diphyllobothrium* species.

5. **Mode of transmission**—Humans acquire the infection by eating raw or inadequately cooked fish. Eggs in mature segments of the worm are discharged in feces into bodies of fresh water, where they mature and hatch; ciliated embryos (coracidium) infect the first intermediate host (copepods of the genera *Cyclops* and *Diaptomus*), and become procercoid larvae. Susceptible species of freshwater fish (pike, perch, turbot, salmon) ingest infected copepods and become second intermediate hosts, in which the worms transform into the plerocercoid (larval) stage, which is infective for people and fish eating mammals, e.g. foxes, mink, bears, cats, dogs, pigs, walruses and seals. The egg-to-egg cycle takes at least 11 weeks. For species such as *D. pacificum*, the life cycle is similar, excepting that marine fishes serve as the second intermediate host.

6. **Incubation period**—3 to 6 weeks from ingestion to passage of eggs in the stool.

7. **Period of communicability**—No direct person-to-person transmission. Humans and other definitive hosts disseminate eggs into the environment as long as worms remain in the intestine, sometimes for many years.

8. **Susceptibility**—Humans are universally susceptible. No apparent resistance follows infection.

9. **Methods of control**—

   A. *Preventive measures:* Thorough heating of freshwater fish (56°C/133°F for 5 minutes), freezing for 24 hours at −18°C (0°F), or irradiation.

   B. *Control of patient, contacts and the immediate environment:*

   1) Report to local health authority: Official report not ordinarily justifiable, Class 5 (see *Reporting*). Report indicated if a commercial source is implicated.
   2) Isolation: Not applicable.
   3) Concurrent disinfection: Sanitary disposal of feces.
   4) Quarantine: Not applicable.
   5) Immunization of contacts: Not applicable.
   6) Investigation of contacts and source of infection: Not usually justified.

7) Specific treatment: Drugs of choice are either praziquantel (10–25 mg/kg single dose) or niclosamide (children under 2 years: 500 mg; children 2–6 years: 1 g; children over 6 years and adults: 2 g; half the dose may be taken after breakfast and the remainder 1 hour later followed by a purgative 2 hours after last dose). Hydroxocobalamin (a natural analog of vitamin B12) and folic acid (a form of vitamin B9) supplements may also be administered.

C. Epidemic measures: None.

D. Disaster implications: None.

E. International measures: None.

DRACUNCULIASIS   ICD-9 125.7; ICD-10 B72
(Guinea worm disease, Dracontiasis)
[CCDM19: M. Eberhard, M. Karam]
[CCDM18: M. Karam]

1. Identification—An infection of the subcutaneous and deeper tissues by a large nematode. A blister appears, usually on a lower extremity (especially the foot) when the gravid, 60–100 cm long adult female worm is ready to discharge its larvae. Burning and itching of the skin in the area of the lesion, and frequently fever, nausea, vomiting, diarrhea, dyspnea, generalized urticaria and eosinophilia, may accompany or precede vesicle formation. After the vesicle ruptures, the worm discharges larvae whenever the infected part is immersed in fresh water. The prognosis is good unless bacterial infection of the lesion occurs; such secondary infections may produce arthritis, synovitis, ankylosis and contractures of the involved limb, and may be life-threatening. Tetanus infections may occur via the site of the lesion.

Diagnosis is made by visual recognition of the adult worm protruding from a skin lesion, or by microscopic identification of larvae.

2. Infectious agent—*Dracunculus medinensis*, a nematode.

3. Occurrence—In Africa, in five countries south of the Sahara: Ghana, Mali, Niger, Nigeria, and Sudan. As of 2007, infection has been eliminated from 15 formerly endemic countries, via a Guinea worm eradication campaign. Local prevalence varies greatly. In some locales, nearly all inhabitants are infected; in others, only a few, mainly young adults.

4. Reservoir—Humans; there are no other known animal reservoirs.

5. Mode of transmission—Larvae discharged by the female worm into stagnant fresh water are ingested by minute crustacean copepods (*Cyclops* spp). In about 2 weeks, the larvae develop into the infective stage. People swallow the infected copepods in drinking water from infested step wells, ponds, and other surface water. The larvae are liberated in the stomach, cross the duodenal wall, migrate through the viscera, and become adults. The female, after mating, grows and develops to full maturity, then migrates to the subcutaneous tissues (most frequently of the legs).

6. Incubation period—About 12 months.

7. Period of communicability—From rupture of vesicle until larvae have been completely evacuated from the uterus of the gravid worm, usually 2–3 weeks. In water, the larvae are infective for the copepods for about 5 days. After ingestion by copepods, the larvae become infective for people after 12–14 days at temperatures above 25°C (77°F), and remain infective in the copepods for about 3 weeks, the life span of an infected copepod. No direct person-to-person transmission.

8. Susceptibility—Susceptibility is universal. No acquired immunity; multiple and repeated infections may occur in the same person.

9. Methods of control/eradication—The provision of safe, filtered drinking water, treatment of stagnant sources of drinking water with the insecticide temephos, and health education of the populations at risk is leading to eradication of the disease. Foci of disease formerly present in some parts of the Middle East and the Indian subcontinent have been eliminated in this manner.

A. Preventive measures:

1) Provide health education programs in endemic communities to convey three messages: 1) that guinea worm infection comes from drinking unsafe water; 2) that villagers with blisters or ulcers should not enter any source of drinking water; and 3) that drinking water should be filtered through fine mesh cloth (such as nylon gauze with a mesh size of 100 micrometers) to remove copepods.
2) Provide potable water. Abolish step wells or, where possible, convert ground water sources to draw wells. Construction of protected wells or rainwater catchments can provide noninfected water.
3) Control copepod populations in ponds, tanks, reservoirs and step wells by use of the temephos, which is effective and safe.
4) Immunize high-risk populations against tetanus.

B. Control of patient, contacts and the immediate environment:

1) Report to local health authority: Case report required wherever the disease occurs, as part of the WHO eradication program, Class 2 (see *Reporting*).

2) Isolation: Cases are contained and advised not to enter drinking water sources while worm is emerged.

3) Concurrent disinfection: Not applicable.

4) Quarantine: Not applicable.

5) Immunization of contacts: Not applicable.

6) Investigation of contacts and source of infection: Obtain information as to source of drinking water at probable time of infection (about 1 year previously). Search for other cases.

7) Specific treatment: Tetanus toxoid and local treatment with antibiotic ointment and occlusive bandage. Aseptic surgical extraction just prior to worm emergence is only possible on an individual basis, but not applicable as a public health measure of eradication. Drugs, such as thiabendazole, albendazole, ivermectin and metronidazole, have no therapeutic value.

C. Epidemic measures: Wherever cases are identified—field survey to determine prevalence, discover sources of infection and guide control/eradication measures as described under 9A.

D. Disaster implications: None.

E. International measures: The World Health Assembly adopted a resolution (WHA 44.5, May 1991) to eradicate dracunculiasis by 1995. As of March 2008, the disease remains endemic only in five sub-Saharan countries: Ghana, Mali, Niger, Nigeria, and Sudan.

EBOLA-MARBURG VIRAL
  DISEASES   ICD-9 078.8; ICD-10 A98.4, A98.3
(African hemorrhagic fever, Ebola virus hemorrhagic fever,
Marburg virus hemorrhagic fever)
[CCDM18: P. Formenty]

1. Identification—Severe acute viral illnesses, usually with sudden onset of fever, malaise, myalgia and headache, followed by pharyngitis, vomiting, diarrhea and maculopapular rash. In severe and fatal forms, the hemorrhagic diathesis is often accompanied by hepatic damage, renal failure, CNS involvement and terminal shock with multi-organ dysfunction. Laboratory findings usually show lymphopenia, severe thrombocyto-penia and transaminase elevation (AST greater than ALT), sometimes with hyperamylasemia, elevated creatinine and blood urea nitrogen levels during the final renal failure phase. Case-fatality rates for Ebola infections in well-studied outbreaks in Africa have ranged from 50% to nearly 90%; 25%–80% of reported cases of Marburg virus infection have been fatal.

Diagnosis is usually through a combination of assays detecting antigen or RNA and antibody IgM or IgG. RT-PCR or ELISA antigen detection can be used on blood, serum or organ homogenates (the presence of IgM antibody suggests recent infection). Virus isolation attempts in cell culture or suckling mice must be undertaken in a BSL-4 laboratory. ELISA is used for specific IgM and IgG antibody detection in serum (the presence of IgM antibody suggesting recent infection). Virus may sometimes be visualized in liver, spleen, skin and other tissue sections by EM. Post-mortem diagnosis through immunohistochemical examination of formalin-fixed skin biopsy or autopsy specimens is possible. IFA tests for antibodies have often been misleading, particularly in serological surveys for past infec-tion. Laboratory studies represent an extreme biohazard, and should be carried out only where protection against infection of the staff and community is available (BSL-4 containment).

2. Infectious agents—Virions are 80 nanometers in diameter and 970 (Ebola) or 790 nanometers (Marburg) in length, and are respectively members of *Ebolavirus* and *Marburgvirus* genus in the family Filoviridae. Pleomorphic virions with branched, circular or coiled shapes are frequent on electron microscopy preparation, and may reach micrometers in length. The Ebola and Marburg viruses are antigenically distinct. In the Republic of Congo, Côte d'Ivoire, the Democratic Republic of Congo (DRC), Gabon, Sudan and Uganda, 3 different subtypes of *Ebolavirus* (Côte d'Ivoire, Sudan and Zaire) have been associated with human disease. A fourth Ebola subtype, Reston, which causes fatal hemorrhagic disease in non-human primates, originated in the Philippines: human infections in workers in laboratories where primates were being held have been documented; these were clinically asymptomatic.

3. Occurrence—Ebola disease was first recognized in 1976 in the western Equatoria province of the Sudan, and 800 kilometers away in what was then Zaire (now DRC). More than 600 cases were identified in rural hospitals and villages; case-fatality rates for these near-simultaneous out-breaks were approximately 55% and 90% respectively. A second outbreak occurred in the same area of DRC in 1977, and in the same area of Sudan in 1979. A new subtype of Ebola virus was recovered from one person, probably infected while dissecting an infected chimpanzee, in Côte d'Ivoire in 1994. In 1995, a major Ebola outbreak with 315 cases and 244 deaths was centered on Kikwit, DRC. Between 1994 and 1996, three outbreaks reported in Gabon resulted in 150 cases and 98 deaths. A fatal secondary infection occurred in a nurse in South Africa.

Between August 2000 and January 2001, an epidemic (425 cases, 224 deaths) occurred in northern Uganda. From October 2001 to April 2003, several outbreaks were reported in Gabon and DRC, with a total of 278 cases and 235 deaths; high numbers of deaths were reported among wild animals in the region, particularly non-human primates. Antibodies have been found in residents of other areas of sub-Saharan Africa; their relation to the Ebola virus is unknown. In 2003, an outbreak in DRC with high case-fatality, thought to be related to contact with non-human primates, was rapidly controlled. In 2004 Russia and the USA reported 2 laboratory infections (1 fatal). The most recent outbreaks of Ebola occurred in Sudan in 2005 (20 cases, five deaths); in DRC in 2007 (249 cases, 183 deaths); and in Uganda in 2007–2008 (1 491 cases, 37 deaths).

Ebolavirus, Reston subtype, has been isolated from cynomolgus monkeys (*Macaca fascicularis*) imported to the USA in 1989, 1990 and 1996, and to Italy in 1992, all from the same export facility in the Philippines; many of these monkeys died. In Reston, in 1989 four animal handlers with daily exposure to these monkeys developed specific antibodies.

Marburg disease has been recognized occasionally: in 1967, in Germany and what was then the Federal Republic of Yugoslavia, 31 humans (seven fatalities) were infected following exposure to African green monkeys (*Cercopithecus aethiops*) imported from Uganda; in 1975, the fatal index case of three cases diagnosed in South Africa had been infected in Zimbabwe; in 1980, two linked cases, one of which fatal, were confirmed in Kenya; in 1987, a fatal case occurred in Kenya. From 1998 to 2000, in DRC, at least 12 cases were confirmed among more than 145 suspected cases (case-fatality rate 80%) of Marburg viral hemorrhagic fever; in 2005, a major outbreak occurred in Angola (351 cases, 312 deaths); and in 2007 an outbreak occurred in Uganda, among several workers in a gold mine.

4. Reservoir—Unknown, despite extensive studies—though increasing evidence suggests a role of non-human primates (that have similar disease to humans) and/or bats in the transmission chain to humans. In Africa, Ebola infections of human index cases were linked to contact with gorillas, chimpanzees, monkeys, forest duikers and porcupines found dead or killed in the rainforest. So far, Ebola virus has been detected in the wild in carcasses of chimpanzees (in Côte d'Ivoire and DRC), gorillas (Gabon and Republic of Congo), and duikers (Republic of Congo) found dead in the rainforest. Large numbers of deaths amongst chimpanzees and gorillas can serve as sentinels for virus activity. In 2007, African fruit bats were shown to have antibody and the Marburg RNA genome in serum taken during field study of various potential Marburg reservoirs.

Evidence also indicates bats as reservoirs, through detection of antibodies and RT-PCR products in bats, and association of human antibody production with handling of bats.

5. Mode of transmission—Ebola infection of index cases seems to occur as follows:

i) In Africa, while manipulating infected wild mammals found dead in the rainforest

ii) For Ebola Reston, while handling infected cynomolgus monkeys, through direct contact with their infected blood or fresh organs.

Person-to-person transmission occurs through direct contact with infected blood, secretions, organs or semen. Risk is highest during the late stages of illness, when the patient is vomiting, having diarrhea or hemorrhaging, and during funerals with unprotected body preparation. Risk during the incubation period is low. Under natural conditions, airborne transmission among humans has not been documented. Nosocomial infections have been frequent; virtually all patients who acquired infection from contaminated syringes and needles died. Transmission through semen has occurred seven weeks after clinical recovery. Risk factors for Marburg transmission are less well understood.

6. Incubation period—Probably 2 to 21 days for both Ebola and Marburg virus disease.

7. Period of communicability—Not before the febrile phase, and increasing with stages of illness, as long as blood and secretions contain virus. Ebola virus was isolated from the seminal fluid on the 61st, but not on the 76th, day after onset of illness in a laboratory-acquired case.

8. Susceptibility—All ages are susceptible.

9. Methods of control—No vaccine and no specific treatment available as yet for either Ebola or Marburg. For control measures, see *Lassa fever* 9B, C, D and E. In addition: protection of sexual intercourse for 3 months or until semen can be shown to be free of virus.

ECHINOCOCCOSIS
ICD-9 122; ICD-10 B67

[CCDM19: M. Eberhard, F. Meslin, P. Kern, P. Schantz]
[CCDM18: F. Meslin]

The larval stages (hydatid cyst or solid/multivesiculated lesions) of *Echinococcus* spp. produce disease in humans and animals; disease characteristics depend upon the infecting species. Cysts/lesions usually develop in the liver (in two-thirds of cases) or the lungs (one-fourth of cases), but also develop in other viscera, nervous tissue, or bone. They can be a) cystic, b) alveolar, and/or c) polycystic.

I. ECHINOCOCCOSIS DUE TO *ECHINOCOCCUS GRANULOSUS*

ICD-9 122.4;
ICD-10 B67.0-B67.4

(Cystic echinococcosis, Cystic hydatid disease)

1. Identification—Larval stages of the tapeworm *Echinococcus granulosus*, the most common *Echinococcus*, cause cystic echinococcosis or hydatid disease. Hydatid cysts enlarge slowly and require several years for development. Developed cysts range from 1–15 cm in diameter, but may be larger. Infections may be asymptomatic until cysts cause noticeable mass effect; signs and symptoms vary according to location, cyst size, cyst type and numbers. Ruptured or leaking cysts can cause severe anaphylactoid reactions and may release protoscolices that can produce secondary echinococcosis. One or several cysts, typically spherical, thick-walled and consisting of a single cavity (unilocular), are most frequently found in the liver and lungs, although they may occur in other organs.

Clinical diagnosis is based on signs and symptoms compatible with a slowly growing tumor, a history of residence in an endemic area, and association with canines. Differential diagnoses include benign tumor, malignancies, amebic abscesses, and congenital cysts. Ultrasonography, computerized tomography and serological testing are useful for supporting diagnosis, with ultrasonography the method of first choice. WHO has developed a classification of ultrasound images of liver cystic echinococcosis for diagnostic and prognostic purposes and determination of the type of intervention required (see Specific treatment, 9B7). Definitive diagnosis in seronegative patients, however, requires microscopic identification from specimens obtained at surgery or by percutaneous aspiration; the potential risks of this (anaphylaxis, spillage) can be avoided by ultrasound guidance and anthelminthic coverage. Species identification is based on finding thick laminated cyst walls and protoscolices as well as on the structure and measurements of protoscolex hooks. Molecular techniques are now available to identify the species from biopsies.

2. Infectious agent—*Echinococcus granulosus*, a small tapeworm of dogs and other canids.

3. Occurrence—All continents except Antarctica; depends on close association of humans and infected dogs. Especially common in grazing countries where dogs eat viscera containing cysts. Transmission has been eliminated in Iceland and greatly reduced in Tasmania (Australia), Cyprus and New Zealand. Control programs exist in Argentina, Brazil, China, Kenya (Turkana district), Spain, Uruguay and other countries, including those of the Mediterranean basin.

4. Reservoir—The domestic dog and other canids, definitive hosts for *E. granulosus*, may harbor thousands of adult tapeworms in their intestines without signs of infection. Felines and most other carnivores are normally not suitable hosts for the parasite. Intermediate hosts include herbivores, primarily sheep, cattle, goats, pigs, horses, camels and other animals.

5. Mode of transmission—Human infection often takes place directly with hand-to-mouth transfer of eggs after association with infected dogs or indirectly through contaminated food, water, soil or fomites. In some instances, flies have dispersed eggs after feeding on infected feces.

Adult worms in the small intestines of canines produce eggs containing infective embryos (oncospheres); these are passed in feces and may survive for several months in pastures or gardens. When ingested by susceptible intermediate hosts, including humans, eggs hatch, releasing oncospheres that migrate through the mucosa and are bloodborne to organs, primarily the liver (first filter), then the lungs (second filter), where they form cysts. Strains of *E. granulosus* vary in their ability to adapt to infect various hosts as well as their infectivity to humans.

Canines become infected by eating animal viscera containing hydatid cysts. Sheep and other intermediate hosts are infected while grazing in areas contaminated with dog feces containing parasite eggs.

6. Incubation period—12 months to years, depending on number and location of cysts and how rapidly they grow.

7. Period of communicability—Not directly transmitted from person to person or from one intermediate host to another. Infected dogs begin to pass eggs 5 to 7 weeks after infection. Most canine infections resolve spontaneously by 6 months; however some adult worms may survive up to 2-3 years. Dogs may become infected repeatedly.

8. Susceptibility—Children, who are more likely to have close contact with infected dogs and less likely to have adequate hygienic habits, are at greater risk of infection, especially in rural areas. There is no evidence that they are more susceptible to infection than adults.

9. Methods of control—

   A. Preventive measures:

   1) Avoid ingestion of raw vegetables and water that may have been contaminated with the feces of infected dogs. Emphasize basic hygiene practices such as handwashing and washing fruits and vegetables. Educate those at risk on avoidance of exposure to dog feces and possibly infected dogs.
   2) Interrupt transmission from intermediate to definitive hosts by preventing access of dogs to potentially contaminated (uncooked) viscera, and through inspection of livestock carcasses and organs after slaughter, and condemnation and safe disposal of infected viscera. Disposal should be by incineration or deep burial.

3) Periodically treat high-risk dogs and all dogs in high-risk areas; encourage responsible dog ownership and implement programs for the reduction of dog populations, in compliance with principles of animal welfare.

4) Field and laboratory personnel must observe strict safety precautions to avoid ingestion of tapeworm eggs.

B. **Control of patient, contacts and the immediate environment:**

1) Report to the local health authority: Not normally a reportable disease, Class 3 (see *Reporting*).

2) Isolation: Not applicable.

3) Concurrent disinfection: Not applicable.

4) Quarantine: Not applicable.

5) Immunization of contacts: Not applicable.

6) Investigation of contacts and source of infection: Examine families and associates for suspicious cysts or tumors using ultrasound, chest X-ray, and other imaging techniques. Check dogs kept in and around houses for infection, by autopsy, coproantigen or copro PCR techniques. Determine beliefs, practices and behaviors affecting risk of infection.

7) Specific treatment: Must be based on WHO classification of liver cysts. In some instances, surgical resection of isolated cysts is the most common treatment. Other cysts types may first be treated by percutaneous techniques such as PAIR (Puncture, Aspiration, Injection, Re-aspiration). PAIR consists of the percutaneous drainage of echinococcal cysts located in the abdomen with a fine needle or a catheter, followed by the killing of remaining protoscolices with a protoscolicide and by the re-aspiration of protoscolicide solution. It is a minimally invasive technique of lesser risk than surgery, and WHO recommends it for certain cysts (see *Puncture, Aspiration, Injection, Re-aspiration: An Option for the Treatment of Cystic Echinococcosis,* <http://whqlib doc.who.int/>. Treatment with mebendazole and albendazole has also proved successful and may be the preferred treatment in many cases. If a primary cyst ruptures, praziquantel, a protoscolicidal agent, reduces the probability of secondary cysts. Other cyst types may not need a surgical, percutaneous or medical intervention, and can be followed for a long period of time ("wait and watch").

C. **Epidemic measures:** In hyperendemic areas, educate those at risk on avoidance of exposure to dog feces and possibly-infected dogs. Periodic treatment of owned and community dogs with praziquantel. Strict control of livestock slaughtering in abattoirs, and mandatory condemnation and destruction of infested organs.

Improvement of infrastructure and inspection in rural abattoirs. Promote destruction and safe disposal of infested organs on farms.

D. *Disaster implications:* None.

E. *International measures:* Control the movement of dogs from known enzootic areas.

II. ECHINOCOCCOSIS DUE TO *ECHINOCOCCUS MULTILOCULARIS*

ICD-9 122.7;
ICD-10 B67.5-B67.7

(Alveolar echinococcosis)

1. Identification—A highly invasive, destructive disease caused by the larval stage of *E. multilocularis*. Lesions are usually found in the liver; because their growth is not restricted by a thick laminated cyst wall, they expand at the periphery to produce solid, tumor-like masses. Metastases can result in secondary cysts and larval growth in other organs. Clinical manifestations depend on the size and location of cysts, but are often confused with hepatic carcinoma and cirrhosis. The disease is often fatal, although spontaneous cure through calcification has been observed.

Diagnosis is often based on histopathology, i.e. evidence of the thin host layer and multiple microvesicles formed by external proliferation. Humans are an abnormal host, and the lesions rarely produce brood capsules, protoscolices or calcareous bodies. Serodiagnosis using purified or recombinant *E. multilocularis* antigen is highly sensitive and specific. A staging and classification system recently proposed by WHO, named PNM, is based on a) Hepatic localization of the parasite (P); b) extrahepatic involvement of neighboring organs (N); and c) metastases (M).

2. Infectious agent—*Echinococcus multilocularis*.

3. Occurrence—Distribution is limited to areas of the Northern Hemisphere: China, Turkey, Canada, central Europe, China, Russia, northern Japan, Alaska, and rarely the north central USA. The disease is usually diagnosed in adults.

4. Reservoir—Adult tapeworms are largely restricted to wild animals such as foxes, and *E. multilocularis* is commonly maintained in nature in fox-rodent cycles. Dogs and cats can be sources of human infection if hunting wild (and rarely domestic) intermediate hosts such as rodents, including voles, lemmings and mice.

5. Mode of transmission—Ingestion of eggs passed in the feces of Canidae and Felidae that have fed on infected rodents. Fecally soiled dog hair, harnesses and environmental fomites also serve as vehicles of infection.

6., 7., 8. and **9. Incubation period, Period of communicability, Susceptibility, Methods of control**—As in section I, *Echinococcus granulosus*; radical surgical excision is less often successful and must be followed by chemotherapy. Mebendazole or albendazole for a limited period after surgery, or long-term (several years) for inoperable patients, may prevent progression of the disease; pre-surgical chemotherapy is indicated in rare cases.

III. ECHINOCOCCOSIS DUE TO *ECHINOCOCCUS VOGELI* AND *E. OLIGARTHRUS*

ICD-9 122.9;
ICD-10 B67.9

(Polycystic hydatid disease)

This disease occurs in the liver, lungs and other viscera. Symptoms vary depending on cyst size and location. This species is distinguished by its rostellar hooks. The polycystic hydatid is unique, in that the germinal membrane proliferates externally to form new cysts, and internally to form septae that divide the cavity into numerous microcysts. Brood capsules containing many protoscolices develop in the microcysts. The causal agents are *Echinococcus vogeli* (over 100 cases) and *E. oligarthrus* (a few cases), encountered in Central and South America. Immunodiagnosis using a purified antigen of *E. vogeli* does not always allow differentiation from alveolar echinococcosis (which is not co-occurring in South America). Albendazole has been used for chemotherapy.

EHRLICHIOSES

ICD-9 083.8; ICD-10 A79.8

(Human monocytotropic ehrlichiosis, Ehrlichiosis *ewingii*, Human granulocytotropic anaplasmosis, Sennetsu fever)
[CCDM19: G. Dasch, M. Eremeeva]
[CCDM18: D. H. Walker, J. S. Dumler]

1. Identification—Acute, febrile, bacterial illnesses caused by a group of small, obligate intracellular, pleomorphic bacteria of the family *Anaplasmataceae*, which survive and reproduce in the phagosomes of mononuclear or polymorphonuclear leukocytes of the infected host. The organisms are sometimes observed within these cells in the peripheral blood. The agents persist in animal reservoirs and are transmitted to humans by different species of ticks.

Ehrlichia chaffeensis affects primarily mononuclear phagocytes; the disease is known as human monocytotropic ehrlichiosis and occurs in both North and South America. *Ehrlichia ewingii* infects neutrophils of patients and causes the disease called ehrlichiosis *ewingii* in North America. *Ehrlichia muris* is present in ticks in Japan, Russia and China; however, only serologic evidence is available to suggest that *E. muris* may be an agent of human monocytic ehrlichiosis in those regions.

The clinical spectrum of ehrlichioses infections ranges from mild illness to severe, life-threatening or fatal disease, with a 2.7% case-fatality rate. Ehrlichiosis due to *E. ewingii* infection has not been associated with fatalities. Symptoms are usually nonspecific; commonly fever, headache, anorexia, nausea, myalgia and vomiting. About 20% of patients have meningoencephalitis. Human monocytotropic ehrlichiosis may be confused clinically with Rocky Mountain spotted fever, although rash occurs less often in the former. Laboratory findings include leukopenia, thrombocytopenia and elevation of one or more hepatocellular enzymes. *Ehrlichia canis*, the agent of tropical canine pancytopenia, infects monocytes and can cause both fatal and persistent chronic infection in dogs; but it has only been described as a cause of human infections resembling human monocytotropic ehrlichiosis in Venezuela.

Anaplasma phagocytophilum, which infects neutrophils, causes human granulocytotropic anaplasmosis, an emerging infectious disease in Asia, Europe and North America, characterized by acute and usually self-limited fever, headache, malaise, myalgia, thrombocytopenia, leukopenia, and increased hepatic transaminases. Meningoencephalitis is rare. The illness ranges from mild to severe, with less than 1% case-fatality. Co-infections with *Borrelia burgdorferi*, *Babesia* spp. and tick-borne encephalitis viruses may occur, since all these organisms are transmitted by *Ixodes* ticks. There is no current evidence for persistent infection in humans. Blood transfusions donated during the eclipse phase of infections with both *A. phagocytophilum* and *E. chaffeensis* have caused infections in blood recipients.

Sennetsu fever caused by *Neorickettsia sennetsu* is characterized by the sudden onset of fever, chills, malaise, headache, muscle and joint pain, sore throat, and sleeplessness. Generalized lymphadenopathy with tenderness of the enlarged nodes is common. Atypical lymphocytosis with postauricular and posterior cervical lymphadenopathy is similar to that seen in infectious mononucleosis. The course is usually benign; fatal cases have not been reported.

Differential diagnosis includes various viral syndromes, Rocky Mountain spotted fever, sepsis, toxic shock syndrome, gastroenteritis, meningoencephalitis, tularemia, Colorado tick fever, tick-borne encephalitis, babesiosis, Lyme borreliosis, leptospirosis, hepatitis, typhoid fever, murine typhus, and blood malignancies. Diagnosis is based on clinical and laboratory findings and 4-fold rise or fall in titer antibody detection using organism-specific antigens or *E. chaffeensis* as surrogate antigen for the uncultivated agent, *E. ewingii*. Blood smears or buffy coat smears should be examined for characteristic inclusions (morulae) during the acute stage of illness; however, the percentage of infected cells is generally low (<1%). Other diagnostic techniques include DNA amplification methods (e.g. PCR), culture, and immunohistochemistry of blood marrow or necropsy tissues for fatal cases.

2. Infectious agents—The agent of human monocytotropic ehrlichiosis, *E. chaffeensis*, is named after Fort Chaffee AK, USA, the site of infection of the first patient from whom an isolate was obtained. Human granulocytotropic anaplasmosis is caused by *A. phagocytophilum,* described in animals in 1932 and in humans in 1994. *E. ewingii*, which like *E. chaffeensis* is commonly found in deer and dogs, was identified in 1999 as another of the ehrlichiae causing human granulocytotropic ehrlichiosis. *E. canis* is commonly present in dogs and the brown dog tick, *Rhipicephalus sanguineus*. *Neorickettsia sennetsu* is the causal agent of sennetsu fever. These organisms are members of the family *Anaplasmataceae*, though they were classified as members of the family *Rickettsiaceae* until 1984. The agent of sennetsu fever was classified as *Ehrlichia sennetsu* until 2001, when it was moved to the genus *Neorickettsia*.

3. Occurrence—In the USA, active prospective surveillance for human monocytotropic ehrlichiosis detects 10 cases per 100 000 population in rural and suburban areas south of New Jersey to Kansas, as well as in California. Human monocytotropic ehrlichiosis has also been described in Brazil. Human granulocytotropic anaplasmosis occurs in areas of the USA endemic for Lyme disease, as well as in Asia and Europe. Sennetsu fever appears confined to western Japan and perhaps Malaysia.

4. Reservoirs—The major reservoirs of *E. chaffeensis* and *E. ewingii* are white-tailed deer and dogs, and for *A. phagocytophilum,* ruminants, cervids, and field rodents. *E. muris* is found in association with small rodents and *E. canis* in dogs. *Neorickettsia* generally parasitize trematodes that live in aquatic hosts such as snails, insects, and fish. The trematode and aquatic hosts of *N. sennetsu* have not been identified.

5. Mode of transmission—Feeding ticks, mostly *Amblyomma americanum* in Northern America and likely *A. cajenennse* in Southern and Central America, transmit *E. chaffeensis* and *E. ewingii*. *E. canis* is transmitted by *Rhipicephalus sanguineus*. *E. muris* has been identified in *Ixodes persulcatus* and *Haemaphysalis flava* ticks. The vectors of *A. phagocytophilum* are *Ixodes* spp., including *I. scapularis*, *I. ricinus*, *I. pacificus*, *I. trianguliceps*, *I. spinipalpis* and *I. persulcatus* ticks. The means of transmission are not known for sennetsu fever, although ingestion of an uncooked trematode-parasitized aquatic host by patients is suspected.

6. Incubation period—For sennetsu fever, 14 days; 7-10 days for human ehrlichioses; and 7-14 days for human granulocytotropic anaplasmosis.

7. Period of communicability—No evidence of person-to-person transmission other than by blood transfusion.

8. Susceptibility—Susceptibility is believed to be general; older or immunocompromised individuals are likely to suffer a more serious illness. No data are available on protective immunity in humans due to infections caused by these organisms; re-infection is rare, but has been reported.

9. Methods of control—

A. Preventive measures:

1) None established for sennetsu fever; however, consumption of raw fish and fish products should be avoided in endemic areas.
2) Measures against ticks (see *Lyme disease*, 9A) should be employed to prevent other ehrlichioses and human granulocytotropic anaplasmosis.

B. Control of patient, contacts and the immediate environment:

1) Report to local health authority: Case report required in most countries, Class 2 (see *Reporting*).
2) Isolation: Not applicable.
3) Concurrent disinfection: Remove any attached ticks. Effective transmission of agents probably requires 24 hours of attachment.
4), 5) and 6) Quarantine, Immunization of contacts and Investigation of contacts and source of infection: Not applicable.
7) Specific treatment: Doxycycline is the drug of choice for adults and children over eight years of age (it should not be used in children of lesser age). Rifampicin has been used for human granulocytotropic anaplasmosis in pregnant and pediatric patients. There is no established alternative drug for human monocytotropic ehrlichiosis. *E. chaffeensis* and *A. phagocytophilum* have shown resistance to chloramphenicol.

C. Epidemic measures: Not applicable.

D. Disaster implications: Not applicable.

E. International measures: Not applicable.

ENCEPHALOPATHY, TRANSMISSIBLE SPONGIFORM ENCEPHALOPATHIES, PRION-RELATED ENCEPHALOPATHIES   ICD-9 046; ICD-10 A81

(Slow virus infections of the CNS)
[CCDM19: E. Belay, R. Knight, F. Meslin]
[CCDM18: F. Meslin]

A group of diseases of the brain characterized by a degenerative neuropathology and the tissue deposition of an abnormal form of a normal protein (the prion protein). Human prion diseases comprise:

- The Creutzfeldt-Jakob disease complex (CJD) and its four known variants: sporadic CJD (sCJD); genetic CJD (gCJD); variant CJD (vCJD); and iatrogenic CJD (iCJD).
- Gerstmann-Staussler-Scheinker syndrome (GSSS).
- Kuru.
- Fatal familial insomnia (FFI).

Most instances of the human transmissible encephalopathies are idiopathic and sporadic in occurrence (sCJD). Some, however, are genetically associated, such as gCJD, FFI and GSSS (related to an underlying mutation of the prion protein gene, PRNP), and some are acquired by diet (vCJD, kuru), medical treatment, surgery or blood transfusion (iCJD). Even those diseases thought not to be primarily acquired—such as sCJD—and even some that are genetically associated, may be transmissible to others in certain settings.

The infectious agent, unconventional and filterable, has been termed the "prion." It has not yet been fully characterized, but the most widely held view is that it is comprised, or largely comprised, of abnormally folded prion protein (PrP). When the infection is acquired, incubation periods are generally long (many years), and there is no demonstrable inflammatory or immune response.

I. CREUTZFELDT-JAKOB DISEASE   ICD-9 046.1; ICD-10 A81.0

(Jakob-Creutzfeldt syndrome, Subacute spongiform encephalopathy)

1. Identification—CJD presents with subacute onset of confusion, progressive dementia, and variable ataxia, usually in patients aged 55 to 75 years. Myoclonic jerks appear later, together with a variable spectrum of other neurological signs. Characteristically, routine laboratory studies and the CSF cell count are normal and there is no fever. Typical periodic high-voltage complexes are present in the electroencephalogram (EEG) in about 75% of patients, and the CSF 14-3-3 protein is elevated in most patients. Symptomatic disease is limited to the CNS, but there can be pathological changes in other tissues in some instances—essentially, in lymphoreticular tissues in vCJD.

CJD must be differentiated from other forms of dementia (especially Alzheimer's disease), other infections (including encephalitis), and toxic and metabolic encephalopathies. More conventional CNS infections (encephalitis), inflammatory disorders (including cerebral vasculitis), and toxic, metabolic, endocrine or autoimmune encephalopathies all also need consideration.

Sporadic CJD typically presents as a subacute illness in the middle-aged and elderly (median duration around 4 months): a rapidly progressive encephalopathy with confusion, dementia and other features, especially cerebellar ataxia and myoclonic jerking. However, there is some clinical heterogeneity in sCJD, and there can be atypical presentations. There are no systemic features such as pyrexia, and routine laboratory studies are normal, with a normal CSF cell count. Typical periodic high-voltage complexes are present in the electroencephalogram (EEG) in about 70% of cases, and the CSF 14-3-3 protein is elevated in about 90%. The cerebral MRI shows signal hyperintensity in the caudate/putamen in many (but not all) cases (especially on FLAIR sequences). Sometimes there is high signal seen in some cerebral cortical regions.

Variant CJD was first identified in 1996, and has been linked causally to bovine spongiform encephalopathy, with human cases thought due to dietary exposure to BSE-contaminated tissues. vCJD typically affects a younger age group than sCJD (mean age at death 29 versus 68 years), has a longer clinical course (mean 14 months vs. 7 months), and usually presents with psychiatric or behavioral disturbance. The typical EEG changes of sCJD are not seen in vCJD, but the MRI scan in vCJD shows high signal in the pulvinar area of the posterior thalamus in about 90% of cases. The pulvinar sign occurs in the majority of cases, especially on FLAIR sequences. The CSF 14-3-3 may be elevated, but in only around 45% of cases. All tested cases of vCJD to date have been homozygous for methionine at codon 129 of the PRNP gene. It is unclear whether vCJD will occur in non-MM individuals who may be infected at present, however, because MM individuals are thought to have a shorter incubation period than other genotypes. Tonsil biopsy may show the abnormal disease-related prion protein.

There have been three humans with vCJD in the UK who are thought to have become infected from blood from pre-clinical vCJD donors. Although the incidence of vCJD cases in the UK is falling, there remain concerns about secondary transmission by blood, surgery and dentistry.

Genetic CJD accounts for some 10–15% of cases and is associated with one of several mutations in the PRNP gene on chromosome 20 that encodes for PrP. The pattern of inheritance is autosomal dominant, but up to 40% of cases may have no family history of CJD. The clinical picture is highly variable, and traditionally it has been classified as familial CJD, GSS, and FFI. GSS is used to describe a heterogeneous group of inherited spongiform encephalopathies that are characterized by long illness duration and the presence of amyloid plaques, primarily in the cerebellum. FFI predominantly involves the thalamus, resulting in an illness characterized by intractable insomnia and autonomic nervous system dysfunction.

Iatrogenic CJD occurs when sCJD or vCJD is inadvertently transmitted to another person in the course of medical/surgical treatment. It has occurred following the use of contaminated cadaver-derived human pituitary hormone, *dura mater* and corneal grafts, EEG depth electrodes, and neurosurgical instruments, as well as after blood transfusion in the case of vCJD.

Diagnosis of all forms of CJD is based on clinical features together with investigations, including EEG, CSF 14-3-3 assay, and neuro-imaging, to differentiate from structural disease including tumors and vascular disease. In vCJD, tonsil biopsy can be very helpful, but is probably best reserved for those cases with atypical features and/or without the MRI pulvinar sign. A definite diagnosis of all prion diseases depends on neuropathological examination of brain tissue, and is usually undertaken at postmortem examination. Genetic testing on a simple blood sample is of importance in the diagnosis of suspect genetic prion disease. Brain biopsy can provide antemortem diagnosis, but this is an invasive procedure and is arguably best reserved for those cases in which an alternative diagnosis is otherwise not possible.

2. Infectious agent—CJD is believed to be caused by an abnormal form of the self-replicating host-encoded protein, or prion protein (PrP). Many prion diseases are transmissible in the laboratory to other species, including wild and transgenic mice and non-human primates.

3. Occurrence—sCJD has been reported worldwide. The annual mortality rate for sCJD is around 1–2 per million, with the highest age-specific average mortality rate (more than 5 cases/million) occurring in the 65–79 age group. Foci of gCJD have been reported in familial clusters in Chile, Israel and Slovakia. As of March 2008, 206 vCJD cases had been identified worldwide, including in the UK (166), France (23), Ireland (4), USA (3), the Netherlands (2), Portugal (2), Spain (2), Canada (1), Japan (1), Italy (1), and Saudi Arabia (1).

4. Reservoir—Human cases constitute the only known reservoir for sCJD. The original reservoir for vCJD is believed to be BSE-infected cattle. Because of its long incubation period, it is thought that subclinical infection with BSE is present in human populations (especially in the UK). The magnitude of this is unknown, but it represents a potential reservoir of infection for secondary, human-to-human spread by blood transfusion, organ transplantation or infected medical implements.

5. Mode of transmission—There is no firm evidence that sCJD is an acquired disease; de novo spontaneous generation of the self-replicating protein has been hypothesized. There are two recent studies suggesting that surgery may be a risk factor for sCJD, and it is conceivable that there are other iatrogenic causes as well. Iatrogenic transmission of CJD has occurred following the use of contaminated cadaver-derived human pituitary hormone, *dura mater* and corneal grafts, EEG depth electrodes, and neurosurgical instruments. In all these cases it is presumed that infection from a case or cases of sCJD was inadvertently transmitted to another person in the course of medical/surgical treatment.

The mechanism of transmission of BSE from cattle to humans has not been established, but the favored hypothesis is that humans are infected through dietary consumption of the BSE agent, probably beginning in the 1980s, and now thought to have ended because of human dietary protection measures and changes in animal feeding and slaughtering practices. Three cases of vCJD have resulted from blood transfusion. To date, blood has not been shown to be a risk factor for other forms of prion disease.

6. Incubation period—Iatrogenic cases: 15 months to over 30 years. The route of exposure influences incubation period: 15–120 months with direct CNS exposure (depth electrode, neurosurgical instruments); and 4.5–30 years with peripheral exposure (human pituitary hormones given by injection). The incubation period for 3 patients with vCJD infected by blood transfusion ranged from 6.6–8.5 years. Incubation periods in men exceeding 50 years have been reported in Kuru. Incubation period is not yet known in naturally occurring sCJD and vCJD. The concept of incubation period is not applicable to gCJD.

7. Period of communicability—In prion diseases generally, the highest levels of infectivity are associated with CNS and related tissues (e.g. parts of the eye) during, and throughout, the clinical illness. In sCJD, infectivity may be present in non-CNS tissues, but at much lower levels and probably essentially during the period of clinical illness. In vCJD, infection is present in lymphoid tissues and blood during the incubation period and during clinical illness. The level of infectivity in the CNS rises late in the incubation period, and high levels of infectivity occur in the CNS throughout symptomatic illness.

8. Susceptibility—Mutations of the prion protein gene (PRNP) are associated with genetic or familial forms of human prion disease. Polymorphic regions of the PRNP influence susceptibility to infection and incubation period in animal species, including sheep and mice. In human disease, the genotype at codon 129 of the PRNP influences susceptibility to sCJD (70% methionine homozygous), vCJD (100% methionine homozygous) and iatrogenic CJD (an excess of homozygotes for either valine or methionine). It also has potential effects on the incubation period in acquired forms (kuru, iCJD and potentially also vCJD). Finally, it has potential effects on the phenotype of the subsequent illness; for example, sCJD varies in its expression in MM, MV and VV individuals.

9. **Methods of control—**

A. *Preventive measures:*

Absolute avoidance of organ or tissue transplants from infected patients, and of reuse for potentially contaminated surgical instruments. WHO guidelines to minimize the risk of transmission of CJD (WHO/CDS/CSR/APH/2000.3) are available at:

<http://whqlibdoc.who.int/hq/2000/WHO_CDS_CSR_APH_2000.3.pdf>

The guidelines identify categories of individuals at higher risk of human prion diseases (such as those with family history of CJD, or who have experienced prior treatment with human pituitary hormones, or neurosurgery). Blood transfusion has not been shown to have resulted in the transmission of sCJD as have other tissues used in transplantation and human growth hormone, but three incidents of vCJD transmission via blood transfusion have been reported in the UK.

Avoid iatrogenic exposures:

- Specific precautions should be taken in the management of persons with confirmed or suspected transmissible spongiform encephalopathy (TSEs) and their tissues.
- The following persons have been regarded as "at risk" for developing TSE: recipients of human *dura mater*, human cadaver-derived pituitary hormones (especially human cadaver-derived growth hormone), and cornea transplants; persons undergoing neurosurgery; and members of families with heritable TSE.
- When determining the risk of iatrogenic transmission, infectivity of a given tissue should be considered together with the route of exposure. Infectivity is found most often, and in the highest concentration, in the central nervous system. Precautions have been proposed when performing certain interventions (dental, diagnostic, surgical procedures), and when handling instruments or cleaning and decontaminating instruments, work surfaces and waste.

Blood transfusion has been shown to have resulted in the transmission of vCJD. This has not been demonstrated for other forms of prion disease, but as a precautionary measure to reduce the risk of transmission of vCJD through blood or blood products, some countries—including Canada and the USA and some continental European countries—have requested that blood centers exclude potential blood donors who have resided for a specified period in the UK.

<u>Avoid exposures to BSE-causing agent in food of bovine origin:</u>

- BSE is a risk to animal and public health; it is transmissible to humans, and food is considered the most likely source of exposure. Bovines, bovine products and byproducts potentially carrying the BSE agent have been traded worldwide, giving this risk a global dimension, with possible repercussions for public health, animal health, and trade. At this time, protecting public health from exposure through food is primarily accomplished by preventing and eliminating BSE in livestock populations. For further information consult the report of the Joint WHO/FAO/OIE technical consultation on *BSE: Public Health, Animal Health and Trade*.

B. Control of patient, contacts and the immediate environment:

1) Report to local health authority: Official case report not ordinarily justifiable, Class 5 (see *Reporting*). Many countries have made CJD (including vCJD) a notifiable disease.
2) Isolation: Universal precautions.
3) Concurrent disinfection: Prions are remarkably resistant to standard disinfection and sterilization methods, but a combination of sodium hydroxide (2M for 1 hour) or sodium hypochlorite (20 000 ppm for 1 hour) with porous load autoclaving can be used to inactivate prions. If they cannot be discarded, one of the three most stringent chemical and autoclave sterilization methods recommended by the WHO should be used to reprocess heat-resistant instruments that come in contact with high infectivity tissues (brain, spinal cord, and eyes) or low infectivity tissues (cerebrospinal fluid, kidneys, liver, lungs, lymph nodes, spleen, olfactory epithelium, and placenta) of patients with suspected or confirmed CJD. These and the necessary precautions that need to be followed are available at:
<http://www.cdc.gov/ncidod/dvrd/cjd/qa_cjd_infection_control.htm#sterilization>
4) Quarantine: Not applicable.
5) Immunization of contacts: None.
6) Investigation of contacts and source of infection: Obtain detailed history of past surgical procedures, exposure to human pituitary hormones or human *dura mater* grafts, family history, and blood transfusion donation history.
7) Specific treatment: None.

C. D., and **E. Epidemic measures, Disaster Implications,** and **International measures:** None, except for control of transborder passage of cattle and bovine meat from areas where cattle are infected with BSE.

International measures for the prevention of vCJD:

Avoiding human exposures to BSE-causing agent in food of bovine origin:

- No part or product of any animal that has shown signs of a TSE should enter the human; countries should not permit tissues that are likely to contain the BSE agent to enter any (human or animal) food chain.

Managing BSE in cattle:

- All countries should determine the BSE risk status of their cattle population through the outcome of an annual risk assessment identifying all potential factors for BSE introduction, recycling and amplification. A BSE surveillance system fitting the estimated level of risk should be put into place.
- Whenever a risk of BSE is identified, countries must take immediate steps to define the specific risk material (SRM): all tissues that have been shown to contain infectivity should be removed and destroyed. If the BSE risk is considered higher, other tissues that under certain conditions may carry infectivity should be added to the SRM list for removal and destruction. Additional precautions may be taken, such as prohibiting cattle over a certain age from entering food or feed chains. WHO, FAO and OIE continuously review this approach specifically in relation to public health issues.
- Countries must monitor the effective application of the regulatory measures that have been decided upon, in particular the effectiveness of their ban (if in place) on feeding ruminant tissues to ruminants.
- International trade in food products may disseminate tissues containing BSE. WHO, FAO and OIE continue to work together to mitigate the risk of dissemination of BSE agents.

Prevention of bloodborne transmission:

- As a precautionary measure to reduce theoretical risk of transmission of vCJD through blood or blood products, some countries—including Canada, the USA and some continental European countries—have requested that blood centers exclude potential blood donors who have resided for a specified period in the UK.

II. KURU   ICD-9 046.0; ICD-10 A81.8

A fatal disease of the CNS presenting with cerebellar ataxia, malcoordination, tremor and rigidity in patients aged 4 years or older. The disease occurs exclusively in the Fore language group in the highlands of Papua

New Guinea, and is caused by a self-replicating prion. Kuru was transmitted by traditional burial practices involving consumption or smearing on the skin and mucous membranes of infected tissues, including the brain. Formerly very common, the annual incidence of kuru has declined, and only occasional cases now occur.

ENTEROBIASIS ICD-9 127.4; ICD-10 B80
(Pinworm infection, Oxyuriasis)
[CCDM19: M. Eberhard, A. Gabrielli, L. Savioli]
[CCDM18: L. Savioli]

1. Identification—A common intestinal helminthic infection that may be asymptomatic. There may be perianal itching, disturbed sleep, irritability and sometimes secondary infection of scratched skin. Other clinical manifestations include vulvovaginitis, salpingitis, and pelvic and liver granulomata. Appendicitis and enuresis have, rarely, been reported as possible associated conditions.

Diagnosis is made by applying transparent adhesive tape (tape swab or pinworm paddle) to the perianal region and examining the tape or paddle microscopically for eggs; the material is best obtained in the morning before bathing or passage of stools. Examination should be repeated 3 or more times before accepting a negative result. Eggs are sometimes found on microscopic stool and urine examination. Female worms may be found in feces and in the perianal region during rectal or vaginal examinations.

2. Infectious agent—*Enterobius vermicularis*, a small (<12 mm) intestinal nematode.

3. Occurrence—Worldwide, affecting all socioeconomic classes, with high rates in some areas. It is the most common worm infection in North America and other countries of temperate climate; prevalence is highest in school-age children (in some groups near 50%), followed by preschoolers, and is lowest in adults except for mothers of infected children. Infection often occurs in more than one family member. Prevalence is often high in domiciliary institutions.

4. Reservoir—Humans. Pinworms of other animals are not transmissible to people.

5. Mode of transmission—Direct transfer of infective eggs by hand from anus to mouth of the same or another person, or indirectly through clothing, bedding, food or other articles contaminated with parasite eggs. Dust-borne infection is possible in heavily contaminated households and institutions. Eggs become infective within a few hours after being deposited on perianal skin by migrating gravid females; eggs survive less than 2 weeks outside the host. Larvae from ingested eggs hatch in the small intestine; young worms mature in the cecum and upper portions of the colon. Gravid worms usually migrate actively from the rectum and may enter adjacent orifices.

6. **Incubation period**—The life cycle requires 2–6 weeks. Symptomatic disease with high worm burdens results from successive re-infections occurring within months after initial exposure.

7. **Period of communicability**—As long as gravid females discharge eggs on perianal skin. Eggs remain infective in an indoor environment for about 2 weeks.

8. **Susceptibility**—Universal. Differences in frequency and intensity of infection are due primarily to differences in exposure.

9. **Methods of control**—

   A. *Preventive measures:*

   1) Educate the public in personal hygiene, particularly the need to wash hands before eating or preparing food. Keep nails short; discourage nail biting and scratching anal area.
   2) Remove sources of infection through treatment of cases.
   3) Daily morning bathing, with showers (or stand-up baths) preferred to tub baths.
   4) Change to clean underclothing, nightclothes and bedsheets frequently, preferably after bathing.
   5) Clean and vacuum house daily for several days after treatment of cases.
   6) Reduce overcrowding in living accommodations.
   7) Provide adequate toilets; maintain cleanliness in these facilities.

   B. *Control of patient, contacts and the immediate environment:*

   1) Report to local health authority: Official report not ordinarily justifiable, Class 5 (see *Reporting*).
   2) Isolation: Not applicable.
   3) Concurrent disinfection: Change bed linen and underwear of infected person daily for several days after treatment, avoiding aerial dispersal of eggs. Use closed sleeping garments. Eggs on discarded linen are killed by exposure to temperatures of 55°C (131°F) for a few seconds; either boil bed clothing or use a washing machine on the "hot" cycle, and dry on "hot" setting. Clean and vacuum sleeping and living areas daily for several days after treatment. Sunlight and ultraviolet destroy eggs in the environment.
   4) Quarantine: Not applicable.

5) Immunization of contacts: Not applicable

6) Investigation of contacts and source of infection: Examine all members of an affected family or institution.

7) Specific treatment: Pyrantel pamoate (10 mg/kg), mebendazole (500 mg), or albendazole (400 mg). Treatment to be repeated after 2 weeks; concurrent treatment of the whole family may be advisable if several members are infected.

C. Epidemic measures: Multiple cases in schools and institutions can best be controlled through systematic treatment of all infected individuals and household contacts.

D. Disaster implications: None.

E. International measures: None.

ERYTHEMA INFECTIOSUM
HUMAN PARVOVIRUS
INFECTION
(Fifth Disease)   ICD-9 057.0; ICD-10 B08.3

1. Identification—Erythema infectiosum is a mild, usually non-febrile, viral disease with an erythematous eruption that occurs sporadically or in epidemics, especially among children. Characteristic is a striking erythema of the cheeks (slapped face appearance), frequently associated with a lace-like rash on the trunk and extremities, which fades but may recur for 1–3 weeks or longer on exposure to sunlight or heat (e.g. bathing). Mild constitutional symptoms may precede onset of rash. In adults, the rash is often atypical or absent, but arthralgias or arthritis lasting days to months or even years may occur. Arthropathy is uncommon in children, and occurs in 50% of adults, more commonly in women; distribution is symmetric with involvement of small joints of hands and occasionally ankles, knees and wrists. Twenty-five percent or more of infections may be asymptomatic. Differentiation from rubella, scarlet fever and erythema multiforme is often necessary. Chikungunya fever should also be considered as a differential diagnosis, especially in adults and people with dark skins.

Severe complications of infection with the causal virus are unusual, but persons with anemia that requires increased red cell production (e.g. sickle cell disease) may develop transient aplastic crisis, often in the absence of a preceding rash. Intrauterine infection in the first half of pregnancy has resulted in fetal anemia with hydrops fetalis and fetal death in less than 10% of such infections. Immunosuppressed people may develop severe, chronic anemia. Several diseases (e.g. rheumatoid arthritis, systemic vasculitis, fulminant hepatitis and myocarditis) have been reported in association with erythema infectiosum, but no causal link has been established.

Diagnosis, usually on clinical and epidemiological grounds; can be confirmed by detection of specific IgM antibodies against parvovirus B19 (B19), or by a rise in B19 IgG antibodies. IgM titers begin to decline 30–60 days after the onset of symptoms. Diagnosis of B19 infection can also be made by detecting viral antigens of DNA. PCR for B19 DNA is the most sensitive of these tests, and will often be positive during the first month of an acute infection, and for prolonged periods in some people.

2. Infectious agent—Human parvovirus B19, a 20-25-nanometer DNA virus belonging to the family Parvoviridae. The virus replicates primarily in erythroid precursor cells.

3. Occurrence—Worldwide, common in children; both sporadic and epidemic. In temperate zones, epidemics tend to occur in winter and spring, with a periodicity of 3–7 years in a given community.

4. Reservoir—Humans.

5. Mode of transmission—Primarily through contact with infected respiratory secretions; also from mother to fetus, and parenterally through transfusion of blood and blood products. B19 is resistant to inactivation by various methods, including heating to 80°C (176°F) for 72 hours.

6. Incubation period—Variable; 4–20 days to development of rash or symptoms of aplastic crisis.

7. Period of communicability—In people with rash illness alone, greatest before onset of rash and probably not communicable thereafter. People with aplastic crisis are infectious up to 1 week after onset of symptoms; immunosuppressed people with chronic infection and severe anemia are infectious for months to years.

8. Susceptibility—Universal susceptibility in persons with blood group P antigen, the receptor for B19 erythroid cells; protection appears to be conferred with development of B19 antibodies. Attack rates among susceptibles can be high: 50% in household contacts, and 10%-60% in the day care or school setting over a 2-6 month outbreak period. In the USA, 50%-80% of adults have serological evidence of past infection, depending on age and location.

9. Methods of control—

   A. Preventive measures:

      1) Since the disease is generally benign, prevention should focus on those most likely to develop complications (e.g. those with underlying anemia or immunodeficiency, and pregnant women not immune to B19), who should avoid exposure to potentially

infectious people in hospital or outbreak settings. Immunoglobulin (IG) has not yet had a trial for efficacy.

2) Susceptible women who are pregnant or who might become pregnant, and have continued close contact to people with B19 infection (e.g. at school, home, or in health care facilities), should be advised of the potential for acquiring infection and of the potential risk of complications to the fetus. Pregnant women with sick children at home are advised to wash hands frequently and to avoid sharing eating utensils.

3) Health care workers should be advised of the importance of following good infection control measures. Rare nosocomial outbreaks have been reported. Transmission can occur as a result of transfusion, most commonly pooled components; plasma pools should be screened by NAAT and high titer pools should be discarded.

B. _Control of patient, contacts and the immediate environment:_

1) Report to local health authority: Community-wide outbreaks, Class 4 (see _Reporting_).

2) Isolation: Impractical in the community at large. Cases of transient aplastic crisis in the hospital setting should be placed on droplet precautions. Although children with B19 infection are most infectious before onset of illness, it may be prudent to exclude them from school or day care attendance while fever is present.

3) Concurrent disinfection: Strict handwashing after patient contact.

4) Quarantine: Not applicable.

5) Immunization of contacts: A recombinant B19 capsid vaccine is in development at time of writing.

6) Investigation of contacts and source of infection: Exposed pregnant women should be offered B19 IgG and IgM antibody testing to determine susceptibility, and to assist with counseling regarding risks to their fetuses.

7) Specific treatment: Intravenous immunoglobulin (IGIV) has been successfully used to treat chronic anemia in persistent infections, but relapses can occur and require additional IGIV therapy.

C. _Epidemic measures:_ During outbreaks in school or day care settings, those with anemia or immunodeficiency and pregnant women should be informed of the possible risk of acquiring and transmitting infection.

D. _Disaster implications:_ None.

E. _International measures:_ None.

EXANTHEMA SUBITUM   ICD-9 057.8; ICD-10 B08.2
(Sixth disease, Roseola infantum)
[CCDM19: Editorial Board]

1. Identification—Exanthema subitum is an acute, febrile rash illness of viral etiology, which occurs usually in children aged less than four but is most common before the age of two. It is one manifestation of illnesses caused by human herpesvirus-6B (HHV-6B). A fever, sometimes as high as 41°C (106°F), appears suddenly and lasts 3–5 days. A maculopapular rash on the trunk, and later on the remainder of the body, ordinarily follows lysis of the fever, and the rash usually fades rapidly. Symptoms are generally mild, but febrile seizures have been reported.

The spectrum of clinical illness in children includes high fever without rash, inflamed tympanic membranes, and—rarely—meningoencephalitis, recurrent seizures, or fulminant hepatitis. In immunocompetent adults, a mononucleosis-like syndrome has been described, and in immunocompromised hosts, pneumonitis has been noted. HHV-6 also causes asymptomatic and latent infection. Differentiation from similar vaccine-preventable exanthems (e.g. measles, rubella) is often necessary.

Diagnosis can be confirmed by testing of paired sera for antibodies to HHV-6 by IFA, or by isolation of HHV-6. Practical IgM tests are not available; an IgM response is usually not detectable until at least 5 days following the onset of symptoms. Detection of HHV-6 DNA in blood by PCR in the absence of concurrent IgG antibody shows promise as a future practical method for rapid diagnosis.

2. Infectious agent—Human herpesvirus-6 (subfamily betaherpesvirus, genus Roseolovirus) is the most common cause of exanthema subitum. HHV-6 can be divided into HHV-6A and HHV-6B by using monoclonal techniques. Most HHV-6 infections in humans are now known to be caused by HHV-6B. Cases of exanthema subitum due to human herpesvirus 7 also occur.

3. Occurrence—Worldwide. In Hong Kong (China), Japan, the UK and USA, where the sero-epidemiology of HHV-6 has been best described, incidence peaks in 6–12 month olds, with 65%–100% seroprevalence by age two years. Seroprevalence in childbearing women ranges from 80%–100% in most of the world, although rates as low as 20% have been observed in Morocco, and 49% in Malaysia. Distinct outbreaks of exanthema subitum or HHV-6 are rarely recognized; a seasonal predilection (late winter, early spring) has been described only in Japan.

4. Reservoir—Humans appear to be the main reservoir of infection.

5. Mode of transmission—In children, the rapid acquisition of early childhood infection that follows the waning of maternal antibodies and the high prevalence of HHV-6 viral DNA in salivary glands of adults suggest that salivary contact with care givers and parents is the most likely mode of infection. However, in one study, the age-specific infection rate increased when there was more than one sibling in the household, which suggests that children may also be important reservoirs for transmission. Renal and hepatic transplants from HHV-6-infected donors can cause primary infection in seronegative transplant recipients.

6. Incubation period—Ten days, with a usual range of 5–15 days. Onset of illness is usually 2–4 weeks after transplantation in susceptible transplant recipients.

7. Period of communicability—In acute infection, unknown. Following acute infection, the virus may establish latency in lymph nodes, kidney, liver, salivary glands and monocytes. The duration of potential communicability from these latent infections is unknown, but may be lifelong.

8. Susceptibility—Susceptibility is general. Infection rates in infants under 6 months are low but increase rapidly thereafter, which suggests that temporary protection is conferred by transplacentally acquired maternal antibodies. Second cases of exanthema subitum are rare. Latent infection appears to be established in most persons, but is of uncertain clinical significance, notably in persons who are immunosuppressed, among whom primary disease may be more severe, and in whom symptoms last longer.

9. Methods of control—Effective measures are not available.

   A. Preventive measures:

   1) Transplantation of organ tissues from HHV-6 seropositive donors to seronegative recipients is better avoided.

   B. Control of patient, contacts and the immediate environment:

   1) Report to local health authority: Official report not ordinarily justifiable, Class 5 (see *Reporting*).
   2) Isolation: In hospitals and institutions, patients suspected of having exanthema subitum should preferably be managed under contact isolation precautions.
   3) Concurrent disinfection: Not applicable.
   4) Quarantine: Not applicable.
   5) Immunization of contacts: Not applicable. Sustained immunity against re-infection following primary infections appears to occur, and there is potential for a vaccine.
   6) Investigation of contacts and source of infection: None, because of the high prevalence of asymptomatic shedders in the population.
   7) Specific treatment: None.

    C. Epidemic measures: None.

    D. Disaster implications: None.

    E. International measures: None.

FASCIOLIASIS   ICD-9 121.3; ICD-10 B66.3
[CCDM19: M. Eberhard]
[CCDM18: D. Engels]

    1. Identification—A zoonotic disease of the liver caused by a large trematode that is a natural parasite of sheep, cattle and related animals worldwide. Flukes measuring up to about 3 cm live in the bile ducts; the young stages live in the liver parenchyma and cause tissue damage and enlargement of the liver. During the early period of parenchymal invasion, there may be right upper quadrant pain, liver function abnormalities and eosinophilia. After migration to the biliary ducts, the flukes may cause biliary colic or obstructive jaundice. Ectopic infection, especially by *Fasciola gigantica*, may produce transient or migrating areas of inflammation in the skin over the trunk or other areas of the body.

    Diagnosis is based on finding eggs in feces or in bile aspirated from the duodenum. Serodiagnostic tests, available in some centers, suggest the diagnosis when positive. "Spurious infection" may be diagnosed when nonviable eggs appear in the feces after consumption of liver from infected animals.

    2. Infectious agents—*Fasciola hepatica* and *F. gigantica.*

    3. Occurrence—Human infection has been reported from 61 countries, mainly in sheep- and cattle-raising areas. Sporadic cases are reported in the USA. The infection is a public health problem in countries such as Bolivia, Ecuador, Egypt, Georgia, Peru, Russia and Viet Nam. Outbreaks have occurred in Cuba, the Islamic Republic of Iran, and to a lesser extent in Bolivia.

    4. Reservoir—Traditionally humans are considered accidental hosts. The infection in nature is known to be maintained in a cycle between other animal species, mainly sheep, cattle, water buffalo and other large herbivorous mammals and snails of the family Lymnaeidae. In certain areas humans may also act as reservoir.

    5. Mode of transmission—Eggs passed in the feces develop in water; in about 2 weeks a motile ciliated larva (miracidium) hatches. On entering a snail (lymnaeid), larvae develop to produce large numbers of free-swimming cercariae that attach to aquatic plants and encyst; these encysted forms (metacercariae) resist drying. Infection is acquired by eating uncooked aquatic plants (such as watercress) bearing metacercariae. Free-floating metacercariae in drinking water can also transmit the disease. On reaching the intestine, larvae migrate through the wall into the peritoneal cavity, enter the liver, and, after development, enter the bile ducts to lay eggs 3–4 months after initial exposure.

6. Incubation period—Variable.

7. Period of communicability—Infection is not transmitted directly from person to person.

8. Susceptibility—People of all ages are susceptible; infection persists indefinitely.

9. Methods of control—

A. Preventive measures:

1) Educate the public in endemic areas to abstain from eating watercress or other aquatic plants of wild or unknown origin, especially from grazing areas or places where the disease is known to be endemic.
2) Avoid using livestock feces to fertilize water plants.
3) Drain the land or use chemical molluskicides to eliminate mollusks where this is technically and economically feasible.

B. Control of patient, contacts and the immediate environment:

1) Report to local health authority: Official report not ordinarily justifiable, Class 5 (see *Reporting*).
2) Isolation: Not applicable.
3) Concurrent disinfection: Not applicable.
4) Quarantine: Not applicable.
5) Immunization of contacts: Not applicable.
6) Investigation of contacts and source of infection: Identification of the source of infection may be useful in preventing additional infections in the patient or others.
7) Specific treatment: Triclabendazole is the treatment of choice. Bithionol was formerly the drug of choice, but cure rates with this or praziquantel are not dependable. During the migratory phase, symptomatic relief may be provided by dehydroemetine, chloroquine or metronidazole. Nitazoxanide is under investigation.

C. Epidemic measures: Determine source of infection and identify plants and snails involved in transmission. Prevent the consumption of aquatic plants from contaminated areas.

D. Disaster implications: None.

E. International measures: None.

FASCIOLOPSIASIS   ICD-9 121.4; ICD-10 B66.5
[CCDM19: M. Eberhard]
[CCDM18: D. Engels]

1. Identification—A zoonotic trematode infection of the small intestine, particularly the duodenum. Symptoms result from local inflammation, ulceration of intestinal wall, and systemic toxic effects. Diarrhea usually alternates with constipation; vomiting and anorexia are frequent. Large numbers of flukes may produce acute intestinal obstruction. Patients may show edema of the face, abdominal wall and legs within 20 days after massive infection; ascites is common. Eosinophilia is usual; secondary anemia may occur. Death is rare; light infections are usually asymptomatic. Diagnosis is made by finding the large flukes or characteristic eggs in feces; worms are occasionally vomited.

2. Infectious agent—*Fasciolopsis buski*, a large trematode reaching lengths up to 7 cm.

3. Occurrence—Widely distributed in rural southeastern Asia, especially central and south China, parts of India, and Thailand. Prevalence is often high in pig-rearing areas.

4. Reservoir—Swine and humans are definitive hosts of adult flukes; dogs less commonly.

5. Mode of transmission—Eggs passed in feces, most often of swine, develop in water within 3–7 weeks under favorable conditions; miracidia hatch and penetrate planorbid snails as intermediate hosts; cercariae develop, are liberated and encyst on aquatic plants to become infective metacercariae. Human infections result from eating these plants uncooked. In China, chief sources of infection are the nuts of the red water caltrop (*Tapa bicornis*, *T. natans*), grown in enclosed ponds, and tubers of the so-called water chestnut (*Eliocharis tuberosa*) and water bamboo (*Zizania aquatica*); infection frequently results when the hull or skin is peeled off with teeth and lips; less often from metacercaria in pond water.

6. Incubation period—Eggs appear in feces about 3 months after infection.

7. Period of communicability—As long as viable eggs are discharged in feces; without treatment, probably for 1 year. No direct person-to-person transmission.

8. Susceptibility—Susceptibility is universal. In malnourished individuals, ill effects are pronounced; the number of worms influences severity of disease.

9. **Methods of control—**

A. *Preventive measures:*

1) Educate the population at risk in endemic areas on the mode of transmission and life cycle of the parasite.
2) Treat night soil to destroy eggs.
3) Bar swine from contaminating areas where water plants are growing; do not feed water plants to pigs.
4) Dry suspected plants, or if plants are to be eaten fresh, dip them in boiling water for a few seconds; both methods kill metacercariae.

B. *Control of patient, contacts and the immediate environment:*

1) Report to local health authority: In selected endemic areas; in most countries, not a reportable disease, Class 3 (see *Reporting*).
2) Isolation: Not applicable.
3) Concurrent disinfection: Safe disposal of feces.
4) Quarantine: Not applicable.
5) Immunization of contacts: Not applicable.
6) Investigation of contacts and source of infection: In the individual case, of little value. A community problem (see 9C).
7) Specific treatment: Praziquantel is the drug of choice.

C. *Epidemic measures:* Identify aquatic plants that harbor encysted metacercariae and are eaten fresh; identify infected snail species living in water with such plants; and prevent contamination of water with human and pig feces.

D. *Disaster implications:* None.

E. *International measures:* None.

FILARIASIS
ICD-9 125; ICD-10 B74
[CCDM19: M. Eberhard, P. Lammie]
[CCDM18: G. Biswas]

The term filariasis denotes infection with any of several nematodes belonging to the family Filarioidea. However, as used here, the term refers only to the lymphatic-dwelling filariae listed below. For others, refer to the specific disease.

FILARIASIS DUE TO *WUCHERERIA BANCROFTI*   ICD-9 125.0; ICD-10 B74.0
(Bancroftian filariasis)

FILARIASIS DUE TO *BRUGIA MALAYI*   ICD-9 125.1; ICD-10 B74.1
(Malayan filariasis, Brugian filariasis)

FILARIASIS DUE TO *BRUGIA TIMORI*   ICD-9 125.6; ICD-10 B74.2
(Timorean filariasis)

1. Identification—Bancroftian filariasis is an infection with the nematode *Wuchereria bancrofti*, which normally resides in the lymphatics in infected people. Female worms produce microfilariae that reach the bloodstream 6–12 months after infection. Two biologically different forms occur: in one, the microfilariae circulate in the peripheral blood at night (nocturnal periodicity) with greatest concentrations between 10 pm and 2 am; in the other, microfilariae circulate continuously in the peripheral blood, but occur in greater concentration in the daytime (diurnal subperiodicity). The latter form is endemic in the South Pacific and in small rural foci in southeastern Asia, where the principal vectors are day-biting *Aedes* mosquitoes.

Parasites primarily cause lymphatic damage; the subsequent lymphoedema and its progression are due to secondary bacterial infections. Clinical manifestations in regions of endemic filariasis include a) a symptomatic and parasitologically negative form; b) asymptomatic microfilaremia; c) filarial fevers manifested by high fever, acute recurrent lymphadenitis and retrograde lymphangitis with or without microfilaremia; d) lymphostasis associated with chronic signs, including hydrocele, chyluria, lymphoedema and elephantiasis of the limbs, breasts and genitalia, with low-level or undetectable microfilaremia; and e) tropical pulmonary eosinophilic syndrome, manifested by paroxysmal nocturnal asthma, chronic interstitial lung disease, recurrent low-grade fever, profound eosinophilia, and degenerating microfilariae in lung tissues but not in the bloodstream (occult filariasis).

Brugian and Timorean filariasis are caused by the nematodes *Brugia malayi* and *B. timori*, respectively. The nocturnally periodic form of *B. malayi* occurs in rural populations living in open rice-growing areas throughout much of southeastern Asia. The sub-periodic form infects humans, monkeys and wild and domestic carnivores in the forests of Malaysia and Indonesia. Clinical manifestations are similar to those of Bancroftian filariasis, except that the recurrent acute attacks of adenitis and retrograde lymphangitis associated with fever are more severe, while chyluria is uncommon and elephantiasis is usually confined to the distal extremities, most frequently to the legs below the knees. Hydrocele and breast lymphoedema are rarely if ever seen.

Brugia timori infections have been described in Timor-Leste and on southeastern islands of Indonesia. Clinical manifestations are comparable to those seen in *B. malayi* infections.

Microfilariae are best detected during periods of maximal microfilaremia. Live microfilariae can be seen under low power in a drop of peripheral blood (finger prick) on a slide or in hemolyzed blood in a counting chamber. Giemsa-stained thick and thin smears permit species identification. Microfilariae may be concentrated by filtration of anti-coagulated blood through a Nuclepore® filter (2–5 micrometer pore size), in a Swinnex® adapter, by the Knott technique (centrifugal sedimentation of 2 ml of anti-coagulated blood mixed with 10 ml of 2% formalin), or by the Quantitative Buffy Coat (QBC) acridine orange/microhematocrit tube technique. More sensitive techniques to detect circulating filarial antigen of *W. bancrofti* by ELISA or immunochromatic test cards have recently become available commercially. The adult worms in nests can be visualized on ultrasound by the "filarial dance sign," the random motion of echogenic particles in patients with filariasis caused by the typical movement of these filariae in dilated intrascrotal lymphatic vessels (little is known about the prevalent worm nest locations in women); but the sensitivity of this technique is too low for routine diagnosis.

2. Infectious agents—*Wuchereria bancrofti, Brugia malayi* and *B. timori*; long threadlike worms.

3. Occurrence—*W. bancrofti*, the most commonly prevalent of the 3 parasites responsible for 90% of the lymphatic filariases, is endemic in most of the warm humid regions of the world, including Latin America (scattered foci in Brazil, the Dominican Republic, Guyana, and Haiti), Africa, Asia, and the Pacific Islands. It is common in those urban areas where conditions favor breeding of vector mosquitoes. In general, nocturnal sub-periodicity in *Wuchereria*-infected areas of the Pacific is found West of 140°E longitude, and diurnal sub-periodicity East of 180°E longitude. *B. malayi* is endemic in rural southwestern India and southeastern Asia. *B. timori* occurs in Timor-Leste and on the rural islands of Flores, Alor and Roti in southeastern Indonesia.

4. Reservoir—Humans with microfilariae in the blood for *W. bancrofti*, periodic *B. malayi* and *B. timori*. In Malaysia, southern Thailand, the Philippines, Timor-Leste and Indonesia, cats, civets (*Viverra tangalunga*) and nonhuman primates serve as reservoirs for sub-periodic *B. malayi*, but zoonotic transmission is not of much significance.

5. Mode of transmission—Bite of a mosquito harboring infective larvae. *W. bancrofti* is transmitted by many species, the most important being *Culex quinquefasciatus, Anopheles gambiae, An. funestus, Aedes polynesiensis, Ae. scapularis* and *Ae. pseudoscutellaris. B. malayi* is transmitted by various species of *Mansonia, Anopheles* and *Aedes. B. timori* is transmitted by *An. barbirostris*. In the female mosquito, ingested microfilariae penetrate the stomach wall and develop in the thoracic muscles into elongated, infective filariform larvae that migrate to the proboscis. When the mosquito feeds, the larvae emerge and enter the punctured skin following the mosquito bite. They travel via the lymphatics, where they molt twice before becoming adults.

6. Incubation period—Microfilariae may not appear in the blood until after 3–6 months in *B. malayi* and 6–12 months in *W. bancrofti* infections. This period is described as the pre-patent period.

7. Period of communicability—Not directly transmitted from person to person. Humans may infect mosquitoes when microfilariae are present in the peripheral blood; microfilaremia may persist for 5–10 years or longer after initial infection. The mosquito becomes infective about 12–14 days after an infective blood meal. A large number of infected mosquito bites are required to initiate infection in the host.

8. Susceptibility—Universal susceptibility to infection is probable; there is considerable geographic difference in the type and severity of disease. Repeated infections may occur in endemic regions.

9. Methods of control—

A. Preventive measures:

1) Educate the inhabitants of endemic areas on the mode of transmission and methods of mosquito control.
2) Identify the vectors by detecting infective larvae in mosquitoes caught; identify times and places of mosquito biting and locate breeding places. If indoor night biters are responsible, screen houses or use bed nets (preferably impregnated with synthetic pyrethroid) and insect repellents. Eliminate breeding places (e.g. open latrines, tires, coconut husks) and treat with polystyrene beads or larvicides. Where *Mansonia* species are vectors, clear ponds of vegetation (*Pistia*) that serve as sources of oxygen for the larvae.
3) Long-term vector control may involve changes in housing construction to include screening, and environmental control in order to eliminate mosquito-breeding sites.
4) Mass treatment with diethylcarbamazine citrate (DEC), especially when followed by monthly treatment with a low dose of DEC for 1–2 years or the use of DEC-medicated cooking salt for 6 months to 2 years, has proven effective. However, DEC cannot be used in areas where onchocerciasis is co-endemic due to possible adverse reactions (see also *Onchocerciasis*, Mazzotti reaction). In areas co-endemic for onchocerciasis, ivermectin is used; albendazole in multiple and single doses also has anti-filarial properties. In lymphatic filariasis where onchocerciasis is not endemic, WHO cur-

rently recommends mass drug administration, as an annual single dose, of combinations of DEC with albendazole for 4–6 years, or the regular use of DEC-fortified salt for 1–2 years. In areas where onchocerciasis is co-endemic, the use of ivermectin and albendazole is recommended. Certain groups of individuals, such as pregnant women, children below 2 years (DEC and albendazole co-administration), children under 90 cm height and lactating women in the first week (ivermectin and albendazole co-administration), as well as severely ill persons, should not receive the drugs. Mass drug administration is contraindicated at present in areas with concurrent loiasis, due to the risk of severe adverse reactions in patients with high density *Loa loa* infections.

B. Control of patient, contacts and the immediate environment:

1) Report to local health authority: In selected endemic regions; in most countries, not a reportable disease, Class 3 (see *Reporting*). Reporting of cases with demonstrated microfilariae or circulating filarial antigen provides information on areas of transmission.
2) Isolation: Not practicable. As far as possible, patients with microfilaremia should be treated with anti-filarial drugs and protected from mosquitoes to reduce transmission.
3) Concurrent disinfection: Not applicable.
4) Quarantine: Not applicable.
5) Immunization of contacts: Not applicable.
6) Investigation of contacts and source of infection: Only as part of a general community effort (see 9A and 9C).
7) Specific treatment: Diethylcarbamazine citrate (DEC) is generally effective; ivermectin in combination with albendazole results in rapid and sustained suppression of most or all microfilariae from the blood, but may not destroy all the adult worms. Low-level microfilaremia may reappear after treatment with any drug. Therefore, treatment must usually be repeated at yearly intervals. Low-level microfilaremia can be detected only by concentration techniques. DEC may cause acute generalized reactions during the first 24 hours of treatment because of death and degeneration of microfilariae; these reactions are mostly self-limiting and often controlled by paracetamol and antihistamines. Localized lymphadenitis and lymphangitis may follow the death of the adult worms and usually occurs 5–7 days after taking the drugs. Care of the skin to prevent entry lesions; exercise; elevation of affected limbs; and use of topical anti-fungal or antibiotics when infected all help prevent acute dermato-adenolymphangitis and subsequent progression to lympho-

edema. Management of lymphoedema includes local limb care; surgical decompression may be required. Hydroceles can be surgically repaired.

C. *Epidemic measures:* Because of low infectivity and long incubation period, epidemics of filariasis are unlikely.

D. *Disaster implications:* None.

E. *International measures:* WHO Collaborating Centres provide support as required. More information can be found at http://www.who.int/collaboratingcentres/database/en/.

WHO has launched a global program subsequent to the Resolution of the 1997 World Health Assembly calling for the elimination of lymphatic filariasis as a public health problem, through an alliance of endemic countries and partners from the public and private sectors. Further information can be found on <http://www.filariasis.org> and <http://www.who.int/tdr/diseases/lymphfil/default.htm>.

DIROFILARIASIS
(Zoonotic filariasis)

ICD-9 125.6; ICD-10 B74.8

Certain species of filariae commonly seen in wild or domestic animals occasionally infect humans, but microfilaremia occurs rarely. The genus *Dirofilaria* causes pulmonary and cutaneous disease in humans. Infection with *D. immitis*, the dog heartworm, has been reported from most parts of the world, including Australia, Europe, Canada, the USA, Japan, and other parts of Asia. Transmission to humans is by mosquito bite. The worm lodges in a pulmonary artery, where it may form the nidus of a thrombus; this can then lead to vascular occlusion, coagulation, necrosis and fibrosis. Symptoms are chest pain, cough and hemoptysis. Eosinophilia is infrequent. A fibrotic nodule, 1–3 cm in diameter, which is most commonly asymptomatic, is recognizable by X-ray as a "coin lesion."

Various species cause cutaneous lesions, including *D. tenuis*, a parasite of the raccoon in the USA; *D. ursi*, a parasite of bears in Canada; and *D. repens*, a parasite of dogs and cats in Europe, Africa and Asia. The worms develop in or migrate to the conjunctivae and the subcutaneous tissues of the scrotum, breasts, arms and legs, but microfilaremia is rare. Animal species of *Brugia* cause zoonotic infections, localize in lymph nodes, and have been reported from North and South America and Africa. Diagnosis is usually made by the finding of worms in tissue sections of surgically excised lesions.

OTHER NEMATODES PRODUCING MICROFILARIAE IN HUMANS

Several other nematodes may infect humans and produce microfilariae. These include *Onchocerca volvulus* and *Loa loa*, which cause onchocerciasis and loiasis, respectively (see under each disease listing). Other infections are forms of mansonellosis (ICD-9 125.4 and 125.5; ICD-10 B74.4): *Mansonella perstans* is widely distributed in western Africa and northeastern South America; the adult is found in the body cavities, and the unsheathed microfilariae circulate with no regular periodicity. Infection is usually asymptomatic, but eye infection from immature stages has been reported.

In some countries of western and central Africa, infection with *M. streptocerca* (ICD-9 125.4-125.6; ICD-10 B74.4) is common and is suspected of causing cutaneous edema and thickening of the skin, hypo-pigmented macules, pruritus and papules. Adult worms and unsheathed microfilariae occur in the skin as in onchocerciasis. *M. ozzardi* (ICD-9 125.5; ICD-10 B74.4) occurs from the Yucatan Peninsula in Mexico to northern Argentina and in the West Indies; diagnosis is based on demonstration of the circulating unsheathed non-periodic microfilariae. Infection is generally asymptomatic but may be associated with allergic manifestations such as arthralgia, pruritus, headaches and lymphadenopathy.

Culicoides midges are the main vectors for *M. streptocerca*, *M. ozzardi* and *M. perstans*; in the Caribbean area, blackflies also transmit *M. ozzardi*. *M. rodhaini*, a parasite of chimpanzees, was found in 1.7% of skin snips taken from humans in Gabon.

Diethylcarbamazine is effective against *M. streptocerca* and occasionally against *M. perstans* and *M. ozzardi*. Ivermectin is effective against *M. ozzardi*.

FOOD-BORNE INTOXICATIONS (Food poisoning)
[CCDM19: J. Schlundt
[CCDM18: H. Toyofuku]

Food-borne diseases, including food-borne intoxications and food-borne infections, are terms applied to illnesses acquired through consumption of contaminated food; they are frequently and inaccurately referred to as food poisoning. These diseases include those caused by chemical contaminants such as heavy metals and many organic compounds. The more frequent causes of food-borne illnesses are: 1) Toxins elaborated by bacterial growth in the food before consumption (*Clostridium botulinum*, *Staphylococcus aureus* and *Bacillus cereus*; scombroid fish poisoning is associated not with a specific toxin but with elevated histamine levels), or in the intestines (*Clostridium perfringens*); 2) Bacterial, viral, or parasitic infections (amebiasis, brucellosis, *Campylobacter* enteritis, diarrhea caused by *Escherichia coli*, hepatitis A, listeriosis, salmonellosis, shigellosis, toxoplasmosis, viral gastroenteritis, teniasis, trichinosis, and infection with vibrios); 3) Toxins produced by harmful algal species (ciguatera fish poisoning, paralytic, neurotoxic, diarrheic or amnesic shellfish poisoning) or present in specific species (puffer fish poisoning, azaspiracid poisoning [AZP]).

This chapter deals specifically with toxin-related food-borne illnesses (with the exception of botulism, elaborated in a separate chapter). Food-borne illnesses associated with infection by specific agents are covered in chapters dealing with these agents.

Food-borne disease outbreaks are recognized by the occurrence of illness within a variable but usually short time period (a few hours to a few weeks) after a meal, among individuals who have consumed foods in common. Prompt and thorough laboratory evaluation of cases and implicated foods is essential. Single cases of food-borne disease are difficult to identify unless, as in botulism, there is a distinctive clinical syndrome. Food-borne disease may be one of the most common causes of acute illness; many cases and outbreaks are unrecognized and unreported.

Prevention and control of these diseases, regardless of specific cause, are based on the same principles: avoiding food contamination, destroying or denaturing contaminants, and preventing further spread or multiplication of these contaminants. Specific problems and appropriate modes of intervention may vary from one country to another, and depend on environmental, economic, political, technological and sociocultural factors. Ultimately, prevention also depends on educating food handlers about proper practices in cooking and storage of food, and personal hygiene. To this end, the WHO document, *Five Keys to Safer Food* (at <http://www.who.int/fsf/Documents/5keys-ID-eng.pdf>) sets out five steps to ensuring safer food:

1. Keep clean;
2. Separate raw and cooked;
3. Cook thoroughly;
4. Keep food at safe temperatures;
5. Use safe water and raw materials.

I. STAPHYLOCOCCAL FOOD INTOXICATION

9 005.0; ICD-10 A05.0

1. Identification—An intoxication (not an infection) of abrupt and sometimes violent onset, with severe nausea, cramps, vomiting and prostration, often accompanied by diarrhea and sometimes with subnormal temperature and lowered blood pressure. Deaths are rare; illness commonly lasts only a day or two, but can take longer in severe cases; in rare cases, the intensity of symptoms may require hospitalization and unnecessary surgical exploration has sometimes been done in pursuit of a diagnosis. Diagnosis is easier when a group of cases presents the characteristic acute, predominantly upper GI symptoms, and a short interval between eating a common food item and the onset of symptoms (usually within 4 hours).

Differential diagnosis includes other recognized forms of food poisoning as well as chemical poisons.

In the outbreak setting, recovery of large numbers of staphylococci (10^5 organisms or more/gram of food) on routine culture media, or detection of enterotoxin from an epidemiologically implicated food item, confirms the diagnosis. Absence of staphylococci on culture from heated food does not rule out the diagnosis; a Gram stain of the food may disclose the organisms that have been heat killed. It may be possible to identify enterotoxin or thermonuclease in the food in the absence of viable organisms. Isolation of organisms of the same phage type from stools or vomitus of two or more ill persons confirms the diagnosis. Recovery of large numbers of enterotoxin-producing staphylococci from stool or vomitus from a single person supports the diagnosis. Phage typing and enterotoxin tests may help epidemiological investigations, but are not routinely available or indicated; in outbreak settings, pulsed field gel electrophoresis may be more useful in subtyping strains.

2. Toxic agent—Several enterotoxins of *Staphylococcus aureus* are stable at the boiling point, and resist some thermal processing procedures. Staphylococci multiply in food and produce the toxins even when water content is too low for the growth of many other competing bacteria.

3. Occurrence—Widespread and relatively frequent; one of the principal acute food intoxications worldwide.

4. Reservoir—Humans in most instances (about 25% of healthy people are carriers of *Staphylococcus aureus*); occasionally cows with mastitis, as well as dogs and fowl.

5. Mode of transmission—Ingestion of a food product containing staphylococcal enterotoxin, particularly those foods that come in contact with food handlers' hands, either without subsequent cooking or with inadequate heating or refrigeration. Pastries, custards, salad dressings, sandwiches, sliced meat, and meat products are at great risk of contamination. Toxin has also developed in inadequately cured ham and salami, and in unprocessed or inadequately processed cheese. When these foods remain at room temperature for several hours before being eaten, toxin-producing staphylococci multiply and elaborate the heat-stable toxin.

Organisms may be of human origin from purulent discharges of an infected finger or eye, abscesses, acneiform facial eruptions, nasopharyngeal secretions, or apparently normal skin; or of bovine origin, from products originating from contaminated milk, especially cheese.

6. Incubation period—Interval between eating food and onset of symptoms is 30 minutes to 8 hours, usually 2-4 hours.

7. Period of communicability—Not applicable.

8. Susceptibility—Most people are susceptible.

9. Methods of control—

A. Preventive measures:

1) Educate food handlers about: (a) strict food hygiene, sanitation and cleanliness of kitchens, proper temperature control, handwashing, and cleaning of fingernails; (b) the danger of working with exposed skin, nose or eye infections, and uncovered wounds.
2) Reduce food-handling time (from initial preparation to service) to a minimum, no more than 4 hours at ambient temperature. If foods are to be stored for more than 2 hours, keep those that are perishable hot (above 60°C/140°F) or cold (below 5°C/41°F), in shallow containers, and covered.
3) Temporarily exclude people with boils, abscesses and other purulent lesions of hands, face or nose from food handling.

B. Control of patient, contacts and the immediate environment:

1) Report to local health authority: Obligatory report of outbreaks of suspected or confirmed cases in some countries, Class 4 (see *Reporting*).
2), 3), 4), 5) and 6) Isolation, Concurrent disinfection, Quarantine, Immunization of contacts and Investigation of contacts and source of infection: Not pertinent. Control is of outbreaks; single cases are rarely identified.
7) Specific treatment: Fluid replacement when indicated.

C. Epidemic measures:

1) Through quick review of reported cases, determine time and place of exposure and population at risk; obtain a complete listing of the foods served and embargo, under refrigeration, all foods still available. The prominent clinical features, coupled with an estimate of the incubation period, provide useful leads to the most probable causal agent. Collect specimens of feces and vomitus for laboratory examination; alert the laboratory to suspected causal agents. Conduct an epidemiological investigation, including interviews of ill and well persons, to determine the association of illness with consumption of a given food. Compare attack rates for specific food items eaten and not eaten;

implicated food item(s) will usually have the greatest difference in attack rates, and most of the sick will remember having eaten the contaminated food.

2) Inquire about the origin of incriminated food and the manner of its preparation and storage before serving. Look for possible sources of contamination and periods of inadequate refrigeration and heating that would permit growth of staphylococci. Submit leftover suspected foods promptly for laboratory examination; failure to isolate staphylococci does not exclude the presence of the heat-resistant enterotoxin if the food has been heated.

3) Search for food handlers with skin infections, particularly of the hands. Culture all purulent lesions and collect nasal swabs from all food handlers. Antibiograms and/or phage typing of representative strains of enterotoxin-producing staphylococci isolated from foods and food handlers and from patient vomitus or feces may be helpful.

D. Disaster implications: A potential hazard in situations involving mass feeding and lack of refrigeration facilities, including feeding during air travel.

E. International measures: WHO Collaborating Centres provide support as required. More information can be found at: <http://www.who.int/collaboratingcentres/database/en>

II. CLOSTRIDIUM PERFRINGENS FOOD INTOXICATION ICD-9 005.2; ICD-10 A05.2
(C. welchii food poisoning, Enteritis necroticans, Pigbel)

1. Identification—An intestinal disorder characterized by sudden onset of colic followed by diarrhea; nausea is common, vomiting and fever are usually absent. Generally a mild disease of short duration—1 day or less—and rarely fatal in previously healthy people. Outbreaks of severe disease with high case-fatality rates associated with necrotizing enteritis have been documented in postwar Germany and in Papua New Guinea (pigbel).

In the outbreak setting, diagnosis is confirmed by demonstration of *Clostridium perfringens* in semiquantitative anerobic cultures of food (10^5/g or more) or patients' stool (10^6/g or more), in addition to clinical and epidemiological evidence. Detection of enterotoxin in patients' stool also confirms the diagnosis. When serotyping is possible during outbreaks, the same serotype is usually demonstrated in different specimens; serotyping is done routinely only in Japan and the United Kingdom.

2. Infectious agent—Type A strains of *C. perfringens* (*C. welchii*) cause typical food poisoning outbreaks (they also cause gas-gangrene);

type C strains cause necrotizing enteritis. Disease is produced by toxins elaborated by the organisms.

3. Occurrence—Widespread and relatively frequent in countries with cooking practices that favor multiplication of clostridia to high levels.

4. Reservoir—GI tract of healthy people and animals (cattle, fish, pigs and poultry).

5. Mode of transmission—Ingestion of food containing soil or feces and then held under conditions that permit multiplication of the organism. Almost all outbreaks are associated with inadequately heated or (especially) reheated meats, usually stews, meat pies, and gravies made of beef, turkey or chicken. Spores survive normal cooking temperatures, germinate, and multiply during slow cooling, storage at ambient temperature, and/or inadequate re-heating. Outbreaks are usually traced to catering firms, restaurants, cafeterias and schools with inadequate cooling and refrigeration facilities for large-scale service. Illness results from the release of toxin by cells undergoing sporulation in the lower intestinal tract. Heavy bacterial contamination (more than 10^5 organisms/gram of food) is usually required to produce toxin in the human intestine for clinical disease.

6. Incubation period—From 6 to 24 hours, usually 10–12 hours.

7. Period of communicability—Not applicable.

8. Susceptibility—Most people are probably susceptible. In volunteer studies, no resistance was observed after repeated exposures.

9. Methods of control—

    A. Preventive measures:

        1) Educate food handlers about the risks inherent in large-scale cooking, especially of meat dishes. Where possible, encourage serving hot dishes (above 60°C/140°F) while still hot from initial cooking.

        2) Serve meat dishes hot, as soon as cooked, or cool them rapidly in a properly designed chiller and refrigerate until serving time; reheating, if necessary, should be thorough (internal temperature of at least 70°C/158°F, preferably 75°C/167°F or higher) and rapid. Meat and poultry should not be partially cooked one day and reheated the next, unless it can be stored at a safe temperature. Large cuts of meat must be thoroughly cooked; for more rapid cooling of cooked foods, divide stews and similar dishes prepared in bulk into many shallow containers, and place in a rapid chiller.

B., C. and **D. Control of patient, contacts and the imme-diate environment, Epidemic measures** and **Disaster im-plications:** See *Staphylococcal food intoxication* (I, 9B, 9C and 9D).

E. International measures: None.

III. *BACILLUS CEREUS* FOOD INTOXICATION   ICD-9 005.8; ICD-10 A05.4

1. Identification—An intoxication characterized in some cases by sudden onset of nausea and vomiting, and in others by colic and diarrhea. Illness generally persists no longer than 24 hours and is rarely fatal. In outbreak settings, diagnosis is confirmed through quantitative cultures on selective media to estimate the number of organisms present in the suspected food (generally more than 10^5 to 10^6 organisms per gram of the incriminated food are required). Isolation of organisms from the stool of 2 or more ill persons and not from stools of controls also confirms the diagnosis. Enterotoxin testing is valuable but may not be widely available.

2. Toxic agent—*Bacillus cereus*, an aerobic spore former. Two enterotoxins have been identified: one (heat stable), causing vomiting, is produced in food when *B. cereus* levels reach 10^5 colony-forming units/gram of food; and one (heat labile), causing diarrhea, is formed in the small intestine of the human host.

3. Occurrence—A well-recognized cause of food-borne disease throughout the world.

4. Reservoir—A ubiquitous organism in soil and environment, commonly found at low levels in raw, dried and processed foods.

5. Mode of transmission—Ingestion of food kept at ambient temperatures after cooking, with multiplication of the organisms. Outbreaks associated with vomiting have been most commonly associated with cooked rice held at ambient room temperatures before reheating. Various mishandled foods have been implicated in outbreaks associated with diarrhea.

6. Incubation period—From 0.5 to 6 hours in cases where vomiting is the predominant symptom; from 6 to 24 hours where diarrhea predominates.

7. Period of communicability—Not communicable from person to person.

8. Susceptibility—Unknown.

9. **Methods of control—**

A. **Preventive measures:** Foods should not remain at ambient temperature after cooking, since the ubiquitous *B. cereus* spores can survive boiling, germinate, and multiply rapidly at room temperature. The emetic toxin is also heat-resistant. Refrigerate leftover food promptly (toxin formation is unlikely at temperatures below 10°C/50°F); reheat thoroughly and rapidly to avoid multiplication of microorganisms.

B., C. and D. **Control of patient, contacts and the immediate environment, Epidemic measures** and **Disaster implications:** See *Staphylococcal food intoxication* (I, 9B, 9C and 9D).

E. **International measures:** None.

IV. SCOMBROID FISH POISONING
(Histamine poisoning)

ICD-9 988.0; ICD-10 T61.1

A syndrome of tingling and burning sensations around the mouth, facial flushing and sweating, nausea and vomiting, headache, palpitations, dizziness and rash occurring within a few hours after eating fish containing high levels of free histamine (more than 20 mg/100 grams of fish); this occurs when the fish undergoes bacterial decomposition after capture. Symptoms resolve spontaneously within 12 hours and there are no long-term sequelae.

Occurrence is worldwide; the syndrome was initially associated with fish in the families Scombroidea and Scomberesocidae (tuna, mackerel, skipjack and bonito) containing high levels of histidine that can be decarboxylated to form histamine by histidine-decarboxylase-producing bacteria in the fish. Scombroid fish poisoning is not solely caused by excess histamine ingestion—other substances that facilitate histamine absorption and urocanic acid add to the histamine-related symptoms. Nonscombroid fish, such as mahi-mahi (*Coryphaena hippurus*) and bluefish (*Pomatomus saltatrix*), are also associated with illness. Risks appear to be greatest for fish imported from tropical or semitropical areas and fish caught by recreational or artisanal fishermen, who may lack appropriate storage facilities for large fish. Detection of histamine in epidemiologically implicated fish confirms the diagnosis.

Adequate and rapid refrigeration, with evisceration and removal of the gills in a sanitary manner, prevents this spoilage. Symptoms usually resolve spontaneously. In severe cases, antihistamines may be effective in relieving symptoms.

While this is most often associated with fish, any food (such as certain cheeses) that contains the appropriate amino acids and is subjected to certain bacterial contamination and growth may lead to scombroid poisoning when ingested, especially in patients taking isoniazid or other drugs interfering with histamine metabolism.

The cornerstone of treatment is with antihistamines, preferably intravenously; inhalators can be useful in special cases.

V. CIGUATERA FISH POISONING   ICD-9 988.0; ICD-10 T61.0

A characteristic GI and neurological syndrome may occur within 1 hour after eating tropical reef fish. GI symptoms (diarrhea, vomiting, abdominal pain) occur first, usually within 24 hours of consumption. In severe cases, patients may also become hypotensive, with a paradoxical bradycardia. Neurological symptoms, including pain and weakness in the lower extremities and circumoral and peripheral paresthesias, may occur at the same time as the acute symptoms or follow 1–2 days later; they may persist for weeks or months.

Symptoms such as temperature reversal (ice cream tastes hot, hot coffee seems cold) and "aching teeth" are frequently reported. In very severe cases, neurological symptoms may progress to coma and respiratory arrest within the first 24 hours of illness. Most patients recover completely within a few weeks; intermittent recrudescence of symptoms can occur over a period of months to years.

This syndrome is caused by the presence in the fish of toxins elaborated by the dinoflagellate *Gambierdiscus toxicus* and algae growing on underwater reefs. Fish eating the algae become toxic, and the effect is magnified through the food chain so that large predatory fish become the most toxic; this occurs worldwide in tropical areas.

Ciguatera poisoning is the most commonly reported marine food poisoning. Ciguatera is a significant cause of morbidity where consumption of reef fish is common (Australia, the Caribbean, southern Florida, Hawaii and the South Pacific). Incidence has been estimated at 500 cases/100 000 population/year in the South Pacific, with rates 50 times higher reported for some island groups. More than 400 fish species may have the potential for becoming toxic. Worldwide, 50 000 cases of ciguatera are estimated to occur per year. Evidence of ciguatoxin in epidemiologically implicated fish confirms the diagnosis.

The consumption of large predatory fish should be avoided, especially in the reef area, and particularly the barracuda, snapper and sea bass. Where assays for toxic fish are available, screening all large "high-risk" fish before consumption can reduce risk. The occurrence of toxic fish is sporadic and not all fish of a given species or from a given locale will be toxic. Intravenous infusion of mannitol (1 gram/kg of a 20% solution over 45 minutes) may have a dramatic effect on acute symptoms of ciguatera fish poisoning, particularly in severe cases, and may be lifesaving in severe cases that have progressed to coma.

VI. PARALYTIC SHELLFISH
POISONING   ICD-9 988.0; ICD-10 T61.2
(PSP)

Classic paralytic shellfish poisoning (PSP) is a characteristic syndrome (predominantly neurological) starting within minutes to several hours after eating bivalve mollusks. Initial symptoms include paresthesias of the mouth and extremities, accompanied by GI symptoms, and usually resolving within a few days. In severe cases, ataxia, dysphonia, dysphagia and muscle paralysis with respiratory arrest and death may occur within 12 hours. Symptoms usually resolve completely within hours to days after shellfish ingestion.

This syndrome is caused by the presence in shellfish of saxitoxins and gonyautoxins produced by *Alexandrium* species and other dinoflagellates. Concentration of these toxins occurs during massive algal blooms known as "red tides," but also in the absence of recognizable algal bloom. PSP is common in shellfish harvested from colder waters above 30°N and below 30°S latitude, but may also occur in tropical waters. In North America, PSP is primarily a problem in northern latitudes. Blooms of the causative *Alexandrium* species occur several times each year, primarily from April through October. Shellfish remain toxic for several weeks after the bloom subsides; some shellfish species remain toxic constantly. Most cases occur in individuals or small groups who gather shellfish for personal consumption. Detection of toxin in epidemiologically implicated food confirms the diagnosis. On an experimental basis, saxitoxins have been demonstrated in serum during acute illness, and in urine after acute symptoms resolve.

PSP neurotoxins are heat-stable. Surveillance of high-risk harvest areas is routine in Canada and the European Union. Japan and the USA use a standard mouse bioassay; when toxin levels in shellfish exceed 80 micrograms of saxitoxin equivalent/100 grams, areas are closed to harvesting and warnings posted in shellfish-growing areas, on beaches, and in the media.

VII. NEUROTOXIC SHELLFISH
POISONING   ICD-9 988.0; ICD-10 T61.2

Neurotoxic shellfish poisoning is associated with algal blooms of *Gymnodinium breve*, which produce brevetoxin. Red tides caused by *G. breve* have long occurred along the Florida coast, where the syndrome has been most studied, with associated mortality in fish, seabirds and marine mammals. Symptoms after eating toxic shellfish—including circumoral paresthesias and paresthesias of the extremities, dizziness and ataxia, myalgia and GI symptoms—tend to be mild and resolve quickly and completely. Respiratory and eye irritation also occur in association with

G. breve blooms, apparently through aerosolization of the toxin through wind and wave action.

VIII. DIARRHETIC SHELLFISH POISONING ICD-9 988.0; ICD-10 T61.2

Diarrhetic shellfish poisoning (DSP) was first reported in Japan in 1978, and thereafter worldwide. The causative toxins, dinophysistoxin-1 (DTX1), dinophysistoxin-2 (DTX2), dinophysistoxin-3 (DTX3), okadaic acid (OA), 7-O-acylDTX2 (acylDTX2), and 7-O-acylOA (acylOA) have been isolated. Illness results from eating mussels, scallops, or clams that have fed on *Dinophysis fortii* or *Dinophysis acuminata*. Symptoms include diarrhea, nausea, vomiting, and abdominal pain.

In scallops, the distribution of toxins was localized in the hepatopancreas (midgut gland), the elimination of which renders scallops safe to eat. Ordinary cooking such as boiling in water or steaming cannot reduce OAs in this gland, because of their chemical stability and lipophilic properties. Methods of detection of DSP in shellfish include mouse bioassay, ELISA and liquid chromatography-mass spectrometry. The USA has established the action level for DSP at 0.2 ppm okadaic acid (OA) plus 35-methyl okadaic acid (DXT1).

IX. AMNESIC SHELLFISH POISONING ICD-9 988.0; ICD-10 T61.2

Amnesic shellfish poisoning (ASP) results from ingestion of shellfish containing domoic acid produced by the diatom *Pseudonitzschia pungens*. Cases were first reported in the Atlantic provinces of Canada in 1987, with vomiting, abdominal cramps, diarrhea, headache and loss of short-term memory. When tested several months after acute intoxication, patients show antegrade memory deficits with relative preservation of other cognitive functions, together with clinical and electromyographical evidence of pure motor or sensorimotor neuropathy and axonopathy. Canadian authorities now analyse mussels and clams for domoic acid, and close shellfish beds to harvesting when levels exceed 20 ppm domoic acid. In 1991, domoic acid was also identified in razor clams and Dungeness crabs on the Oregon and Washington coast (USA), and in the marine food web along the Texas coast. The clinical significance of ingestion of low levels of domoic acid (in persons eating shellfish and anchovies harvested from areas where *Pseudonitzschia* species are present) is unknown. EC-directive 91/492/EEC and amendments for the safety of shellfish (Amendment 97/61/EC) state that: "total Amnesic Shellfish Poison (ASP) content in the edible part of mollusks (the entire body or any part edible separately) must not exceed 20 micrograms of domoic acid per gram using HPLC [high pressure liquid chromatography]."

X. PUFFER FISH POISONING (TETRODOTOXIN)   ICD-9 988.0; ICD-10 T61.2

Puffer fish poisoning is characterized by onset of paresthesias, dizziness, GI symptoms and ataxia, often progressing to paralysis and death within several hours after eating. Case-fatality rate approaches 60%. The causative toxin is tetrodotoxin, a heat-stable, non-protein neurotoxin concentrated in the skin and viscera of puffer fish, porcupine fish, ocean sunfish, and species of newts and salamanders. More than 6 000 cases have been documented, mostly in Japan. Toxicity can be avoided by not consuming any of the tetrodotoxin-producing species of fish or amphibians. Some fish species contain no or little tetrodotoxin in the muscle. Japan implements control measures such as species identification and adequate removal of toxic parts (e.g. ova, intestine) by qualified cooks.

XI. AZASPIRACID POISONING (AZP)   ICD-9 988.0; ICD-10 T61.2

Occurrence of azaspiracid poisoning (AZP) was first reported when mussels harvested in Ireland caused diarrhea in humans in the Netherlands in 1995. Since 1996 several AZP incidents have been identified in several European countries, mainly through mussels. Symptoms occur 12 to 24 hours after consumption and persist for up to 5 days: they include severe diarrhea and vomiting with abdominal pain and occasional nausea, chills, headaches, and stomach cramps. Azaspiracid poisoning can cause necrosis in the intestine, thymus, and liver.

GASTRITIS CAUSED BY *HELICOBACTER PYLORI*   ICD-9 535; ICD-10 K29
[CCDM19: J. Schlundt, A. Sheth, D. Swerdlow]
[CCDM18: I. Lejnev]

1. Identification—A bacterial infection causing acute and chronic gastritis, primarily in the antrum of the stomach, and peptic ulcer disease. Infection with *Helicobacter pylori* is epidemiologically associated with gastric adenocarcinoma and gastric mucosa-associated lymphoid tissue (MALT) type lymphoma. Most of those infected with H. pylori remain asymptomatic. The key pathophysiological event in *H. pylori* infection is initiation and continuance of an inflammatory response. Development of atrophy and intestinal metaplasia of the gastric mucosa are strongly associated with *H. pylori* infection. Oxidative and nitrosative stress in combination with inflammation plays an important role in gastric carcinogenesis.

Diagnosis may be made from a gastric biopsy specimen through detection of *H. pylori* urease, using commercially available kits, histology, or bacterial culture. The organism requires nutrient media for growth, and cultures should be incubated at 37°C (98.6°F) in microaerophilic conditions for 48–72 hours. Selective media have been developed to prevent contaminating growth when culturing gastric biopsy material. Noninvasive tests include urea-based breath tests, which are based on the organism's extremely high urease activity, stool antigen tests, and serum antibody tests. Serum antibody tests may remain positive for months after treatment. Testing for *H. pylori* infection is indicated in patients with active peptic ulcer disease, a past history of documented peptic ulcer disease, or gastric MALT lymphoma.

2. Infectious agent—*Helicobacter pylori* is a Gram-negative, "S" and "U" spirally shaped bacillus, catalase-, oxidase- and urease-positive. Many different *Helicobacter* species have been identified in other animals; *H. cinaedi* and *H. fennelliae* have been associated with diarrhea in men who have sex with men.

3. Occurrence—*H. pylori* has an estimated rate of infection of over half of the world population, and could reach up to 70% in developing countries and up to 20%–30% in industrialized countries. Only a minority of those infected develop duodenal ulcer disease. Although individuals infected with the organism often have histological evidence of gastritis, the vast majority are asymptomatic. *H. pylori* infection is usually acquired during childhood, and atrophy of the gastric mucosa progresses during aging. Cross-sectional serological studies demonstrate increasing prevalence with increasing age. Low socio-economic status, especially in childhood, is associated with infection.

4. Reservoir—Mainly humans, though recently *H. pylori* has been found in other primates. Most infected persons are asymptomatic, and without treatment infection is often lifelong. Isolation of *H. pylori* from non-gastric sites such as oral secretions and stool has been reported, but is infrequent.

5. Mode of transmission—Not clearly established, but infection is almost certainly a result of ingesting organisms. Transmission is presumed to be either oral-oral and/or fecal-oral. There is some evidence that *H. pylori* may be transmitted through vomitus from an infected person, inadequately treated drinking water, and incompletely decontaminated gastroscopes and pH electrodes.

6. Incubation period—Data collected from two volunteers who ingested 10^6–10^9 organisms indicate that the onset of gastritis occurred within 5–10 days. No other information about inoculum size or incubation period is available.

7. Period of communicability—Not known. Since infection may be lifelong, those infected are potentially infectious for life. It is not known whether acutely infected patients are more infectious than those with long-standing infection. There is some evidence that persons with low stomach acidity may be more infectious.

8. Susceptibility—All individuals are presumed to be susceptible to infection. Although poor socio-economic conditions are an important risk factor for infection, there are scant data on individual susceptibility. A variety of cofactors may be required for the development of disease. No protective immunity is apparent after infection.

9. Methods of control—

A. *Preventive measures:*

1) Persons living in uncrowded, clean environments are less likely to acquire *H. pylori*.
2) Complete disinfection of gastroscopes, pH electrodes and other instruments entering the stomach.
3) Use of appropriately treated drinking water.

B. *Control of patient, contacts and the immediate environment:*

1) Report to local health authority: Official report not ordinarily justifiable, Class 5 (see *Reporting*).
2) Isolation: Not applicable.
3) Concurrent disinfection: Of intragastric instruments.
4) Quarantine: Not necessary.
5) Immunization of contacts: Prototype protein-based vaccines have shown promising results, but have not cleared infection and/or prevented reinfection.
6) Investigation of contacts and source of infection: Testing is recommended only if the intention is to treat. Patients with asymptomatic infection should not undergo testing.
7) Specific treatment: Treatment for asymptomatic infection remains controversial. There is a wide variety of treatment regimens available for eradicating infections in individuals with symptoms of disease attributable to *H. pylori*, such as gastritis, peptic ulcer disease, or MALT lymphoma. Regimens for first and second line treatment include: a) combinations of proton-pump inhibitor (PPI) drugs with clarithromycin and amoxicillin or metronidazole; or b) bismuth subsalicylate with tetracycline and metronidazole, each for one week (eradication rates may be higher with 2 week treatment courses; tetracycline cannot be used in children less than eight years of age). Cure rates of up to 90% have been reported with these regimens. Follow-up testing with a breath test or stool antigen test may be used to document eradication. Some patients may require an additional 2 week treatment course. If infection persists, isolates should be

checked for resistance to the antibiotics. Ulcers relapse in those patients in whom cure was not achieved. In industrialized countries, reinfection following cure is infrequent.

C. Epidemic measures: None.

D. Disaster implications: None

E. International measures: None.

GASTROENTERITIS, ACUTE VIRAL
[CCDM18 & 19: O. Fontaine]

ICD-9 008.6; ICD-10 A08

Viral gastroenteritis presents as an endemic or epidemic illness in infants, children and adults. Several viruses (rotaviruses, enteric adenoviruses, astroviruses and caliciviruses, including Norwalk-like viruses) infect children in their early years, causing a diarrheal illness that may be severe enough to produce dehydration. Viral agents such as Norwalk-like viruses are also common causes of epidemics of gastroenteritis among children and adults. The epidemiology, natural history and clinical expression of enteric viral infections are best understood for type A rotavirus in infants and Norwalk agent in adults.

I. ROTAVIRAL ENTERITIS ICD-9 008.61; ICD-10 A08.0
(Sporadic viral gastroenteritis, Severe viral gastroenteritis of infants and children)

1. Identification—A sporadic, seasonal, often severe gastroenteritis of infants and young children, characterized by vomiting, fever and watery diarrhea. Rotaviral enteritis is occasionally associated with severe dehydration and death in young children. Secondary symptomatic cases among adult family contacts can occur, although subclinical infections are more common. Rotavirus infection has occasionally been found in pediatric patients with a variety of other clinical manifestations, but the virus is probably coincidental rather than causative in these conditions. Rotavirus is a major cause of nosocomial diarrhea of newborns and infants. Although rotavirus diarrhea is generally more severe than acute diarrhea due to other agents, illness caused by rotavirus is not distinguishable from that caused by other enteric viruses for any individual patient.

EM, ELISA, LA and other immunological techniques for which commercial kits are available can identify rotavirus in stool specimens or rectal swabs. Evidence of rotavirus infection can be demonstrated by serological techniques, but diagnosis is usually based on the demonstration of rotavirus antigen in stools. False-positive ELISA reactions are common in newborns; positive reactions require confirmation by an alternative test.

2. Infectious agent—The 70-nanometer rotavirus belongs to the Reoviridae family. Group A is common; group B is uncommon in infants but has caused large epidemics in adults in China; and group C appears to be uncommon in humans. Groups A, B, C, D, E and F occur in animals. There are 4 major and at least 10 minor serotypes of group A human rotavirus, based on antigenic differences in the viral protein 7 (VP7) outer capsid surface protein, the major neutralization antigen. Another outer capsid protein, called VP4, is associated with virulence and also plays a role in virus neutralization.

3. Occurrence—In both industrialized and developing countries, rotavirus is associated with about one-third of hospitalized cases of diarrheal illness in infants and young children under 5. Neonatal rotaviral infections are frequent in certain settings but are usually asymptomatic. Essentially all children are infected by rotavirus in their first 2–3 years of life, with peak incidence of clinical disease in the 6- to 24-month age group. Outbreaks occur among children in day care settings. Rotavirus is more frequently associated with severe diarrhea than other enteric pathogens; in developing countries, it is responsible for an estimated 600 000–870 000 diarrheal deaths each year.

In temperate climates, rotavirus diarrhea occurs in seasonal peaks during cooler months; in tropical climates, cases occur throughout the year, often with a moderate peak in the cooler dry months. Infection of adults is usually subclinical, but outbreaks of clinical disease occur in geriatric units. Rotavirus occasionally causes travelers' diarrhea in adults and diarrhea in immunocompromised persons (including those with HIV infection), parents of children with rotavirus diarrhea, and the elderly.

4. Reservoir—Probably humans. The animal viruses do not produce disease in humans; group B and group C rotaviruses identified in humans appear to be quite distinct from those found in animals.

5. Mode of transmission—Probably fecal-oral with possible contact or respiratory spread. Although rotaviruses do not effectively multiply in the respiratory tract, they may be encountered in respiratory secretions. There is some evidence that rotavirus may be present in contaminated water.

6. Incubation period—Approximately 24–72 hours.

7. Period of communicability—During the acute stage, and later while virus shedding continues. Rotavirus is not usually detectable after about the eighth day of infection, although excretion of virus for 30 days or more has been reported in immunocompromised patients. Symptoms last for an average of 4–6 days.

8. Susceptibility—Susceptibility is greatest between 6 and 24 months of age. By age 3, most children have acquired rotavirus antibodies. Diarrhea is uncommon in infected infants under 3 months. Immunocompromised individuals are at particular risk for prolonged rotavirus antigen excretion and intermittent rotavirus diarrhea.

9. Methods of control—

A. Preventive measures

1) Regulatory authorities recognized by the World Health Organization (WHO) have licensed two new vaccines against rotavirus in 2006: Rotarix® (licensed in the USA in 2008) and Rota Teq®. Clinical trials in Europe, Latin America and the US demonstrated their safety and efficacy towards preventing rotavirus-associated severe gastroenteritis.

   In early 2007, WHO granted prequalification to Rotarix® and Rota Teq® is under review at time of writing in early 2008. Preliminary vaccine usage data during recent rotavirus seasons in the developed world suggests promising results for long-term protection.

2) The effectiveness of other preventive measures is undetermined. Hygienic measures applicable to diseases transmitted via the fecal-oral route may not be effective in preventing transmission. The virus survives for long periods on hard surfaces, in contaminated water and on hands. It is relatively resistant to some commonly used disinfectants, but is inactivated by chlorine.

3) In day care, dressing infants with overalls to cover diapers has been demonstrated to decrease transmission of the infection.

4) Prevent exposure of infants and young children to individuals with acute gastroenteritis in family and institutional (day care or hospital) settings by maintaining a high level of sanitary practices; exclusion from day care centers is not necessary.

5) Passive immunization by oral administration of IG has been shown to protect low birthweight neonates and immunocompromised children. Breastfeeding does not affect infection rates, but may reduce the severity of the gastroenteritis.

B. Control of patient, contacts and the immediate environment:

1) Report to local health authority: Obligatory report of epidemics in some countries; no individual case report, Class 4 (see *Reporting*).

2) Isolation: Enteric precautions, with frequent handwashing by caretakers of infants.

3) Concurrent disinfection: Sanitary disposal of diapers; place overalls over diapers to prevent leakage.
4) Quarantine: Not applicable.
5) Immunization of contacts: Not applicable.
6) Investigation of contacts and source of infection: Sources of infection should be sought in certain high-risk populations and antigen excretors.
7) Specific treatment: None. Oral rehydration therapy with oral glucose-electrolyte solution is adequate in most cases. Parenteral fluids are needed in cases with vascular collapse or uncontrolled vomiting (see *Cholera*, 9B7). In children aged less than five, give 20 mg elemental zinc per day for 10 to 14 days. Antibiotics and anti-motility drugs are contraindicated.

C. *Epidemic measures:* Search for vehicles of transmission and source on epidemiological bases.

D. *Disaster implications:* A potential problem with dislocated populations.

E. *International measures:* WHO Collaborating Centers provide support as required. More information can be found at:

<http://www.who.int/collaboratingcentres/database/en/>

II. EPIDEMIC VIRAL GASTROENTEROPATHY
ICD-9 008.6, 008.8;
ICD-10 A08.1

(Norwalk agent disease, Norwalk-like disease, Viral gastroenteritis in adults, Epidemic viral gastroenteritis, Acute infectious nonbacterial gastroenteritis, Viral diarrhea, Epidemic diarrhea and vomiting, Winter vomiting disease, Epidemic nausea and vomiting)

1. Identification—Usually a self-limited, mild to moderate disease that often occurs in outbreaks, with clinical symptoms of nausea, vomiting, diarrhea, abdominal pain, myalgia, headache, malaise, low grade fever or a combination of these symptoms. GI symptoms characteristically last 24–48 hours.

The virus may be identified in stools through direct or immune EM or, for the Norwalk virus, through RIA or reverse transcription polymerase chain reaction (RT-PCR). Serological evidence of infection may be demonstrated by IEM or, for the Norwalk virus, by RIA. Diagnosis requires collection of a large volume of stools, with aliquots stored at 4°C (39°F) for EM, and at 20°C (4°F) for antigen assays. Acute and convalescent sera (3–4-week interval) are essential to link particles observed by EM with disease etiology. RT-PCR seems to be more sensitive than IEM, and can be used to examine links among widely scattered clusters of disease.

2. Infectious agents—Norwalk-like viruses are small (27–32-nanometers), structured RNA viruses classified as caliciviruses; they have been implicated as on of the most common causal agents of nonbacterial gastroenteritis outbreaks. Several morphologically similar but antigenically distinct viruses have been associated with gastroenteritis outbreaks; these include Hawaii, Taunton, Ditchling or W, Cockle, Parramatta, Oklahoma and Snow Mountain agents.

3. Occurrence—Worldwide and common; most often in outbreaks but also sporadically; all age groups are affected. Outbreaks in industrialized countries are usually associated with consumption of raw shellfish. In one study in the USA, antibodies to Norwalk agent were acquired slowly; by the fifth decade of life, more than 60% of the population had antibodies. In most developing countries studied, antibodies are acquired much earlier. Seroresponse to Norwalk virus has been widely detected in infants and young children from Bangladesh and Finland.

4. Reservoir—Humans are the only known reservoir.

5. Mode of transmission—Probably by the fecal-oral route, although contact or airborne transmission from fomites has been suggested to explain rapid spread in hospital settings. Several recent outbreaks have strongly suggested primary community foodborne, waterborne and shellfish transmission, with secondary transmission to family members.

6. Incubation period—Usually 24–48 hours; in volunteer studies with Norwalk agent, the range was 10–50 hours.

7. Period of communicability—During acute stage of disease and up to 48 hours after Norwalk diarrhea stops.

8. Susceptibility and resistance—Susceptibility is widespread. Short-term immunity lasting up to 14 weeks has been demonstrated in volunteers after induced Norwalk illness, but long-term immunity was variable; some individuals became ill on rechallenge 27–42 months later. Levels of pre-existing serum antibody to Norwalk virus did not correlate with susceptibility or resistance.

9. Methods of control—

A. Preventive measures: Use hygienic measures applicable to diseases transmitted via fecal-oral route (see *Typhoid fever*, 9A). In particular, cooking shellfish and surveillance of shellfish breeding waters can prevent infection from that source.

B. Control of patient, contacts and the immediate environment:

1) Report to local health authority: Obligatory report of epidemics in some countries; no individual case report, Class 4 (see *Reporting*).

2) Isolation: Enteric precautions.
3) Concurrent disinfection: Not applicable.
4) Quarantine: Not applicable.
5) Immunization of contacts: Not applicable.
6) Investigation of contacts and source of infection: Search for means of spread of infection in outbreak situations.
7) Specific treatment: Fluid and electrolyte replacement in severe cases (see *Cholera*, 9B7). In children aged less than five, give 20 mg elemental zinc per day for 10 to 14 days.

C. Epidemic measures: Search for vehicles of transmission and source; determine course of outbreak to define epidemiology.

D. Disaster implications: Large-scale outbreaks could be a potential problem in any disaster where water supplies or food preparation do not meet accepted hygiene standards.

E. International measures: None.

GIARDIASIS · ICD-9 007.1; ICD-10 A07.1
(*Giardia* enteritis)
[CCDM19: M. Eberhard, A. Gabrielli, L.Savioli]
[CCDM18: A. Montresor]

1. Identification—A protozoan infection, principally of the upper small intestine; it can a) remain asymptomatic; b) bring on acute, self-limited diarrhea; c) lead to intestinal symptoms such as chronic diarrhea; steatorrhea; abdominal cramps; bloating; frequent loose and pale greasy stools; fatigue; malabsorption (of fats and fat-soluble vitamins); and weight loss. There is usually no extraintestinal invasion, but reactive arthritis and, in severe giardiasis, damage to duodenal and jejunal mucosal cells may occur.

Diagnosis is traditionally made through identification of cysts or trophozoites in feces (to rule out the diagnosis at least 3 negative results are needed). Because *Giardia* infection is often asymptomatic, the presence of *G. lamblia* (in stool or duodenum) does not necessarily indicate that *Giardia* is the cause of illness. Tests using ELISA or direct fluorescent antibody methods to detect antigens in the stool, generally more sensitive than direct microscopy, are commercially available. Where results of stool examination and antigen assays are questionable, it may be useful to examine for trophozoites from duodenal fluid (aspiration or string test) or mucosa obtained by small intestine biopsy.

2. Infectious agent—*Giardia lamblia* (*G. intestinalis*, *G. duodenalis*), a flagellate protozoan.

3. Occurrence—Worldwide. Children are infected more frequently than adults. Prevalence is higher in areas of poor sanitation and in institutions with children not toilet-trained, including day care centers. The prevalence of stool positivity in different areas may range between 1% and 30%, depending on the community and age group surveyed. Endemic infection in Mexico, the UK and the USA most commonly occurs in July–October among children under 5 and adults aged 25–39. It is associated with drinking water from unfiltered surface water sources or shallow wells, swimming in bodies of freshwater, and having a young family member in day care. Large community outbreaks have occurred from drinking treated but unfiltered water. Smaller outbreaks have resulted from contaminated food, person-to-person transmission in day care centers, and contaminated recreational waters (including swimming and wading pools).

4. Reservoir—Humans; possibly beaver and other wild and domestic animals.

5. Mode of transmission—Person-to-person transmission occurs by hand-to-mouth transfer of cysts from the feces of an infected individual, especially in institutions and day care centers; this is probably the principal mode of spread. Anal intercourse also facilitates transmission. Localized outbreaks may occur from ingestion of cysts in fecally contaminated drinking and recreational water more often than from fecally contaminated food. Concentrations of chlorine used in routine water treatment do not kill *Giardia* cysts, especially when the water is cold; unfiltered stream and lake waters open to contamination by human and animal feces are a source of infection.

6. Incubation period—Usually 3–25 days or longer; median 7–10 days.

7. Period of communicability—Entire period of infection, often months.

8. Susceptibility—Asymptomatic carrier rate is high; infection is frequently self-limited. Pathogenicity of *G. lamblia* for humans has been established by clinical studies. Persons with HIV infection may have more serious and prolonged giardiasis.

9. Methods of control—

    A. Preventive measures:

        1) Educate families, personnel and inmates of institutions—and especially adult personnel of day care centers—in personal hygiene and the need for washing hands before handling food, before eating, and after toilet use.

        2) Filter public water supplies exposed to human or animal fecal contamination.

3) Protect public water supplies against contamination with human and animal feces.

4) Dispose of feces in a sanitary manner.

5) Boil emergency water supplies. Chemical treatment with hypochlorite or iodine is less reliable; use 0.1 to 0.2 ml (2 to 4 drops) of household bleach or 0.5 ml of 2% tincture of iodine per liter for 20 minutes (longer if water is cold or turbid).

B. Control of patient, contacts and the immediate environment:

1) Report to local health authority: Case report in selected areas, Class 3 (see *Reporting*).

2) Isolation: Enteric precautions.

3) Concurrent disinfection: Of feces and articles soiled therewith. In communities with a modern and adequate sewage disposal system, feces can be discharged directly into sewers without preliminary disinfection. Terminal cleaning.

4) Quarantine: Not applicable.

5) Immunization of contacts: Not applicable.

6) Investigation of contacts and source of infection: Microscopic examination of feces of household members and other suspected contacts, especially if symptomatic.

7) Specific treatment: Metronidazole or tinidazole are the drugs of choice: metronidazole one daily dose of 2 grams for 3 days (children 15 mg/kg daily in divided doses for 5–10 days), or tinidazole 2 grams in a single dose (children 50–75 mg/kg). Nitazoxanide may be effective; paromomycin, furazolidone or quinacrine are alternatives. Furazolidone is available in pediatric suspension for young children and infants (2 mg/kg 3 times daily for 7–10 days). Paromomycin can be used during pregnancy, but when disease is mild, delay of treatment until after delivery is recommended. Drug resistance and relapses may occur with any drug.

C. Epidemic measures: Institute an epidemiological investigation of clustered cases in an area or institution to determine source of infection and mode of transmission. A common vehicle, such as water, food or association with a day care center or recreational area must be sought; institute applicable preventive or control measures. Control of person-to-person transmission requires special emphasis on personal cleanliness and sanitary disposal of feces.

D. Disaster implications: None.

E. International measures: None.

GONOCOCCAL INFECTIONS   ICD-9 098; ICD-10 A54
[CCDM19: L. Newman]
[CCDM18: S. Resnikoff]

Urethritis, epididymitis, proctitis, cervicitis, Bartholinitis, pelvic inflammatory disease (salpingitis and/or endometritis) and pharyngitis of adults; vulvaginitis of children; and conjunctivitis of the newborn and adults are localized inflammatory conditions caused by *Neisseria gonorrhoeae*. Gonococcal bacteremia can result in the arthritis-dermatitis syndrome, occasionally associated with endocarditis or meningitis. Other complications include perihepatitis and neonatal sepsis. Infection with gonorrhea increases risk of both acquisition and transmission of HIV infection.

Clinically similar infections of the same genital structures may be caused by *Chlamydia trachomatis* and other infectious agents. Simultaneous infections are not uncommon.

I. GONOCOCCAL INFECTION   ICD-9 098.0-098.3; ICD-10 A54.0-A54.2

(Gonorrhea, Gonococcal urethritis, Gonococcal vulvovaginitis, Gonococcal cervicitis, Gonococcal Bartholinitis, Clap, Strain, Gleet, Dose, GC)

1. Identification—A sexually transmitted bacterial disease limited to columnar and transitional epithelium, which differs in males and females in course, severity and ease of recognition. In males, gonococcal infection generally presents as an acute purulent discharge from the anterior urethra with dysuria within 2–7 days after exposure. Urethritis can be documented by a) the presence of mucopurulent or purulent discharge and b) Gram stain of urethral discharge showing 5 or more WBC per oil immersion field. The Gram stain is highly sensitive and specific for documenting urethritis and the presence of gonococcal infection in symptomatic males. A small percentage of gonococcal infections in males are asymptomatic.

In females, infection is followed by the development of mucopurulent cervicitis (MPC), often asymptomatic, although some women have abnormal vaginal discharge and vaginal bleeding after intercourse. In about 20% there is also uterine invasion, often timed with menstruation, with resultant endometritis, salpingitis or pelvic peritonitis and subsequent risk of infertility and ectopic pregnancy. Prepubescent girls may develop gonococcal vulvovaginitis through direct genital contact with exudate from infected people during sexual abuse.

In females and homosexual males, pharyngeal and anorectal infections are not uncommon. While infection of the pharynx and rectum often are asymptomatic, anorectal infections may cause pruritus, tenesmus and discharge. Conjunctivitis occurs in newborns and rarely in adults, with resultant blindness if not rapidly and adequately treated. Septicemia (also known as disseminated gonococcal infection, or DGI) may occur in

0.5%–1% of all gonococcal infections, and can result in arthritis, skin lesions and (rarely) endocarditis and meningitis. Arthritis can produce permanent joint damage if appropriate antibiotherapy is delayed. Death is rare except among persons with endocarditis or underlying health conditions such as complement deficiency.

Nongonococcal urethritis (NGU) and MPC are caused by other sexually transmitted agents and seriously complicate the clinical diagnosis of gonorrhea; the organisms that cause these diseases often coexist with gonococcal infections. In many populations, the incidence of NGU exceeds that of gonorrhea. *Chlamydia trachomatis* (see *Chlamydial infections*) causes about 30%–40% of NGU in most industrialized countries.

Diagnosis of gonococcal infection is made by Gram stain of discharge, bacteriological culture on selective media (e.g. modified Thayer-Martin agar), or tests that detect gonococcal nucleic acid. Typical Gram-negative intracellular diplococci can be considered diagnostic in male urethral smears; they are nearly diagnostic when seen in cervical smears (specificity 90%–97%), but are not considered sufficiently sensitive in women to reliably rule out infection. Cultures on selective media, plus presumptive identification based on both macroscopic and microscopic examination and biochemical testing, are sensitive and specific, as are nucleic acid detection tests. In cases with potential legal implications, specimens should be cultured and isolates confirmed as *N. gonorrhoeae* by at least 2 different methods.

2. Infectious agent—*Neisseria gonorrhoeae*, the gonococcus.

3. Occurrence—Worldwide, the disease affects both men and women, especially sexually active adolescents and younger adults. Prevalence is highest in communities of lower socioeconomic status. In most industrialized countries, incidence has decreased for over 20 years, but in recent years incidence has reached a plateau and is still at unacceptably high levels in many countries. New infections tend to be concentrated in population subgroups at increased risk, such as men who have sex with men and minority racial and ethnic groups.

N. gonorrhoeae readily develops resistance to common antimicrobials, either through chromosomal mutations or acquisition of plasmids. Resistance to penicillin and tetracycline is widespread. Quinolone-resistant *N. gonorrhoeae* (QRNG) continues to spread, and has become common in parts of Europe, Asia, Central Asia, the South Pacific, and North America. For many regions there are inadequate susceptibility data available. Resistance to azithromycin and spectinomycin has been documented in many countries, but is rarely greater than 5% of tested isolates. Although clinical failure to recommended cephalosporins has not been documented, reports from Asia, Europe, North America, and the Western Pacific have identified strains with decreased susceptibility to cephalosporins.

4. Reservoir—Strictly a human disease.

5. Mode of transmission—Contact with exudates from mucous membranes of infected people, almost always as a result of sexual activity. Can be transmitted perinatally. In children over 1 year, it is considered an indicator of sexual abuse.

6. Incubation period—Generally 1–14 days; can be longer.

7. Period of communicability—May extend for months in untreated individuals. Effective treatment ends communicability within hours.

8. Susceptibility—Susceptibility is general. Humoral and secretory antibodies have been demonstrated, but gonococcal strains are antigenically heterogeneous and re-infection is common. Individuals deficient in complement components are uniquely susceptible to bacteremia. In women, use of hormonal contraception may increase the risk of acquiring gonorrhea, and use of the diaphragm has a protective influence. Only columnar and transitional epithelium is susceptible to the gonococcus. Transmission by fomites is extremely rare.

9. Methods of control—

A. *Preventive measures:*

1) Same as for syphilis (see *Syphilis*, 9A), except for measures that apply specifically to gonorrhea—i.e. the use of prophylactic agents in the eyes of the newborn (see section II, 9A2), and special attention (presumptive treatment) to contacts of infected patients (see 9B6).
2) Prevention is based primarily on safer sexual practices; i.e. consistent and correct use of condoms with all partners not known to be infection-free, avoiding multiple sexual encounters or anonymous/casual sex, and mutual monogamy with a noninfected partner.

B. *Control of patient, contacts and the immediate environment:*

1) Report to local health authority: Case report is required in many countries, Class 2 (see *Reporting*).
2) Isolation: Contact isolation for all newborn infants and prepubertal children with gonococcal infection, until effective parenteral antimicrobial therapy has been administered for 24 hours. Effective antibiotics in adequate dosage promptly render discharges noninfectious. Patients should refrain from sexual intercourse until antimicrobial therapy is completed, and, to avoid re-infection, abstain from sex with previous sexual partners until these have been treated.
3) Concurrent disinfection: Care in disposal of discharges from lesions and contaminated articles.
4) Quarantine: Not applicable.

5) Immunization of contacts: Not applicable.

6) Investigation of contacts and source of infection: Interview patients and notify sexual partners. With uncooperative patients, trained interviewers obtain the best results, but clinicians can motivate most patients to help arrange treatment for their partners. Sexual contacts of cases should be examined, tested and treated if their last sexual contact with the case was within 60 days before the onset of symptoms or diagnosis in the case. Even outside these time limits the most recent sexual partner should be examined, tested and treated. All infants born to infected mothers must receive prophylactic treatment.

7) Specific treatment: On clinical, laboratory or epidemiological grounds (contacts of a diagnosed case), adequate treatment must be given as follows:

For uncomplicated gonococcal infections of the cervix, rectum and urethra in adults, recommended treatments include ceftriaxone IM (125 mg single dose) and cefixime PO (400 mg single dose). Quinolones— ciprofloxacin PO (500 mg single dose), ofloxacin PO (400 mg single dose) or levofloxacin PO (250 mg single dose)—should not be used in any area where the prevalence of quinolone resistance is >5%. Patients who can take neither cephalosporins nor quinolones may be treated with spectinomycin IM (2 grams single dose), but spectinomycin has poor efficacy in eradicating infections of the pharynx. If chlamydial infection is not ruled out, patients infected with *N. gonorrhoeae* must also be treated orally with azithromycin (1 gram single dose) or doxycyline (100 mg twice daily for 7 days)—though doxycyline cannot be used in children less than eight years of age.

Providing patients under treatment for gonorrhea with a treatment effective against genital chlamydial infection is recommended routinely because chlamydial infection is common among patients diagnosed with gonorrhea. This may also inhibit the emergence of antimicrobial-resistant gonococci.

Gonococcal infections of the pharynx are more difficult to eliminate than infections of the urethra, cervix or rectum. Recommended regimens for this infection include ceftriaxone IM (125 mg single dose), or ciprofloxacin PO (500 mg single dose) in areas without widespread QRNG.

Treatment failure following any of the anti-gonococcal regimens listed above is rare, and routine culture as a test of cure is unnecessary. If symptoms persist, re-infection is most likely, but specimens should be obtained for culture and antimicrobial susceptibility testing to rule out treatment failure. Retesting of high-risk patients after 3 months is advisable to detect asymptomatic infections. Patients with gonococcal infections are at increased risk of HIV infection and should be offered confidential counseling and testing.

C. *Epidemic measures:* Intensify routine procedures, especially treatment of contacts on epidemiological grounds.

D. *Disaster implications:* None.

E. *International measures:* See *Syphilis*, 9E.

II. GONOCOCCAL CONJUNCTIVITIS (NEONATORUM)   ICD-9 098.4; ICD-10 A54.3
(Gonorrheal ophthalmia neonatorum, Gonococcal neonatal ophthalmia)

1. Identification—Acute redness and swelling of conjunctiva in one or both eyes, with mucopurulent or purulent discharge, typically occurring within 1–5 days of birth. Gonococci may be identified by microscopic or culture methods. Corneal ulcer, perforation and blindness may occur if antimicrobial treatment is not given promptly.

Gonococcal ophthalmia neonatorum is only one of several acute inflammatory conditions of the eye or the conjunctiva occurring within the first 3 weeks of life, collectively known as ophthalmia neonatorum. The gonococcus is the most serious, but not the most frequent, infectious cause of ophthalmia neonatorum. The most common infectious cause is *Chlamydia trachomatis*, which produces inclusion conjunctivitis that tends to be less acute than gonococcal conjunctivitis and usually appears 5–14 days after birth (see *Conjunctivitis, chlamydial*). Any purulent neonatal conjunctivitis should be considered gonococcal until proven otherwise.

2. Infectious agent—*Neisseria gonorrheae*, the gonococcus.

3. Occurrence—Varies widely according to prevalence of maternal infection, prenatal screening coverage, and use of infant eye prophylaxis at delivery; it is infrequent where infant eye prophylaxis is adequate. The disease continues to be an important cause of blindness throughout the world. Ocular prophylaxis of all infants at birth is warranted because it can prevent sight-threatening gonococcal ophthalmia, and because it is safe, easy to administer, and inexpensive.

4. Reservoir—Infection of the maternal cervix.

5. Mode of transmission—Contact with the infected birth canal during childbirth.

6. **Incubation period**—Usually 1-5 days.

7. **Period of communicability**—While discharge persists if untreated; for 24 hours following initiation of specific treatment.

8. **Susceptibility and resistance**—Susceptibility is general.

9. **Methods of control**—

A. Preventive measures:

1) Prevent maternal infection (see section I, 9A and *Syphilis*, 9A). Diagnose gonorrhea in pregnant women and treat the woman and her sexual partners. Routine culture of the cervix and rectum for gonococci should be considered prenatally, especially in the third trimester in populations where infection is prevalent.

2) Use an established effective preparation for protection of babies' eyes within one hour of birth, regardless of whether they are delivered vaginally or by cesarean section. Erythromycin (0.5%) and tetracycline (1%) ophthalmic ointments are both effective options. Instillation of 1% silver nitrate aqueous solution is also effective and widely used, but may be associated with an increased risk of chemical irritation. Prophylaxis with 2.5% ophthalmic solution of povidone-iodine has not yet been studied adequately. Single use tubes or ampoules are preferable to multiple-use tubes.

3) Infants born to mothers who have untreated gonorrhea are at high risk for infection. The recommended regimen for such infants in the absence of signs of gonococcal infection is a single dose of ceftriaxone 25-50 mg/kg (not to exceed 125 mg) IV or IM.

B. Control of patient, contacts and the immediate environment:

1) Report to local health authority: Case report is required in many countries, Class 2 (see *Reporting*).

2) Isolation: Contact isolation for the first 24 hours after administration of effective therapy. Hospitalize patients if possible. Bacterial cure after therapy should be confirmed by culture.

3) Concurrent disinfection: Care in disposal of conjunctival discharges and contaminated articles.

4) Quarantine: Not applicable.

5) Immunization of contacts: Not applicable; prompt treatment on diagnosis or clinical suspicion of infection.

6) Investigation of contacts and source of infection: Examination and treatment of mothers and their sexual partners.

7) Specific treatment: A single dose of ceftriaxone, 25-50 mg/kg (not to exceed 125 mg) IV or IM, is recommended for the

treatment of uncomplicated ophthalmia neonatorum. Mother and infant should also be treated for chlamydial infection. Infants who have gonococcal ophthalmia should be hospitalized and evaluated for signs of disseminated infection (e.g. sepsis, arthritis, and meningitis). Treatment of disseminated gonococcal infection in the newborn should be with ceftriaxone 25–50 mg/kg (not to exceed 125 mg) IV or IM in a single daily dose for 7 days, with a duration of 10–14 days if meningitis is documented, **OR** cefotaxime 25 mg/kg IV or IM every 12 hours for 7 days, with a duration of 10–14 days, if meningitis is documented.

C. Epidemic measures: None.

D. Disaster implications: None.

E. International measures: None.

GRANULOMA INGUINALE   ICD-9 099.2; ICD-10 A.58
(Donovanosis)
[CCDM18 & 19: F. Ndowa]

1. Identification—A chronic and progressively destructive, but poorly communicable bacterial disease of the skin and mucous membranes of the external genitalia, inguinal and anal regions. One or more indurated nodules or papules lead to a slowly spreading, nontender, exuberant, granulomatous, ulcerative or cicatricial lesions. The lesions are characteristically non-friable, beefy red granulomas that extend peripherally with characteristic rolled edges and eventually form fibrous tissue. Lesions occur most commonly in warm, moist surfaces such as the folds between the thighs, the perianal area, the scrotum, or the vulvar labia and vagina. The genitalia are involved in close to 90% of cases, the inguinal region in close to 10%, the anal region in 5%–10% and distant sites in 1%–5%. If neglected, the process may result in extensive destruction of genital organs and may spread by autoinoculation to other parts of the body. Laboratory diagnosis is based on demonstration of intracytoplasmic rod-shaped organisms (Donovan bodies) in Wright- or Giemsa-stained smears of granulation tissue, or on histological examination of biopsy specimens; the presence of large infected mononuclear cells filled with deeply staining Donovan bodies is pathognomonic. Culture is difficult and unreliable. Serological tests are not useful for confirmation of diagnosis and use of the polymerase chain reaction (PCR) remains a research tool; further validation studies of these nucleic acid amplification tests are needed. *Haemophilus ducreyi* should be excluded by culture on appropriate selective media.

2. Infectious agent—The causal agent is *Klebsiella granulomatis* (*Donovania granulomatis*, *Calymmatobacterium granulomatis*), a Gram-negative bacillus.

3. Occurrence—Rare in industrialized countries, but cluster outbreaks occasionally occur. Endemic in tropical and subtropical areas, such as central and northern Australia, southern India, Papua New Guinea, and Viet Nam; occasionally in Latin America, the Caribbean islands and central, eastern and southern Africa. It is more frequently seen among males than females and among people of lower socioeconomic status; it may occur in children aged 1–4 years but is predominantly seen at ages 20–40.

4. Reservoir—Humans.

5. Mode of transmission—Presumably by direct contact with lesions during sexual activity, but in various studies only 20%–65% of sexual partners were infected, thus not quite fulfilling the criteria for sexual transmission. Donovanosis occurs in sexually inactive individuals and the very young, suggesting that some cases are transmitted non-sexually.

6. Incubation period—Unknown; probably between 1 and 16 weeks.

7. Period of communicability—Unknown; probably for the duration of open lesions on the skin or mucous membranes.

8. Susceptibility and resistance—Susceptibility is variable; immunity apparently does not follow attack.

9. Methods of control—

A. *Preventive measures:* Preventive measures are the same as those for *Syphilis*, 9A, with the exception of those measures applicable only to syphilis. Educational programs in endemic areas should stress the importance of early diagnosis and treatment.

B. *Control of patient, contacts and the immediate environment:*

1) Report to local health authority: A reportable disease in most states and countries, Class 3 (see *Reporting*).
2) Isolation: Avoid close personal contact until lesions are healed.
3) Concurrent disinfection: Care in disposal of discharges from lesions and articles soiled therewith.
4) Quarantine: Not applicable.
5) Immunization of contacts: Not applicable; prompt treatment upon recognition or clinical suspicion of infection.

6) Investigation of contacts and source of infection: Examination of sexual contacts.

7) Specific treatment: Azithromycin is effective and its long tissue half-life allows a flexible dosing regimen and short course treatment. Erythromycin, trimethoprim-sulfamethoxazole and doxycycline have been reported to be effective but drug-resistant strains of the organism occur (and doxycycline cannot be used in children less than eight years of age). Treatment is continued for 3 weeks or until the lesions have resolved; recurrence is not rare but usually responds to a repeat course unless malignancy is present. Single-dose treatment with ceftriaxone IM or ciprofloxacin PO is anecdotally reported to be effective.

C. Epidemic measures: Not applicable.

D. Disaster implications: None.

E. International measures: See *Syphilis,* 9E.

HANTAVIRAL DISEASES
[CCDM19: J. Mackenzie]
[CCDM18: J. Mackenzie, A. Plant]

Hantaviruses infect rodents worldwide. Several species are known to infect humans, with varying severity. Primary impact effect is on the vascular endothelium, resulting in increased vascular permeability, hypotensive shock and hemorrhagic manifestations. Many of these agents have been isolated from rodents but are not associated with human cases. In 1993, an outbreak of disease caused by a previously unrecognized hantavirus occurred in the USA; the principal target organ was not the kidney (the usual target organ in human hantaviral infections), but the lung. Because they are caused by related organisms and have similar features of epidemiology and pathology (febrile prodrome, thrombocytopenia, leukocytosis and capillary leakage), both the renal and the pulmonary syndrome are presented under hantaviral diseases.

I. HEMORRHAGIC FEVER WITH
 RENAL SYNDROME   ICD-9 078.6; ICD-10 A98.5
(Epidemic hemorrhagic fever, Korean hemorrhagic fever,
Nephropathia epidemica, Hemorrhagic nephrosonephritis, HFRS)

1. Identification—Acute zoonotic viral disease with abrupt onset of fever, lower back pain, varying degrees of hemorrhagic manifestations, and renal involvement. Severe illness is associated with Hantaan (primarily in Asia) and Dobrava viruses (in the Balkans). Disease is characterized by 5 clinical phases that frequently overlap:

a) Febrile
b) Hypotensive
c) Oliguric
d) Diuretic
e) Convalescent.

The febrile phase, which lasts 3–7 days, is characterized by high fever, headache, malaise and anorexia, followed by severe abdominal or lower back pain, often accompanied by nausea and vomiting, facial flushing, petechiae and conjunctival injection. The hypotensive phase lasts from several hours to 3 days and is characterized by defervescence and abrupt onset of hypotension, which may progress to shock and more apparent hemorrhagic manifestations. Blood pressure returns to normal or is high in the oliguric phase (3–7 days); nausea and vomiting may persist, severe hemorrhage may occur and urinary output falls dramatically.

The case-fatality rate ranges from 5% to 15%, and the majority of deaths occur during the hypotensive and oliguric phases. Diuresis heralds the onset of recovery in most cases, with polyuria of 3–6 liters per day. Convalescence takes weeks to months.

A less severe illness (case-fatality rate 1%) caused by Puumala virus, and referred to as nephropathia epidemica, is predominant in Europe. Infections caused by Seoul virus, carried by brown or Norway rats, are clinically milder, although severe disease may occur with this strain. They show less clear distinction between clinical phases.

Diagnosis is through demonstration of specific antibodies using ELISA or IFA; most patients have IgM antibodies at the time of hospitalization. The presence of proteinuria, leukocytosis, hemoconcentration, thrombocytopenia and elevated blood urea nitrogen supports diagnosis. Hantaviruses can be propagated in a limited range of cell cultures and laboratory rats and mice, mainly for research purposes. Leptospirosis and rickettsioses must be considered in differential diagnosis.

2. Infectious agent—Hantaviruses (a genus of the family Bunyaviridae, the only genus without an arthropod vector); 3-segmented RNA viruses with spherical to oval particles, 95–110 nanometers in diameter. More than 25 antigenically distinguishable viral species exist, each associated primarily with a single rodent species. Seoul virus is found worldwide; Puumala virus in Europe; Hantaan virus principally in Asia, and less often in Europe; and Dobrava (Belgrade) virus in Serbia and Montenegro.

3. Occurrence—Prior to World War II, Japanese and Soviet authors described the disease in Manchuria along the Amur River. In 1951, it was recognized among United Nations troops in Asia and later in both military personnel and civilians—the virus was first isolated from a field rodent (*Apodemus agrarius*) in 1977 near the Hantaan River. The disease is considered a major public health problem in China and the Republic of Korea. Occurrence is seasonal, with most cases occurring in late autumn and early winter, primarily among rural populations. In the Balkans, a severe form of the disease due to Dobrava virus affects a few hundred people annually, with fatality rates at least as high as those in Asia (5%-15%). Most cases there are seen during spring and early summer.

Nephropathia epidemica, due to Puumala virus, is found in most of Europe, including the Balkans and Russia west of the Ural Mountains. It is often seen in summer and in the autumn and early winter. Seasonal occupational and recreational activities probably influence the risk of exposure, as do climate and other ecological factors of rodent population densities. Among medical research personnel and animal handlers in Asia and Europe, the disease has been traced to laboratory rats infected with Seoul virus, which has been identified in captured urban rats worldwide, including in Argentina, Brazil, Thailand and the USA; only in Asia has it been regularly associated with human disease. The availability of newer diagnostic techniques has led to increasing recognition of hantaviruses and hantaviral infections.

4. Reservoir—Field rodents (*Apodemus* spp. for Hantaan and Dobrava-Belgrade viruses in Asia and the Balkans; *Clethrionomys* spp. for Puumala in Europe; *Rattus* spp. for Seoul virus worldwide). Humans are accidental hosts.

5. Mode of transmission—Presumed aerosol transmission from rodent excreta (aerosol infectivity has been demonstrated experimentally), though this may not explain all human cases or all forms of inter-rodent transmission. Virus occurs in urine, feces and saliva of persistently infected asymptomatic rodents, with maximal virus concentration in the lungs. Nosocomial transmission of hantaviruses has been documented, but is believed rare.

6. Incubation period—From a few days to nearly 2 months, usually 2-4 weeks.

7. Period of communicability—Not well defined. Person-to-person transmission is rare.

8. Susceptibility—Persons without serological evidence of past infection appear to be uniformly susceptible. Unapparent infections occur; second attacks have not been documented.

9. Methods of control—

  A. Preventive measures:

    1) Exclude rodents from, and prevent rodent access to, houses and other buildings.

2) Store human and animal food in rodent-proof conditions.
3) Disinfect rodent-contaminated areas by spraying a disinfectant solution (e.g. diluted bleach) prior to cleaning. Do not sweep or vacuum rat-contaminated areas; use a wet mop or towels moistened with disinfectant. As far as possible, avoid inhalation of dust by using approved respirators when cleaning previously unoccupied areas.
4) Trap rodents and dispose of them using suitable precautions. Live trapping is not recommended.
5) In enzootic areas, minimize exposure to wild rodents and their excreta.
6) Laboratory rodent colonies, particularly *Rattus norvegicus*, must be tested to ensure freedom from asymptomatic hantavirus infection.

B. Control of patient, contacts and the immediate environment:

1) Report to local health authority: In endemic countries where reporting is required, Class 3 (see *Reporting*).
2) Isolation: Not applicable.
3) Concurrent disinfection: Not applicable.
4) Quarantine: Not applicable.
5) Immunization of contacts: Not applicable.
6) Investigate contacts and source of infection: Exterminate rodents in and around households where feasible.
7) Specific treatment: Bed rest and early hospitalization are critical. Jostling and the effect of lowered atmospheric pressures during airborne evacuation of cases can be deleterious to patients critically ill with hantavirus. Careful attention to fluid management is important in order to avoid overload and minimize the effects of shock and renal failure. Dialysis is often required. Administering ribavirin IV as early as possible during the first few days of illness has shown benefit.

C. Epidemic measures: Rodent control; surveillance for hantavirus infections in wild rodents. Laboratory-associated outbreaks call for evaluation of the associated rodents and, if positive, elimination of the rodents and thorough disinfection.

D. Disaster implications: Natural disasters and wars often result in increased numbers of rodents and rodent contact with humans.

E. International measures: Control transport of exotic reservoir rodents.

II. HANTAVIRUS PULMONARY SYNDROME ICD-9 480.8; ICD-10 B33.4
(Hantavirus adult respiratory distress syndrome, Hantavirus cardiopulmonary syndrome)

1. Identification—An acute zoonotic viral disease characterized by fever, myalgias and GI complaints, followed by the abrupt onset of respiratory distress and hypotension. The illness progresses rapidly to severe respiratory failure and shock. Most cases show an elevated hematocrit, hypoalbuminemia and thrombocytopenia. The fatality rate can be as high as 35-50%. In survivors, recovery from acute illness is rapid, but full convalescence may require weeks to months. Restoration of normal lung function generally occurs, but pulmonary function abnormalities may persist in some individuals. Renal and hemorrhagic manifestations are usually absent except in some severe cases.

Diagnosis is through demonstration of specific IgM antibodies using ELISA, Western blot or strip immunoblot techniques. Most patients have IgM antibodies at the time of hospitalization. PCR analysis of autopsy or biopsy tissues and immunohistochemistry in specialized laboratories are also established diagnostic techniques.

2. Infectious agents—Many hantaviruses have been identified in the Americas: Andes virus (Argentina, Chile); Laguna Negra virus (Bolivia, Paraguay); Juquitiba virus (Brazil); Black Creek Canal and Bayou viruses (southeastern USA); and New York-1 and Monongahela viruses (eastern USA); Sin Nombre virus was responsible for the 1993 epidemic in southwestern USA and many other cases in North America.

3. Occurrence—The disease was first recognized in the spring and summer of 1993 among resident Native American populations; cases have been confirmed in Canada and in many eastern and western regions of the USA. Sporadic cases and several outbreaks have been reported in South America (Argentina, Bolivia, Brazil, Chile, Panama, and Paraguay). The disease is not restricted to any ethnic group. Incidence appears to coincide with the geographic distribution and population density of infected carrier rodents and their infection levels.

4. Reservoir—The major reservoir of Sin Nombre virus appears to be the deer mouse, *Peromyscus maniculatus*. Antibodies have also been found in other *Peromyscus* species, pack rats, the chipmunk, and other rodents. Other hantavirus strains have been associated mainly with other rodent species of the subfamily Sigmodontinae.

5. Mode of transmission—As with hantaviral hemorrhagic fever with renal syndrome, aerosol transmission from rodent excreta is presumed. The natural history of viral infections of host rodents has not been characterized. Indoor exposure in closed, poorly ventilated homes, vehicles, and outbuildings with visible rodent infestation is especially important.

6. Incubation period—Incompletely defined, but thought to be approximately 2 weeks, with a range of a few days to 6 weeks.

7. Period of communicability—Person-to-person spread of hantaviruses appears to be rare, but further study is required.

8. Susceptibility—All persons without prior infection are presumed to be susceptible. No unapparent infections have been documented to date, but milder infections without frank pulmonary edema have occurred. No second cases have been identified, but the protection and duration of immunity conferred by previous infection is unknown.

9. Methods of control—

   A. Preventive measures: See section I, 9A.

   B. Control of patient, contacts and the immediate environment:

      1), 2), 3), 4), 5) and 6) Report to local health authority, Isolation, Concurrent disinfection, Quarantine, Immunization of contacts, and Investigation of contacts and source of infection—See section I, 9B1–9B6.

      7) Specific treatment: Provide respiratory intensive care management. Carefully avoid over-hydration that might lead to exacerbation of pulmonary edema. Cardiotonic drugs and pressors given early under careful monitoring help prevent shock. Strictly avoid hypoxia, particularly if transfer is contemplated. Ribavirin is under investigation and as yet is of no proven benefit. Extracorporeal membrane oxygenation has been used with some success.

   C. Epidemic measures: Public education regarding rodent avoidance and rodent control in homes is desirable in endemic situations, and should be intensified during epidemics. Monitoring of rodent numbers and infection rates is desirable, but as yet of unproven value. See section I, 9C.

   D. Disaster implications: See section I, 9D.

   E. International measures: Control transport of exotic reservoir rodents.

HENIPAVIRUSES: HENDRA AND NIPAH VIRAL DISEASES   ICD-9 078.8; ICD-10 B33.8

[CCDM19: J. Mackenzie]
[CCDM18: A. Plant]

1. Identification—Hendra and Nipah viral diseases are recently recognized zoonotic viral diseases named for the locations in Australia and Malaysia where the first human isolates were confirmed, in 1994 and 1999, respectively. Nipah virus manifests primarily as encephalitis. Hendra virus manifests as a respiratory illness (five recorded cases at time of writing in early 2008) and as a prolonged and initially mild meningoencephalitis (one case).

The full course and spectrum of these diseases is now becoming clearer: symptoms range in severity, from mild to coma and/or respiratory failure and death, and include fever and headaches, sore throat, dizziness, drowsiness and disorientation, or influenza-like symptoms and atypical pneumonitis. Sub-clinical cases also occur. Pneumonitis was prominent in the two initial Hendra cases—one of which was fatal—whereas Nipah virus (NiV) cases have been largely encephalitic, and were initially misdiagnosed as Japanese encephalitis, although a proportion of patients displayed pulmonary involvement with atypical pneumonitis. Most patients who survived acute NiV encephalitis made a full recovery, but approximately 20% had residual neurologic deficits. Cases of late onset and relapse encephalitis were observed several months after initial infection, the former usually in mild or sub-clinical cases. The case-fatality rate for clinical cases was approximately 40%, but lower in late-onset and relapsed cases of encephalitis.

Serological diagnosis is available through detection of IgM and IgG with an antibody capture ELISA or serum neutralization. Virus isolation from infected tissues confirms the diagnosis.

2. Infectious agent—Hendra and Nipah viruses are members of a new genus, *Henipaviruses*, of the Paramyxoviridae family.

3. Occurrence—Hendra virus has caused severe respiratory disease in horses in Queensland, Australia; in 1994, three human cases followed close contact with sick horses, the first two during the initial outbreak in Hendra, the third occurring 13 months after an initially mild meningitic illness, when the virus reactivated to cause a fatal encephalitis. Sporadic cases of disease in horses have continued to occur in coastal Queensland and northern New South Wales, from 1999 to time of writing in 2008. A mild human case occurred in 2004 in a veterinarian, following an autopsy on a euthanized horse in Cairns, north Queensland, and two further human cases occurred during an outbreak in horses at a veterinary clinic in Brisbane in 2008, all presenting with a moderate to severe influenza-like illness requiring hospitalization. All human infections have been associated with contact with infected horses.

Nipah virus has caused severe and highly contagious disease in domestic swine in the pig-farming provinces of Perak, Negeri Sembilan, and Selangor in Malaysia. Asymptomatic infection in the pigs was common, and the case-fatality rate was generally low (5%). The first human case is believed to have occurred in 1996, although the disease became apparent in late 1998, and most cases were identified in the first months of 1999 (with 105 confirmed deaths). During 1999, 11 abattoir workers in Singapore developed Nipah virus infection following contact with pigs imported from Malaysia, with one fatality. In 2001, Nipah virus emerged for the first time in Bangladesh and West Bengal, India. In all, there have been eight outbreaks of Nipah virus infection in Bangladesh between 2001 and 2008, with over 120 cases and a fatality rate of about 75%. In the same period there have been two confirmed outbreaks in India, with over 70 cases and a fatality rate of about 70%. The outbreaks in India and Bangladesh differed in a number of significant ways from that in Malaysia: there was no evidence of involvement of the intermediate host, swine; a number of cases presented with an acute respiratory distress syndrome, suggesting that transmission could be by inhalation of large droplets; there was strong suggestive evidence of human-to-human transmission for the first time, including nosocomial infections; and there was evidence to suggest that some of the cases were food-borne, due to ingestion of contaminated date palm juice.

4. **Reservoir**—Fruit bats, particularly members of the genus *Pteropus*, are the major reservoir hosts of Hendra and Nipah viruses, but the viruses do not cause overt disease in their hosts. Hendra virus has been isolated from all four Australian members of the genus *Pteropus*, and Nipah virus has been isolated from *Pteropus hypomelanus* in Malaysia. Elsewhere, Nipah virus has also been isolated from Pteropid bats in Cambodia, and antibodies to a Nipah-like virus have been found in sera from fruit bats collected in Timor Leste, Indonesia, Thailand, India, and Madagascar. Antibodies to a Hendra-like virus have been found in sera from fruit bats collected in Papua New Guinea and Madagascar. It is therefore probable that related viruses exist throughout the range of Pteropid bats, spanning a geographic area stretching from Oceania to the Middle East, and including islands off the east coast of Africa.

The major spillover hosts are horses for Hendra virus, and domestic swine for Nipah virus (in Malaysia). The viruses cause an acute febrile illness that may lead to severe respiratory and CNS involvement, and death. Dogs infected with Nipah virus show a distemper-like manifestation, but their epidemiological role has not been defined. Nipah-sero-positive horses have been identified, but their role is also undetermined. Testing of other animals is under way; susceptibility testing suggests that cats and guinea pigs can be infected, sometimes with fatal outcomes. Mice, rabbits and rats appear refractory to infection.

5. Mode of transmission—Primarily through direct contact with infected horses (Hendra) or swine (Nipah), or contaminated tissues. Oral and nasal routes of infection, or infection through contaminated body fluid entering into cuts and abrasions, are suspected in most cases in Australia and Malaysia. In Bangladesh and India, it is believed that transmission can occur as a result of ingestion of contaminated fruit juice, and possibly from droplet infection; but modes of transmission remain to be determined in many instances.

6. Incubation period—From 4 to 18 days.

7. Period of communicability—Unknown.

8. Susceptibility—Undetermined—recurrent infection appears to occur.

9. Methods of control

  A. *Preventive measures:* Health education about measures to be taken, and the need to avoid contact with fruit bats and infected animals such as pigs and horses. Ensure that fruit bats are not able to roost close to pig pens or stables.

  B. *Control of patient, contacts, and the immediate environment:*

  1) Report to local authority: Case report should be obligatory wherever these diseases occur; Class 2 (see *Reporting*).
  2) Isolation: Of infected horses or swine; as evidence for person-to-person transmission continues to be accumulated, isolation appears warranted for humans with infections, as well as strict care when handling body fluids and excreta.
  3) Concurrent disinfection: Slaughter of infected horses or swine, with burial or incineration of carcasses under government supervision.
  4) Quarantine: Restrict movement of horses or pigs from infected farms to other areas.
  5) Immunization of contacts: Not applicable.
  6) Investigation of contacts and source of infection: Search for missed cases.
  7) Specific treatment: None at present, although there is some research evidence that ribavirin may decrease mortality from Nipah virus.

  C. *Epidemic measures:*

  1) Precautions by animal handlers: protective clothing, including boots, gloves, gowns, goggles and face shields; washing of hands and body parts with soap before leaving pig farms.

2) Slaughter of infected horses or swine, with burial or incineration of carcasses, under government supervision.
3) Restrict movement of horses or pigs from infected farms to other areas.
4) Isolate infected humans if person-to-person transmission appears to be a possibility.

D. *Disaster implications:* None

E. *International measures:* Prohibit exportation of horses or pigs and horse/pig products from infected areas.

HEPATITIS, VIRAL ICD-9 070; ICD-10 B15-B19
[CCDM19: M. Klevens, D. Lavanchy. P. Spradling]
[CCDM18: D. Lavanchy]

Several distinct infections are grouped as the viral hepatitides; they are primarily hepatotrophic and have similar clinical presentations, but differ in etiology and in some epidemiological, immunological, clinical and pathological characteristics. Their prevention and control vary greatly. Each will be presented below in a separate section.

I. VIRAL HEPATITIS A ICD-9 070.1; ICD-10 B15

(Infectious hepatitis, Epidemic hepatitis, Epidemic jaundice, Catarrhal jaundice, Type A hepatitis, HA)

1. Identification—In most developing countries, infection occurs in childhood asymptomatically, or with a mild illness. The latter infections may be detectable only through laboratory tests of liver function. Onset of illness in adults in non-endemic areas is usually abrupt, with fever, malaise, anorexia, nausea and abdominal discomfort, followed within a few days by jaundice. The disease varies in clinical severity from a mild illness lasting 1-2 weeks to a severely disabling disease lasting several months. Prolonged, relapsing hepatitis for up to 1 year occurs in 15% of cases; no chronic infection is known to occur. Convalescence is often prolonged. In general, severity increases with age, but complete recovery without sequelae or recurrences is the rule. Reported case fatality is normally low, 0.1%–0.3%; it can reach 1.8% for adults over 50. Persons with chronic liver disease have an elevated risk of death from fulminant hepatitis A.

Demonstration of IgM antibodies against hepatitis A virus (IgM anti-HAV) in the serum of acutely or recently ill patients establishes the diagnosis. IgM anti-HAV becomes detectable 5-10 days after exposure. A 4-fold or greater rise in specific antibodies in paired sera, detected by commercially available EIA, also establishes the diagnosis. If laboratory tests are not available, epidemiological evidence may provide support for the diagnosis. HAV RNA can be detected in blood and stools of most persons during the acute phase of infection through nucleic acid amplification methods, but these are not generally used for diagnostic purposes.

2. Infectious agent—Hepatitis A virus (HAV), a 27-nanometer picornavirus (positive-strand RNA virus). It has been classified as a member of the family Picornaviridae.

3. Occurrence—Worldwide, geographic areas can be characterized by high, intermediate, or low levels of endemicity. Levels of endemicity are related to hygienic and sanitary conditions. In areas of high endemicity, adults are usually immune and epidemics of HA are uncommon. Improved sanitation in many parts of the world is leaving many young adults susceptible, and the frequency of outbreaks is increasing. In industrialized countries, disease transmission is most frequent among household and sexual contacts of acute cases, and occurs sporadically in day care centers with children in diapers/nappies, among travelers to countries where the disease is endemic, among injecting drug users, and among men who have sex with men. Because most children have asymptomatic or unrecognized infections, they play an important role in HAV transmission and serve as a source of infection for others. Where environmental sanitation is poor, infection is common and occurs at an early age. In some southeastern Asian areas, over 90% of the general population has serological evidence of prior HAV infection, *vs.* a rate of 33% in industrialized countries.

Epidemics often evolve slowly, cover wide geographic areas, and last many months; common source epidemics may evolve rapidly. During some outbreaks, day care center employees or attenders, men with multiple male sex partners and injecting drug users may be at higher risk than the general population. In about half the cases no source of infection is identified. The disease is most common among school-age children and young adults. In recent years, community-wide outbreaks have accounted for most disease transmission, although common source outbreaks due to food contaminated by food handlers and contaminated produce continue to occur and require intensive public health efforts to control. These outbreaks are usually associated with contamination of food by an HAV-infected food handler during preparation, or with food (e.g. shellfish, raw produce) contaminated before entering the food chain. Outbreaks have been reported among susceptible persons working with nonhuman primates raised in the wild.

4. Reservoir—Humans, rarely chimpanzees and other primates.

5. Mode of transmission—Person-to-person by the fecal-oral route. The infectious agent is found in feces, reaches peak levels the week or two before onset of symptoms, and diminishes rapidly after liver dysfunction or symptoms appear, which is concurrent with the appearance of circulating antibodies to HAV.

Common source outbreaks have been related to contaminated water; food contaminated by infected food handlers, including foods not cooked or handled after cooking; raw or undercooked mollusks harvested from contaminated waters; and contaminated produce such as lettuce and strawberries. Several outbreaks have been associated with injecting and non-injecting drug use. Transmission through transfusion of blood and clotting factor concentrates obtained from viremic donors during incubation has been reported, albeit rarely.

6. **Incubation period**—Average 28–30 days (range 15–50 days).

7. **Period of communicability**—Studies of transmission in humans and epidemiological evidence indicate that maximum infectivity occurs during the latter half of incubation and continues for a few days after onset of jaundice (or during peak aminotransferase activity in anicteric cases). Most cases are probably noninfectious after the first week of jaundice, although prolonged viral excretion (up to 6 months) has been documented in infants and children. Chronic shedding of HAV in feces does not occur.

8. **Susceptibility**—General. Low incidence of manifested disease in infants and preschool children suggests that mild and anicteric infections are common. Homologous immunity after infection probably lasts for life.

9. **Methods of control**—

    A. *Preventive measures:*

       1) Educate the public about proper sanitation and personal hygiene, with special emphasis on careful hand-washing and sanitary disposal of feces.

       2) Provide proper water treatment and distribution systems and sewage disposal.

       3) There are at least 4 inactivated vaccines on the market, all in line with the WHO recommendations. The dose of vaccine, vaccination schedule, ages for which the vaccine is licensed, and whether there is a pediatric and adult formulation all vary by manufacturer, and no vaccine is licensed for use in children under 1. Clinical trials have shown these vaccines to be safe, immunogenic and efficacious. Protection against clinical hepatitis A may begin in some persons as soon as 14–21 days after a single dose of vaccine, and nearly all have protective levels of antibody by 30 days after receiving the first dose of vaccine. A second dose is felt to be necessary for long-term protection. Depending on the level of HAV endemicity, it may in some cases be cost-effective to screen for HAV antibody prior to immunization.

       4) WHO has issued recommendations for the use of hepatitis A vaccine. In industrialized countries with low endemicity and

with high rates of disease in specific high-risk populations, vaccination of these populations against hepatitis A may be recommended. High-risk groups include the following: a) persons at increased risk for HAV infection or its consequences (chronic liver disease or clotting factor disorders; men who have sex with men; injecting drug users; all susceptible persons traveling to or working in countries where HAV is endemic; persons who work with HAV infected primates or with HAV in research laboratory settings); b) children in communities with consistently elevated rates of hepatitis A.

Close personal contacts (e.g. household, sexual) of hepatitis A patients should be given post-exposure prophylaxis with hepatitis A vaccine, preferably simultaneously with IG within 2 weeks of last exposure given at a separate injection site. Recommendations for hepatitis A vaccination in outbreak situations depend on the epidemiology of hepatitis A in the community and the feasibility of rapid implementation of a widespread vaccination program. The use of hepatitis A vaccine to control community-wide outbreaks has been most successful when vaccination is started early in the course of the outbreak and with high coverage of multiple-age cohorts.

5) Although day care centers can be the source of outbreaks of hepatitis A in some communities, disease within those centers commonly reflects extended transmission in the community. Management of day care centers should stress measures to minimize the possibility of fecal-oral transmission, including thorough hand-washing after every diaper/nappy change and before eating. If one or more hepatitis A cases are associated with a center, or if cases are recognized in two or more households of attenders, hepatitis A vaccine, possibly in combination with IG, should be administered to the staff and attenders. The same should be considered for family contacts of children in diapers/nappies attending centers where outbreaks occur and cases are recognized in 3 or more families.

6) All susceptible travelers to intermediate or highly endemic areas, including Africa, the Middle East, Asia, eastern Europe and Central and South America should be given hepatitis A vaccine prior to departure, possibly together with IG if departure takes place in less than 1 week. If used, IG in a single dose of 0.02 ml/kg, or 2 ml for adults, is recommended for expected exposures of up to 3 months; for more prolonged exposures, 0.06 ml/kg or 5 ml should be given and repeated every 4–6 months if exposure continues (only if vaccine administration is contraindicated).

7) Hepatitis A vaccine should be considered for all populations with increased risk of hepatitis A infection, such as men who

have sex with men, injecting drug users and persons who work with HAV-infected primates or HAV in a research laboratory setting.

8) Raw oysters, clams and other shellfish are risky for a variety of infections including hepatitis, and should only be consumed if it can be ascertained that they are from a non-contaminated area. Otherwise, all such items should be heated to a temperature of 85°–90°C (185°–194°F) for 4 minutes or steamed for 90 seconds before eating. In endemic areas, travelers should take only hot or bottled beverages and hot, well-cooked food.

B. *Control of patient, contacts and the immediate environment:*

1) Report to local health authority: Obligatory in some countries, although not required in many others; Class 2 (see *Reporting*).

2) Isolation: For proven hepatitis A, enteric precautions during the first 2 weeks of illness, but no more than 1 week after onset of jaundice; the exception is an outbreak in a neonatal intensive care setting, where prolonged enteric precautions must be considered.

3) Concurrent disinfection: Sanitary disposal of feces, urine and blood.

4) Quarantine: Not applicable.

5) Immunization of contacts: Active immunization should be given as soon as possible, but no later than 2 weeks after exposure. Passive immunization with IG (IM), 0.02 ml/kg of body weight, should be given as soon as possible after exposure, but also within 2 weeks. Because hepatitis A cannot be reliably diagnosed on clinical presentation alone, serological confirmation of HAV infection in index patients by IgM anti-HAV testing should be obtained before post-exposure prophylaxis of contacts. Persons who have received 1 dose of hepatitis A vaccine at least 1 month prior to exposure do not need IG.

Hepatitis A vaccine and IG are not indicated for contacts in the usual office, school or factory settings. Hepatitis A vaccine should be given to previously unimmunized persons in the situations listed below, preferably together with IG administered concurrently at a separate injection site:

a) Close personal contacts, including household, sexual, drug using and other close personal contacts

b) Attenders at day care centers if one or more cases of hepatitis A are recognized in children or employees or if cases are recognized in 2 or more households of attenders—prophylaxis may be given to classroom contacts of an index case

c) In a common source outbreak, if a food handler is diagnosed with hepatitis A, hepatitis A vaccine and IG should be administered to other food handlers in the same establishment. Hepatitis A vaccine and IG is usually not offered to patrons; this may be considered if (i) food handlers were involved in the preparations of foods that were not heated; (ii) deficiencies in personal hygiene are noted or the food handler has had diarrhea; and (iii) the hepatitis A vaccine and IG can be given within 2 weeks after last exposure.

6) Investigation of contacts and source of infection: Search for missed cases and maintain surveillance of contacts in the patient's household or, in a common source outbreak, surveillance of people exposed to the same risk.

7) Specific treatment: None.

C. Epidemic measures:

1) Determine mode of transmission (person-to-person or common vehicle) through epidemiological investigation; identify the population exposed. Eliminate common sources of infection.

2) Effective use of hepatitis A vaccine in community-wide outbreak situations requires the initiation of immunization early in the course of the outbreak and the rapid achievement of high (approximately 70% at least) first-dose vaccine coverage levels. Specific outbreak control measures must be tailored to the characteristics of hepatitis A epidemiology and of the existing hepatitis A immunization program, if any, in the community. Immunization of older children who have not previously received vaccine should be accelerated in communities with ongoing programs of routine hepatitis A immunization for young children; target immunization should be undertaken for groups or areas (age groups, risk groups, census tracts) where local surveillance and epidemiological data show the highest rates. In outbreak settings such as day care, hospitals, institutions and schools, routine use of hepatitis A vaccine is not warranted. These immunization programs may reduce disease incidence only in the group(s) targeted.

3) Make special efforts to improve sanitary and hygienic practices to eliminate fecal contamination of foods and water.

4) Outbreaks in institutions may warrant mass prophylaxis with hepatitis A vaccine and IG.

    D. Disaster implications: Hepatitis A is a potential problem in large collections of susceptible people with overcrowding, inadequate sanitation and water supplies; if cases occur, increased efforts should be exerted to improve sanitation and safety of water supplies. Mass administration of hepatitis A vaccine, which should be carefully planned, is not a substitute for environmental measures.

    E. International measures: None.

II. VIRAL HEPATITIS B   ICD-9 070.3; ICD-10 B16

(Type B hepatitis, Serum hepatitis, Homologous serum jaundice, Australia antigen hepatitis, HB)

    1. Identification—A small proportion of acute hepatitis B virus (HBV) infections may be clinically recognized; less than 10% of children and 30%–50% of adults with acute hepatitis B virus (HBV) infection show icteric disease. In those with clinical illness, the onset is usually insidious, with anorexia, vague abdominal discomfort, nausea and vomiting, sometimes arthralgias and rash, often progressing to jaundice. Fever may be absent or mild. Severity ranges from unapparent cases detectable only by liver function tests to fulminating, fatal cases of acute hepatic necrosis. The case-fatality rate is about 1%; higher in those over 40. Fulminant HBV infection also occurs in pregnancy and among newborns of infected mothers.

    Chronic HBV infection is found in 0.5% of adults in North America and in 0.1%–20% in other parts of the world. After acute HBV infection, the risk of developing chronic infection varies inversely with age; chronic HBV infection occurs among about 90% of infants infected at birth, 20%–50% of children infected from 1 to 5 years, and 1%–10% of persons infected as older children and adults. Chronic HBV infection is common in persons with immunodeficiency. Persons with chronic infection may or may not have a history of clinical hepatitis. About one-third have elevated aminotransferases; biopsy findings range from normal to severe necro-inflammatory hepatitis, with or without cirrhosis. An estimated 15%–25% of persons with chronic HBV infection will die prematurely of either cirrhosis or hepatocellular carcinoma. HBV is the cause of up to 80% of all cases of hepatocellular carcinoma worldwide.

    Demonstration in sera of specific antigens and/or antibodies confirms diagnosis. Three clinically useful antigen-antibody systems are identified for hepatitis B:

    1) Hepatitis B surface antigen (HBsAg) and antibody to HBsAg (anti-HBs)
    2) Hepatitis B core antigen (HBcAg) and antibody to HBcAg (anti-HBc)
    3) Hepatitis B e antigen (HBeAg) and antibody to HBeAg (anti-HBe).

Commercial kits are available for all markers except HBcAg. HBsAg can be detected in serum from several weeks before onset of symptoms to days, weeks or months after onset; it is present in serum during acute infections and persists in chronic infections. The presence of HBsAg indicates that the person is infectious. Anti-HBc appears at the onset of illness and persists indefinitely. Demonstration of anti-HBc in serum indicates HBV infection, current or past; high titers of IgM anti-HBc occur during acute infection—IgM anti-HBc usually disappears within 6 months but can persist in some cases of chronic hepatitis; this test may reliably diagnose acute HBV infection. The presence of HBeAg is associated with relatively high infectivity.

2. Infectious agent—Hepatitis B virus (HBV), a hepadnavirus, is a 42-nanometer partially double-stranded DNA virus composed of a 27-nanometer nucleocapsid core (HBcAg), surrounded by an outer lipoprotein coat containing the surface antigen (HBsAg). HBsAg is antigenically heterogeneous, with a common antigen (designated a) and 2 pairs of mutually exclusive antigens (d, y, w (including several subdeterminants) and r), resulting in 4 major subtypes: adw, ayw, adr and ayr. The distribution of subtypes varies geographically; because of the common "a" determinant, protection against one subtype appears to confer protection against the other subtypes, and no differences in clinical features have been related to subtype. Genotype classification based on sequencing of genetic material has been introduced and is becoming the standard: HBV is currently classified into 8 main genotypes (A–H). There is growing evidence of differences in severity of liver disease between some HBV genotypes.

3. Occurrence—Worldwide; endemic with little seasonal variation. WHO estimates that more than 2 billion persons have been infected with HBV (including 350 million chronically infected). Each year approximately 600 000 to 1 million persons die as a result of HBV infections, and over 4 million new acute clinical cases occur. In countries where HBV is highly endemic (HBsAg prevalence 8% or higher), most infections occur during infancy and early childhood. Where HBV endemicity is intermediate (HBsAg prevalence from 2%–7%), infections occur commonly in all age groups, although the high rate of chronic infection is primarily maintained by transmission during infancy and early childhood. Where endemicity is low (HBsAg prevalence under 2%), most infections occur in young adults, especially those belonging to known risk groups. Even in countries with low HBV endemicity, a high proportion of chronic infections may be acquired during childhood because the development of chronic infection is age-dependent. Almost all of these infections would be prevented by perinatal vaccination against hepatitis B of all newborns or infants.

Serological evidence of previous infection may vary depending on age and socioeconomic class. Exposure to HBV may be common in certain high-risk groups, including: injecting drug users; heterosexuals with multiple partners; men who have sex with men; household contacts and sex partners of HBV-infected persons; health care and public safety workers who have exposure to blood in the workplace; clients and staff in institutions for the developmentally disabled; hemodialysis patients; and prisoners. All health care workers performing exposure-prone procedures should be immunized against hepatitis B.

In the past, recipients of blood products were at high risk. In countries where pre-transfusion screening of blood for HBsAg is performed, and where pooled blood clotting factors (especially antihemophilic factor) are processed to destroy the virus, this risk has been virtually eliminated; however, it is still present in many developing countries. Contaminated and inadequately sterilized syringes and needles have resulted in outbreaks of hepatitis B among patients; this has been a major mode of transmission worldwide. Occasionally, outbreaks have been traced to tattoo parlors and acupuncturists. Rarely, transmission to patients from HBsAg-positive health care workers has been documented. Outbreaks have been reported among patients in dialysis centers in many countries through failure to adhere to recommended infection control practices against transmission of HBV and other blood-borne pathogens in these settings.

4. Reservoir—Humans. Chimpanzees are susceptible, but an animal reservoir in nature has not been recognized. Closely-related hepadnaviruses are found in woodchucks, ducks, ground squirrels and other animals, such as snow leopards and German herons; none cause disease in humans.

5. Mode of transmission—Body substances capable of transmitting HBV include: blood and blood products; saliva (although no outbreaks of HBV infection due to saliva alone have been documented); cerebrospinal fluid; peritoneal, pleural, pericardial and synovial fluid; amniotic fluid; semen and vaginal secretions; any other body fluid containing blood; and unfixed tissues and organs. The presence of antigen or viral DNA (HBV-DNA above 10^5 copies/mL) indicates high virus titer and higher infectivity of these fluids.

Transmission occurs by percutaneous (IV, IM, SC, intradermal) and mucosal exposure to infective body fluids. Since HBV is stable on environmental surfaces for at least 7 days, indirect inoculation of HBV can occur via inanimate objects. Fecal-oral or vector-borne transmission has not been demonstrated.

Major modes of HBV transmission include sexual or close household contact with an infected person, perinatal mother-to-infant transmission, injecting drug use and nosocomial exposure. Sexual transmission from infected men to women is about 3 times more efficient than that from infected women to men. Anal intercourse, insertive or receptive, is associated with an increased risk of infection. Transmission of HBV in households primarily occurs from child to child. Communally used razors and toothbrushes have been implicated as occasional vehicles of HBV transmission in this setting. Perinatal transmission is common, especially when HBV-infected mothers are also HBeAg-positive or if they are highly viremic. The rate of transmission from HBsAg-positive, HBeAg-positive mothers is more than 70%; from HBsAg-positive, HBeAg-negative mothers it is less than 10%. Anti-HBe antibody-positive chronic hepatitis B was first described in patients of the Mediterranean Basin, where about 20% of HBsAg carriers were positive for anti-HBe antibodies and showed detectable serum levels of HBV DNA with liver necro-inflammation. The infecting HBV variants show mutations in the precore region that hamper HBeAg production. The HBeAg-negative form of chronic hepatitis B is present worldwide, and has been associated with transmission. Transmission through injecting drug use occurs though transfer of HBV-infected blood by sharing syringes and needles either directly or through contamination of drug preparation equipment. Nosocomial exposures such as transfusion of blood or blood products, hemodialysis, acupuncture and needle-stick or other "sharps" injuries sustained by hospital personnel have all resulted in HBV transmission. IG, heat-treated plasma protein fraction, albumin and fibrinolysin are considered safe.

6. **Incubation period**—Usually 45–180 days, average 60–90 days. As short as 2 weeks to the appearance of HBsAg, and rarely as long as 6–9 months; variation is related in part to amount of virus in the inoculum, mode of transmission, and host factors.

7. **Period of communicability**—All persons who are HBsAg-positive are potentially infectious. Blood from experimentally inoculated volunteers has been shown to be infective weeks before the onset of first symptoms and to remain infective through the acute clinical course of the disease. The infectivity of chronically infected individuals varies from high (HBeAg-positive, HBV-DNA above 10^5 copies/mL) to modest (anti-HBe-positive).

8. **Susceptibility**—Susceptibility is general. Disease is often milder and anicteric in children; in infants it is usually asymptomatic. Protective immunity follows infection if antibodies to HBsAg (anti-HBs) develop and HBsAg is negative. Persons with Down's syndrome, lymphoproliferative disease, HIV infection, immunosuppression and those on hemodialysis appear more likely to develop chronic infection.

9. **Methods of control**—

   A. *Preventive measures:*

   1) Effective hepatitis B vaccines have been available since 1982. Two types of hepatitis B vaccines have been licensed and have been shown to be safe and highly protective against all subtypes of HBV. The first was prepared from plasma from HBsAg-positive persons, and was widely used in the past. The second, from recombinant DNA (rDNA), is produced by using

HBsAg synthesized by yeast or cell-lines, into which a plasmid containing the gene for HBsAg has been inserted; this has now replaced the earlier vaccine. Combined passive-active immunoprophylaxis with hepatitis B immunoglobulin (HBIG) and vaccine has been shown comparable to vaccine alone in stimulating anti-HBs titers, but is expensive and not available in all countries. Several combined vaccines (e.g. hepatitis A & B and tetra- and pentavalent vaccines) have been licensed and show comparable efficacy.

a) In all countries, routine infant immunization should be the primary strategy to prevent HBV infection. Immunization of successive infant cohorts produces a highly immune population and suffices to interrupt transmission. In countries with high endemicity for HBV, routine infant immunization rapidly eliminates transmission because virtually all chronic infections are acquired among young children. Where HBV endemicity is low or intermediate, immunizing infants alone will not substantially lower disease incidence for about 15 years, because most infections occur among adolescents and young adults; vaccine strategies for older children, adolescents and adults may be desirable. Strategies to ensure high vaccine coverage of successive age group cohorts are likely to be most effective in eliminating HBV transmission. In addition, immunization strategies can be targeted to high-risk groups, which account for most cases among adolescents and adults.

b) Testing to exclude adolescent or adult people with pre-existing anti-HBs or anti-HBc is not required prior to immunization, but may be considered as a cost-saving method in countries where the level of preexisting infection is high.

c) Immunity against HBV persists for at least 15 years after successful immunization, and booster injections are not recommended.

d) Vaccines licensed in different parts of the world may have varying dosages and schedules; in the USA they are most commonly administered in 3 IM doses: for infants, the first dose is given at birth or at 1–2 months of age with subsequent doses 1 to 2 and 6 to 18 months later. For infants born to HBsAg positive women, the schedule should be birth, 1–2 and 6 months of age. These infants should also receive 0.5 ml of HBIG (see 9B5a). The dose of vaccine varies by manufacturer. In mid-1999, it was hypothesized that very small infants who receive multiple doses of vaccines containing thiomersal/thimerosal would be at risk of receiving more than the recommended limits for mercury exposure as set out by regulatory guidelines. On the basis of this hypothetical risk of mercury exposure, elimination of thiomersal/thimerosal in vaccines was implemented, although pharmacological and epidemiological data render it highly unlikely that such vaccines give rise to neurological adverse effects. A significant number of hepatitis B vaccines available today are antigen preservative-free.

e) Pregnancy is not a contraindication for receiving hepatitis B vaccine.

2) The current WHO hepatitis B prevention strategy is based on routine universal newborn or infant immunization. The greatest fall in incidence and prevalence of hepatitis B is in countries with high vaccine coverage at birth or in infancy. Vaccination of adolescents is also valuable, as it protects against transmission through sexual contact or injecting drug use. The current hepatitis B prevention strategy in the USA includes the following aspects:

a) Screening of all pregnant women for the presence of HBsAg, providing HBIG and hepatitis B vaccine to infants of HBsAg positive mothers, and providing hepatitis B vaccine to susceptible household contacts

b) Pregnant women who are identified as being at risk for HBV infection during pregnancy (e.g., more than one sex partner during the previous 6 months, previous evaluation or treatment for an STD, recent or current injecting-drug use, or having had an HBsAg-positive sex partner) should be vaccinated

c) Providing routine hepatitis B immunization for all infants

d) Providing catch-up immunization to previously unimmunized children, with highest priority for children aged 11–12 years, in groups with high rates of chronic HBV infection (Alaskan natives, Pacific Islanders, first generation immigrants from countries with high prevalence of chronic HBV infection)

e) Intensified efforts to immunize adolescents and adults in defined risk groups.

3) Persons at high risk who should routinely receive pre-exposure hepatitis B immunization include:

a) Those who are diagnosed as having recently acquired other STDs and people who have a history of sexual activity with more than one partner in the previous 6 months

b) Men who have sex with men
c) Sexual partners and household contacts of HBsAg positive persons
d) Inmates of juvenile detention facilities, prisons and jails
e) Health care and public safety workers who perform tasks involving contact with blood or blood-contaminated body fluids
f) Clients and staff of institutions for the developmentally disabled
g) Hemodialysis patients
h) Patients with bleeding disorders who receive blood products
i) International travelers who plan to spend more than 6 months in areas with intermediate to high rates of chronic HBV infection (2% or greater), and who will have close contact with the local population.

4) Adequately sterilize all syringes and needles (including acupuncture needles) and lancets for finger puncture; use disposable, mono-use equipment whenever possible. A sterile syringe and needle are essential for each individual receiving skin tests, parenteral inoculations or venepuncture. Enforce aseptic sanitary practices in tattoo parlors, including proper disposal of sharp or cutting tools, and discourage traditional tattooing and scarring practices.

5) In blood banks, all donated blood should be tested for HBsAg by sensitive tests; reject as donors all persons with a history of viral hepatitis, those who have a history of injecting drug use or show evidence of drug addiction, or those who have received a blood transfusion or tattoo within the preceding 6 months. Avoid using paid donors.

6) Limit administration of unscreened whole blood or potentially hazardous blood products to those in life-threatening need of such therapeutic measures.

7) Maintain surveillance for all cases of post-transfusion hepatitis; keep a register of all people who donated blood for each case. Notify blood banks of potential carriers so that future donations may be identified promptly.

8) Although few public health authorities have established recommendations for HBV-positive health care workers, there is general consensus that HBeAg-positive HBV carriers should not perform exposure-prone surgery or similar treatment of patients. In several countries (including the USA), medical and dental personnel infected with HBV and who are HBeAg-positive and/or have significant levels of viremia, should not perform invasive procedures unless they have sought counsel from an expert review panel and have been advised under

what circumstances—if any—they may continue to perform these procedures.

B. **Control of patient, contacts and the immediate environment:**

1) Report to local health authority: Official report obligatory in some countries; Class 2 (see *Reporting*).

2) Isolation: Universal precautions to prevent exposures to blood and body fluids.

3) Concurrent disinfection: Of equipment contaminated with blood or infectious body fluids.

4) Quarantine: Not applicable.

5) Immunization of contacts: Products available for post-exposure prophylaxis include hepatitis B vaccine and HBIG. Administer hepatitis B vaccine and, when indicated, HBIG as soon as possible after exposure.

   a) Infants born to HBsAg positive mothers should receive a single dose of vaccine within 12 hours of birth and, where available, HBIG (0.5 ml IM), the first dose of vaccine to be given concurrently with HBIG but at a separate site; second and third doses of vaccine (without HBIG) 1–2 and 6 months later. It is recommended to test the infant for HBsAg and anti-HBs at 9–15 months of age to monitor the success or failure of prophylaxis. Infants who are anti-HBs positive and HBsAg negative are protected and do not need further vaccine doses. Infants found to be anti-HBs negative and HBsAg negative should be re-immunized.

   b) After percutaneous (e.g. needle-stick) or mucous membrane exposures to blood that might contain HBsAg, a decision to provide post-exposure prophylaxis must include consideration of: (i) whether the source of the blood is available; (ii) the HBsAg status of the source; and (iii) the hepatitis B immunization status of the exposed person. For previously unimmunized persons exposed to blood from an HBsAg positive source, a single dose of HBIG (0.06 ml/kg, or 5 ml for adults) should be given as soon as possible, but at least within 24 hours of high-risk needle-stick exposure, and the hepatitis B vaccine series should be started. If active immunization cannot be given, another dose of HBIG should be given 1 month after the first. HBIG is not usually given for needle-stick exposure to blood that is not known or highly suspected to be positive for HBsAg, since the risk of infection in these instances is small; however, initiation of hepatitis B immunization is recommended if the person has not previously been immunized. For previously immunized persons exposed to an HBsAg positive source, post-exposure prophylaxis is not needed in cases with a protective antibody response to immunization (anti-HBs titer of 10 milli-IUs/mL or greater). For persons whose response to immunization is unknown, hepatitis B vaccine and/or HBIG should be administered.

c) After sexual exposure to a person with acute HBV infection, application of hepatitis B vaccine together with a single dose of HBIG (0.06 ml/kg) is recommended if it can be given within 14 days of the last sexual contact. For all exposed sexual contacts of persons with acute and chronic HBV infection, vaccine should be administered.

6) Investigation of contacts and source of infection: See 9C.

7) Specific treatment: No specific treatment is available for acute hepatitis B. In fulminant hepatitis B, uncontrolled reports suggest some efficacy of lamivudine; therefore, it may be tried (as may any other rapidly acting antiviral drug) if there is evidence of ongoing HBV replication. Two major groups of antiviral treatment have been licensed for the treatment of chronic hepatitis B in the USA and many other countries. These include interferon alpha (IFNa, or PEG-IFNa) and nucleoside or nucleotide analogues such as lamivudine, adefovir, entecavir and telbivudine. Many other drugs are being evaluated (e.g. tenofovir, emtricitabine, clevudine, elvucitabine, valtorcitabine, and amdoxovir). Patients who are candidates for therapy should have evidence of severe necroinflammatory disease; treatment is most effective in individuals in the high-replicative phase (HBeAg positive) of infection, because these are the most likely to be symptomatic, infectious, and at risk of long-term sequelae. Although decision to treat and the choice of the appropriate therapy remain challenging, considerable progress has been made in the treatment of chronic hepatitis B. Studies show that alpha interferon is successful in arresting viral replication in about 25%–40% of treated patients. Approximately 10% of patients who respond lose HBsAg 6 months after therapy. Clinical trials of long-term treatment with nucleoside or nucleotide analogues have demonstrated sustained clearance of HBV DNA from serum, followed by improvements in serum aminotransferase levels and histological improvement. The majority of the patients will require prolonged treatment in order to maintain suppression of viral replication. Consequently, treatment costs in both developing and developed countries are currently prohibitively high. The efficacy of combination therapy will have to be studied further, but it is likely to diminish the occurrence of virus mutants resistant to

treatment. These medications have significant side-effects that require careful monitoring.

C. Epidemic measures: When 2 or more cases occur in association with some common exposure, search for additional cases. Institute strict aseptic techniques. If a plasma derivative such as antihemophilic factor, fibrinogen, pooled plasma or thrombin is implicated, withdraw the lot from use and trace all recipients of the same lot in a search for additional cases.

D. Disaster implications: Relaxation of sterilization precautions and emergency use of unscreened blood for transfusions may result in an increased number of cases.

E. International measures: None.

III. VIRAL HEPATITIS C ICD-9 070.5; ICD-10 B17.1

(Parenterally transmitted non-A non-B hepatitis [PT-NANB], Non-B transfusion associated hepatitis, Post-transfusion non-A non-B hepatitis, HCV infection)

1. Identification—Onset is usually insidious, with anorexia, vague abdominal discomfort, nausea and vomiting; progression to jaundice less frequent than with hepatitis B. Although initial infection may be asymptomatic (more than 90% of cases) or mild, a high percentage of cases (50%–80%) develop a chronic infection. Of chronically infected persons, about half will eventually develop cirrhosis or cancer of the liver.

Diagnosis depends on detecting antibody to the hepatitis C virus (anti-HCV). Various tests are available for the diagnosis and monitoring of HCV infection. Tests that detect antibodies against the virus include the enzyme immunoassay (EIA) and the recombinant immunoblot assay. The same HCV antigens are used in both EIAs and the immunoblot assays. These tests do not distinguish between acute, chronic, or resolved infection. Reproducible and inexpensive EIA tests for the diagnosis of HCV are suitable for screening at-risk populations and recommended as the initial test for patients with clinical liver disease. A negative EIA test suffices to exclude a diagnosis of chronic HCV infection in immunocompetent patients. The high sensitivity and specificity of third-generation EIAs obviate the need for a confirmatory immunoblot assay in the diagnosis of individuals with clinical liver disease, particularly those with risk factors for HCV. Immunoblot assays are useful as a supplemental assay for persons screened in non-clinical settings and in persons with a positive EIA who test negative for HCV RNA.

Acute or chronic HCV infection in a patient with a positive EIA test should be confirmed by detection of the presence of HCV RNA in the serum using a sensitive assay. Target amplification techniques using polymerase chain reaction (PCR), transcription-mediated amplification

(TMA) and signal amplification techniques (branched DNA) may be used to measure HCV RNA levels. A single positive qualitative assay for HCV RNA confirms active HCV replication, but a single negative assay does not exclude viremia and may reflect a transient decline in viral level below the level of detection of the assay. Therefore, a follow-up HCV RNA detection should be performed to confirm the absence of active HCV replication. Quantitative determination of HCV RNA levels and of HCV genotype provides information on the likelihood of response to treatment in patients undergoing antiviral therapy. Liver biopsy can provide direct histological assessment of liver injury due to HCV, but cannot be used to diagnose HCV infection.

2. Infectious agent—The hepatitis C virus is an enveloped RNA virus classified as a separate genus (*Hepacivirus*) in the Flaviviridae family. At least 6 different genotypes and approximately 100 subtypes of HCV exist. Evidence is limited regarding differences in clinical features, disease outcome or progression to cirrhosis or hepatocellular carcinoma (HCC) among persons with different genotypes. However, differences do exist in responses to antiviral therapy according to HCV genotypes.

3. Occurrence—Worldwide distribution. HCV prevalence is directly related to the prevalence of persons who routinely share injection equipment, and to the prevalence of unsafe parenteral practices in health care settings. WHO estimates that some 130-170 million people (approximately 2%-3% of world population) are chronically infected with HCV, like HBV one of the most common global causes of chronic hepatitis, cirrhosis, and liver cancer. Most populations in Africa, the Americas, Europe and southeast Asia have anti-HCV prevalence rates under 2.5%. Prevalence rates for the Western Pacific regions average 2.5-4.9%. In the Middle East, the prevalence of anti-HCV ranges from 1% to more than 12%. The number of people with serological manifestation of HCV infection in Europe is estimated at 8.9 million, and at 12.6 million in the Americas; the majority of infected individuals live in Asia (60 million in eastern Asia, 32 million in southeastern Asia) and Africa (28 million).

4. Reservoir—Humans; virus has been transmitted experimentally to chimpanzees.

5. Mode of transmission—HCV is primarily transmitted parenterally. The primary sources of HCV infection include transfusion of blood or blood products from unscreened donors; transfusion of blood products that have not undergone viral inactivation; parenteral exposure to blood through the use of contaminated or inadequately sterilized instruments and needles used in medical and dental procedures; the use of unsterilized objects for rituals (e.g. circumcision, scarification), traditional medicine (e.g. blood-letting) or other activities that break the skin (e.g. tattooing, ear or body piercing); and intravenous drug abuse. Household or sexual contacts of HCV-infected persons are marginally at risk. Sexual and mother-to-child transmissions have both been documented, but appear rare.

6. Incubation period—Ranges from 2 weeks to 6 months; commonly 6–9 weeks. Chronic infection may persist for up to 20 years before the onset of cirrhosis or hepatoma.

7. Period of communicability—From one or more weeks before onset of the first symptoms; may persist in most persons indefinitely. Peaks in virus concentration appear to correlate with peaks in ALT activity.

8. Susceptibility—Susceptibility is general. The degree of immunity following infection is not known; repeated infections with HCV have been demonstrated.

9. Methods of control —

A. *Preventive measures:* General control measures against HBV infection apply (see section II, 9A). Prophylactic IG is not effective. In blood bank operations, all donors should be routinely screened for anti-HCV and all donor units with elevated liver enzyme levels should be discarded. Routine virus inactivation of plasma-derived products, risk reduction counseling for persons uninfected but at high risk (e.g. health care workers) and nosocomial control activities must be maintained.

B. *Control of patient, contacts and the immediate environment:* General control measures against HBV apply. Post-exposure prophylaxis with IG is not effective in preventing infection. For the treatment of chronic hepatitis C, highest response rates (40–80%) have been achieved with a combination therapy of ribavirin and slow-release interferons ("pegylated interferons"), making this the treatment of choice. Genotype determinations influence treatment decisions and treatment duration. These medications have significant side-effects that require careful monitoring. Ribavirin is a teratogen; thus pregnancy should be avoided during treatment. Corticosteroids and acyclovir have not been effective.

C. *Epidemic measures:* Same as for hepatitis B.

D. *Disaster implications:* Same as for hepatitis B.

E. *International measures:* Ensure adequate virus inactivation for all internationally traded biological products.

IV. DELTA HEPATITIS   ICD-9 070.5; ICD-10 B17.0

(Viral hepatitis D, Hepatitis delta virus, Delta agent hepatitis, Delta associated hepatitis)

1. Identification—Onset is usually abrupt, with signs and symptoms resembling those of hepatitis B; may be severe and always associated with a coexistent hepatitis B virus (HBV) infection. Delta hepatitis infection may occur as acute co-infection with hepatitis B virus, or as super-infection in persons with chronic HBV infection. In the former case the infection is usually self-limiting, in the latter it will usually progress to chronic hepatitis, and acute delta hepatitis can be misdiagnosed as an exacerbation of chronic hepatitis B. Children may have a severe clinical course with usual progression to severe chronic hepatitis. In studies throughout Europe and the USA, 25%–50% of fulminant hepatitis cases thought to be caused by HBV were associated with concurrent HDV infection. Fulminant cases occur in super-infections rather than co-infections.

Diagnosis is through detection of total antibody to HDV (anti-HDV) by EIA. A positive IgM titer indicates ongoing replication; reverse transcription PCR is the most sensitive assay for detecting HDV viremia.

2. Infectious agent—HDV is a virus-like particle of 35–37 nanometers consisting of a coat of HBsAg and a unique internal antigen, the delta antigen. Encapsulated with the delta antigen is the genome, a single-stranded RNA that can have a linear or circular conformation. The RNA does not hybridize with HBV DNA. HDV is unable to infect a cell by itself, and requires co-infection with the HBV to undergo a complete replication cycle. Synthesis of HDV, in turn, results in temporary suppression of synthesis of HBV components. HDV is best considered in the new "satellite" family of sub-virions, some of which are pathogens of higher plants. Hepatitis D is the only agent in this family that infects animal species. Three genotypes of HDV have been identified: Genotype I is the most prevalent and widespread; genotype II is represented by 2 isolates from Japan and Taiwan (China); genotype III is reported only in the Amazon basin, causing severe fulminant hepatitis with microvesicular steatosis (spongiocytosis).

3. Occurrence—Worldwide, but prevalence varies widely. An estimated 10 million people are infected with hepatitis D virus and its helper virus HBV. It occurs epidemically or endemically in populations at high risk of HBV infection, such as where hepatitis B is endemic (highest in Africa and South America, Romania, and parts of Russia); among hemophiliacs, injecting drug users and others who come in frequent contact with blood; in institutions for the developmentally disabled; and, to a lesser extent, among men who have sex with men. Severe epidemics have been observed in tropical South America (Brazil, Colombia, Venezuela), in the Central African Republic, and among injecting drug users in the USA. Dramatic changes have occurred in the epidemiology of HDV in the past years. Since HDV requires a concomitant HBV infection, the recent decrease in the prevalence of chronic HBsAg carriers in the general population has led to a rapid decline in both acute and chronic hepatitis D in the Mediterranean area (Greece, Italy, Spain) and in many other parts of the world. Better sanitation and social standards may also have contributed. New foci of high HDV prevalence continue to appear, as in the case of Albania, areas of China, northern India and Japan (Okinawa).

4. Reservoir—Humans. Virus can be transmitted experimentally to chimpanzees and to woodchucks infected with HBV and woodchuck hepatitis virus, respectively.

5. Mode of transmission—Thought to be similar to that of HBV: exposure to infected blood and serous body fluids, contaminated needles, syringes and plasma derivatives such as antihemophilic factor, and through sexual transmission. Intrafamily contacts with HBsAg carriers are a major risk factor for the spreading of HDV.

6. Incubation period—Approximately 2-8 weeks.

7. Period of communicability—Blood is potentially infectious during all phases of active hepatitis infection. Peak infectivity probably occurs just prior to onset of acute illness, when particles containing the delta antigen are readily detected in the blood. Following onset, viremia probably falls rapidly to low or undetectable levels. HDV has been transmitted to chimpanzees from the blood of chronically infected patients in whom particles containing delta antigen could not be detected.

8. Susceptibility—All people susceptible to HBV infection or who have chronic HBV can be infected with HDV. Severe disease can occur even in children.

9. Methods of control—

  A. **Preventive measures:** For people susceptible to HBV infection, same as for hepatitis B. Prevention of HBV infection with hepatitis B vaccine prevents infection with HDV. Among persons with chronic HBV, the only effective measure is avoidance of exposure to any potential source of HDV. HBIG, IG and hepatitis B vaccine do not protect persons with chronic HBV from infection by HDV. Studies suggest that measures decreasing sexual exposure and needle-sharing are associated with a decline in the incidence of HDV infection.

  B, C, D. and E. **Control of patient, contacts and the immediate environment, Epidemic measures, Disaster implications** and **International measures:** See *Hepatitis B*. For treatment, the only approved therapy for chronic hepatitis D is interferon-alpha.

V. VIRAL HEPATITIS E   ICD-9 070.5; ICD-10 B17.2

(Enterically transmitted non-A non-B hepatitis [ET-NANB], Epidemic non-A non-B hepatitis, Fecal-oral non-A non-B hepatitis)

1. Identification—Clinical course similar to that of hepatitis A; no evidence of a chronic form. The case-fatality rate is similar to that of hepatitis A except in pregnant women, where it may reach 20% among those infected during the third trimester of pregnancy. Epidemic and sporadic cases have been described.

Diagnosis depends on clinical and epidemiological features and exclusion of other causes of hepatitis, especially hepatitis A, by serological means. Acute hepatitis E is diagnosed in the presence of IgM anti-HEV. HEV RNA can be detected by PCR in acute phase feces in approximately 50% of cases. Western blot assays to detect anti-HEV IgM and IgG in serum can be used to confirm the results of EIA tests, along with PCR tests for the detection of HEV RNA in serum and feces, immunofluorescent antibody blocking assays to detect antibody to HEV antigen in serum and liver, and immune electron microscopy to visualize viral particles in feces.

2. Infectious agent—The hepatitis E virus (HEV), the only known Hepevirus, is a spherical, non-enveloped, single-stranded RNA virus approximately 32 to 34 nanometers in diameter, classified in the *Hepeviridae* family. HEV is comprised of at least five genotypes.

3. Occurrence—HEV is the major causal agent of enterically transmitted non-A, non-B hepatitis worldwide. In recent years, serological tests for both IgM and IgG anti-HEV have allowed a comprehensive epidemiological survey of the distribution of HEV: the prevalence of HEV antibodies in suspected or documented endemic regions was much lower than expected (3%–26%), and was higher than anticipated (1–3%) in non-endemic regions such as north America. Outbreaks of hepatitis E and sporadic cases occur over a wide geographic area, primarily in countries with inadequate environmental sanitation. HEV infections account for 50% of acute sporadic hepatitis in some highly endemic areas, and hepatitis E virus is the single most important cause of acute clinical hepatitis among adults throughout central and southeast Asia, and the second most important cause, behind hepatitis B virus, in the Middle East and north Africa. The highest rates of clinically evident disease occur in young to middle-aged adults; lower disease rates in younger age groups may be the result of anicteric and/or sub-clinical HEV infection. In most industrialized countries, hepatitis E cases have been documented almost only among travelers returning from HEV endemic areas. Outbreaks often occur as waterborne epidemics, but sporadic cases and epidemics not clearly related to water have been reported. Outbreaks have also been reported from: Algeria; Bangladesh; Chad; China; Côte d'Ivoire; Egypt; Ethiopia; Greece; India; Indonesia; the Islamic Republic of Iran; Jordan; the Libyan Arab Jamahiryia; Mexico; Myanmar; Nepal; Nigeria; Pakistan; southern areas of Russia;

Somalia; eastern Sudan; and The Gambia. A large waterborne outbreak (3 682 cases) occurred in 1993 in Uttar Pradesh, India.

4. Reservoir—Humans are natural hosts for HEV; some non-human primates (e.g. chimpanzees, cynomolgus monkeys, rhesus monkeys, pig-tail monkeys, owl monkeys, tamarins and African green monkeys) are reported as susceptible to infection with HEV. Cows, sheep and goats, particularly the first two, have high prevalences of anti-HEV in some populations. Thus, they may be sources of zoonotic infections of humans.

5. Mode of transmission—Primarily by the fecal-oral route; fecally contaminated drinking-water is the most commonly documented vehicle of transmission. Person-to-person transmission probably also occurs through the fecal-oral route, although secondary household cases are uncommon during outbreaks. Recent studies suggest that hepatitis E may in fact be a zoonotic infection with coincident areas of high human infection.

6. Incubation period—The range is 15 to 64 days; the mean incubation period has varied from 26 to 42 days in various epidemics.

7. Period of communicability—Not known. HEV has been detected in stools 14 days after the onset of jaundice and approximately 4 weeks after oral ingestion of contaminated food or water, where it persists for about 2 weeks.

8. Susceptibility—Unknown. Over 50% of HEV infections may be anicteric; the expression of icterus appears to increase with increasing age. Women in the third trimester of pregnancy are especially susceptible to fulminant disease. The occurrence of major epidemics among young adults in regions where other enteric viruses are highly endemic and most of the population acquires infection in infancy remains unexplained.

9. Methods of control—

A. *Preventive measures:* Provide educational programs to stress sanitary disposal of feces and careful hand-washing after defecation and before handling food; follow basic measures to prevent fecal-oral transmission, as listed under Typhoid fever, 9A. Administration of immune serum globulin from endemic areas has not decreased infection rates during epidemics in India; encouraging advances have occurred in HEV vaccine development.

B. *Control of patient, contacts and the immediate environment:*

1), 2) and 3) Report to local health authority, Isolation and Concurrent disinfection: See *Hepatitis A.*
4) Quarantine: Not applicable.
5) Immunization of contacts: No products are available to prevent hepatitis E. IG prepared from plasma collected in

non- and high-HEV endemic areas was not effective in preventing clinical disease during hepatitis E outbreaks. Prototype hepatitis E vaccines have been shown to prevent significant illness, but despite these successes in field trials, they are not yet marketed.

6) Investigation of contacts and source of infection: Same as for hepatitis A.

7) Specific treatment: None.

C. Epidemic measures: Determine mode of transmission through epidemiological investigation; investigate water supply and identify populations at increased risk of infection; make special efforts to improve sanitary and hygienic practices in order to eliminate fecal contamination of foods and water.

D. Disaster implications: A potential problem where there is mass crowding and inadequate sanitation and water supplies. If cases occur, increased effort should be exerted to improve sanitation and the safety of water supplies.

E. International measures: None.

HERPES SIMPLEX
ICD-9 054; ICD-10 B00
[CCDM19: S. Gottlieb, F. Ndowa]
[CCDM18: D. Lavanchy]

ANOGENITAL HERPESVIRAL INFECTIONS
ICD-10 A60
(Alphaherpesviral disease, Herpesvirus hominis, Human herpesviruses 1 and 2)

1. Identification—Herpes simplex is a viral infection characterized by systemic and local symptoms, latency, and a tendency to localized recurrence. The two causal agents—herpes simplex virus (HSV) types 1 and 2—generally produce distinct clinical syndromes, depending on the portal of entry. Either may infect the genital tract or oral mucosa.

Primary infection with HSV-1 may be mild and inapparent and occur in early childhood. In approximately 10% of primary infections, overt disease may appear as an illness of varying severity, marked by fever and malaise lasting a week or more; it may be associated with gingivostomatitis accompanied by vesicular lesions in the oropharynx, severe keratoconjunctivitis, a generalized cutaneous eruption complicating chronic eczema, meningoencephalitis, or some of the fatal generalized infections in newborn infants (congenital herpes simplex, ICD-9 771.2, ICD-10 P35.2).

HSV-1 causes about 2% of acute pharyngotonsillitis, usually as a primary infection.

Reactivation of latent infection commonly results in herpes labialis (fever blisters, cold sores), manifested usually on the face or lips, by superficial clear vesicles on an erythematous base that crust and heal within days. Reactivation is precipitated by various forms of trauma, fever, physiological changes or intercurrent disease, and may also involve other body tissues; it occurs in the presence of circulating antibodies, which are seldom elevated by reactivation. Severe and extensive spread of infection may occur in those who are immunodeficient or immunosuppressed. The onset of reactivation is heralded by tingling prior to the onset of vesicles; if patients learn this sign, they can prevent or shorten the clinical course of the reactivated infection through the use of antivirals.

CNS involvement may appear in association with either primary infection or recrudescence. HSV-1 is a cause of meningoencephalitis. Fever, headache, leukocytosis, meningeal irritation, drowsiness, confusion, stupor, coma and focal neurological signs may occur, and are frequently referable to one or the other temporal region. The condition may be confused with other intracranial lesions, including brain abscess and tuberculous meningitis. Because antiviral therapy may reduce case fatality, diagnostic PCR for DNA of herpes virus in the CSF or biopsy of cerebral tissue should be considered early in clinically suspected cases.

Genital herpes, usually caused by HSV-2, occurs mainly in adults and is sexually transmitted. Primary and recurrent infections occur, with or without symptoms. In women, the principal sites of primary disease are the cervix and the vulva; recurrent disease generally involves the vulva, perineal skin, legs and buttocks. In men, lesions appear on the glans penis or prepuce, and in the anus and rectum of those engaging in anal sex. Other genital or perineal sites, as well as the mouth, may be involved in men and women, depending on sexual practices. HSV-2 has been associated with aseptic meningitis and radiculitis rather than meningoencephalitis.

Neonatal infections can be divided into 3 clinical presentations: disseminated infections involving the liver; encephalitides; and infections limited to the skin, eyes or mouth. The first two forms are often lethal. Infections are most frequently due to HSV-2, but HSV-1 is also common. Risk to the infant depends on two important maternal factors: stage of pregnancy at which the mother excretes HSV, and whether the infection is primary or secondary. Only excretion at the time of delivery is dangerous to the newborn, with the rare exception of intrauterine infections. Newly acquired infection in the mother raises the risk of infection from about 1% to over 30%, presumably because maternal immunity confers a degree of protection.

Diagnosis of herpes simplex infection is by viral isolation, HSV DNA detection by polymerase chain reaction (PCR), HSV antigen detection by enzyme immunoassay (EIA), or direct immunofluorescence (IFA). This is done with samples from oral or genital lesions, or from spinal fluid in cases of encephalitis. Brain biopsy may be considered in some cases of the latter. A 4-fold titer rise in paired sera in various serological tests confirms the diagnosis of primary infection; the presence of herpes-specific IgM is suggestive but not conclusive evidence of primary infection. Reliable techniques to differentiate type 1 from type 2 antibody are now available in diagnostic laboratories; virus isolates can be distinguished readily from one another by DNA analysis. Type-specific serologic tests are not yet widely available.

2. Infectious agent—Herpes simplex virus in the virus family Herpes-viridae, subfamily Alphaherpesvirinae. HSV types 1 and 2 can be differentiated immunologically (especially when highly specific or monoclonal antibodies are used), and differ with respect to their growth patterns in cell culture, embryonated eggs and experimental animals.

3. Occurrence—Worldwide; 50%–90% of adults possess circulating antibodies against HSV-1; initial infection with HSV-1 usually occurs before the fifth year of life, but more primary infections in adults are now being reported. HSV-2 infection usually begins with sexual activity and is rare before adolescence, except in sexually abused children. HSV-2 antibody occurs in 20%–30% of American adults. The prevalence is greater (up to 60%) in lower socioeconomic groups and in persons with multiple sexual partners.

4. Reservoir—Humans.

5. Mode of transmission—Contact with HSV-1 in the saliva of carriers is probably the most important mode of spread. Infection on the hands of health care personnel (e.g. dentists) from patients shedding HSV results in herpetic whitlow. Transmission of HSV-2 is usually by sexual contact. Both types 1 and 2 may be transmitted to various sites by oral-genital, oral-anal or anal-genital contact. Transmission to the neonate usually occurs via the infected birth canal, less commonly *in utero* or postpartum.

6. Incubation period—From 2–12 days.

7. Period of communicability—HSV can be isolated for 2 weeks and up to 7 weeks after primary stomatitis or primary genital lesions. Both primary and recurrent infections may be asymptomatic. After either, HSV may be shed intermittently from mucosal sites for years and possibly lifelong, in the presence or absence of clinical manifestations. In recurrent lesions, infectivity is shorter than after primary infection, and usually the virus cannot be recovered after 5 days.

8. Susceptibility—Humans are probably universally susceptible.

9. **Methods of control—**

   A. *Preventive measures:*

   1) Health education and personal hygiene directed toward minimizing the transfer of infectious material.
   2) Avoid contaminating the skin of eczematous patients with infectious material.
   3) Health care personnel should wear gloves when in direct contact with potentially infectious lesions.
   4) When primary genital herpes infections occur in late pregnancy, caesarean section is advised before the membranes rupture because of the risk of fatal neonatal infection (30%–50%). The risk of fatal neonatal infection after a recurrent infection is much lower (3%–5%), and caesarean section is advisable only when active lesions are present at delivery.
   5) Use of latex condoms in sexual practice may decrease the risk of infection; no antiviral agent has yet been proved to be practical in prophylaxis of primary infection, although acyclovir or valacyclovir may be used prophylactically to reduce the incidence of recurrences.

   B. *Control of patient, contacts and the immediate environment:*

   1) Report to local health authority: Official case report in adults not ordinarily justifiable, Class 5; neonatal infections reportable in some areas, Class 3 (see *Reporting*).
   2) Isolation: Contact isolation for neonatal and disseminated or primary severe lesions; for recurrent lesions, drainage and secretion precautions. Patients with herpetic lesions should have no contact with newborns, children with eczema or burns, or immunodeficient patients.
   3) Concurrent disinfection: Not applicable.
   4) Quarantine: Not applicable.
   5) Immunization of contacts: Not applicable. Vaccine trials are ongoing.
   6) Investigation of contacts and source of infection: Seldom of practical value.
   7) Specific treatment: The acute manifestations of herpetic keratitis and early dendritic ulcers may be treated with trifluridine or adenine arabinoside as an ophthalmic ointment or solution. Corticosteroids should never be used for ocular involvement unless administered by an experienced ophthalmologist. Intravenous acyclovir is of value in herpes simplex encephalitis, but may not prevent residual neurological problems. Acyclovir used orally or intravenously has been shown to reduce shedding of virus, diminish pain, and accelerate healing time in primary genital and recurrent

herpes, rectal herpes, and herpetic whitlow. The oral preparation is most convenient to use and may benefit patients with extensive recurrent infections. However, mutant strains of herpes virus resistant to acyclovir have been reported. Valacyclovir and famciclovir are more recently licensed congeners of acyclovir that have equivalent efficacy. Prophylactic daily administration of these drugs can reduce the frequency of HSV recurrences in adults. Neonatal infections should be treated with high-dose intravenous acyclovir. Topical creams are not effective in genital herpes.

C. Epidemic measures: Not applicable.

D. Disaster implications: None.

E. International measures: None.

MENINGOENCEPHALITIS DUE TO CERCOPITHECINE HERPES VIRUS 1   ICD-9 054.3; ICD-10 B00.4
(B-virus, Simian B disease)

B-virus infection is a CNS disease caused by cercopithecine herpesvirus 1, a zoonotic virus closely related to HSV. It causes an ascending encephalomyelitis seen in veterinarians, laboratory workers and others in close contact with eastern Hemisphere monkeys or monkey cell cultures. After an incubation of 3 days to 3 weeks, there is acute febrile onset with headache, often local vesicular lesions, lymphocytic pleocytosis, and variable neurological patterns, ending in death in over 70% of cases, 1 day to 3 weeks after onset of symptoms. Occasional recoveries have been associated with considerable residual disability; a few cases, treated with acyclovir, have recovered completely. The virus causes a natural infection of monkeys analogous to HSV infection in humans; 30%–80% of rhesus monkeys (*Macaca mulatta*) are seropositive. During periods of stress (shipping and handling), they have high rates of viral shedding. Human illness, rare but highly fatal, is acquired through the bite of apparently normal monkeys, or exposure of naked skin or mucous membrane to infected saliva or monkey cell cultures. Prevention depends on proper use of protective gauntlets and care taken to minimize exposure to monkeys. All bite or scratch wounds incurred from macaques or from cages possibly contaminated with macaque secretions and that result in bleeding must be immediately and thoroughly scrubbed and cleaned with soap and water. Prophylactic treatment with an antiviral agent such as valacyclovir, acyclovir or famciclovir should be considered when an animal handler sustains a deep, penetrating wound that cannot be adequately cleaned, though it is not clear if this is as effective in humans as it is in rabbits. The B-virus status of the monkey should be determined to evaluate the risk.

The appearance of any skin lesions or neurological symptoms, such as itching, pain, or numbness near the site of the wound, calls for expert medical consultation for diagnosis and possible treatment.

HISTOPLASMOSIS
[CCDM19: M. Brandt]

ICD-9 115; ICD-10 B39

Two clinically different mycoses are designated as histoplasmosis; the pathogens that cause them cannot be distinguished morphologically when grown on culture media as molds. Detailed information is given for the infection caused by *Histoplasma capsulatum* var. *capsulatum*, and a brief summary for that caused by *H. capsulatum* var. *duboisii*.

I. INFECTION BY *HISTOPLASMA CAPSULATUM*
ICD-9 115.0; ICD-10 B39.4
(Histoplasmosis capsulati, Histoplasmosis due to *H. capsulatum* var. *capsulatum*, American histoplasmosis)

1. Identification—A systemic mycosis of varying severity ranging from symptom-free or minor self-limited to life-threatening illnesses. The primary lesion is usually in the lungs. While infection is common, overt clinical disease is not. Five clinical forms are recognized:

1) Asymptomatic: individuals manifest skin test reactivity to histoplasmin, but this reagent is no longer commercially available.
2) Acute respiratory: varies from a mild respiratory illness to temporary incapacity with general malaise, fever, chills, headache, myalgia, chest pains and nonproductive cough; occasional erythema multiforme and erythema nodosum. Multiple, small scattered calcifications in the lung, hilar lymph nodes, spleen and liver may be late findings.
3) Acute disseminated histoplasmosis: with debilitating fever, GI symptoms, evidence of bone marrow suppression, hepatosplenomegaly, lymphadenopathy and a rapid course; most frequent in infants and young children and immunocompromised patients including AIDS cases. Usually fatal unless treated.
4) Chronic disseminated disease: with low-grade intermittent fever, weight loss, weakness, hepatosplenomegaly, mild hematological abnormalities and focal manifestations of disease (e.g. endocarditis, meningitis, mucosal ulcers of mouth, larynx, stomach or bowel, and Addison disease). Subacute course progressing over 10-11 months and usually fatal unless treated.

   5) Chronic pulmonary form: clinically and radiologically resembling chronic pulmonary tuberculosis with cavitation; occurs most often in middle-aged and elderly men with underlying emphysema. Progresses over months or years, with periods of quiescence and sometimes spontaneous cure.

   Clinical diagnosis is confirmed by culture, DNA probe, or by visualizing the fungus in Giemsa- or Wright-stained smears of ulcer exudates, bone marrow, sputum or blood; demonstrating the fungus in biopsies of ulcers, liver, bone marrow, lymph nodes or lung requires special stains. Serology has been a vital instrument in the diagnosis of infection with *H. capsulatum*. The immuno-diffusion test is the most specific and reliable of available serological tests. The M antigen is detected in up to 80% of individuals after exposure to the fungus. A rise in complement fixation titers in paired sera may occur early in acute infection; a titer of 1:32 or greater is suggestive of active disease. Low levels of CF antibodies are detected in approximately 10% of healthy individuals who reside in an endemic region. False-negative tests are common, particularly in HIV-infected patients, and negative serology does not exclude the diagnosis. Detection of antigen in serum or urine is useful in making the diagnosis and following the results of treatment for disseminated histoplasmosis; however there is a high degree of cross-reactivity with patients infected with *Blastomyces dermatitidis*, *Paracoccidioides brasiliensis* and *Penicillium marneffei*.

2. Infectious agent—*Histoplasma capsulatum* (*Ajellomyces capsulatus*), a dimorphic fungus growing as a mold in soil and as a yeast in animal and human tissue.

3. Occurrence—Infections commonly occur in geographic foci over wide areas of the Americas, Africa, eastern Asia and Australia; rare in Europe. Hypersensitivity to histoplasmin (no longer manufactured) indicates antecedent infection and has been noted in as much as 80% of population in parts of eastern and central USA. Clinical disease is less frequent; severe progressive disease is rare. Prevalence increases from childhood to age 15; the chronic pulmonary form is more common in males. Outbreaks have occurred in endemic areas in families, students and workers with exposure to bird, chicken or bat droppings or recently disturbed contaminated soil. Histoplasmosis occurs in dogs, cats, cattle, horses, rats, skunks, opossums, foxes and other animals, often with a clinical picture comparable to that in humans.

4. Reservoir—Soil with high organic content and undisturbed bird droppings, in particular that around and in old chicken houses, in bat-caves, and around starling, blackbird and pigeon roosts.

5. Mode of transmission—Growth of the fungus in soil produces microconidia and tuberculate macroconidia; infection results from inhalation of airborne microconidia. Person-to-person transmission can occur only if infected tissue is inoculated into a healthy person.

6. Incubation period—Symptoms appear within 3–17 days after exposure but this may be shorter with heavy exposure; commonly 10 days.

7. Period of communicability—Not transmitted from person to person.

8. Susceptibility—Susceptibility is general. Inapparent infections are common in endemic areas and usually result in increased resistance to infection. May be an opportunistic infection in those with compromised immunity.

9. Methods of control—

A. *Preventive measures:* Minimize exposure to dust in a contaminated environment, such as chicken coops and surrounding soil. Spray with water or oil to reduce dust; use protective masks.

B. *Control of patient, contacts and the immediate environment:*

1) Report to local health authority: In selected endemic areas; in many countries not a reportable disease, Class 3 (see *Reporting*).
2) Isolation: Not applicable.
3) Concurrent disinfection: Of sputum and articles soiled therewith. Terminal cleaning.
4) Quarantine: Not applicable.
5) Immunization of contacts: Not applicable.
6) Investigation of contacts and source of infection: Household and occupational contacts for evidence of infection from a common environmental source.
7) Specific treatment: Itraconazole approved for pulmonary and disseminated histoplasmosis in non-HIV infected individuals. Amphotericin B followed by itraconazole for at least one year and until resolution of CSF abnormalities for patients with CNS histoplasmosis. For patients with acute disseminated histoplasmosis, IV amphotericin B is the drug of choice. Itraconazole constitutes effective chronic suppres-

sive therapy in AIDS patients previously treated with ampho-tericin B.

C. Epidemic measures: Occurrence of grouped cases of acute pulmonary disease in or outside of an endemic area, particularly with history of exposure to dust within a closed space (caves or construction sites), should arouse suspicion of histoplasmosis. Suspected sites such as attics, basements, caves or construction sites with large amounts of bird droppings or bat guano must be investigated.

D. Disaster implications: None. Possible hazard if large groups, especially from nonendemic areas, are forced to move through, live in, or disturb soil in areas where the mold is prevalent.

E. International measures: None.

II. HISTOPLASMOSIS DUE TO
H. DUBOISII   ICD-9 115.1; ICD-10 B39.5
(Histoplasmosis due to *H. capsulatum* var. *duboisii*, African histoplasmosis)

This usually presents as a subacute granuloma of skin or bone. Infection, though usually localized, may be disseminated in the skin, subcutaneous tissue, lymph nodes, bones, joints, lungs and abdominal viscera. Disease is more common in males and may occur at any age, but especially in the second decade of life. Thus far, the disease has been recognized only in Africa and Madagascar. Diagnosis is made through culture or demonstration of yeast cells of *H. capsulatum* var. *duboisii* in tissue by smear or biopsy. These cells are much larger than the yeast cells of *H. capsulatum* var. *capsulatum*. The true prevalence of *H. duboisii*, its reservoir, mode of transmission and incubation period are unknown. It is not communicable from person to person. Treatment is the same as for histoplasmosis due to *H. capsulatum*.

HOOKWORM DISEASE   ICD-9 126; ICD-10 B76
(Ancylostomiasis, Uncinariasis, Necatoriasis)
[CCDM19: M. Eberhard, A. Gabrielli, L. Savioli]
[CCDM18: L. Savioli]

1. Identification—A common chronic parasitic infection with a variety of symptoms, usually in proportion to the degree of anemia. In heavy infections, the bloodletting activity of the nematode leads to iron deficiency and hypochromic, microcytic anemia, the major cause of disability. Children with heavy long-term infection may have hypoproteinemia and may be retarded in mental and physical development. Occasionally, severe acute pulmonary and GI reactions follow exposure to infective larvae. Death is infrequent and usually can be attributed to other infections. Light hookworm infections generally produce few or no clinical effects. Infection is confirmed by finding hookworm eggs in feces; early stool examinations may be negative until worms mature. Species differentiation requires microscopic examination of larvae cultured from the feces, or examination of adult worms expelled by purgation following a vermifuge. PCR-RFLP techniques allow species differentiation.

2. **Infectious agents**—*Ancylostoma duodenale, A. ceylanicum, A. braziliense, A. caninum* and *Necator americanus*.

3. **Occurrence**—Endemic in tropical and subtropical countries where sanitary disposal of human feces is not practiced and soil, moisture and temperature conditions favor development of infective larvae. Also occurs in temperate climates under similar environmental conditions (e.g. mines). Both *Necator* and *Ancylostoma* occur in many parts of Asia (particularly southeastern Asia), the South Pacific and eastern Africa. *N. americanus* is the prevailing species throughout southeastern Asia, most of tropical Africa and America; *A. duodenale* prevails in North Africa, including the Nile Valley, northern India, northern parts of eastern Asia and the Andean areas of South America. *A. ceylanicum* occurs in southeastern Asia but is less common than either *N. americanus* or *A. duodenale. A. caninum* has been described in Australia as a cause of eosinophilic enteritis syndrome.

4. **Reservoir**—Humans for *A. duodenale* and *N. americanus*; cats and dogs for *A. ceylanicum, A. braziliense* and *A. caninum*.

5. **Mode of transmission**—Eggs in feces are deposited on the ground, embryonate, and hatch; under favorable conditions of moisture, temperature and soil type, larvae develop and become infective in 7-10 days. Human infection occurs when infective larvae penetrate the skin, usually of the foot; in so doing, they produce a characteristic dermatitis (ground itch). The larvae of *A. caninum* and *A. braziliense* die within the skin, having produced cutaneous larva migrans. Normally, the larvae of *Necator, A. duodenale, A. ceylanicum* and other *Ancylostoma* enter the skin and pass via lymphatics and bloodstream to the lungs, enter the alveoli, migrate up the trachea to the pharynx, are swallowed and reach the small intestine, where they attach to the intestinal wall, developing to maturity

in 6-7 weeks (3-4 weeks in the case of *A. ceylanicum*), and typically producing thousands of eggs per day. Infection with *Ancylostoma* may also be acquired by ingesting infective larvae; possible vertical transmission through breastmilk has been reported.

6. Incubation period—Symptoms may develop after a few weeks to many months, depending on intensity of infection and iron intake of the host. Pulmonary infiltration, cough and tracheitis may occur during the lung migration phase of infection, particularly in *Necator* infections. After entering the body, *A. duodenale* may become dormant for up to 8 months, after which development resumes, with a patent infection (stools containing eggs) a month later.

7. Period of communicability—No person-to-person transmission, but infected people can contaminate soil for several years in the absence of treatment. Under favorable conditions, larvae remain infective in soil for several weeks.

8. Susceptibility—Universal; no evidence that immunity develops with infection.

9. Methods of control—

   A. Preventive measures:

1) Educate the public to the dangers of soil contamination by human, cat or dog feces, and in preventive measures, including wearing shoes in endemic areas.
2) Prevent soil contamination by installation of sanitary disposal systems for human feces, especially sanitary latrines in rural areas. Night soil and sewage effluents are hazardous, especially where used as fertilizer.
3) Examine and treat people migrating from endemic to receptive nonendemic areas, especially those who work barefoot in mines, construct dams, or work in the agricultural sector.
4) WHO recommends a "preventive chemotherapy" strategy focused on treatment of high-risk groups at regular intervals, for the control of morbidity due to soil-transmitted helminth (STH) infections, including ascariasis, trichuriasis and hookworm disease. Recommended drugs and dosages are single-dose mebendazole (500 mg) or albendazole (400 mg, half dose for children 12-24 months). Action to be taken is differentiated according to prevalence of any STH infection (infection with at least one STH) among school-age children (aged 6-15 years):

Recommended treatment strategy for STH in preventive chemotherapy[a]

Category	Preva-lence of infection among school-age children	Action to be taken	
High-risk community	≥50%	Treat all school-age children (enrolled and not en-rolled) twice each year[b]	Also treat with the same frequency: • Preschool children (aged 1–5) • Women of childbear-ing age, including women in the 2nd and 3rd trimesters and lactating women • Adults at high risk in certain occupations (e.g. tea pickers and miners)
Low-risk community	≥20% and <50%	Treat all school-age chil-dren (enrolled and not enrolled) once each year	Also treat with the same frequency: • Preschool children (aged 1–5) • Women of childbear-ing age, including women in the 2nd and 3rd trimesters and lactating women • Adults at high risk in certain occupations (e.g. tea pickers and miners)

[a]When prevalence of any STH infection is less than 20%, large-scale preventive chemotherapy interventions are not recommended. Affected individuals should be dealt with on a case-by-case basis.

[b]If resources are available, a third drug distribution intervention might be added. In this case the appropriate frequency of treatment would be every 4 months.

Extensive monitoring has shown no significant ill effects of adminis-tration to pregnant women, but as a precautionary measure, women in the 1st trimester of pregnancy should not be treated. Administration of anthelminthics to very young children (1–2 years old) is safe, but some key recommendations should be followed: a) children should never be forced to swallow tablets; b) tablets should be crushed and mixed with water; c) treatment should be supervised by trained personnel.

B. Control of patient, contacts and the immediate environment:

1) Report to local health authority: Official report not ordinarily justifiable, Class 5 (see *Reporting*).
2) Isolation: Not applicable.
3) Concurrent disinfection: Safe disposal of feces to prevent contamination of soil.
4) Quarantine: Not applicable.
5) Immunization of contacts: Not applicable.
6) Investigate contacts and source of infection: Each infected contact and carrier is a potential or actual indirect spreader of infection.
7) Specific treatment: Single dose oral mebendazole (500 mg), or albendazole (400 mg, half dose for children 12–24 months); on theoretical grounds, both are contraindicated during the first trimester of pregnancy unless there are specific medical or public health indications. Single-dose pyrantel pamoate (10 mg/kg) or levamisole (2.5 mg/kg) are also effective. Adverse reactions are infrequent. Follow-up stool examination is indicated after 2 weeks, and treatment must be repeated if a heavy worm burden persists. Iron supplementation will correct the anemia and should be used in conjunction with de-worming. Transfusion may be necessary for severe anemia.

C. Epidemic measures: Prevalence survey in highly endemic areas: provide periodic mass treatment. Health education in environmental sanitation and personal hygiene, and provide facilities for excreta disposal.

D. Disaster implications: None.

E. International measures: None.

HYMENOLEPIASIS   ICD-9 123.6; ICD-10 B71.0

I. HYMENOLEPIASIS DUE TO *HYMENOLEPIS NANA*

(Dwarf tapeworm infection)
[CCDM19: M. Eberhard, A. Gabrielli, L. Savioli]
[CCDM18: L. Savioli]

1. Identification—An intestinal infection with very small tapeworms; light infections are usually asymptomatic. Massive numbers of worms may cause enteritis with or without diarrhea, abdominal pain and other vague symptoms such as pallor, loss of weight and weakness. Microscope identification of eggs in feces confirms diagnosis.

2. Infectious agent—*Hymenolepis nana* (dwarf tapeworm), the only human tapeworm without an obligatory intermediate host.

3. Occurrence—Cosmopolitan; more common in warm than cold, and in dry than wet climates. Dwarf tapeworm is the most common human tapeworm in the USA and Latin America; it is common in Australia, Mediterranean countries, the Near East and India.

4. Reservoir—Humans; possibly mice.

5. Mode of transmission—Eggs of *H. nana* are infective when passed in feces. Infection is acquired through ingestion of eggs in contaminated food or water; directly from fecally contaminated fingers (autoinfection or person-to-person transmission); or through ingestion of insects bearing larvae that have developed from eggs ingested by the insect. *H. nana* eggs, once ingested, hatch in the intestine, liberating oncospheres that enter mucosal villi and develop into cysticercoids; these rupture into the lumen and grow into adult tapeworms. Some *H. nana* eggs are immediately infectious when released from the proglottids in the human gut, so autoinfections or person-to-person transmission can occur. If eggs are ingested by mealworms, larval fleas, beetles or other insects, they may develop into cysticercoids that are infective to humans and rodents when ingested.

6. Incubation period—Onset of symptoms is variable; the development of mature worms requires about 2 weeks.

7. Period of communicability—As long as eggs are passed in feces. *H. nana* infections may persist for years.

8. Susceptibility—Universal; infection produces resistance to re-infection. Children are more susceptible than adults; intensive infection occurs in immunodeficient and malnourished children.

9. Methods of control—

A. Preventive measures:

1) Educate the public in personal hygiene, especially handwashing, and safe disposal of feces.
2) Provide and maintain clean toilet facilities.
3) Protect food and water from contamination with human and rodent feces.
4) Treat to remove sources of infection.
5) Eliminate rodents from home environment.

B. *Control of patient, contacts and the immediate environment:*

1) Report to local health authority: Official report not ordinarily justifiable, Class 5 (see *Reporting*).
2) Isolation: Not applicable.
3) Concurrent disinfection: Safe disposal of feces.
4) Quarantine: Not applicable.
5) Immunization of contacts: Not applicable.
6) Investigation of contacts and source of infection: Fecal examination of family or institution members.
7) Specific treatment: Drugs of choice are either praziquantel (15-25 mg/kg single dose) or niclosamide (children under 2 years: 500 mg on the first day then 250 mg daily for 6 days; children 2-6 years: 1 g on the first day then 500 mg daily for 6 days; children over 6 years and adults: 2 g on the first day then 1 g daily for 6 days). Nitazoxanide may be effective.

C. *Epidemic measures:* Outbreaks in schools and institutions can best be controlled through treatment of infected individuals and special attention to personal and group hygiene.

D. *Disaster implications:* None.

E. *International measures:* None.

II. HYMENOLEPIASIS DUE TO
HYMENOLEPIS DIMINUTA   ICD-9 123.6; ICD-10 B71.0
(Rat tapeworm infection, Hymenolepiasis diminuta)

The rat tapeworm, *H. diminuta*, occurs accidentally in humans, usually in young children. Eggs passed in rodent feces are ingested by insects such as flea larvae, grain beetles and cockroaches, in which cysticercoids develop in the hemocele. The mature tapeworm develops in rats, mice or other rodents when the insect is ingested. People are rare accidental hosts, usually of a single or few tapeworms; human infections are rarely symptomatic. Definitive diagnosis is based on finding characteristic eggs in the feces; treatment as for *H. nana*.

III. DIPYLIDIASIS   ICD-9 123.8; ICD-10 B71.1
(Dog tapeworm infection)

Toddler-age children are occasionally infected with the dog tapeworm (*Dipylidium caninum*), the adult of which is found worldwide in dogs and cats. It rarely, if ever, produces symptoms in the child, but is disturbing to the parent who sees motile, seed-like proglottids (tapeworm segments) at the anus or on the surface of the stool. Infection is acquired when the child ingests fleas that, in their larval stage, have eaten eggs from proglottids. In 3-4 weeks the tapeworm becomes mature. Infection is prevented by keeping dogs and cats free of fleas and worms; treatment as for *H. nana*.

INFLUENZA   ICD-9 487; ICD-10 J09, J10, J11

I. SEASONAL INFLUENZA ICD-9 487; ICD-10 J10, J11
[CCDM19: C. B. Bridges, A. Fry, K. Fukuda, N. Shindo]
[CCDM18: K. Stöhr]

1. Identification—An acute viral disease of the respiratory tract characterized by fever, cough (usually dry), headache, myalgia, prostration, coryza, and sore throat. Cough is often severe and can last 2 or more weeks; fever and other symptoms generally resolve in 5-7 days. In temperate climates, recognition is commonly based on clinical presentation during winter months with a syndrome consistent with influenza. Diagnosis improves when influenza surveillance information is available to indicate influenza viruses are in circulation. Influenza may be clinically indistinguishable from disease caused by other respiratory viruses, such as rhinovirus, RSV, parainfluenza, adenovirus and other pathogens. Syndromes consistent with influenza include acute upper respiratory illness, croup, bronchiolitis, febrile seizures, and pneumonia. In children, GI tract manifestations (nausea, vomiting, diarrhea) may accompany the respiratory phase, and have been reported in up to 25% of children in school outbreaks of influenza B and A (H1N1). GI manifestations are uncommon in adults. Infants may present with a sepsis-like syndrome. Older adults with influenza can present with worsening of underlying conditions such as congestive heart failure, and may not have an elevated temperature.

Point-of-care rapid testing is increasingly available to assist with diagnosis. Such tests are useful especially in rapidly establishing influenza as the basis for out-of-season outbreaks or outbreaks in remote areas where specimen transportation takes time. Such information can enable timely implementation of control measures. Commercially available point-of-care tests are generally 70% or less sensitive, but approximately 95% specific. Thus, particularly in the setting of a known influenza epidemic, negative results from patients with symptoms consistent with influenza must be interpreted cautiously. If excluding a false-negative result is important, then more sensitive testing should be considered, including viral culture and RT-PCR testing.

Yearly seasonal influenza epidemics impose a substantial health burden on all age groups, but the highest risk of complications occur among children less than 2 years, adults older than 64 years, and persons of any age with certain medical conditions, including chronic cardiovascular, pulmonary, renal, hepatic, hematologic or metabolic disorders (e.g. diabetes); immunosuppression; pregnancy; and neurologic/neuromuscular conditions that can compromise respiratory function or handling of respiratory secretions. Secondary complications of influenza include bacterial pneumonia, including co-infection with MRSA and S. pneumonia; viral pneumonia; worsening of underlying conditions; sinusitis; otitis media; febrile seizures; encephalitis/encephalopathy; myositis; and Reye syndrome in association with use of salicylates. Although seasonal influenza deaths can occur in any age group, over 90% of influenza deaths occur among those aged 65 years and older. Annual epidemics of influenza can be explosive and overwhelm health care services.

Most studies of the epidemiology of influenza have been conducted in developed countries in temperate climates, but more information is now being obtained from developing and tropical countries that have found higher risk of influenza complications and death among children less than 5 years, the elderly, and those with chronic diseases. Reports of influenza outbreak investigations in Africa and Indonesia suggest malnutrition and poor access to health care are likely to contribute to higher rates of complications and death.

Laboratory confirmation of influenza infection can be done by isolation of viruses from throat, nasal, and nasopharyngeal secretions or tracheal aspirate or washings using cell culture or in embryonated eggs; direct identification of viral antigens in nasopharyngeal cells and fluids (FA test or ELISA); rapid diagnostic tests; or viral RNA amplification. Demonstration of a 4-fold or greater rise in specific antibody titer between acute and convalescent sera can also be used to confirm acute infection. Single serological specimens cannot be used to diagnose an acute infection. Ideally, respiratory specimens should be collected as early in the illness as possible. Virus shedding starts to wane by the 3rd day of symptoms, and in most cases virus is not detected after 5 days in adults, though virus shedding can occur longer in children.

2. Infectious agents—Three types of seasonal influenza virus are recognized: A, B and C. The antigenic properties of the two relatively stable internal structural proteins, the nucleoprotein and the matrix protein, determine virus type. Influenza A viruses are further divided into subtypes based on two viral surface glycoproteins: the hemagglutinin (H) and the neuraminidase (N). There are 16 different hemagglutinin subtypes and 9 different neuraminidase subtypes. The current subtypes of influenza A viruses circulating widely among humans are A (H1N1) and A (H3N2). Aquatic birds are the primary reservoir for influenza A viruses and all subtypes of influenza A have been found among birds. Influenza A viruses also circulate among other animals, including pigs, horses, seals, and other animals. Influenza B viruses are not divided into subtypes, but two antigenically distinct lineages of B viruses currently circulate among humans. Humans are the primary reservoir for influenza B. Both influenza A and B viruses can be further classified into strains, and can cause seasonal outbreaks of influenza. Only the emergence and spread of influenza A viruses bearing an H or H/N combination to which most persons have never been exposed are known to cause pandemics. Type C influenza is associated with sporadic cases and minor localized outbreaks and imposes much less of a disease burden than influenza A and B. Only influenza A and influenza B viruses are included in seasonal influenza vaccines.

Levels of antibody against the hemagglutinin are the most important predictor of protection against infection by human influenza viruses. Antibody against the neuraminidase can reduce the severity of illness. Genes encoding these surface glycoproteins are constantly changing through mutations, a process termed "drift" that occurs during virus replication. The constant emergence of new influenza strains through drift requires the annual review and periodic replacement of vaccine strains. Usually, one or more strains are replaced in each year's vaccine. The constant emergence of new strains is the virologic basis for yearly epidemics of seasonal influenza and one of the main reasons why multiple influenza infections can occur in an individual over their lifetime. Influenza virus strains are named based on their type, geographic site of isolation, laboratory number, year of isolation, and subtype (for A viruses only). Examples are A/New Caledonia/20/99(H1N1); A/Brisbane/10/2007 (H3N2); and B/Malaysia/2506/2004.

3. Occurrence—Seasonal influenza results in yearly epidemics of varying severity, with sporadic cases or outbreaks of human disease occurring outside of typical seasonal patterns, and, rarely, as a pandemic. Clinical attack rates during annual epidemics can range from 5% to 20% in the general community to more than 50% in closed populations (e.g. nursing homes, schools). During yearly epidemics in industrialized countries, influenza illness often appears earliest among school-age children. The highest illness rates generally occur in children, with accompanying increases in school absences, physician visits, and pediatric hospital admissions. Influenza illness among adults is associated with increases in workplace absenteeism, adult hospital admissions, and mortality, especially among the elderly. In North America, epidemics generally last from 8–10 weeks. One or more strains, subtypes and/or types of influenza can circulate within a single influenza season in the same area. In temperate zones, epidemics tend to occur in winter months. In some tropical countries, influenza can occur year-round with 2 peaks per year consistent with peak activity in Northern and Southern Hemisphere temperate zones, and/or peaks during the rainy season.

4. Reservoir—Humans are normally infected by human influenza viruses (H3N2, H1N1 and B), and form the primary reservoir for these human viruses. With some notable exceptions, seasonal influenza usually is not a zoonotic disease.

5. Mode of transmission—The relative contribution of large droplet, droplet nuclei (i.e. airborne spread), and contact transmission (direct and indirect) in the spread of seasonal influenza is unknown, although large droplet spread is believed to be the primary means of transmission, through coughing and sneezing by infected persons. Human influenza virus may persist for hours on solid surfaces, particularly in lower temperatures and lower humidity.

6. Incubation period—Average 2 days (range 1–4) for seasonal influenza.

7. Period of communicability—In adults, viral shedding and probable communicability is greatest in the first 3–5 days of illness. In young children, virus shedding can occur for longer, 7–10 days, and may be even longer in severely immunocompromised persons.

8. Susceptibility—The size and relative impact of epidemics and pandemics depend upon several factors, including natural or vaccine-induced levels of protective immunity in the population, the age and condition of the population, strain virulence, and the extent of antigenic variation of new viruses. Infection induces immunity to the infecting virus and antigenically similar viruses. The duration and breadth of immunity depend, in part, upon the degree of antigenic similarity between viruses causing immunity and those causing disease. During seasonal epidemics, much of the population has partial protection, because of earlier infections from related viruses. Vaccines produce serological responses specific for the influenza vaccine virus strains, but can also provide cross-protection against related strains.

Age-specific attack rates during seasonal influenza epidemics reflect persisting immunity from past experience with variant viruses related to the epidemic subtype, so that the incidence of infection is often highest in children who have fewer prior influenza infections and less pre-existing antibody.

9. Methods of control—Detailed recommendations for the prevention and control of annual seasonal influenza epidemics are issued annually by national health agencies and WHO.

A. Preventive measures:

1) Educate the public and health care personnel in basic personal hygiene, including hand hygiene and cough etiquette, and especially transmission via unprotected coughs and sneezes, and from hand to mucous membranes.

2) Immunization with available inactivated influenza vaccines (IIV) and live virus vaccines may provide 70%-90% protection against infection in healthy young adults when the vaccine antigen closely matches the circulating strains of virus. Live attenuated influenza vaccines (LAIV), used in Russia for many years, are now also licensed in other industrialized countries for intranasal application in healthy

individuals aged 2–49. In the elderly, although immunization may be less effective in preventing illness, inactivated vaccines may reduce severity of disease and incidence of complications by 50%–60%, and deaths by approximately 80%. Influenza immunization should preferably be coupled with immunization against pneumococcal pneumonia for groups recommended to receive both vaccines (see *Pneumonia*).

A single dose suffices for those with prior exposures to influenza A and B viruses; 2 doses at least 4 weeks apart are essential for children less than 9 years old who have not previously been vaccinated against influenza. Routine immunization programs should focus efforts on vaccinating those at greatest risk of serious complications or death from influenza (see Identification, above) and those who might spread influenza (health care personnel and household contacts of high-risk persons) to high-risk persons. Immunization of children on long-term aspirin treatment is also recommended to prevent development of Reye syndrome after influenza infection.

The vaccine should be given each year before influenza is expected in the community; the timing of immunization should be based on a country's seasonal patterns of influenza circulation (i.e. winter months in temperate zones, often rainy season in tropical regions). Biannual recommendations for vaccine strain are based on the viral strains currently circulating, as determined by WHO through global surveillance.

Contraindications: Allergic hypersensitivity to egg protein or other vaccine components is a contraindication. During the swine influenza vaccine program in 1976, the USA reported an increased risk of developing Guillain-Barré syndrome (GBS) within 6 weeks after vaccination. Subsequent vaccines produced from other virus strains in other years have not been clearly associated with an increased risk of GBS. However, prior GBS is a contraindication for receiving an LAIV. The development of GBS within the 6 weeks following a dose of IIV is considered a precaution for future IIV use.

3) There are two classes of antiviral agents that are available for prophylaxis and treatment of influenza infections. Antiviral agents are supplemental to vaccine when immediate maximal protection is desired. The use of antiviral agents should be considered in persons at high risk for complications due to influenza, persons hospitalized with influenza, and during facility outbreaks. Antiviral agents are effective at reducing inter-facility transmission during outbreaks, such as among residents of nursing homes for the elderly. The drugs will not

interfere with the response to inactivated influenza vaccine, and should ideally be continued throughout the period of likely exposure to influenza. However, antivirals ideally should not be administered for 2 weeks after receipt of LAIV, and should be stopped for 2 days prior to LAIV vaccination. Treatment with antiviral agents within 48 hours of influenza symptom onset reduces the duration and severity of symptoms, and may reduce complications and deaths associated with influenza infections.

Inhibitors of influenza neuraminidase (oseltamivir and zanamivir) have been shown to be safe and effective for both prophylaxis and treatment of influenza A and B. Oseltamivir is an orally administered medicine; zanamivir is a powder administered via an inhaler. Oseltamivir may be used for persons 1 year and zanamivir is approved for treatment of persons 7 years and for prophylaxis for persons 5 years. Dosing is twice a day for 5 days for treatment and once a day for prophylaxis, with dosing for oseltamivir adjusted by body weight for children. Post-exposure prophylaxis should be continued for 7–10 days after a known exposure to influenza; however, prophylaxis used to prevent exposures throughout an influenza season would extend through the season. Few data, however, are available on the use of antiviral prophylaxis for more than 6 weeks. Reports of resistance to neuraminidase inhibitors have been rare until recently. In 2008, a significant increase in the number of oseltamivir-resistant influenza A (H1N1) viruses was detected in many countries. The proportion of viruses resistant to oseltamivir was variable among countries, and studies to characterize transmission and illness due to these viruses are underway. Resistance to zanamivir is rare. Serious cases of bronchospasm have been reported with zanamivir use in patients with and without underlying airways disease. Zanamivir use should be avoided in patients with underlying lung disease or reactive airway disease.

The adamantanes, amantadine and rimantadine, are effective for prophylaxis and treatment of influenza type A infection, but not influenza type B. Both adamantane agents may be used in persons 1 year of age. During treatment, 15–30% of patients develop resistance to adamantanes and resistant viruses are fully transmissible. Globally, adamantane resistance among influenza type A viruses is high. Therefore, routine use of adamantanes is not recommended. CNS side-effects are reported in 5%–10% of recipients of amantadine, and may be more severe in the elderly or those with impaired kidney function—the latter should receive reduced dosages that reflect the degree of renal impairment. Fewer CNS side effects have been reported with rimantadine use compared with amantadine.

B. *Control of patient, contacts and the immediate environment:*

1) Report to local health authority: Reporting outbreaks or laboratory-confirmed cases assists disease surveillance. Report identity of the infectious agent as determined by laboratory testing if possible, Class 1 (see *Reporting*). Untypable or new subtypes of influenza infections should be further tested by qualified laboratories, and public health authorities should be rapidly notified.

2) Isolation: Ideally, all persons admitted to a hospital with a respiratory illness, including suspected influenza, should be placed in single patient rooms or, if this is not possible, placed in a room with patients with similar illness (cohorting). When cohorting is used, adequate spacing between beds should be provided for droplet precautions. For influenza, isolation should continue for the initial 5–7 days of illness, and possibly longer for patients who are severely immunocompromised who may be infectious for longer periods. Both standard and droplet precautions are recommended.

3) Concurrent disinfection: Not applicable for seasonal influenza.

4) Quarantine: Not applicable for seasonal influenza.

5) Protection of contacts: A specific role has been shown for antiviral chemoprophylaxis (see 9A3). Clinicians should take local antiviral susceptibility information into account when prescribing antivirals.

6) Investigation of contacts and source of infection: Of no practical value during annual seasonal influenza epidemics.

7) Specific treatment: Antiviral agents begun within 48 hours of symptom onset reduce illness duration and may reduce complications associated with influenza (see 9A3).

    Patients should be watched for bacterial complications, including co-infection with MRSA, and antibiotics prescribed accordingly. Because of the association with Reye syndrome, avoid salicylates in children with suspected influenza infection.

C. *Epidemic measures:*

1) The severe and often disruptive effects of epidemic seasonal influenza on community activities may be reduced in part by effective health planning and education, particularly locally organized immunization programs for high-risk patients, their close contacts, and health care providers. Community

surveillance for influenza, use of outbreak control measures, adherence to infection control recommendations, and reporting of surveillance and outbreak findings to the community are all important.

2) Closure of individual schools has not been proven to be an effective measure to reduce the impact of seasonal influenza in a community, possibly because such measures are generally applied late in the course of an epidemic, due to high staff and student absenteeism rather than as an outbreak control measure.

3) Hospital administrators should anticipate increased demand for medical care during epidemic periods and possible absenteeism of health care personnel as a result of influenza. Health care personnel should be immunized annually to minimize absenteeism and transmission of seasonal influenza from health care personnel to patients.

4) Maintaining adequate supplies of appropriate antiviral drugs would be desirable to treat high-risk patients, persons hospitalized with influenza, and essential personnel in the event of the emergence of a new pandemic strain for which no suitable vaccine is available in time for the initial wave.

D. Disaster implications: Aggregations of people in emergency shelters will favor outbreaks of influenza if the virus is introduced.

E. International measures: A disease under surveillance by WHO. The following are recommended:

1) Report regularly on epidemiological situations within each given country to WHO/GISN (http://www.who.int/flunet).

2) Respiratory specimens, throat and nasal swabs, nasopharyngeal swabs or aspirates, and paired blood samples may be sent to any WHO-recognized National Influenza Center (http://www.who.int/csr/disease/influenza/centres/en/index.html). Identify the causative virus in reports, and submit prototype strains to one of the WHO Centers for Reference and Research on Influenza in Atlanta, London, Melbourne or Tokyo (http://www.who.int/influenza).

3) Conduct epidemiological studies; promptly identify and report viruses to national and international health agencies.

4) Ensure sufficient commercial and/or governmental facilities to provide rapid production of adequate quantities of vaccine and antiviral drugs, and maintain programs for vaccine and antiviral drug administration to high-risk persons and essential personnel.

II. INFLUENZA VIRUS INFECTION OF AVIAN AND OTHER ANIMAL ORIGIN

ICD-10 J09

1. Identification—Occasionally, a new subtype of influenza A emerges that is infectious for humans (a process termed shift). If such a virus is able to transmit from person to person efficiently enough to cause community outbreaks, then such a virus has the potential to cause a pandemic. Although most human infections with novel influenza A viruses probably result in sporadic cases or very limited human-to-human transmission, all human cases of novel influenza A infection must be considered a potential pandemic infection and should be investigated to assess the risk of human-to-human transmission. The first laboratory clue of a novel influenza A infection is the inability of available tests to subtype influenza A viruses. Suspicion is heightened if illness has occurred after exposure to birds, pigs or other animals that may be infected with influenza or exposure to their environments. Animal influenza A virus subtypes that have infected humans include H5N1, H7N2, H7N3, H7N7, H9N2, H10N7 and swine and avian H1 viruses, which are antigenically distinct from human H1 viruses. The current situation of widespread outbreaks of highly pathogenic avian influenza (HPAI) A(H5N1) virus infection among poultry is of a great concern because H5N1 virus is now endemic in poultry in some countries, causes high rates of death among infected poultry, and has resulted in a 60% case-fatality ratio among infected humans. Although human-to-human transmission of this H5N1 virus is currently limited and unsustained, continued vigilance is needed to detect changes in H5N1 viruses that might signal a pandemic. H5N1 viruses are dealt with in a separate section on influenza virus infection of avian and other animal origin, below.

New subtypes of influenza A can emerge among humans through direct transmission of an animal influenza virus to humans, or through reassortment of genes derived from an animal influenza virus and a human influenza virus. Such genetic reassortment can create a new virus that combines human and animal influenza properties. The 1918 pandemic virus is hypothesized to have developed from an avian influenza virus that adapted to humans. The 1957 and 1968 pandemic viruses were the result of genetic reassortment between avian and human influenza viruses. Pandemic viruses in the past have spread globally within 4 months of detection; modern air travel may further hasten the spread of a new pandemic virus, leaving little time for vaccine development, manufacturing or administration to the world's population. Planning for responses to pandemics ahead of actual pandemics is therefore critical for preparedness.

Human infections with avian H7 influenza virus have been reported, resulting in subclinical infections, conjunctivitis, and respiratory tract symptoms. In 2003, there were 89 human cases of avian influenza A

(H7N7) virus infection, including 1 death and limited human-to-human transmission in the Netherlands. In 2007, there were 4 cases of human infection with avian influenza A (H7N2) virus in the United Kingdom. In addition, four cases of avian influenza A (H9N2) illness in children in Hong Kong, SAR, China, were reported from 1999-2007. Swine influenza viruses have also caused illness in humans. Earlier, in 1976, the A/New Jersey/76 (Hsw1N1) influenza virus of swine origin caused severe respiratory illness in 13 soldiers, including one death, at Fort Dix, New Jersey, but did not spread beyond Fort Dix. Other human infections with swine influenza viruses have been sporadically identified, including 5 cases of human infection with a swine influenza A (H1N1) virus containing swine, avian, and human influenza virus genes (i.e. a triple reassortant) during 2007 in the United States. In most non-H5N1 cases, including swine influenza, symptoms associated with animal influenza virus infections have been similar to those for seasonal influenza infections. Conjunctivitis has been prominent in many cases of H7N7 and H7N2 infection. Of the animal influenza virus infections of humans, H5N1 has been the most studied and has the most advanced prevention guidance developed; thus this chapter will focus mostly on H5N1.

Diagnosis of animal influenza viruses often requires specialized laboratories, since these viruses cannot be typed by reagents used for seasonal influenza viruses. Detection of viral RNA in respiratory and other clinical specimens by means of conventional or real-time reverse-transcriptase polymerase chain reaction remains the best method for the initial diagnosis. Infection can be also confirmed by documenting seroconversion based upon a rise in antibody titer between an acute and a convalescent serum specimen. Otherwise, point-of-care rapid testing (also sometimes called "rapid tests") used for human influenza viruses have been insensitive for animal influenza viruses, and generally not useful. If an animal influenza virus infection is suspected, a negative test result by a point-of-care test does not exclude the presence of the virus infection.

Avian influenza A(H5N1) virus infection in humans: In 1997, the first avian influenza A(H5N1) outbreak among humans occurred in Hong Kong, SAR, China; since 2003, there has been a resurgence of H5N1 outbreaks, first among poultry in southeast Asia, with subsequent rapid spread to other parts of the world. In association with this panzootic in poultry, sporadic cases and clusters of human infection have been reported. Human H5N1 illness typically manifests as severe pneumonia, and the case fatality has been high (60%). Common initial symptoms are fever (usually higher than 38°C) and cough, plus signs and symptoms of lower respiratory tract involvement including dyspnea. Upper respiratory tract symptoms such as sore throat and coryza are present only sometimes. Gastrointestinal symptoms were frequently reported in cases in Thailand and Vietnam in 2004, but less frequently since 2005, suggesting that clinical presentations may differ depending on the virus (see II.2 for different virus clades). Severe lower respiratory tract manifestations often develop early in the course of illness, and clinically apparent pneumonia with radiological changes has usually been found at presentation. The disease progresses rapidly, and often progresses to an acute respiratory distress syndrome. Median times of 4 days from the onset of illness to presentation at a health care facility and 9 to 10 days until death in fatal cases has been reported. Atypical presentations have included fever and diarrhea without pneumonia, and fever with diarrhea and seizures progressing to coma. Common laboratory findings include leukopenia, lymphopenia, mild-to-moderate thrombocytopenia, and elevated levels of aminotransferases. Lymphopenia and increased levels of lactate dehydrogenase at presentation have been associated with a poor prognosis. Other reported abnormalities include elevated levels of creatine phosphokinase, hypoalbuminemia, and increased D-dimer levels and changes indicative of disseminated intravascular coagulopathy. Of six infected pregnant women, four have died, and the two survivors had spontaneous abortion. Mild illnesses such as upper respiratory illnesses without clinical or radiological signs of pneumonia have been reported more frequently recently in children. Limited seroepidemiologic studies conducted since 2004 suggest that subclinical infection appears uncommon.

2. **Infectious agents**—(See II.2). The first outbreak of highly pathogenic avian influenza (HPAI) A(H5N1) virus infections in humans—in Hong Kong, SAR, China, in 1997—was coincident with local outbreaks in poultry. In the intervening years, reports of limited H5N1 infections among birds in southeast Asia were reported, but starting in 2003, H5N1 infections led to large and recurring outbreaks in poultry. The viruses have spread, and are now entrenched among poultry populations in parts of Eurasia, Africa and the Middle East. In the summer of 2005, outbreaks in migratory birds in China preceded rapid spread of H5N1 through Mongolia and Russia to many European, Middle Eastern and African countries. A(H5N1) virus infections have been associated with high levels of mortality among poultry and substantial economic losses. Based on evolution of the hemagglutinin gene, H5N1 viruses can now be divided into 10 phylogenetically distinct clades that are antigenically distinguishable, and additional subclades; however, only 3 clades have caused human illness since 1997. The influenza A(H5N1) viruses that have infected humans so far have contained only avian influenza virus genes, and generally have been similar to strains circulating among poultry and wild birds in the same general location. Although migratory birds may sometimes spread A(H5N1) viruses to new geographic regions, their importance as a vector for spread is uncertain. Gene sequencing of some viruses isolated from infected humans showed mutations that may reflect some adaptation in humans.

3. **Occurrence**—

Epidemiology of Human infection with HPAI A(H5N1) virus: By the end of February 2008, over 360 cases of Human infection with HPAI

A(H5N1) virus in humans had been reported from Azerbaijan, Cambodia, China, Djibouti, Egypt, Indonesia, Iraq, Lao People's Democratic Republic, Myanmar, Nigeria, Pakistan, Thailand, Turkey and Viet Nam, with an overall case fatality of 64%. Regular updates on case counts are available at:

https://www.who.int/csr/disease/avian_influenza/country/en/index.html

Reasons for national differences in mortality are uncertain, but in all countries, mortality has been high. Potential differences could be differences in patient behaviors, types of viral exposure, time before case recognition, access to health care and/or clinical management, or differences in surveillance. The case fatality is highest among persons 10 to 19 years of age and lowest among persons 50 years of age or older. The median age of patients is approximately 18 years with 90% of patients 40 years of age or younger. In comparison to estimated numbers of poultry infections and human exposures to infected birds, human infections by an influenza A(H5N1) virus remain relatively rare. During situations in which there was close, prolonged and unprotected contact between a severely ill patient and a susceptible person, and most often a family member acting as a care giver, instances of non-sustained human-to-human transmission are thought to have occurred.

4. **Reservoir**—Aquatic birds are natural reservoirs of influenza A subtypes. For some avian influenza viruses, and particularly H5N1, the range of mammals that can be infected from aquatic birds (pigs, whales, seals, horses, ferrets, cats, dogs, tigers, etc.) has been wide. Domestic poultry are also infected, and are the main source of human infections. Swine influenza viruses are endemic in pigs. Influenza infections are also known to occur in other animals besides birds and pigs, including horses and dogs, but with the exception of pigs, influenza viruses have not been shown to transmit from these mammals to humans.

5. **Mode of transmission**—Most human infections by animal influenza viruses are thought to result from direct contact with infected animals. For H5N1 virus infection, the exact mode and sites of the virus entry are incompletely understood, but possibilities include inhalation of small particles to the lower respiratory tract, contamination of facial mucus membranes by self-inoculation or by droplet contact, or ingestion. In about one quarter of patients with influenza A(H5N1) virus infection, the source of exposure is unclear, and infection from exposure to contaminated environments remains possible. Visiting live-poultry markets is a recognized risk factor. Human-to-human transmission is thought to have occurred in some instances when there has been very close and prolonged contact between a very sick patient and care givers who have usually been family members. This observation suggests near-distance aerosol, droplet or direct contact may have been routes of transmission. However, the potential contribution of each route has not been demonstrated. No evidence to support long-distance airborne transmission has

been reported to date. For swine influenza virus infections in humans, close proximity to ill pigs or visiting a place where pigs are exhibited has been reported for most cases, but some human-to-human transmission, such as among soldiers in the 1976 Fort Dix outbreak and transmission to health care workers from an infected pregnant woman, has also occurred. Serologic studies show increased prevalence of swine influenza antibody among persons occupationally exposed to pigs compared to controls.

6. Incubation period—For H5N1 disease associated with poultry exposure, 7 days or less, and often 2–5 days. For swine influenza, 2–7 days has been reported.

7. Period of communicability—For H5N1 disease, limited data suggest that patients may remain infectious as long as 3 weeks, and perhaps even longer in immunosuppressed patients (e.g. those using corticosteroids). The longest documented period has been 27 days after the onset of illness, based upon detection of virus antigen in a patient's respiratory specimens.

8. Susceptibility—H5N1 illness occurs in all age groups, and limited serological studies demonstrate negligible pre-existing immunity in the subjects. Duration of protection from immunity generated by previous infection or immunization by an H5N1 vaccine is unknown. The role of host factors other than acquired immunity is uncertain.

9. Methods of control—

A. Preventive measures:

1) Preventing human exposure to infected animals or contaminated environments and controlling spread of infection among domesticated animal populations are critical elements for protecting humans from animal influenza virus infections. Guidelines for controlling outbreaks in domesticated animals have been issued by relevant national and international agencies (e.g. the Food and Agriculture Organization of the United Nations and the World Organization for Animal Health).

2) Rapid information sharing between animal and/or agricultural sectors and human health authorities is essential for timely implementation of public health actions. Social mobilization and risk communication targeting high-risk populations in affected areas are important measures for raising disease awareness and initiating protective behavioral changes.

3) Use of appropriate personal protective equipment (PPEs) and proper training is recommended for groups considered to be at high risk of exposure to infected birds (e.g. poultry workers, persons involved in mass culling operations, outbreak investigators, etc.). Following a probable exposure,

asymptomatic persons should be followed for signs of illness for at least one week, while symptomatic persons should be tested for infection, administered antiviral medicines, and monitored closely.

4) Immunization: Inactivated H5N1 vaccines for human use have been developed based on WHO recommended strains and licensed in several countries, but are not yet generally available, although this situation is expected to change. Some countries are stockpiling these vaccines as part of pandemic preparedness measures. Although immunogenic, the effectiveness of these vaccines in preventing the H5N1 infection or reducing disease severity is unknown. Use of seasonal influenza vaccination in certain high-risk animal exposure occupational groups is recommended in some countries for reducing influenza-like illness caused by seasonal influenza viruses. Such vaccines will not provide direct protection against animal influenza virus infections, but may prevent seasonal and animal influenza co-infections.

B. Control of patient, contacts and the immediate environment:

1) Report to local health authority: Laboratory-confirmed human infection with a novel subtype of influenza A virus, or influenza A infection where the virus cannot be subtyped, should be reported immediately to the national authority and then to WHO. Reporting to WHO is mandatory under the International Health Regulations (2005).

2) Isolation: When possible, suspected or confirmed cases with H5N1 and other non-human influenza virus infections should be treated using well-ventilated single isolation rooms with implementation of Standard and Droplet Precautions. Use of higher-level precautions such as airborne precautions may be considered when aerosol-generating procedures (e.g. sampling respiratory specimens, suction, use of nebulizers, intubation and mechanical ventilation) are to be performed.

3) Concurrent disinfection: Regular surface cleaning and disinfection with a commonly used detergent or hospital disinfectant is desirable during hospitalization and after removal of a patient from the room. Environmental disinfection should follow guidelines published by relevant agencies (e.g. Food and Agriculture Organization of the United Nations, World Organization for Animal Health).

4) Quarantine: Hospital isolation is recommended for symptomatic patients infected with novel influenza A viruses, including H5N1. In large-scale outbreak settings, voluntary home quarantine of contacts may be used. Symptomatic contacts

with mild illness that do not require hospitalization should be placed in isolation and provided with antiviral treatment.

5) Protection of contacts: A neuraminidase inhibitor drug (oseltamivir or zanamivir) should be administered as chemoprophylaxis for 7–10 days to close contacts (such as household or family members) after the last exposure to a person strongly suspected or confirmed to have a H5N1 infection. This includes pregnant women. Where neuraminidase inhibitors are not available, amantadine or rimantadine might be used for chemoprophylaxis of high-risk exposure groups if the virus is known or likely to be susceptible to these drugs. However, these drugs should not be used as chemoprophylaxis in pregnant women.

6) Investigation of contacts and source of infection: When an influenza infection with H5N1 is suspected, clinical samples (e.g. throat swab and other respiratory specimens) should be collected and tested to confirm infection. Virus isolation or PCR testing will allow further genetic characterization of the virus. When concomitant animal outbreaks are ongoing, co-ordination with the animal and/or agricultural sectors is essential. Epidemiological field investigations should identify the source of infection, identify situation-specific control measures, and determine whether human-to-human transmission has occurred. If a novel influenza virus is associated with efficient spread among people, then rapid containment, using antivirals and vaccines, may be indicated to try and prevent pandemic spread. The WHO protocol for such operation is available, and can be found at:

<http://www.who.int/csr/disease/avian_influenza/guide lines/RapidContProtOct15.pdf>

7) Specific treatment: The efficacy of antiviral drugs for treating non-seasonal influenza infections is uncertain, due to limited opportunities for documentation. For H5N1 disease, early treatment with oseltamivir is recommended, using the standard regimen indicated for treatment of seasonal influenza. Data from uncontrolled clinical studies suggest this improves survival, although the optimal dose and duration of therapy are uncertain and no data from controlled trials are available. Based on in vitro and animal studies suggesting improved outcomes, physicians may consider using higher doses of oseltamivir therapy, longer durations of treatment, or combination therapy (oseltamivir + amantadine). Clade 1 H5N1 viruses and most clade 2 subclade 1 H5N1 viruses from Indonesia are fully resistant to M2 inhibitors, whereas clade 2 subclade 2 H5N1 viruses from the lineages in other parts of

Eurasia and Africa and clade 2 subclade 3 H5N1 viruses from China are usually susceptible. During oseltamivir therapy, the emergence of highly resistant H5N1 variants was observed in Vietnamese patients, with fatal outcomes. Infection by viruses partially resistant to oseltamivir, before treatment, was reported in two Egyptian patients who died. Treatment of H5N1-associated ARDS should follow published national guidelines. In principle, early intervention by intermittent positive pressure ventilation (IPPV) using low tidal volumes and low pressure ventilation may help, and is recommended. Corticosteroid therapy has not been shown to be effective in patients with influenza A(H5N1) virus infection, and it has not been determined whether other immunomodulators and serotherapy are useful.

C. Epidemic measures:

1) Clinicians and local public health officers should be aware that human infections may occur in countries with outbreaks of influenza A(H5N1) among poultry. The clinical presentation of influenza A(H5N1) disease is nonspecific, and has often resulted in an initial misdiagnosis, especially in circumstances in tropical countries where endemic acute febrile diseases are common. Influenza A(H5N1) virus infection should be considered in the differential diagnosis for patients who present with fever, rapidly progressing atypical pneumonia and epidemiologic risk factors.

2) Develop or use a case definition and undertake active surveillance in the appropriate epidemiological setting for early detection of human cases. If an infection occurs or is strongly suspected, family members and household contacts should be placed under medical observation and provided with antiviral chemoprophylaxis or treatment according to national guidelines.

3) Establish a mechanism for rapidly obtaining reliable laboratory testing results. Characterization of the virus and its susceptibility to antivirals are important factors for disease control.

4) Provide information about the disease and preventive measures to at-risk population. Social mobilization including sensitization campaigns may be required for effective message penetration. Timely provision of information to the public is essential.

5) Collect epidemiological, clinical and other information to assess the situation. If efficient human-to-human transmission is observed, a large-scale containment operation should be considered to stop further spread of the infection (see 9B6).

D. Disaster implications: The emergence of an animal virus with the capacity to transmit and spread easily among humans could result in a global pandemic.

E. International measures: Human influenza caused by a new subtype is subject to notification to WHO under IHR (2005), Class 1 (see *Reporting*).

1) Any specimen from a patient suspected of novel influenza A virus infection, including H5N1, should be immediately tested and forwarded to a national reference laboratory or WHO Collaborating Centre/Reference Laboratories for confirmatory testing. WHO Collaborating Centres provide support as required—more information on the Centres can be found at:

    <http://www.who.int/collaboratingcentres/database/en/>

2) Under the 2005 International health regulations, human influenza caused by a new subtype is considered as an event that may constitute a public health emergency of international concern.

3) Continued viral and disease surveillance is critical for identifying human infections caused by influenza viruses of animal origin, including H5N1, and determining their ability to transmit efficiently among humans.

    Pandemic Influenza: The response to an influenza pandemic must be planned at the local, national and international levels; guidance is provided on the WHO website:

    <http://www.who.int/csr/disease/avian_influenza/en/>

    Similar information is available on the websites of many governments, including that of the USA at:

    <www.pandemicflu.gov>

KAWASAKI SYNDROME   ICD-9 446.1; ICD-10 M30.3
(Kawasaki disease, Mucocutaneous lymph node syndrome, Acute febrile mucocutaneous lymph node syndrome)
[CDDM19: Editorial Board]
[CCDM18: H. Yanagawa]

1. Identification—An acute febrile, self-limited, systemic vasculitis of early childhood, presumably of infectious or toxic origin. Clinically characterized by a high, spiking fever, unresponsive to antibiotics, associated with pronounced irritability and mood change; usually solitary and frequently unilateral non-suppurative cervical adenopathy; bilateral non-exudative bulbar conjunctival injection; an enanthem consisting of a "strawberry tongue," injected oropharynx or dry fissured or erythematous lips; limb changes consisting of edema, erythema or periungual/generalized desquamation; and a generalized polymorphous erythematous exanthem that can be truncal or perineal, and which ranges from morbilliform maculopapular rash to urticarial rash or vasculitic exanthem.

Typically there are 3 phases:

a) Acute febrile phase of about 10 days, characterized by high, spiking fever, rash, adenopathy, peripheral erythema or edema, conjunctivitis and enanthem.

b) Sub-acute phase lasting about 2 weeks, with thrombocytosis, desquamation, and resolution of fever.

c) Lengthy convalescent phase, during which clinical signs fade.

The case-fatality rate is 0.1%; half the deaths occur within 2 months of illness.

There is no pathognomonic laboratory test for Kawasaki syndrome, but an elevated ESR, C-reactive protein and platelet counts above 450 000/mm^3 (SI units 450 109/L) are common laboratory features.

According to *Diagnostic Guidelines of Kawasaki Disease* (Japan Kawasaki Disease Research Committee, 2002), at least 5 of the following 6 principal symptoms should be satisfied for diagnosis (although patients with 4 principal symptoms can be diagnosed when coronary aneurysm or dilatation is recognized by two-dimensional echocardiography or coronary angiography):

i) Fever persisting 5 days or more (including cases in whom the fever has subsided before the 5th day in response to treatment).

ii) Bilateral conjunctival congestion.

iii) Changes of lips and oral cavity: reddening of lips, strawberry tongue, diffuse injection of oral and pharyngeal mucosa.

iv) Polymorphous exanthema.

v) Changes of peripheral extremities: reddening of palms and soles, indurative edema in the initial stage, and membranous desquamation from fingertips in the convalescent stage.

vi) Acute non-purulent cervical lymphadenopathy.

2. **Infectious agent**—Unknown. Postulated to be a superantigen bacterial toxin secreted by *Staphylococcus aureus* or group A streptococci, but this has neither been confirmed nor is it generally accepted.

3. Occurrence—Worldwide; most cases (around 170 000) reported from Japan, with nationwide epidemics documented in 1979, 1982 and 1986. In North America, the estimated number of new cases each year is about 2 000. Approximately 80% of cases are diagnosed in children under 5, with a peak incidence at 1–2 years, more in boys than in girls. Cases are more frequent in the winter and spring. In Japan, where the disease has been tracked since 1970, peak incidence occurred in 1984–1985. Since then, the incidence rate has been steady, about 140 per 100 000 children under 5.

4. Reservoir—Unknown, perhaps humans.

5. Mode of transmission—Unknown; no firm evidence of person-to-person transmission, even within families. Seasonal variation, limitation to the pediatric age group and outbreak occurrence in communities are all consistent with an infectious etiology.

6. Incubation period—Unknown.

7. Period of communicability—Unknown.

8. Susceptibility and resistance—In North America, children, especially those of Asian ancestry, are most likely to develop the syndrome, but the majority of cases are reported among Caucasian children and American children of African origin. Recurrences appear infrequent (3% of reported patients in Japan).

9. Methods of control—

   A. Preventive measures: Unknown.

   B. Control of patient, contacts and the immediate environment:

   1) Report to local health authority: Clusters and epidemics should be reported immediately, Class 5 (see *Reporting*).
   2) Isolation: Not applicable.
   3) Concurrent disinfection: Not applicable.
   4) Quarantine: Not applicable.
   5) Immunization of contacts: Not applicable.
   6) Investigation of contacts: Not beneficial except in outbreaks and clusters.
   7) Specific treatment: High-dose IVIG, preferably as a single dose, within 10 days of onset of fever can reduce fever, inflammatory signs and aneurysm formation and should be considered even if the duration of fever exceeds 10 days. About 10% of patients may not respond and may require re-treatment. Recourse to high doses of aspirin is recommended during the acute phase, followed by low doses for at least 2 months. Measles and/or varicella vaccination should usually be deferred following receipt of IVIG.

C. Epidemic measures: Investigate outbreaks and clusters to elucidate etiology and risk factors.

D. Disaster implications: None.

E. International measures: None.

LASSA FEVER   ICD-9 078.8; ICD-10 A96.2
[CCDM19: P. Rollin]
[CCDM18: C. Roth]

1. Identification—Acute viral illness of 1–4 weeks duration. Onset is gradual, with malaise, fever, headache, sore throat, cough, nausea, vomiting, diarrhea, myalgia and chest and abdominal pain; fever is persistent or spikes intermittently. Inflammation and exudation of the pharynx and conjunctivae are common. About 80% of human infections are mild or asymptomatic; the remaining cases have severe multisystem disease. Disease is more severe in pregnancy; fetal loss occurs in more than 80% of cases and maternal death is frequent. In severe cases, hypotension or shock, pleural effusion, hemorrhage, seizures, encephalopathy and edema of the face and neck are frequent, often with albuminuria and hemoconcentration. Early lymphopenia may be followed by late neutrophilia. Platelet counts are moderately depressed, and platelet function is abnormal. Transient alopecia and ataxia may occur during convalescence, and eighth cranial nerve deafness occurs in 25% of patients, of whom only half recover some function, after 1–3 months. The overall case-fatality rate is about 1%, as high as 15% among hospitalized cases, and even higher in some epidemics. The mortality rate is particularly high among women in the third trimester of pregnancy, and fetuses. Aspartate aminotransferase (AST) levels above 150 and high viremia are poor prognosis indicators for the patient. Unapparent infections, diagnosed serologically, are common in endemic areas.

Diagnosis is through IgM antibody capture and antigen detection (ELISA), or detection of the viral genome by PCR; isolation of virus from blood, urine or throat washings; and IgG seroconversion by ELISA. Laboratory specimens must be handled with extreme care, including BSL-4 containment for virus isolation attempts, if available. Heating serum at 60°C (140°F) for 1 hour will inactivate the virus, and the serum can then be used to measure heat-stable substances such as electrolytes, blood urea nitrogen or creatinine. Specific immunohistochemistry assay could be used for Lassa fever diagnostic on fixed tissues.

2. Infectious agent—Lassa virus, an arenavirus, serologically related to lymphocytic choriomeningitis (Old World arenavirus group), and arenaviruses from the New World (Machupo, Junín, Guanarito and Sabiá viruses).

3. Occurrence—Endemic in Guinea, Liberia, regions of Nigeria, and Sierra Leone. Serologically related viruses of lesser virulence for laboratory hosts in Central African Republic (Mobala) Mozambique and Zimbabwe (Mopeia) have not yet been associated with human infection or disease.

4. Reservoir—Wild rodents; in western Africa, the multimammate mouse of the *Mastomys* species complex.

5. Mode of transmission—Primarily through aerosol or direct contact with excreta of infected rodents deposited on surfaces such as floors and beds or in food and water. Laboratory infections occur, especially in the hospital environment, through inoculation with contaminated needles and through the patient's pharyngeal secretions or urine. Infection can also spread from person to person by sexual contact through semen for up to three months after infection.

6. Incubation period—Commonly 6-21 days.

7. Period of communicability—Person-to-person spread may theoretically occur during the acute febrile phase when virus is present in secretions and excretions. Virus may be excreted in urine of patients for 3-9 weeks from onset of illness. Infection can also spread from person to person by sexual contact through semen for up to three months after infection.

8. Susceptibility—All ages are susceptible; the duration of immunity following infection is unknown.

9. Methods of control —

    A. **Preventive measures:** Specific rodent control.

    B. **Control of patient, contacts and the immediate environment:**

       1) Report to local health authority: Individual cases should be reported, Class 2 (see *Reporting*).

       2) Isolation: Institute immediate strict isolation in a private hospital room away from traffic patterns. Entry of non-essential staff and visitors should be restricted. Nosocomial transmission has occurred, and strict procedures for isolation of body fluids and excreta must be maintained. Recourse to a negative pressure room and respiratory protection is desirable. Male patients should refrain from unprotected sexual activity. To reduce infectious exposure, laboratory tests should be kept to the minimum necessary for proper diagnosis and patient care, and only performed where full infection control measures are correctly implemented. Technicians must be alerted to the nature of the specimens and supervised to ensure application of appropriate specimen inactivation/isolation procedures. Dead

bodies should be sealed in leak-proof material and cremated or buried promptly in a sealed casket.

3) Concurrent disinfection: Patient's excreta, sputum, blood and all objects with which the patient has had contact, including laboratory equipment used to carry out tests on blood, must be disinfected with 0.5% sodium hypochlorite solution or 0.5% phenol with detergent, and, as far as possible, effective heating methods—such as autoclaving, incineration, boiling or irradiation—should be used as appropriate. Laboratory testing must be carried out in special high containment facilities; if there is no such facility, tests should be kept to a minimum and specimens handled by experienced technicians using all available personal protective equipment, such as gloves, gowns, masks, goggles and biological safety cabinets. When appropriate, serum may be heat-inactivated at 60°C (140°F) for 1 hour. Thorough terminal disinfection with 0.5% sodium hypochlorite solution or a phenolic compound is adequate; formaldehyde fumigation can be considered.

4) Quarantine: Surveillance is recommended for close contacts (see 9B6).

5) Immunization of contacts: Not applicable.

6) Investigation of contacts and source of infection: Identify all close contacts (people living with, caring for, testing laboratory specimens from, or having non-casual contact with the patient) in the 3 weeks after the onset of illness. Establish close surveillance of contacts as follows: body temperature checks at least 2 times daily for at least 3 weeks after last exposure. In case of temperature above 38.3°C (101°F), hospitalize immediately in strict isolation facilities. Determine patient's place of residence during 3 weeks prior to onset; search for unreported or undiagnosed cases.

7) Specific treatment: Ribavirin, most effective within the first 6 days of illness, should be given IV, 30 mg/kg initially, followed by 15 mg/kg every 6 hours for 4 days and 8 mg/kg every 8 hours for 6 additional days.

C. *Epidemic measures:* Rodent control; storing of grains and other food in rodent-proof containers; adequate infection control and barrier nursing measures in hospitals and health facilities; availability of ribavirin; contact tracing and follow-up.

D. *Disaster implications: Mastomys* may become more numerous in homes and food storage areas and increase the risk of human exposures.

E. *International measures:* Notification of source country and to receiving countries of possible exposures by infected travelers.

Lassa fever is listed as one of the etiologic agents that need to be assessed in terms of their potential to cause Public Health Emergencies of International Concern under the IHR (2005) (Annex 2). For more information on the IHR (2005), see the chapter on *Communicable Disease Control and the International Health Regulations (2005)*. WHO Collaborating Centres provide support as required. More information can be found at: <http://www.who.int/collaboratingcentres/database/en/>

LEGIONELLOSIS ICD-9 482.8; ICD-10 A48.1
(Legionnaires' disease; Legionnaires' pneumonia)

NONPNEUMONIC LEGIONELLOSIS ICD-10 A48.2
(Pontiac fever)
[CCDM19: L. Hicks]

1. Identification—An acute bacterial disease with two distinct clinical manifestations: Legionnaires' disease (ICD-10 A48.1) and Pontiac fever (ICD-10 A48.2). Both conditions present with anorexia, malaise, myalgia, headache, and fever. Abdominal pain and diarrhea are also common. Legionnaires' disease is a common cause of pneumonia and is characterized by a nonproductive cough. Chest radiograph findings are variable and may show patchy or focal areas of consolidation or bilateral involvement. The illness can be quite severe, and may ultimately progress to respiratory failure. Despite improvements in diagnostics and treatment options, case fatality rates remain at approximately 15%. Pontiac fever is a self-limited febrile illness that does not progress to pneumonia or death. Cough may or may not be present. Patients recover spontaneously in 2–5 days without treatment. This clinical syndrome may represent reaction to inhaled *Legionella* antigen rather than bacterial invasion.

Diagnosis of Legionnaires' disease depends on isolating the causative organism on special media (BCYE), detecting *Legionella pneumophila* serogroup 1 antigens in the urine, or measuring a 4-fold rise in immunofluorescent antibody titer to *L. pneumophila* serogroup 1 between acute phase serum and serum drawn 3–6 weeks later. Urine antigen and serologic testing is specific to *L. pneumophila* serogroup 1, so disease due to other serogroups or species will be missed, emphasizing the importance of culture. Direct immunofluorescent antibody stain of involved tissue or respiratory secretions may be used, but sensitivity and specificity are highly variable and dependent upon the experience of laboratory personnel. Diagnosis of Pontiac fever is usually made by identifying symptoms consistent with the disease in the appropriate epidemiologic setting. Urine antigen and serologic testing can be used to confirm the diagnosis, but the sensitivity of diagnostic testing is lower than for Legionnaires' disease.

2. Infectious agent—*Legionellae* are poorly staining, Gram-negative bacilli. Of the 18 serogroups of *L. pneumophila* currently recognized, *L. pneumophila* serogroup 1 is most commonly associated with disease. Related organisms, including *L. micdadei*, *L. bozemanii*, *L. longbeachae* and *L. dumoffii* have been isolated, predominantly from immunosuppressed patients with pneumonia. Currently, 48 species of *Legionella* and at least 70 distinct serogroups are recognized.

3. Occurrence—The disease has been identified throughout North America, as well as in Asia, Africa, Australia, Europe and South America. Although cases occur throughout the year, both sporadic cases and outbreaks are recognized more commonly in summer and autumn. In the few locations studied, antibodies to *L. pneumophila* serogroup 1 occur at a titer of 1:128 or greater in 1%-20% of the general population. The proportion of community-acquired pneumonia cases that are due to *Legionella* ranges between 0.5% and 5.0%. Outbreaks of Legionnaires' disease may be difficult to detect due to low attack rates (0.1%-5%). Epidemic Pontiac fever tends to have an explosive presentation; attack rates as high as 95% have been documented.

4. Reservoir—Legionellosis is a waterborne disease. In certain conditions potable water systems (showers), air conditioning cooling towers, evaporative condensers, humidifiers, whirlpool spas, respiratory therapy devices and decorative fountains can harbor *Legionella*. Conditions that are conducive to *Legionella* growth include warm water temperatures (25-42°C), stagnation, scale and sediment, and low biocide levels.

5. Mode of transmission—Epidemiological evidence supports airborne transmission; other modes are possible, including aspiration of water.

6. Incubation period—Legionnaires' disease 2-10 days, most often 5-6 days; Pontiac fever 5-72 hours, most often 24-48 hours.

7. Period of communicability—Person-to-person transmission has not been documented.

8. Susceptibility—Risk factors for illness include increasing age (most cases are >50 years), cigarette smoking, diabetes mellitus, chronic lung disease, renal disease, malignancy; and compromised immunity, particularly patients who are receiving corticosteroids or who have had an organ transplant. Male:female ratio is about 2.5:1. The disease is rare in people aged less than 20. Several outbreaks have occurred among hospitalized patients.

9. **Methods of control—**

A. *Preventive measures:* Man-made water supplies are the primary sources for legionellosis; therefore conditions known to enhance *Legionella* growth need to be avoided. Cooling towers should be drained when not in use and mechanically cleaned periodically to remove scale and sediment. Appropriate biocides should be used to limit the growth of *Legionella* and the formation of protective biofilms. Maintaining hot water system temperatures at 50°C or higher may reduce the risk of transmission. Tap water should not be used in respiratory therapy devices.

B. *Control of patient, contacts and the immediate environment:*

1) Report to local health authority: In many countries, not a reportable disease, Class 3 (see *Reporting*).
2) Isolation: Not applicable.
3) Concurrent disinfection: Not applicable.
4) Quarantine: Not applicable.
5) Immunization of contacts: Not applicable.
6) Investigation of contacts and source of infection: Search (households, business, and health care settings) for additional cases that have shared water exposures. Two or more cases of legionellosis occurring among travelers to the same destination should trigger additional case finding and an environmental assessment. When a case of laboratory-confirmed health care-associated Legionnaires' disease is identified, an epidemiologic investigation should be conducted to identify additional cases. The threshold for initiating environmental sampling and remediation varies among published guidelines, but sampling should be considered for any cluster of health care-associated legionellosis.
7) Specific treatment: Pontiac fever is self-limited and does not require antimicrobial therapy. The recommended treatment for Legionnaires' disease is either a respiratory fluoroquinolone, such as levofloxacin, or a newer macrolide (azithromycin). Observational studies suggest that levofloxacin may be more effective than macrolides, especially in severe cases. Rifampicin has been used as an adjunct in patients failing standard therapy, but data to support this approach are lacking. Penicillin, the cephalosporins and the aminoglycosides are ineffective.

C. *Epidemic measures:* Identify common exposures and review maintenance logs for water systems that are potential sources of infection. Culture of the potential source(s) may be necessary to determine the cause for the outbreak. Remediation by super-chlorination and/or superheating implicated water supplies has been effective. Other remediation methods are under investigation. Proper maintenance and disinfection of whirlpool spas, cooling towers, and potable water supplies are the most effective measures to prevent outbreaks.

D. Disaster implications: None known.

E. International measures: None.

LEISHMANIASIS   ICD-9 085; ICD-10 B55
[CCDM19: C. Bern, M. Eberhard]
[CCDM18: P. Desjeux]

I. CUTANEOUS AND MUCOSAL LEISHMANIASIS

ICD-9 085.1-085.5;
ICD-10 B55.1, B55.2

(Aleppo evil, Baghdad boil, Delhi boil, Oriental sore; in the Americas, Espundia, Uta, Chiclero ulcer)

1. Identification—A polymorphic protozoan disease of skin and mucous membranes caused by several species of the genus *Leishmania*. These protozoa exist as obligate intracellular parasites in humans and other mammalian hosts. The disease starts with a macule, then a papule that enlarges and typically becomes an indolent ulcer in the absence of bacterial infection. Lesions may be single or multiple, occasionally non-ulcerative and diffuse. Lesions may heal spontaneously within weeks to months, or last for a year or more. In some individuals, certain strains (mainly from the Western Hemisphere) can disseminate to cause mucosal lesions (espundia), even years after the primary cutaneous lesion has healed. In the eastern hemisphere, a chronic granulomatous legion occurs, called the recidivans form. These sequelae, which involve nasopharyngeal tissues, are characterized by progressive tissue destruction and often scanty presence of parasites, and can be severely disfiguring. Recurrence of cutaneous lesions after apparent cure may occur as ulcers, papules or nodules, at or near the healed original ulcer.

Diagnosis is through microscope identification of the non-motile, intracellular form (amastigote) in stained specimens from lesions, and through culture of the motile, extra-cellular form (promastigote) on suitable media. An intradermal (Montenegro) test with leishmanin, an antigen derived from promastigotes, is usually positive in established disease; it is not helpful with very early lesions, anergic disease, or immunosuppressed patients. Serological (IFA or ELISA) testing can be done, but antibody levels are typically low or undetectable; this may not be helpful in diagnosis (except for mucosal leishmaniasis). Species identification is based on biological (development in sandflies, culture media and animals), immunological (monoclonal antibodies), molecular (DNA techniques) and biochemical (isoenzyme analysis) criteria. The WHO operational case definition is "a person showing clinical signs [of leishmaniasis] with parasitological confirmation and/or, *for mucosal leishmaniasis only*, serological diagnosis."

2. Infectious agents—Eastern hemisphere: *Leishmania tropica*, *L. major*, *L. aethiopica*. Western hemisphere: *L. braziliensis* and *L. mexicana* complexes. Members of the *L. braziliensis* complex are more likely to produce mucosal lesions; *L. tropica* is the usual cause of "leishmaniasis recidivans" cutaneous lesions. Members of *L. donovani* complex usually cause visceral disease in the eastern hemisphere; in the western hemisphere the responsible organism is *L. infantum/chagasi*. Both may cause cutaneous leishmaniasis without concomitant visceral involvement, as well as post-kala-azar dermal leishmaniasis cases, which are considered residual reservoirs for the maintenance and dissemination of the parasite.

3. Occurrence—2 million new cases per year: China (recently); India; Pakistan; southwestern Asia, including Afghanistan and Iran; southern regions of the former Soviet Union; the Mediterranean littoral; the sub-Saharan African savanna; Sudan; the highlands of Ethiopia and Kenya; Namibia; the Dominican Republic, Mexico (especially Yucatan); south central Texas; all of central America; and every country of South America except Chile and Uruguay. Leishmania have also recently been reported among kangaroos in Australia. A non-ulcerative, keloid-like form due to *L. infantum/chagasi* (atypical cutaneous leishmaniasis) has been observed with increasing frequency in central America, especially Honduras and Nicaragua. Numerous cases of diffuse cutaneous leishmaniasis have been reported in the past from the Dominican Republic and Mexico. In some areas in the eastern hemisphere, urban population groups, including children, are at risk for anthroponotic cutaneous leishmaniasis due to *L. tropica*. In rural areas, people are at risk for zoonotic cutaneous leishmaniasis due to *L. major*. In the western hemisphere, disease is usually restricted to special groups, such as those working in forested areas, those whose homes are in or next to a forest, and visitors to such areas from non-endemic countries. Cutaneous leishmaniasis is generally more common in rural than urban areas, with the exception of *L. tropica*, which can cause large urban outbreaks—such as that in Kabul, Afghanistan, in the late 1990s.

4. Reservoir—Locally variable; humans (in anthroponotic cutaneous leishmaniasis); wild rodents (gerbils); hyraxes; edentates (sloths); marsupials; and domestic dogs (considered victims more than real reservoirs). Unknown hosts in many areas.

5. Mode of transmission—In zoonotic foci, from the animal reservoir through the bite of infective female phlebotomines (sandflies). Motile promastigotes develop and multiply in the gut of the sandfly after it has fed on an infected mammalian host; in 8–20 days, infective parasites develop and are injected during biting. In humans and other mammals, the organisms are taken up by macrophages and transform into amastigote forms, which multiply within the macrophages until the cells rupture, enabling spread to other macrophages. In anthroponotic foci, indirect person-to-person transmission occurs through sandfly bites and, very rarely, through transfusion.

6. Incubation period—At least a week, up to many months.

7. Period of communicability—Not directly transmitted from person to person, but infectious to sandflies as long as parasites remain in lesions in untreated cases, usually a few months to 2 years. Eventual spontaneous healing occurs in most cases, but the rate of healing varies by species. A small proportion of patients infected with *L. amazonensis* or *L. aethiopica* may develop diffuse parasite-rich cutaneous lesions that do not heal spontaneously. A small proportion of infections with parasites of the *L. braziliensis* complex are followed, months or years later, by metastatic mucosal lesions.

8. Susceptibility—Susceptibility is probably general. Lifelong immunity may be present after lesions due to *L. tropica* or *L. major* heal, but may not protect against other leishmanial species. Factors responsible for late mutilating disease are still poorly understood, although nutritional and immunogenetic factors have been implicated; occult infections may be activated years after the primary infection. The most important factor in immunity is the development of an adequate cell-mediated response.

9. Methods of control—

    A. Preventive measures: No vaccine is currently available, although candidate vaccines are in development. Control measures vary according to the habits of mammalian hosts and phlebotomine vectors, and include the following:

        1) Case management: Detect cases systematically and treat rapidly. This applies to all forms of leishmaniasis, and is an important measure in preventing development of destructive mucosal lesions in the western hemisphere and recidivans forms in the eastern hemisphere, particularly where the reservoir is largely or solely human.

        2) Vector control: Apply residual insecticides periodically. Phlebotomine sandflies have a relatively short flight range and are highly susceptible to control by systematic spraying with residual insecticides. Spraying must cover exteriors and interiors of doorways and other openings if transmission occurs

in dwellings. Possible breeding places of eastern hemisphere sandflies, such as stone walls, animal houses and rubbish heaps, must be sprayed.

Exclude vectors by screening with a fine mesh screen (10–12 holes per linear cm or 25–30 holes per linear inch, with an aperture of not more than 0.89 mm or 0.035 inches). Insecticide-treated bed nets are a good vector control alternative, especially in anthroponotic foci. In the focus of Aleppo (Syrian Arab Republic), they appeared particularly efficient, reducing yearly incidence drastically (by 50% to 75%).

3) Eliminate rubbish heaps and other breeding places for eastern hemisphere phlebotomines.

4) Destroy gerbils (and their burrows) implicated as reservoirs in local areas by deep plowing and removal of the plants they feed on (chenopods).

5) In the western hemisphere, avoid sandfly-infested and thickly forested areas, particularly after sundown; use insect repellents and protective clothing if exposure to sandflies is unavoidable.

6) Apply appropriate environmental management and forest clearance.

B. Control of patient, contacts and the immediate environment:

1) Report to local health authority: Official report not ordinarily justifiable, Class 5 (see *Reporting*).

2) Isolation: Not applicable, only of theoretical value.

3) Concurrent disinfection: Not applicable.

4) Quarantine: Not applicable.

5) Immunization of contacts: Not applicable.

6) Investigation of contacts and source of infection: interrupt the local transmission cycle in the most practical fashion.

7) Specific treatment: Mainly pentavalent antimonials: either sodium stibogluconate or meglumine antimonate (used in South America and some other areas). Pentamidine is used as a second line drug for cutaneous leishmaniasis. The imidazoles, ketoconazole and itraconazole, may have moderate antileishmanial activity against some leishmanial species. Liposomal or conventional amphotericin B may be required in South American mucosal disease if it does not respond to antimonial therapy. Miltefosince, an alkylphospholipid and the first oral drug active against visceral leishmaniasis, has had variable efficacy for New World cutaneous leishmaniasis in clinical trials; its efficacy may be dependent on the leishmanial species. Topical formulations of 15% aminosidine (paromomycin) plus 10% urea have reduced the time to

healing in cases due to *L. major.* Although spontaneous healing of simple cutaneous lesions occurs, infections acquired in geographic regions where mucosal disease has been reported should be treated promptly.

C. *Epidemic measures:* In areas of high incidence, use intensive efforts to control the disease by provision of diagnostic facilities and appropriate measures directed against phlebotomine sand-flies and the mammalian reservoir hosts.

D. *Disaster implications:* None.

E. *International measures:* WHO Collaborating Centres provide support as required. More information can be found at: <http://www.who.int/collaboratingcentres/database/en/>

II. VISCERAL LEISHMANIASIS

ICD-9 085.0; ICD-10 B55.0

(Kala-azar)

1. Identification—A chronic systemic disease caused by intracellular protozoa of the genus *Leishmania.* The disease is characterized by fever, hepatosplenomegaly, lymphadenopathy, anemia, leukopenia, thrombocytopenia and progressive emaciation and weakness. Untreated clinically evident disease is usually fatal. Fever may have gradual or sudden onset, is persistent and irregular, and may alternate with periods of apyrexia or low-grade fever. Post-kala-azar dermal leishmaniasis consists of macular, papular and/or nodular skin lesions that occur weeks to years after apparent cure of systemic disease. Post-kala-azar dermal leishmaniasis occurs in up to 50% of visceral leishmaniasis cases in Sudan, and 10–20% of cases in the Indian subcontinent. *Leishmania*/HIV co-infection is a well-known entity in southern Europe, and is currently emerging in eastern Africa and in Asia.

Parasitological diagnosis, based on invasive methods, is based preferably on culture of the organism from a biopsy specimen or aspirated material, or on demonstration of intracellular amastigotes in stained smears from bone marrow, spleen, liver, lymph nodes or blood (the latter is preferable in HIV-co-infected patients). The PCR technique is the most sensitive, but remains expensive.

Serological diagnosis was traditionally based on IFA and ELISA, tests that are expensive and difficult to decentralize. Recently, inexpensive, reliable rapid tests, such as the recombinant k39 immunochromatographic strip test, have become available for field use, and have quickly become the primary diagnostic modality for uncomplicated cases. An antigen detection test in urine is also under evaluation. Serologic testing has poor sensitivity in HIV-co-infected patients; parasitological diagnosis is recommended.

2. Infectious agents—Typically *Leishmania donovani*, *L. infantum* and *L. infantum/chagasi*.

3. Occurrence—Visceral leishmaniasis occurs in 62 countries, with an estimated annual incidence of 500 000 cases and a population at risk of 120 million. Usually a rural disease, occurring in foci in Asia, Africa and the Americas. More than 90% of the global disease burden occurs in India, Nepal, Bangladesh, Sudan, and Brazil. In Brazil, many cases now occur in peri-urban areas. Foci also occur in China, Pakistan, southern regions of eastern Europe, the Middle East including Turkey, the Mediterranean basin, Mexico, central and South America, and in Ethiopia, Kenya, Uganda and sub-Saharan savanna parts of Africa. In many affected areas, the disease occurs as scattered cases among infants, children and adolescents, but occasionally in epidemic waves. Incidence is modified by the use of antimalarial insecticides. Where zoonotic transmission was predominant and dog populations have been drastically reduced (e.g. China), human disease has also been reduced.

4. Reservoir—Known or presumed reservoirs include humans, wild Canidae (foxes and jackals), and domestic dogs. Humans are the only known reservoir in Bangladesh, India and Nepal.

5. Mode of transmission—Through the bite of infected phlebotomine sandflies. In foci of anthroponotic visceral leishmaniasis, humans with visceral leishmaniasis or post-kala-azar dermal leishmaniasis (especially the highly infectious nodular form) comprise the sole reservoir, and transmission occurs from person to person through the sandfly bite. In foci of zoonotic visceral leishmaniasis, dogs, the domestic animal reservoir, constitute the main source of infection for sandflies. Person-to-person transmission has been reported in *Leishmania*/HIV co-infected intravenous drug users, through exchange of syringes. HIV co-infected patients are highly infectious to sandflies, acting as human reservoirs even in zoonotic foci.

6. Incubation period—Generally 2–6 months; range is 10 days to years.

7. Period of communicability—Not usually transmitted from person to person, but infectious to sandflies as long as parasites persist in the circulating blood or skin of the mammalian reservoir host. Infectivity for phlebotomines may persist after clinical recovery of human patients.

8. Susceptibility—Susceptibility is general. Kala-azar apparently induces lasting homologous immunity. Evidence indicates that asymptomatic and sub-clinical infections are common, and that malnutrition increases the likelihood of progression to clinical disease. Manifest disease occurs among AIDS patients, presumably as reactivation of latent infections.

9. **Methods of control—**

A. **Preventive measures:** See corresponding section I, 9A for cutaneous leishmaniasis. The effectiveness of dog control in zoonotic foci remains unknown. In industrialized countries, dogs are usually treated, but they often relapse. In many developing countries, massive culling of infected dogs has failed, except in China. A recent approach based on insecticide-impregnated collars has proved effective in the Islamic Republic of Iran, reducing canine and human incidence of visceral leishmaniasis.

B. **Control of patient, contacts and the immediate environment:**

1) Report to local health authority: In selected leishmaniasis-endemic areas, Class 3 (see *Reporting*).
2) Isolation: Blood and body fluid precautions.
3) Concurrent disinfection: Not applicable.
4) Quarantine: Not applicable.
5) Immunization of contacts: Not applicable.
6) Investigation of contacts and source of infection: Ordinarily none.
7) Specific treatment: The most effective drug is liposomal amphotericin B, but its high cost has generally restricted its use to industrialized countries. Recently introduced preferential pricing for non-profit organizations in developing countries may increase its use.

   Pentavalent antimonials (Sb5) remain the first-line treatment in most countries. Sodium stibogluconate and meglumine antimonate are effective. Cases that do not respond to antimony may be treated with amphotericin B or pentamidine; however, these are not used routinely, because of toxicity.

   In Bihar State, India, and southern Nepal, there is a high prevalence of primary resistance to antimonial drugs, and one of the alternative drugs must be used.

   Recently developed or tested drugs include:
   a) Miltefosine, an alkylphospholipid, the first oral drug active against visceral leishmaniasis. It is licensed in India, Colombia and Germany, and licensing is underway in several other countries. Efficacy was high in India, but the drug is teratogenic, and the long half-life and practice of unsupervised oral administration raises the possibility of rapid development of resistance in India.
   b) Aminosidine (paromomycin), now in phase IV trials in India and Phase III trials in Africa. In the Indian Phase III trials, efficacy was high and toxicity low. The dosage required in Africa appears to be higher than that effective in India.

c) Sitamaquine, a lepidine, is still under phase III development. Experts agree that trials of combination regimens are urgently needed, to prevent the development of resistance to newly developed drugs.

C. *Epidemic measures:* Effective control must include an understanding of the local ecology and transmission cycle, followed by adoption of practical measures to reduce mortality, stop transmission, and avoid geographic extension of the epidemic, especially in anthroponotic foci.

In Sudan, massive distribution of insecticide-treated bed nets is thought to have helped to control the epidemic in the 1990s. In the Indian subcontinent, an elimination campaign is underway; essential components include rapid visceral leishmaniasis and post kala-azar dermal leishmaniasis case detection and effective treatment, vector control through indoor residual spraying and the use of insecticide treated nets, and institution of more effective disease surveillance and program monitoring.

D. *Disaster implications:* None.

E. *International measures:* Institute coordinated programs of control among neighboring countries where the disease is endemic. WHO Collaborating Centres provide support as required. More information can be found at:

<http://www.who.int/collaboratingcentres/database/en/>

Further information can be found at:

<http://www.who.int/tdr/diseases/leish/default.htm>

LEPROSY   ICD-9 030; ICD-10 A30
(Hansen's disease)
[CCDM19: D. Daumerie, K. Glynn]
[CCDM18: D. Daumerie]

1. Identification—A chronic bacterial disease of the skin, peripheral nerves, and in some cases upper airway. The skin involvement can be either nodular/papular or restricted to the level of the skin. Clinical diagnosis is based on complete skin examination. Search for signs of peripheral nerve involvement (hyperesthesia, anesthesia, paralysis, muscle wasting or trophic ulcers) with bilateral palpation of peripheral nerves (ulnar nerve at the elbow, peroneal nerve at the head of the fibula and the great auricular nerve) for enlargement and tenderness. Test skin lesions for sensation (light touch, pinprick, temperature discrimination). Laboratory criteria include the presence of alcohol-acid-fast bacilli in skin smears (scrape-incision method). Clinical manifestations can include acute adverse episodes, termed erythema nodosum leprosum (ENL) or "reversal reactions." Leprosy may be masked in patients with advanced HIV disease, and only seen after immune reconstitution while under antiretroviral treatment. Differential diagnosis includes many infiltrative skin diseases, including lymphomas, lupus erythematosus, psoriasis, scleroderma and neurofibromatosis. Diffuse cutaneous leishmaniasis, some mycoses, myxedema, contact dermatitis, and pachydermoperiostosis may resemble lepromatous leprosy, but acid-fast bacilli are not present. Several skin conditions, such as vitiligo, tinea versicolor, pityriasis alba, nutritional dyschromia, nevus and scars may resemble leprosy of the skin surface. Sometimes the bacilli may be so few that they are not demonstrable. In view of the increasing prevalence of HIV and hepatitis B infection in many countries where leprosy is endemic, the number and frequency of skin smear sites and collection should be limited to the minimum necessary. In practice, laboratories are not essential for the diagnosis of leprosy.

Case definition (WHO operational definition)

A case of leprosy is a person having one or more of the following features, who has yet to complete a full course of treatment:

- Hypopigmented or reddish skin lesion(s) with definite loss of sensation.
- Involvement of the peripheral nerves (definite thickening with loss of sensation).
- Skin smear positive for acid-fast bacilli. The operational case definition includes retrieved defaulters with signs of active disease and relapsed cases who have previously completed a full course of treatment. It does not include cured persons with late reactions or residual disabilities.

2. Infectious agent—*Mycobacterium leprae*. This organism cannot be grown in bacteriological media or cell cultures.

3. Occurrence—The incidence of leprosy is declining worldwide, due to a combination of factors such as economic development, BCG immunization, and high coverage with multidrug therapy. During 2006, approximately 260 000 persons were diagnosed with leprosy, over half of them in India. Control has improved with the introduction of multidrug therapy (MDT). WHO has targeted the disease for elimination (less than 1 case/10 000 population), and this has been achieved in all but three (Brazil, Nepal and United Republic of Tanzania) of the 122 countries endemic in 1985.

Newly recognized cases in the USA are few, diagnosed principally in California, Florida, Hawaii, Louisiana, Texas, New York City, and Puerto Rico. Most of these cases are in immigrants and refugees whose disease was acquired in their native countries; however, the disease remains endemic in California, Hawaii, Louisiana, Texas, and Puerto Rico.

4. Reservoir—Humans are thought to be the only reservoir of proven significance. Feral armadillos in Louisiana and Texas (USA) have been found naturally affected with a disease identical to experimental leprosy in armadillos, and there have been reports suggesting that disease in armadillos has been naturally transmitted to humans. Naturally acquired leprosy has been observed in a mangabey monkey and in a chimpanzee, captured in Nigeria and Sierra Leone, respectively.

5. Mode of transmission—This remains contentious. *M. leprae* transmitted from the nasal mucosa of an affected individual to the skin and respiratory tract of another person is likely to play an important role in most endemic communities. Transmission is favored by close contact. Although the bacillus can survive up to 7 days in dried nasal secretions, indirect transmission is unlikely.

6. Incubation period—Incubation ranges from 9 months to 20 years. The disease is rarely seen in children under age 3; however, more than 50 cases have been identified in children under one year of age, the youngest at 10 weeks.

7. Period of communicability—Clinical and laboratory evidence suggest that infectiousness is lost in most instances within a day of beginning treatment with multidrug therapy (MDT).

8. Susceptibility—The persistence and form of leprosy depend on the patient's ability to develop effective cell-mediated immunity. The high prevalence of *M. leprae*-specific lymphocyte transformation and antibodies specific for *M. leprae* among close contacts of leprosy patients suggests that infection is frequent, yet clinical disease occurs in only a small proportion of such close contacts. The immunological lepromin test, used in the past to classify patients, should be reserved for research activities.

9. Methods of control—The availability of effective and time-limited treatment, with rapid elimination of infectiousness, has changed the management of the leprosy patient from societal isolation with attendant despair to ambulatory treatment without the need for hospitalization, Hospitalization should now be limited only to those in need of procedures such as surgical correction of deformities, and treatment of ulcers resulting from anesthesia.

  A. *Preventive measures:* Early detection and treatment of cases. Dapsone chemoprophylaxis is not recommended (limited effectiveness and danger of resistance).

  1) Health education and counseling of patients and relatives must stress the availability of effective MDT, the absence of infectivity of patients under continuous treatment, and the prevention of physical and social disabilities.

2) Routine BCG vaccination can induce protection against the both the lepromatous and tuberculoid forms of the disease; the vaccine is part of tuberculosis control in many countries (not the USA), but is not undertaken specifically to prevent leprosy.

B. Control of patient, contacts and the immediate environment:

1) Report to local health authority: Case reporting is obligatory in many countries and desirable in all, Class 2 (see *Reporting*).
2) Isolation: Unnecessary. Reducing contact with known leprosy patients is of dubious value and can lead to stigmatization. No restrictions in employment or attendance at school are indicated.
3) Quarantine: Not applicable.
4) Immunization of contacts: Not recommended
5) Investigation of contacts and source of infection: The initial examination of close contacts can be useful.
6) Specific treatment: Combined chemotherapy regimens are essential; a single lesion can be treated with a single dose. Patients under treatment should be monitored for drug side effects, for leprosy reactions, and for development of trophic ulcers. Some complications may need to be treated in a referral center. Ambulatory treatment with MDT is given according to case classification.

   The number of skin lesions is taken as an indicator of bacillary load in the patient, and is used to guide drugs used for therapy as well as its duration.

   Adults with more than 5 skin lesions: the standard WHO regimen is an oral combination of the following for 12 months:
   • Rifampicin: 600 mg once a month.
   • Dapsone: 100 mg once a day.
   • Clofazimine: 50 mg once a day and 300 mg once a month.

   Adults with 2-5 skin lesions: the standard WHO regimen is an oral combination of the following for 6 months:

   • Rifampicin: 600 mg once a month.
   • Dapsone: 100 mg once a day.

   Adults with a single lesion: the standard WHO regimen is an oral combination of the following, given once:

   • Rifampcin: 600 mg.
   • Ofloxacin 400 mg.
   • Minocycline 100 mg.

Children must receive appropriately scaled-down doses (in child blister packs).

Patients must be advised to complete the full course of treatment and to seek care in the event of drug side effects (allergic reaction) and immunological reactions (neuritis leading to damage of the peripheral nerve trunks).

MDT is available free of charge through WHO. MDT drugs must be given in blister packs, free of charge, to all patients.

Treatment of reactions: Corticosteroids are the drugs of choice in the management of reactions associated with neuritis. During the 1960s, thalidomide was reintroduced as treatment for Erythema nodosum leprosum (ENL). In view of the risk of deformed births among users, and despite its possible usefulness for other conditions, thalidomide has no current place in the treatment of leprosy. Clofazimine is the drug of choice for the management of recurrent ENL reactions. Its use in MDT has significantly reduced the frequency and severity of ENL reactions worldwide.

C. Epidemic measures: Not applicable.

D. Disaster implications: Any interruption of treatment schedules is serious. During wars, diagnosis and treatment of leprosy patients has often been neglected.

E. International measures: Further information can be found at <http://www.who.int/lep> and <http://www.who.int/tdr/diseases/leprosy/ default.htm>.

LEPTOSPIROSIS ICD-9 100; ICD-10 A27
(Weil disease, Canicola fever, Hemorrhagic jaundice, Mud fever, Swineherd disease)
[CCDM19: K. Glynn, R. Hartskeel, A. Ko, F. Meslin]
[CCDM18: F. Meslin]

1. Identification—A bacterial zoonotic disease with varied manifestations. Severity of illness ranges from asymptomatic, to a mild self-limiting febrile illness, to fulminant fatal disease. The disease typically presents as one of the following four clinical categories: mild, influenza-like illness; Weil's syndrome characterized by jaundice, renal failure, hemorrhage and myocarditis with arrhythmias; meningitis or meningoencephalitis; and pulmonary hemorrhage with respiratory failure.

Clinical illness lasts from a few days to 3 weeks or longer. Generally, there are two phases in the illness: the leptospiremic or febrile stage, lasting 5 to 7 days, followed by the convalescent or immune phase, which generally lasts 4 to 30 days. The two phases may be separated by a 3- to 4-day abatement of fever; however the distinction between the phases may not be apparent, and patients may present only in the second phase. Recovery of untreated cases can take several months.

Early-phase illness is characterized by the abrupt onset of high fever, myalgias (calves and lumbar region) and headache (retro-orbital and frontal). Other early-phase manifestations that may be present are nausea, vomiting, abdominal pain, diarrhea, cough, photophobia and rash with a truncal or pre-tibial distribution. Conjunctival suffusion (redness of the conjunctiva), a pathognomonic finding of leptospirosis, is observed in about 30% of patients. Late-phase illness occurs 4–9 days after onset of symptoms and is characterized by prolonged fever and systemic complications such as jaundice, renal failure, bleeding, respiratory insufficiency with or without hemoptysis, hypotension, myocarditis, meningitis, mental confusion and depression. Unilateral or bilateral uveitis, characterized by iritis, iridocyclitis and chorioretinitis, may develop up to 18 months after acute illness and persist for years.

Leptospirosis is a self-limiting and often clinically inapparent illness in the majority of cases. However, 5–15% of clinical infections progress to develop the severe late-phase manifestations. Cases with icteric leptospirosis generally have poorer prognosis, yet severe complications may occur in patients without jaundice. Other prognostic predictors for death are older age (>40 years), oliguria, respiratory insufficiency, pulmonary hemorrhage, cardiac arrhythmias, and altered mental status. Clinical outcome is poorest among patients who develop a pulmonary hemorrhage syndrome, which is characterized by massive pulmonary bleeding and acute respiratory distress syndrome. Deaths are due predominantly to renal failure, cardiopulmonary failure, widespread hemorrhage, and— rarely—liver failure. The case-fatality rate is reported to range from <5% to 30%. Case-fatality rates are >10% and >50% in patients who develop acute renal failure or pulmonary hemorrhage syndrome, respectively.

The icteric form (Weil's disease) is the most severe presentation of the disease, and is associated with severe hepatic dysfunction and hemorrhage, cardiac, pulmonary, and neurological involvement, and high mortality. Cases are often under-recognized or misdiagnosed as dengue, malaria and influenza due to the non-specific manifestations of early-phase leptospirosis. Leptospirosis appears to be the cause of a significant proportion (10%) of undiagnosed aseptic meningitis. Severe leptospirosis must be differentiated from other causes of acute jaundice and renal failure, such as rickettsial disease, hantaviral infection, enteric fevers, viral hepatitis and Gram-negative sepsis. Late sequelae may occur, e.g. chronic fatigue, neuropsychiatric symptoms (paresis, depression), and occasionally uveitis. Leptospirosis during pregnancy may result in fetal death, abortion, stillbirth, or congenital infection.

Cases are often misdiagnosed as meningitis, encephalitis or influenza, and outbreaks may be confused with, or occur concurrently with, outbreaks of dengue or other viral hemorrhagic diseases, typhoid, rickettsial infection, malaria, or other febrile illnesses. Difficulties in diagnosis may compromise disease control and result in increased severity and elevated mortality. The severity of illness tends to vary with the infecting serovar; the same serovar may cause mild or severe disease in different hosts. Seroconversion may occur as early as 5 to 7 days after disease onset, but may not develop until after 10 days or longer, especially if antimicrobial therapy is initiated. IgM-class antibodies may remain detectable for months to years at low titers. Patients may develop cross-reactive antibodies to several serovars during acute infection; these gradually disappear weeks to months later.

Clinical diagnosis is by isolation of leptospires from blood (first 7 days), from cerebrospinal fluid (days 4–10) during acute illness, or from urine beginning in the second week of illness (7 days or more after onset). Culture and isolation can be very difficult, requiring special media and incubation for up to 16 weeks, and the sensitivity of culture for diagnosis is low. Diagnosis is most frequently confirmed by seroconversion demonstrated by 4-fold or greater increase in serum leptospira agglutination titer on the microscopic agglutination test (MAT), the confirmatory serologic test, using acute and convalescent specimens obtained at least 10 days apart. Different serovars of leptospires may occur in different regions. Therefore, the MAT preferably uses a panel of locally occurring leptospire serovars. However, antibody titer increase may be delayed or absent in some patients, and seroconversion may occur asymptomatically, especially in endemic areas. IgG assays, ELISA assays, and anti-whole *Leptospira* IgM detection kits in enzyme-linked immunosorbent assay or rapid formats are used to provide presumptive confirmation for leptospirosis. However, sensitivity is low (39–72%) during acute-phase illness. Immunofluorescence, immunohistochemical and nucleic acid detection techniques are used for the demonstration of leptospires in clinical and autopsy specimens.

Immunohistochemical techniques can detect leptospire antigens in clinical and autopsy tissue specimens to confirm diagnosis. Polymerase chain reaction (PCR) assays for detection of leptospire DNA have been developed for use on clinical samples such as blood. These tests are available in reference and research laboratories. Direct examination of blood or urine using dark-field microscopy has poor sensitivity and specificity. Inoculation of experimental animals such as golden hamsters, guinea pigs or gerbils can also confirm diagnosis, but is rarely used.

2. Infectious agent—Leptospires are poorly staining spirochetes that require dark-field microscopy or silver staining procedures for identification. Pathogenic leptospires belong to seven main *Leptospira* species, which are subdivided into serovars. More than 250 pathogenic serovars have been identified, and these fall into 26 serogroups based on serologic relatedness. Serologic classification provides more useful epidemiologic information, since serogroups and serovars are often associated with specific animal reservoirs. Commonly identified serovars in North America are *Icterohaemorrhagiae, Australis, Sejroe, Canicola, Tarassovi, Gryppotyphosa* and *Bataviae*; in Australia, serovar *Arborea* has recently emerged as a significant source of leptospirosis.

3. Occurrence—Worldwide; in all except polar regions. The disease is most prevalent in tropical and subtropical regions, with the highest incidence of human leptospirosis reported in island countries or low-lying countries with frequent flooding. Leptospirosis is an endemic disease in rural subsistence farming areas and urban slum settlements in tropical regions, because of the high density of domestic and wild reservoirs and poor underlying sanitation infrastructure in these environments. The disease is also an occupational hazard for rice and sugarcane field workers; farmers; fish workers; miners; veterinarians; workers in animal husbandry, dairies and abattoirs; sewer workers; and military troops. Males are proportionally more heavily affected due to occupational exposures. Outbreaks occur among those exposed to fresh river, stream, canal and lake water contaminated by the urine of domestic and wild animals, particularly during flooding, and to the urine, body fluids and tissues of infected animals. Outbreaks may occur following excessive rainfall or flooding, especially in endemic areas. The disease is a recreational hazard for persons engaged in activities with water exposures such as swimming, boating and caving, and for bathers, campers and sportsmen in contaminated waters. Disease clusters have been associated with these activities (especially immersion and swallowing water), particularly after flooding. Rodent-borne leptospirosis due to work-related exposures appears to be increasing as an urban hazard, especially during heavy rains when floods occur. The disease is increasingly associated with travel, recreation and water sports in affluent populations. Large epidemics are often in association with heavy seasonal rainfall and flooding and disaster events. A major outbreak in Nicaragua in 1995 caused extensive mortality; and in recent years outbreaks have been reported from Asia, Europe, Australia and the Americas.

4. Reservoir—Pathogenic leptospires are maintained in the genital tract and renal tubules of wild and domestic animals, which serve as natural maintenance hosts and can remain asymptomatic shedders for years or even for life. Serovars are adapted to one or more reservoir animal species, e.g. rats (*Copenhageni* and *Icterohaemorrhagiae*), swine (*Pomona*), cattle (*Hardjo*), dogs (*Canicola*) and raccoons (*Autumnalis*). The leptospires may be shed in infected urine, amniotic fluid, or placental tissue, and contaminate soil and water. They can remain viable for weeks or months under favorable conditions in moist soil or water, especially where temperatures are between 28 and 32°C, with the pH range 6.2 to 8.0.

A high proportion of both stray and domestic canine populations in urban and suburban areas may show evidence of infection and shed leptospires in the urine. Other animal hosts, some with a shorter carrier state, include feral rodents, insectivores, badgers, deer, squirrels, foxes, skunks, raccoons and opossums. Reptiles and amphibians (frogs) have been found to carry pathogenic leptospires, but are unlikely to play an important epidemiological role.

5. Mode of transmission—Contact of the skin (especially if abraded) or mucous membranes with moist soil or vegetation—especially sugar-cane—contaminated with the urine of infected animals; with contaminated waters, e.g. through swimming, wading in floodwaters, accidental immersion or occupational abrasion; with urine, fluids, or tissues of infected animals; and occasionally through drinking of water and ingestion of food contaminated with urine of infected animals, often rats, or through inhalation of droplet aerosols of contaminated fluids.

6. Incubation period—Usually 5–14 days, with a range of 2–30 days.

7. Period of communicability—Direct person-to-person transmission is rare. Leptospires may be excreted in the urine, usually for 1 month, although leptospiruria has been observed in humans and in animals for months, even years, after acute illness.

8. Susceptibility—Susceptibility of humans is general; serovar-specific immunity follows infection or (occasionally) immunization, but this may not protect against infection with a different serovar.

9. Methods of control—

    A. Preventive measures:

        1) Educate the public on modes of transmission, avoidance of swimming or wading in potentially contaminated waters, and the of use proper protection when work requires such exposure.

        2) Protect workers in hazardous occupations by providing protective clothing and equipment such as boots, gloves and aprons. Covering wounds with waterproof dressings may reduce the risk of infection in persons with potential occupational or recreational exposure.

        3) Recognize potentially contaminated waters and soil; drain such waters and when possible create physical barriers, such as closing open sewers, to prevent exposures to potential transmission sources. Small environmental areas such as human habitations that become contaminated may be cleaned and disinfected; leptospires are rapidly killed by disinfectants and desiccation.

        4) Control rodents in human habitations, urban or rural, and recreational areas; removal of refuse and improved sanitation around human habitations may reduce rodent infestation.

Management of sugarcane fields, such as through controlled pre-harvest burning, reduces risks in harvesting.

5) Segregate infected domestic animals; prevent contamination by the urine of infected animals for humans living, working or playing in potentially contaminated areas. Maintain hygienic measures during care and handling of animals and avoid contact with urine or other bodily fluids.

6) Immunization of farm and pet animals prevents illness from infecting serovars contained within the vaccine, but not necessarily infection and renal shedding. Any vaccine must contain the dominant local strains.

7) Immunization of people has been carried out against occupational exposures to specific serovars with varying degrees of success, but is not available in most countries at present. Immunization provides protection only against the particular serovars included in the vaccine.

8) A systematic review concludes that doxycycline (e.g. 200 mg in one weekly oral dose in adults for the duration of the exposure) provides effective prophylaxis against clinical disease and could be considered for preventing leptospirosis among high-risk groups with short-term exposure; however infection may not be prevented. Doxycyline cannot be used in children less than eight years of age.

B. Control of patient, contacts and the immediate environment:

1) Report to local health authority: Obligatory case report in many countries, Class 2 (see *Reporting*).

2) Isolation: Blood and body fluid precautions.

3) Concurrent disinfection: Articles soiled with urine.

4) Quarantine: Not applicable.

5) Immunization of contacts: Not applicable.

6) Investigation of contacts and source of infection: Search for exposure to infected animals and potentially contaminated waters.

7) Specific treatment: Treatment with antimicrobial agents should be given as early in the course of illness as possible. Penicillin G and doxycycline have been shown in double-blind, placebo-controlled trials to be effective in reducing morbidity from leptospirosis. Penicillin G (1.5 million units IV every 6 hours) is recommended for the treatment of severe leptospirosis. Third generation cephalosporins (ceftriaxone, 1 g IV once a day; cefotaxime, 1 g IV every 6 hours) are an alternative, since randomized clinical trials have shown that these agents have equivalent effectiveness to penicillin. Doxycycline (100 mg every 12 hours), ampicillin or amoxicillin (500 mg every 6 hours) can be used as oral

regimens for the treatment of mild leptospirosis. Although their efficacy is not proven, quinolone agents, azithromycin and clarithromycin are inhibitory *in vitro* and may be considered in patients with a history of adverse reactions to penicillin. NB: doxycycline should not be used in pregnant women or children younger than 8 years of age. Jarisch-Herxheimer reactions may occur following initiation of antimicrobial therapy. Prompt triage of high-risk patients and aggressive supportive care is required for the treatment of hypotension, renal and respiratory distress, and hemorrhage associated with severe leptospirosis. Timely initiation of dialysis and mechanical ventilation are essential to preventing mortality from oliguric renal insufficiency and pulmonary hemorrhage syndrome, respectively.

C. *Epidemic measures:* Search for source of infection, such as sewers, contaminated wells and swimming pools, or other contaminated water sources; eliminate the contamination or prohibit use. Investigate industrial and occupational sources, including potential animal exposures.

D. *Disaster implications:* A potential problem following heavy rainfall, monsoons and extreme climactic events such as hurricanes or flooding in endemic areas. Outbreaks may be confused with, or occur concurrently with, outbreaks of other febrile illnesses.

E. *International measures:* WHO Collaborating Centres provide support as required. More information can be found at <http://www.who.int/collaboratingcentres/database/en/>.

LISTERIOSIS   ICD-9 027.0; ICD-10 A32
[CCDM19: M. Iwamoto, C. Olson, J. Schlundt]
[CCDM18: P. Martin]

1. Identification—A bacterial infection that usually causes a mild febrile illness, but that can cause meningoencephalitis and/or septicemia in newborns and adults. The healthy host acquiring infection may exhibit only an acute mild febrile illness; in pregnant women infection can cause preterm delivery and fetal infection, with infection most likely resulting from transplacental transmission, although some infection may be the result of ascending infection from vaginal colonization. Infants may be stillborn or born with septicemia, or may develop meningitis in the neonatal period even though the mother may be asymptomatic at delivery.

Listeria can also cause spontaneous abortions, although the incidence is difficult to estimate since bacterial cultures are not routinely obtained from spontaneously aborted fetuses or products of conception. Spontaneous abortions occur more commonly in the second half of pregnancy; perinatal infection is acquired during the third trimester or possibly from nosocomial infection in the case of late-onset neonatal disease. *Listeria* has not been associated with recurrent pregnancy loss. The postpartum course of the mother is usually uneventful, but the case-fatality rate is 30% in newborns and approaches 50% when onset occurs in the first 4 days. Listeriosis is associated with a higher mortality rate than other common foodborne pathogens such as *Salmonella*. In pregnancy-related cases, the postpartum course of the mother is usually uneventful, but the case-fatality rate is 20-30% in infected newborns. The overall case-fatality rate among non-pregnant adults is approximately 30%, with the case-fatality rate higher among patients ≥50 years old (24%) than in other age groups (14%). In a recent epidemic, the overall case-fatality rate among non-pregnant adults was 35%: 11% in those below 40 and 63% in those over 60.

Those at highest risk are neonates, the elderly, immunocompromised individuals, pregnant women, and alcoholic, cirrhotic or diabetic adults. Non-pregnant adults frequently present with sepsis, meningitis, or meningoencephalitis. The onset of meningoencephalitis (rare in pregnant women) can be sudden—with fever, intense headache, nausea, vomiting and signs of meningeal irritation—or subacute, particularly in immunocompromised or elderly hosts. Rhomboencephalitis may rarely occur. Delirium and coma may appear early; occasionally there is collapse and shock. Endocarditis, granulomatous lesions in the liver and other organs, localized internal or external abscesses, and pustular or papular cutaneous lesions may occur on rare occasions. In pregnant women, symptoms may be mild and nonspecific: fever, headache, myalgia, or gastrointestinal symptoms.

Diagnosis is confirmed only after isolation of the infectious agent from CSF, blood, amniotic fluid, placenta, meconium, lochia, gastric washings, and other sites of infection. *Listeria monocytogenes* can be isolated readily from normally sterile sites on routine media, but care must be taken to distinguish this organism from other Gram-positive rods, particularly diphtheroids. Selective enrichment media improve rates of isolation from contaminated specimens. Microscopic examination of CSF or meconium permits presumptive diagnosis; serological tests are unreliable, and not recommended at the present time.

2. Infectious agent—*Listeria monocytogenes*, a Gram-positive rod-shaped bacterium; human infections are usually (95%) caused by serotypes 1/2a, 1/2b, 1/2c and 4b.

3. Occurrence—An uncommonly diagnosed infection that occurs worldwide; in the USA, the incidence of illness reported in areas under active surveillance requiring hospitalization is about 3.1 cases per 1 million.

Although *Listeria* accounts for a small fraction of all foodborne illnesses, in Europe it is an important contributor to severe illness and accounts for approximately 4% of hospitalizations and 28% of deaths due to foodborne disease. It is often associated with consumption of non-pasteurized milk or milk products, including cheese and ready-to-eat meats. Infection often occurs sporadically; several outbreaks have been recognized in recent years. About 30% of clinical cases occur within the first 3 weeks of life; in non-pregnant adults, remaining infections occur mainly after 40 years of age. Nosocomial acquisition has been reported. Asymptomatic infections probably occur at all ages, although they are of clinical importance only during pregnancy, because of the risk of fetal loss.

4. Reservoir—The organism mainly occurs in soil, forage, water, mud, livestock food, and silage. The seasonal use of silage as fodder is frequently followed by an increased incidence of listeriosis in animals. Animal reservoirs include infected domestic and wild mammals, fowl, and people. Asymptomatic fecal carriage is common in humans without known exposure (up to 5%), and can be much higher in slaughterhouse workers and laboratory workers who work with *Listeria monocytogenes* cultures, and in asymptomatic household contacts of persons with invasive listeriosis. Soft cheeses may support the growth of *Listeria* during ripening, and have caused outbreaks. Unlike most other foodborne pathogens, *Listeria* can multiply in refrigerated foods that are contaminated; it is extremely hardy in comparison to most bacteria. Studies have shown that Listeria can form—and exist in—biofilm, enabling attachment to, for example, stainless steel surfaces in food production systems. Bacteria in biofilm can show increased resistance to sanitizers, disinfectants and antimicrobial agents. Listeria growing or surviving in biofilm in production facilities can be transferred to food products.

5. Mode of transmission—Outbreaks have been reported in association with ingestion of raw or contaminated milk, soft cheeses, vegetables, and ready-to-eat meats such as hot dogs, pâté, and deli meats. A substantial proportion of sporadic infections results from foodborne transmission. Papular lesions on hands and arms may occur from direct contact with infectious material. In neonatal infections, the organism can be transmitted from mother to fetus *in utero*, or during passage through the infected birth canal. There are rare reports of nursery outbreaks attributed to contaminated equipment or materials.

The question of the dose-response relationship for *Listeria* is debated. Newer risk assessment modeling has enabled the preparation of dose-response curves, reflecting the fact that the infection process should be viewed as a probability of infection related to the dose ingested. These models seem to suggest a 10^{-9} to 10^{-13} probability for infection with a dose of 100 organisms, and a 10^{-6} to 10^{-9} probability for infection at 1 000 000 organisms.

6. Incubation period—Variable, and longer than most common foodborne pathogens; cases have occurred 3-70 days after a single exposure to an implicated product. Estimated median incubation is 3 weeks.

7. Period of communicability—Mothers of infected newborn infants can shed the infectious agent in vaginal discharges and urine for 7-10 days after delivery, rarely longer. While fecal-oral transmission from mother to child during vaginal birth may account for some infections in newborns and nosocomial transmission has been documented in newborn nurseries, the primary modes of transmission are transplacental in neonatal cases and foodborne in others. Asymptomatic carriage of *Listeria monocytogenes* has been well documented; infected individuals can shed the organisms in their stools for several months. Secondary infections among household contacts have not been identified.

8. Susceptibility—Fetuses and newborns are highly susceptible. Infection in children and young adults generally cause less severe disease than in the immunocompromised and the elderly. There is a strong association between decreased immunity (particularly cell-mediated) and invasive listeriosis, and disease is often superimposed on other debilitating illnesses or conditions such as malignancy, organ transplantation, diabetes, cirrhosis, renal disease, heart disease, HIV infection, and in those on corticosteroids. In immunocompetent hosts, *Listeria* may be more likely to manifest as febrile gastroenteritis. There is little evidence of acquired immunity, even after prolonged severe infection.

9. Methods of control—

A. Preventive measures:

1) Pregnant women and immunocompromised individuals should avoid ready-to-eat meats and other foods (unless heated until steaming hot); smoked fish; and soft cheeses made with unpasteurized milk. They should cook leftovers or foods such as hot dogs until steaming hot. They should also avoid contact with potentially infectious materials, such as aborted animal fetuses on farms.

2) Ensure safety of all foods of animal origin. Pasteurize all dairy products where possible. Irradiate soft cheeses after ripening or monitor non-pasteurized dairy products, such as soft cheeses, by culturing for *Listeria*.

3) Processed foods found to be contaminated by *Listeria monocytogenes* (e.g. during routine bacteriological surveillance) should be recalled.

4) Thoroughly wash raw vegetables before eating.

5) Thoroughly cook raw food from animal sources such as beef, pork, or poultry.

6) Wash hands, knives, and cutting boards after handling uncooked foods.

7) Avoid the use of untreated manure on vegetable crops.

8) Veterinarians and farmers must take proper precautions in handling aborted fetuses and sick or dead animals, especially sheep that died of encephalitis.

B. Control of patient, contacts and the immediate environment:

1) Report to local health authority: Obligatory case report required in many countries, Class 2; in others, report of clusters required, Class 4 (see *Reporting*).

2) Isolation: Enteric precautions.

3) Concurrent disinfection: Not applicable.

4) Quarantine: Not applicable.

5) Immunization of contacts: Not applicable.

6) Investigation of contacts and source of infection: Case surveillance data—especially strain characteristics—should be analyzed frequently (weekly) for possible clustering. Patients in all suspected clusters should be interviewed promptly to identify common-source exposures, for rapid outbreak identification. Relatively low incidence and long incubation periods can make identifying *Listeria* outbreaks difficult; therefore, prompt and thorough investigation of all cases is important.

7) Specific treatment: Penicillin or ampicillin alone or together with aminoglycosides. For penicillin-allergic patients, trimethoprim-sulfamethoxazole or erythromycin is preferred. Cephalosporins, including third-generation cephalosporins, are not effective in the treatment of clinical listeriosis. Tetracycline resistance has been observed. A Gram-stain smear of meconium from clinically suspected newborns should be examined for short Gram-positive rods resembling *L. monocytogenes*. If positive, prophylactic antibiotics should be administered as a precaution.

C. Epidemic measures: Investigate suspected outbreaks to identify a common source of infection, and prevent further exposure to that source.

D. Disaster implications: None.

E. International measures: WHO Risk assessment of Listeria monocytogenes in ready-to-eat food:
http://www.who.int/foodsafety/publications/micro/en/mra4.pdf

LOIASIS
ICD-9 125.2; ICD-10 B74.3

(*Loa loa* infection, Eyeworm disease of Africa, Calabar swelling)
[CCDM19: A. Gabrielli, L. Savioli]
[CCDM18: M. Karam]

1. Identification—A chronic filarial disease characterized by migration of the adult worm through subcutaneous or deeper tissues of the body, causing transient swellings several centimeters in diameter, located on any part of the body. The swellings may be preceded by localized pain with pruritus. Pruritus localized on arms, thorax, face and shoulders is a major symptom. Migration of the adult worm under the bulbar conjunctivae may be accompanied by pain and edema. Allergic reactions with giant urticaria (large urticaria with severe edema of the skin) and fever may occur occasionally.

Infections with other filariae, such as *Wuchereria bancrofti*, *Onchocerca volvulus*, *Mansonella (Dipetalonema) perstans* and *M. streptocerca* (common in areas where *Loa loa* is endemic) should be considered in the differential diagnosis.

Larvae (microfilariae) are present in peripheral blood during the daytime and can be demonstrated in stained thick blood smears, stained sediment of blood where erythrocytes and hemoglobin have been separated (laking), or through membrane filtration. Eosinophilia is frequent. *Loa loa*-specific DNA can be detected in blood from asymptomatic infected individuals. A travel history is essential for diagnosis in non-Africans.

2. Infectious agent—*Loa loa*, a filarial nematode.

3. Occurrence—Widely distributed in African rain forests, especially in central Africa. In the Congo River basin, up to 90% of indigenous inhabitants of some villages are infected.

4. Reservoir—Humans. Primate *Loa loa* occur but the two have different transmission complexes and the disease is therefore not a zoonosis.

5. Mode of transmission—Transmitted by a deer fly of the genus *Chrysops*. *Chrysops dimidiata*, *C. silacea* and other species ingest blood containing microfilariae; the larvae develop to their infectious stage within 10–12 days in the fly and migrate to the proboscis, from where they are transferred to a human host by the bite of the infective fly.

6. Incubation period—Symptoms usually appear several years after infection but may occur as early as 4 months. Microfilariae may appear in the peripheral blood as early as 6 months after infection.

7. Period of communicability—The adult worm may persist in humans, shedding microfilariae into the blood for as long as 17 years; in the fly, "communicability" starts from 10–12 days after its infection until all infective larvae have been released, or until the fly dies.

8. Susceptibility—Susceptibility is universal; with repeated infections, immunity has not been demonstrated.

9. Methods of control—

A. Preventive measures:

1) Measures directed against the fly larvae are effective but have not proven practical, because their moist, muddy breeding areas are usually too extensive.
2) Diethyltoluamide or dimethyl phthalate applied to exposed skin are effective fly repellents.
3) Wear protective clothing (long sleeves and trousers), screen houses.
4) For temporary residents of endemic areas whose risk of exposure is high or prolonged, a weekly dose of diethylcarbamazine (300 mg) is prophylactic.

B. Control of patient, contacts and the immediate environment:

1) Report to local health authority: Official report not ordinarily required, Class 5 (see *Reporting*).
2) Isolation: As far as possible, patients with microfilaraemia should be protected from deer fly (*Chrysops*) bites to reduce transmission.
3) Concurrent disinfection: Not applicable.
4) Quarantine: Not applicable.
5) Immunization of contacts: Not applicable.
6) Investigation of contacts and source of infection: None; a community problem.
7) Specific treatment: Diethylcarbamazine (DEC) 1 mg/kg as a single dose on the first day, doubled on two successive days then adjusted to 2–3 mg/kg 3 times daily for further 18 days, causes disappearance of microfilariae, and may kill the adult worm with ensuing cure. During treatment, hypersensitivity reactions (sometimes severe) are common.

   Ivermectin (200 to 400 micrograms/kg) also reduces microfilaraemia, and adverse reactions may be milder than with DEC. When microfilaraemia is heavy (greater than 2 000/mL blood), there is a risk of meningoencephalitis and the advantages of treatment must be weighed against the risk of life-threatening encephalopathy.

   Treatment with either drug must be individualized and undertaken under close medical supervision; corticosteroid and antihistaminic cover should be provided for the first 2 to

3 days, and treatment stopped at the first sign of cerebral involvement. Surgical removal of the migrating adult worm under the bulbar conjunctivae is indicated when feasible. *Loa loa* encephalopathy has been reported following ivermectin treatment for onchocerciasis, which is why the drug is not recommended for mass treatment of onchocerciasis in areas where loiasis is endemic.

C. Epidemic measures: Not applicable.

D. Disaster implications: None.

E. International measures: None.

LYME DISEASE

ICD-9 104.8, 088.81;
ICD-10 A69.2, L90.4

(Lyme borreliosis, Tick-borne meningopolyneuritis)
[CCDM19: B. Chomel]
[CCDM18: D. Húlínska]

1. Identification—A tick-borne, spirochetal, zoonotic disease characterized by a distinctive skin lesion, systemic symptoms and neurological, rheumatological and cardiac involvement occurring in varying combinations over months to years. Recent reports state that the optic nerve may be affected because of inflammation or increased intracranial pressure. Early symptoms are intermittent and changing. The illness more frequently occurs in late spring or in the summer following a tick bite, when nymphs are most active. The first manifestation in about 70 to 80% of patients is a red macule or papule that expands slowly in an annular manner, often with central clearing. This lesion is called *erythema migrans* or EM (formerly "erythema chronicum migrans"). EM may be single or multiple; to be considered significant for case surveillance purposes, the EM lesion must reach at least 5 cm in diameter. With or without EM, early systemic manifestations may include malaise, fatigue, fever, headache, stiff neck, myalgia, migratory arthralgias and/or lymphadenopathy, all of which may last several weeks in untreated patients. In central Europe and Scandinavia skin lesions called lymphadenosis benigna cutis and acrodermatitis chronica atrophicans are almost exclusively caused by *Borrelia afzelii*.

Within weeks to months after onset of the EM lesion, neurological abnormalities such as aseptic meningitis and cranial neuritis may develop in approximately 5% of untreated patients—including facial palsy, chorea, cerebellar ataxia, motor or sensory radiculoneuritis, myelitis and encephalitis. Symptoms fluctuate and may become chronic. Cardiac abnormalities (including atrioventricular block and, rarely, acute myopericarditis or cardiomegaly) may occur within weeks after onset of EM. Weeks to years after onset (mean, 6 months), intermittent episodes of swelling and pain in large joints (especially the knees) may develop in 60% of untreated patients, leading to chronic arthritis; this may recur for several years. Treatment-resistant Lyme arthritis is a rare complication that may be the result of cross reactivity between OspA and the human leukocyte function associated antigen-1 (hlFA-1) following natural infection with *B. burgdorferi*. Similarly, following latent infection, chronic neurological manifestations may develop and include encephalopathy, polyneuropathy or leukoencephalitis; the CSF often shows lymphocytic pleocytosis and elevated protein levels, while the electromyogram is usually abnormal.

Diagnosis is currently based on clinical findings supported by two-stage serological tests, IFA, ELISA and then Western immunoblotting. Serological tests are poorly standardized and must be interpreted with caution. They are insensitive during the first weeks of infection and may remain negative in people treated early with antibiotics. An ELISA for IgM antibodies that uses a recombinant outer surface protein C (rOspC) is more sensitive for early diagnosis than whole cell ELISA. VlsE (Vls locus expression site) or C6 recombinant antigens increase the sensitivity of IgG immunoblot. Test sensitivity increases when patients progress to later stages, but some chronic Lyme disease patients may remain seronegative. Cross-reacting IFA and ELISA antibodies may cause false-positive reactions in patients with syphilis, relapsing fever, leptospirosis, HIV infection, Rocky Mountain spotted fever, infectious mononucleosis, lupus or rheumatoid arthritis. The specificity of serological testing is enhanced by immunoblot testing of specimens that are positive or equivocal on IFA or ELISA. Diagnosis of nervous system Lyme disease requires demonstration of intrathecal antibody production. The causal agent is *Borrelia burgdorferi sensu lato*. The genotype present in North America, *Borrelia burgdorferi sensu stricto*, grows at 33°C (91.4°F) in the Barbour, Stoenner, Kelly (BSK) medium; other species causing Lyme-like disease may not grow well in this medium. Isolation from blood and tissue biopsies is difficult, but biopsies of the EM lesions may yield the organism in 80% of cases or more. PCR has identified *B. burgdorferi* genetic material *sensu lato* in synovial fluid, CSF, blood and urine, skin, and other tissues; the usefulness of PCR in routine management of Lyme disease cases has yet to be verified. Recent real-time assays combining DNA amplification with species-specific probes allow single step identification of spirochetal DNA to the species level.

2. **Infectious agents**—The causative spirochete for Lyme disease in North America is *B. burgdorferi*, which was identified in 1982. Three genomic groups of *B. burgdorferi* have now been identified in Europe and

named *B. burgdorferi sensu stricto*, *B. garinii* and *B. afzelii*. A few *B. bissettii*-like strains as well as *B. valaisiana* strains and one atypical A14S strain have been cultured from European patients with EM lesions.

3. Occurrence—In the USA, endemic foci exist along the Atlantic coast, in Wisconsin and Minnesota, and in some areas of California and Oregon; increasing recognition of the disease has led to reports from 47 states and from Ontario and British Columbia in Canada, as well as from Europe, Russia, China and Japan.

The distribution of most cases coincides with the distribution of the black-legged tick, *Ixodes scapularis* (formerly *I. dammini*), in the eastern and midwestern USA; the western black-legged tick, *I. pacificus*, in western USA; *I. ricinus* (sheep tick) in Europe; and *I. persulcatus* in Asia. Initial infection occurs primarily during late spring or summer, with a peak in June and July, but may occur throughout the year, depending on the seasonal abundance of the tick locally. Dogs, cattle and horses develop systemic disease that may include the articular and cardiac manifestations seen in human patients. The explosive repopulation of the eastern USA by white-tailed deer, on which adult ticks feed, has been linked to the spread of Lyme disease in this region.

4. Reservoir—Some ixodid ticks through trans-stadial transmission (no or very limited trans-ovarial transmission). Wild rodents, especially *Peromyscus* spp. in the northeastern and midwestern USA and *Neotoma* spp. and gray squirrels in the western USA, maintain the enzootic transmission cycle. Deer serve as important mammalian maintenance hosts for vector tick species. Larval and nymphal ticks feed on small mammals, and adult ticks feed primarily on deer. The majority of Lyme disease cases result from bites by infected nymphs. Research in Europe supports the possible role of birds in dispersing *B. garinii* and *B. valaisiana*. Other studies support a relationship between *B. afzelii* and European rodents, notably *Clethrionomys* voles.

5. Mode of transmission—Tick-borne; in experimental animals, transmission by *I. scapularis* and *I. pacificus* usually does not occur until the tick has been attached for 24 hours or more; this may also be true in humans. Borrelia survives in blood products: no blood donation should be accepted from people suspected to have Lyme disease.

6. Incubation period—For EM, 3 to 32 days after tick exposure (mean 7 to 10 days); early stages of the illness may be unapparent and the patient may present with later manifestations.

7. Period of communicability—No evidence of natural person-to-person transmission. Despite rare case reports of congenital transmission, epidemiological studies have not shown a link between maternal Lyme disease and adverse outcomes of pregnancy.

8. Susceptibility—All persons are probably susceptible. Re-infection has occurred in those treated with antibiotics for early-stage disease.

9. Methods of control—

A. Preventive measures:

1) Educate the public about the mode of tick transmission and the means for personal protection.

2) Avoid tick-infested areas when feasible. To minimize exposure, wear light-colored clothing that covers legs and arms so that ticks may be more easily seen; tuck trousers into socks and apply tick repellent such as diethyltoluamide to the skin and/or permethrin (repellent and contact acaricide) to sleeves and trouser legs.

3) If working or playing in an infested area, examine the total body area daily. Do not neglect hairy areas. Remove ticks promptly; these may be very small, especially larvae or nymphs. Remove ticks by using gentle, steady traction with forceps (tweezers) applied close to the skin, so as to avoid leaving mouth parts in the skin; protect hands with gloves, cloth or tissue when removing ticks. Following removal, cleanse the attachment site with soap and water.

4) Measures designed to reduce tick populations on residential properties (host management, habitat modification, chemical control) are usually impractical on a large-scale basis.

5) During the late 1990s, two Lyme disease vaccines were developed for protection of humans using recombinant *B. burgdorferi stricto sensu* lipidated outer-surface protein A (rOspA) as an immunogen. In late 1999, one of these vaccines was licensed in the USA for administration on a 3-dose schedule of 0, 1, and 12 months, and was found to be safe and 76% effective in preventing overt Lyme disease after 3 doses. After license of the vaccine, anecdotal reports of joint reactions associated with vaccination, accompanied by lawsuits, led to discontinuation of distribution in February 2002 due to low demand and sales.

   a) Vaccine-induced anti-rOspA antibodies routinely cause false-positive ELISA results for Lyme disease. Experienced laboratory workers can usually discriminate between *B. burgdorferi* infection and previous rOspA immunization, because anti-OspA antibodies do not develop after natural infection.

   b) Lyme disease vaccine did not protect all recipients against infection with *B. burgdorferi* and offers no protection against other tick-borne borrelioses.

c) Risk assessment should include consideration of the geographic distribution of Lyme disease. The areas of highest risk in North America are concentrated within some northeastern and north-central states and provinces. In Europe, sporadic areas of transmission occur in areas where animal vectors are found. However, risk for Lyme disease differs even within counties and townships. Detailed information about the distribution of Lyme disease risk within specific areas is best obtained from public health authorities.

d) In areas of moderate to high risk, immunization had until 2002 been considered for persons aged 15–70 years who engaged in activities (recreational, property maintenance, occupational or leisure) resulting in frequent or prolonged exposure to tick-infested habitats. Future availability of vaccines against Lyme disease is uncertain.

B. Control of patient, contacts and the immediate environment:

1) Report to local health authority: Case report obligatory in some countries, Class 3 (see *Reporting*).
2) Isolation: Not applicable.
3) Concurrent disinfection: Carefully remove all ticks from patients.
4) Quarantine: Not applicable.
5) Immunization of contacts: Not applicable.
6) Investigation of contacts and source of infection: Studies to determine source of infection when cases occur outside a recognized endemic focus.
7) Specific treatment: For adults, the EM stage can usually be treated effectively with doxycycline (100 mg twice daily) or amoxicillin (500 mg 3–4 times daily)—though tetracycline and doxycycline cannot be used in children less than eight years of age. For localized EM, 2 weeks of treatment usually suffice; for early disseminated infection, 3–4 weeks. Children under 9 can be treated with amoxicillin, 50 mg/kg/day in divided doses, for the same period of time as adults. Cefuroxime axetil or erythromycin can be used in those allergic to penicillin or who cannot receive tetracyclines. Lyme arthritis can usually be treated successfully with a 4-week course of the oral agents. However, objective neurological abnormalities, with the possible exception of isolated facial palsy, are best treated with IV ceftriaxone, 2 grams once daily, or IV penicillin, 20 million units in 6 divided doses, for 3–4 weeks. Treatment failures may occasionally occur with any of these regimens and retreatment may be necessary.

C. Epidemic measures: In hyper-endemic and infested areas, identify tick species involved, if possible. See recommendations 9A1 through 9A3.

D. Disaster implications: None.

E. International measures: WHO Collaborating Centres provide support as required. More information can be found at: <http://www.who.int/collaboratingcentres/database/en/>

LYMPHOCYTIC
CHORIOMENINGITIS   ICD-9 049.0; ICD-10 A87.2
(LCM, Benign [or serous] lymphocytic meningitis)
[CCDM19: Editorial Board]

1. Identification—A viral infection of animals—especially mice—transmissible to humans, in whom it produces diverse clinical manifestations. There may be influenza-like symptoms, with myalgia, retro-orbital headache, leukopenia and thrombocytopenia, followed by complete recovery; in some cases, the illness may begin with meningeal or meningo-encephalomyelitic symptoms, or these symptoms may appear after a brief remission. Orchitis, parotitis, arthritis, myocarditis and rash occur occasionally. The acute course is usually short, very rarely fatal, and even with severe manifestations (e.g. coma with meningoencephalitis), prognosis for recovery without sequelae is usually good—although convalescence with fatigue and vasomotor instability may be prolonged. The CSF in cases with neurological involvement typically shows a lymphocytic pleocytosis and, at times, a low glucose level. The primary pathological finding in the rare human fatality is diffuse meningoencephalitis. Fatal cases of hemorrhagic fever-like disease have been reported. Transplacental infection of the fetus leading to hydrocephalus and chorioretinitis occurs, and should be tested for in such cases.

Laboratory diagnostic methods include isolation of virus from blood or CSF early in the course of illness by intracerebral inoculation of LCM-free mice (3 to 5 weeks old) or in cell cultures. Specific IgM in serum or CSF, as evidenced by IgM capture ELISA, or rising antibody titers by IFA in paired sera, are considered diagnostic. LCM requires differentiation from other aseptic meningitides and viral encephalitides.

2. Infectious agent—Lymphocytic choriomeningitis virus, an arenavirus, serologically related to Lassa, Machupo, Junín, Guaranito and Sabiá viruses.

3. Occurrence—Not uncommon in Europe and the Americas; underdiagnosed. Antibody prevalence of 5–10% has been reported among adults from the USA, Argentina and endemic areas of Germany. Loci of infection among feral mice often persist over long periods and result in sporadic clinical disease. Outbreaks have occurred from exposure to pet hamsters and laboratory animals. Nude mice, now extensively used in many research laboratories, are susceptible to infection, and may be prolific chronic excreters of virus.

4. Reservoir—The infected house mouse, *Mus musculus*, is the natural reservoir; infected females transmit infection to the offspring, which become asymptomatic persistent viral shedders. Infection also occurs in mouse and hamster colonies, and in transplantable tumor lines.

5. Mode of transmission—Virus excreted in urine, saliva and feces of infected animals, usually mice. Transmission to humans is probably through oral or respiratory contact with virus-contaminated excreta, food or dust, or through contamination of skin lesions or cuts. Handling articles contaminated by naturally infected mice may place individuals at a high risk of infection.

6. Incubation period—Probably 8-13 days; 15-21 days until meningeal symptoms appear.

7. Period of communicability—Person-to-person transmission not demonstrated, and unlikely.

8. Susceptibility—Recovery from the disease probably indicates immunity of long duration. Cell-mediated mechanisms are important, and antibodies may play a secondary role.

9. Methods of control—

    A. Preventive measures: Clean home and workplace environment; eliminate mice and use caution with diseased pets such as hamsters and mice. Keep foods in closed containers. Virological surveillance of commercial rodent breeding establishments, especially those producing hamsters and mice, is helpful. Ensure that laboratory mice are not infected and that personnel handling mice follow established procedures to prevent transmission from infected animals.

    B. Control of patient, contacts and the immediate environment:

        1) Report to local health authority: Reportable in selected endemic areas, Class 3 (see *Reporting*).
        2) Isolation: Not applicable
        3) Concurrent disinfection: Of discharges from the nose and throat, urine, feces and articles soiled therewith during acute febrile period. Terminal cleaning.
        4) Quarantine: Not applicable
        5) Immunization of contacts: Not applicable

6) Investigation of contacts and source of infection: Search home and place of employment for presence of house mice or sick or infected rodent pets.
7) Specific treatment: None.

C. Epidemic measures: Not applicable.

D. Disaster implications: None.

E. International measures: None.

LYMPHOGRANULOMA
VENEREUM   ICD-9 099.1; ICD-10 A55
(Lymphogranuloma inguinale, Climatic or tropical bubo, LGV)
[CCDM19: R. Ballard, F. Ndowa, Ye Tun]
[CCDM18: F. Ndowa]

1. Identification—A sexually acquired chlamydial infection characterized by a small, painless, evanescent erosion, papule, nodule or herpetiform lesion on the penis or within the urethra in men, or on the vulva, vaginal wall or cervix in women. The primary lesion may remain unnoticed. The regional lymph nodes may undergo suppuration followed by extension of the inflammatory process to the adjacent tissues. In men, inguinal and/or femoral buboes are seen that may become adherent to the skin, fluctuate, and result in sinus formation. In women, these external nodes are less frequently affected and involvement is mainly of the pelvic nodes with extension to the rectum and rectovaginal septum; the result is proctitis, stricture of the rectum and fistulae. Proctitis may result from rectal intercourse; and proctitis or proctocolitis is the most common acute manifestation of lymphogranuloma venereum among men who have sex with men. Common presentations include rectal discharge, pain, constipation and tenesmus. Elephantiasis of the genitalia may occur in both men and women. Fever, chills, headache, joint pains and anorexia are usually present during the bubo phase, and are due to systemic spread. If left untreated, the course of the disease is often prolonged with scar formation and associated severe disability. The disease is generally not fatal. Generalized sepsis with arthritis and meningitis is a rare occurrence.

Diagnosis is made by demonstration of chlamydial organisms in swabs from lesions or bubo aspirates by IF, EIA, DNA probe, PCR or culture. Additional tests such as genotyping or LGV-specific PCR are required to differentiate LGV from non-LGV chlamydial infections. Complement Fixation (CF) and micro-IF (MIF) serological tests could be used to support the diagnosis. A single titer of equal or more than 1:64 and 1:256, in the CF and MIF tests, respectively, is highly suggestive of LGV.

2. Infectious agent—The invasive *Chlamydia trachomatis*, genotypes L-1, L-2 and L-3, related to but distinct from those genotypes that cause trachoma and oculogenital chlamydial infections.

3. Occurrence—Worldwide, especially in tropical and subtropical areas; more common than ordinarily believed. Endemic in parts of Africa, southeast Asia, Latin America and the Caribbean. Outbreaks of LGV have been reported recently in western Europe and the USA in men who have sex with men (MSM) and bisexual men. Most of these cases have been in HIV-infected persons practicing receptive rectal intercourse. Age incidence corresponds with sexual activity. The disease is less commonly diagnosed in women, probably as a result of the frequency of asymptomatic infections. Though acute LGV is reported more frequently in men than in women, late complications, such as hypertrophy of the genitalia and rectal strictures, are reported more frequently in women, probably because of the non-specific or poorly symptomatic nature of early infection in women. All races are affected. In temperate climates, LGV is seen predominantly among MSM. Clusters of cases among MSM have been reported in Europe, Canada, and the USA.

4. Reservoir—Humans; often asymptomatic (particularly in females).

5. Mode of transmission—Direct contact with open lesions of infected people, usually during sexual intercourse.

6. Incubation period—Variable, with a range of 3–30 days for a primary lesion; if a bubo is the first manifestation, 10–30 days to several months.

7. Period of communicability—Variable, from weeks to years during presence of active lesions.

8. Susceptibility and resistance—Susceptibility is general; status of natural or acquired resistance is unclear.

9. Methods of control—

    A. Preventive measures: Except for measures that are specific for syphilis, preventive measures are those for sexually transmitted diseases. See *Syphilis*, 9A, and *Granuloma inguinale*, 9A.

    B. Control of patient, contacts and the immediate environment:

        1) Report to local health authority: A reportable disease in selected endemic areas; not a reportable disease in most countries, Class 3 (see *Reporting*).

        2) Isolation: Refrain from sexual contact until all lesions are healed.

        3) Concurrent disinfection: Exercise care in disposal of discharges from lesions and of articles soiled therewith.

4) Quarantine: Not applicable.

5) Immunization of contacts: Not applicable; prompt treatment on recognition or clinical suspicion of infection.

6) Investigation of contacts and source of infection: Search for infected sexual contacts of patient. Recent contacts of confirmed active cases should receive specific therapy.

7) Specific treatment: Tetracycline and doxycycline, administered orally for at least 2 weeks, are effective for all stages, including buboes and ulcerative lesions. Tetracycline and doxycyline cannot be used in children less than eight years of age. Erythromycin may be used when tetracycline is contraindicated, or if chancroid is a possible diagnosis. Fluctuant buboes should not be incised, but rather drained by aspiration through healthy tissue after initiation of therapy, to minimize formation of sinuses. Although oral azithromycin in a single 1-gram dose has been proven effective for chlamydial urethritis and cervicitis, its effectiveness in treatment of LGV is not known.

C. Epidemic measures: Not applicable.

D. Disaster implications: None.

E. International measures: See *Syphilis*, 9E.

MALARIA ICD-9 084; ICD-10 B50-B54
[CCDM19: K. Mendis, A. Rietveld, L. Slutsker]
[CCDM18: A. Schapira]

1. Identification— Malaria in humans is a parasitic disease caused by infection with one or more of four species of intracellular protozoan parasite: *Plasmodium falciparum*, *P. vivax*, *P. ovale*, and *P. malariae*. *P. falciparum* and *P. vivax* infections are the more common worldwide, but *P. falciparum* malaria represents the most serious public health problem, because of its tendency toward severe or fatal infections.

The early clinical manifestations of malaria are non-specific and similar enough among species to make differentiation impossible without laboratory studies. Moreover, the clinical syndrome in the first few days of infection resembles that in early stages of many other febrile illnesses due to bacterial, viral or parasitic causes, and requires the demonstration of parasites or their products in blood for confirmation. *P. falciparum* malaria (ICD-9 084.0, ICD-10 B50) typically presents a protean clinical picture, including fever, chills, myalgias and arthralgias, headache, diarrhea, vomiting and other nonspecific signs. Splenomegaly, anemia, and thrombocytopenia often develop after a few days. Later, if treatment is delayed, severe malaria may develop. Severe malaria may be characterized by acute encephalopathy (cerebral malaria), severe anemia, icterus, renal failure (black water fever), hypoglycemia, respiratory distress, lactic acidosis and, more rarely, coagulation defects and shock. Severe malaria is a possible cause of coma and other CNS symptoms in any partially immune or non-immune person recently returned from an endemic tropical area. Prompt treatment of *falciparum* malaria is essential, even in mild cases, since irreversible complications may rapidly appear. Case fatality rates of children and non-immunes with uncomplicated malaria are circa 0.1%. This increases to 15%–20% once complications appear. Untreated severe malaria is almost always fatal.

The other human malarias, *vivax* (ICD-9 084.1, ICD-10 B51), *malariae* (ICD-9 084.2, ICD-10 B52) and *ovale* (ICD-9 084.3, ICD-10 B53.0), are not usually life-threatening. Illness may begin with malaise and fever for several days, followed by shaking chills and rapidly rising temperature, accompanied by headache and nausea. Profuse sweating occurs with defervescence. After a fever-free interval, the cycle of chills, fever and sweating recurs daily, every other day or every third day. An untreated primary infection may last from a week to a month or longer and be accompanied by prostration, anemia and splenomegaly. True relapses following periods with no parasitemia can occur in *vivax* and *ovale* infections at irregular intervals for up to 5 years, due to a relapsing parasite stage sequestered in the liver (hypnozoites). Infections with *P. malariae* may persist for life with or without recurrent febrile episodes; however, as with *P. falciparum*, there is no relapsing liver stage.

Persons who have grown up in endemic areas and acquired partial immunity, or non-immune persons who have been taking prophylactic antimalarial drugs, may show an atypical clinical picture and a prolonged incubation period.

The diagnosis of malaria must be considered in all febrile patients who have traveled to or lived in malaria-endemic areas or who have received blood products, tissues or organs from persons who have been to such areas. There are several diagnostic methods, including microscopic diagnosis, antigen detection tests, PCR-based assays, and serological tests. Direct microscopic examination of intracellular parasites on stained blood films is the current standard for definitive diagnosis in nearly all settings. In non-immune persons, symptoms may develop before there are detectable levels of parasitemia. For this reason, several blood smear examinations taken at 12–24 hour intervals may be needed to rule out a diagnosis of malaria in a symptomatic patient.

Laboratory confirmation is possible through:

    a) Demonstration of malaria parasites in a blood film. Repeated microscopic examinations every 12–24 hours may be necessary because the blood density of parasites varies, and parasites are often not demonstrable in films from patients recently or actively under treatment.

b) Detection of parasite antigens by means of rapid diagnostic tests. There are several tests for the routine detection of *falciparum* malaria as well as malaria in general (genus *Plasmodium*), based on the antigens HRP2, pLDH or Aldo-lase. Tests available for the detection of *vivax* malaria are fewer in number, and performance is more limited.

Diagnosis by PCR is the most sensitive method, but this is not generally available in diagnostic laboratories.

Antibodies, demonstrable by IFA or other tests, may appear after the first week of infection but may persist for years, indicating past malarial experience; thus antibody determinations are not helpful for diagnosis of current illness. Guidelines for laboratory diagnosis are summarized elsewhere and are available online at:

<http://www.cdc.gov/malaria/>

2. Infectious agents—*Plasmodium falciparum*, *P. vivax*, *P. ovale* and *P. malariae*; protozoan parasites with asexual and sexual phases that occur in humans and in the mosquito. Mixed species infections are not infrequent in endemic areas.

3. Occurrence—Endemic malaria no longer occurs in most temperate-zone countries and in many areas of subtropical countries; it is still, however, a major cause of ill health in many tropical and other subtropical areas. The disease is responsible for an estimated 1 million deaths per year globally, mostly in young children in Africa; high transmission areas occur throughout tropical Africa, in the southwestern Pacific, in forested areas of South America (e.g. Brazil), in southeastern Asia, and in parts of the Indian sub-continent. *Ovale* malaria occurs mainly in sub-Saharan Africa, where *vivax* malaria is much less frequent.

The development and the rapid spread of antimalarial drug resistance in *Plasmodium falciparum* has been one of the greatest threats to malaria control. Resistance to chloroquine, previously the most widely used anti-malarial drug, is widespread, with a few exceptional areas where chloroquine remains effective (Central America west of the Panama Canal, Haiti and the Dominican Republic). Resistance in *P. falciparum* has also developed to sulfadoxine-pyrimethamine (Amazon Region, southeast Asia, sub-Saharan Africa) and mefloquine (parts of southeast Asia). Resistance has affected all the other antimalarial drugs to different degrees, and is aggravated by cross-resistance between medicines. Sulfadoxine-pyrimethamine, which replaced chloroquine, became almost totally ineffective in Thailand and neighboring countries at the beginning of the 1980s, and this resistance spread rapidly to South America and east Africa. Resistance to quinine and mefloquine is found mainly in Thailand and Cambodia. Sporadic cases of prophylactic failure of mefloquine in travelers and therapeutic failure with amino-alcohols have been reported in Africa,

South America, and in other Asian countries. So far, no resistance to artemisinin or artemisinin derivative has been reported, although some decrease in *in vitro* sensitivity has been reported in China and increased parasite clearance time after treatment with artemisinin-based combination therapy or artesunate monotherapy has been reported at the Thai-Cambodian border.

Most *P. vivax* malaria infections remain sensitive to chloroquine. However, in recent years, chloroquine resistance of *P. vivax* has been reported in southeast Asia, in South America, and even in Africa. The relapsing hepatic stages of some *P. vivax* strains may also be relatively tolerant to primaquine, but its optimum regimen has not been fully defined.

Current information on drug-resistant malaria is published annually by CDC (*Health Information for International Travel*), and can be found at:
 <http://www.cdc.gov/travel/yb/index.htm>
- or on the CDC Malaria website, at:
 <http://www.cdc.gov/malaria>
- and by WHO, at:
 <http://www.who.int/malaria/resistance.html>
- and in *International Travel and Health*, at:
 <http://www.who.int/ith/en/>

4. Reservoir—Humans are the most important reservoir of human malaria, except as regards *P. malariae*, which is common to man, the African apes and probably some South American monkeys. Non-human primates are naturally infected by malaria parasite species, some of which are closely related to the human malarias, and which therefore can infect humans experimentally. Natural transmission of these non-human primate malarias to humans occurs sporadically. Recently, *P. knowlesi*, a parasite of Old World monkeys, has been documented as a cause of hundreds of human infections and some fatalities in Malaysia. Investigations are ongoing to determine the extent of transmission to humans; it is suggested that non-human primates may be a more important source for malaria in humans in certain geographical situations than previously thought.

5. Mode of transmission—Most malaria is transmitted by the bite of an infective female *Anopheles* sp. mosquito. Most species feed at night; some important vectors also bite at dusk or in the early morning.

Malaria infection begins when an infective female mosquito injects *Plasmodium* sp. sporozoites into the bloodstream while feeding. The sporozoites pass almost immediately into the cells of the liver parenchyma, where they undergo asexual reproduction (exo-erythrocytic schizogony) and mature into schizonts. In 6 to 14 days, these schizonts mature and rupture, releasing merozoites into the bloodstream. Merozoites subsequently invade red blood cells and then undergo a second phase of asexual reproduction (erythrocytic schizogony). Once the erythrocytic schizonts mature, the infected red blood cells rupture, releasing more merozoites into the bloodstream, and beginning another cycle of asexual development and multiplication. Clinical symptoms occur with the rupture of erythrocytic schizonts, usually after several cycles of erythrocytic schizogony. The classical clinical presentation of periodic fever and shaking chills occurs when the cycles of erythrocytic schizogony are synchronized.

Some merozoites develop into sexual forms called gametocytes. Male and female gametocytes circulate in the blood without causing symptoms, and can then be ingested by a mosquito during a subsequent blood meal. Sexual reproduction occurs within the mosquito midgut, where male and female gametes unite to form an ookinete; the ookinete then penetrates the midgut wall and forms an oocyst. After maturation for days to weeks, the oocyst ruptures, releasing sporozoites, which migrate through the coelomic cavity to the salivary glands. The life cycle starts again when the infective mosquito bites another human.

The period between an infective bite and detection of the parasite in a thick blood smear is the "prepatent period," which is typically 6–12 days for *P. falciparum*; 8–12 days for *P. vivax* and *P. ovale*; and 12–16 days for *P. malariae*. The period between the infective bite and the appearance of clinical symptoms is called the incubation period. Delayed primary attacks by some *P. vivax* strains may occur 6–12 months after exposure. Gametocytes usually appear in the bloodstream within 3 days of overt parasitemia with *P. vivax* and *P. ovale*, and after about 10 days with *P. falciparum*. Unlike *P. vivax* and *P. ovale*, relapses do not occur with *falciparum* or *malariae* malaria. Reappearance of *P. falciparum* (recrudescence) occurs due to inadequate treatment or infection with drug-resistant strains. With *P. malariae*, low levels of erythrocytic parasites may persist for many years, to be activated at some future time to a level that may result again in clinical illness.

Induced malaria refers to infection that is passed directly from one individual to another through contaminated blood or blood products, injection equipment, or organ transplant. Congenital malaria refers to infection passed from mother to infant *in utero*. Pregnant women in endemic areas, especially primi- and secundigravidae, are at increased risk of infection with *P. falciparum* and *vivax* malaria due to partial loss of immunity during pregnancy. In areas of intense transmission, *P. falciparum* may infect the placenta and contribute to low birth-weight as well as maternal anemia. In low transmission areas, pregnant women are at high risk of severe *falciparum* malaria, abortion and premature delivery. *Vivax* malaria in pregnancy in these areas has been associated with maternal anemia and low birthweight.

6. Incubation periods—The incubation period is approximately 9–14 days for *P. falciparum*; 12–18 days for *P. vivax* and *P. ovale*; and 18–40 days for *P. malariae*. Some strains of *P. vivax*, mostly from temperate areas, may have an incubation period of 6–12 months. With infection through blood transfusion, incubation periods depend on the number of parasites infused and are usually short, but may range up to 2 months. Because there is no liver stage with transfusion-transmitted malaria, *vivax* or *ovale* relapses cannot occur. Suboptimal suppression from suboptimal prophylaxis may result in prolonged incubation periods.

7. Period of communicability—Humans may infect mosquitoes as long as infective gametocytes are present in the blood; this varies with parasite species and with response to therapy. Untreated or insufficiently treated patients may be a source of mosquito infection for several years in *malariae*, up to 5 years in *vivax*, and generally not more than 1 year in *falciparum* malaria; the mosquito remains infective for life. Transfusional transmission may occur as long as asexual forms remain in the circulating blood (with *P. malariae,* up to 40 years or longer). Stored blood can remain infective for at least a month.

8. Susceptibility—Susceptibility is universal except in humans with specific genetic traits. Clinical disease is present but often attenuated in adults in highly endemic communities who have acquired partial immunity following repeated exposure to infective anophelines over many years. Most indigenous populations of West Africa show a natural resistance to infection with *P. vivax*, which is associated with the absence of the Duffy antigen on their erythrocytes. Persons with the inherited sickle cell trait (heterozygotes) show relatively low parasitemia when infected with *P. falciparum*, and thus are relatively protected from severe disease. Homozygotes suffering from sickle cell disease are at increased risk of severe or fatal *falciparum* malaria, especially anemia. Other genetic traits that may modify disease expression include other hemoglobinopathies (HbC, HbE), thalassemias, and glucose-6-phosphate dehydrogenase (G6PD) deficiency. HIV-infected immunosuppressed persons living in endemic areas appear to be at increased risk of more frequent and higher density infections, and may show decreased response to antimalarial therapy.

9. Methods of control—The control of malaria in endemic areas is based on early, effective treatment of all cases and a selection of preventive measures appropriate to the local situation.

Prompt and effective treatment of all cases is essential in order to reduce the risk of severe disease and prevent death. In areas of low transmission, this will also help reduce transmission. In areas of intense transmission, where children are the main risk group, formal health services may not be sufficiently accessible; in these situations, community-based treatment programs may increase access. The increasing problems of drug resistance highlight the importance of selecting a locally effective drug. For *falciparum* malaria, it is now recommended to use artemisinin-based combination therapy, to protect against the development of resistance and thus achieve rapid and effective cure and prolong the useful life of the treatments used.

A confirmatory diagnosis by microscopy or using a Rapid Diagnostic Test is recommended before treatment. However, in high transmission areas young children (under five years of age) with fever or a history of fever and no other obvious cause are often treated presumptively. *P. falciparum* malaria is the most likely cause of their illness and there is as yet no evidence to show that a young child with a negative parasitological diagnosis should not be treated. Similarly, starting treatment on clinical grounds can be justifiable for non-immune travelers.

A. Preventive measures:

I. Local community measures in endemic areas

1) Insecticide-treated mosquito nets (ITNs) are the most universally useful measure for the prevention of malaria. Although people may go to bed after mosquitoes have started biting, the partial protection is still useful; children, who are usually the most susceptible, generally go to bed earlier. If ITN coverage in a community is very high, a community-level or mass effect may be seen, whereby even those who do not have or sleep under ITNs are relatively protected. The use of mosquito nets has been uncommon or absent among most affected populations, but recently, availability, distribution, and coverage have increased in many countries. The nets must be carefully tucked under the sleeping mattress or mat. Conventional ITNs have to be systematically re-treated after 3 washes or at least once a year, which can be quite difficult to achieve; recently, long-lasting insecticidal nets (LLINs) incorporating or coated with pyrethroid insecticides during manufacture have obviated the need for re-treatment of nets, and these are now the preferred products; estimated life span of these nets is 2–5 years. Information on WHO-recommended nets can be found at: <http://www.who.int/whopes/en/>

   In order to obtain the best benefit of this highly cost-effective intervention, information on how nets should be used and maintained must be communicated to the people who will be using them. Other long-lasting nets, including some treated with two insecticides to prevent the development of resistance, are under development.

2) Indoor residual spraying with insecticides (IRS) is another preventive method, targeting adult mosquitoes. IRS is most effective where mosquitoes rest indoors on sprayable surfaces, where people are exposed in or near the home, and when it is applied before the transmission season or period of peak transmission. Coverage rates in the target area must be high: in contrast to ITNs, IRS is a community public health intervention and not a personal protection measure. The susceptibility of vectors to the insecticide applied must be ascertained. When correctly applied on the basis of epidemiological and entomological data, IRS is very effective in reducing transmission by reducing the survival of malaria

vectors entering houses or sleeping units. The most important constraints are operational: IRS requires a complex logistical effort involving teams of sprayers that need to be moved from community to community, and a certain number of households must be covered in a given time period. Thus, IRS becomes increasingly difficult in areas with low or very high human density, and where terrain is difficult. In addition, previous experience has shown that IRS, which may need to be carried out up to twice a year depending on the insecticide chosen and the transmission pattern, may become less popular over time: after repeated spray operations, community acceptance of intervention decreases. There are currently 12 insecticides recommended by WHO for IRS. The choice of insecticide is guided by insecticide susceptibility and vector behavior, safety for humans and the environment, efficacy, and cost-effectiveness. DDT is still needed and used for disease vector control because of its efficacy and operational feasibility. The use of DDT for IRS is closely monitored in the context of the Stockholm Convention on Persistent Organic Pollutants, which bans the use of DDT except for public health purposes. For further information on this, please consult: <http://www.who.int/malaria/ddtandmalariavectorcontrol.html>

3) Control of larval stages by elimination of mosquito breeding sites—for example, by filling and draining, or by increasing the speed of water flow in natural or artificial channels—is of limited use in most areas where malaria transmission persists today. Similarly, chemical and biological control methods (bacterial larvicides, larvivorous fish) applied to impounded water bodies may be difficult to implement in rural areas; however, some success with these methods has recently been documented in urban African settings, and such methods may be useful adjuncts in situations such as arid, coastal and urban areas, or to maintain low receptivity of areas where malaria elimination has been achieved.

4) Intermittent preventive treatment with a full curative dose of an effective antimalarial at predefined intervals during the 2nd and 3rd trimester of pregnancy is a highly effective measure for reducing the malaria burden among pregnant women in areas of stable, moderate to intense *P. falciparum* transmission. This is promoted in Africa, but is of limited use in other parts of the world where transmission is often unstable and of low intensity. ITNs or LLINs should also be made available to pregnant women in endemic areas to help reduce the deleterious effects of malaria in pregnancy.

5) In epidemic-prone areas, malaria surveillance should be based on weekly reporting and combined with monitoring of

locally important factors regarding the genesis of epidemics, such as meteorological and environmental conditions and human population movements. The case definition for surveillance recommended within the national malaria control program should be used. As a minimum, laboratory test-confirmed cases must be distinguished from non-confirmed (probable) cases.

II. Personal protective measures and treatment for non-immune travelers

Because of the severity of malaria, increasing risks for non-immune travelers, and the large number of such travelers who visit endemic regions, personal protective measures taken by travelers are of utmost importance and are presented in detail.

Physicians should realize that all people who visit an endemic area during the transmission season and who are exposed to mosquito bites between dusk and dawn are at risk of developing clinical malaria. *Falciparum* malaria may be fatal if treatment is delayed beyond 24 hours after the onset of clinical symptoms. *Falciparum* malaria is part of the differential diagnosis in all cases of unexplained fever starting at any time between 7 days after the first possible exposure to malaria and 3 months (or, rarely, later) after the last possible exposure. All non-immune persons, but especially young children, pregnant women, people living with HIV/AIDS, the immunosuppressed, and the elderly, are highly susceptible to development of severe and complicated malaria when infected. Ask for a travel history.

Travelers to malarious areas must realize that protection from biting mosquitoes is of paramount importance; no antimalarial prophylactic regimen can give complete protection, but such regimens do reduce the risk of fatal disease; prophylaxis with antimalarial drugs should not automatically be prescribed for all travelers to malarious areas; and "standby" emergency self-treatment is recommended when a febrile illness occurs in a *falciparum* malaria area where professional medical care is not readily available.

1) **Measures to reduce the risk of mosquito bites** include the following:

a) Avoid being outdoors between dusk and dawn, when anopheline mosquitoes commonly bite. Wear long-sleeved clothing and long trousers when going out at night. The thickness of the material used for protective clothing is critical.

b) Systematic use of insect repellent on exposed skin as well as clothing (especially socks and trousers). Choose a repellent containing DEET (*N,N*-diethyl-*m*-toluamide),

IR3535® (3-[N-acetyl-N-butyl]-aminopropionic acid ethyl ester), or Bayrepel®/Picaridin® (1-piperidinecarboxylic acid, 2-(2-hydroxyethyl), 1-methylpropylester). Repellents should be used in strict accordance with the manufacturers' instructions, and dosage must not be exceeded, especially for young children and pregnant women.

c) Stay in a well-constructed building, if possible air-conditioned, in the most developed part of town.

d) Use screens over doors and windows; if no screens are available, close windows and doors at night.

e) Use a mosquito net over the bed, with edges tucked in under the mattress; ensure that the net is not torn and that there are no mosquitoes inside it; sleep in the middle of the bed, avoiding contact between body and net. Use an ITN or LLIN to increase protection.

f) Use anti-mosquito sprays or insecticide dispensers (mains- or battery-operated) that contain tablets impregnated with pyrethroids in bedrooms at night (or mosquito coils if there is no electricity and batteries are unavailable). Different protective measures should be used in combination, especially when staying in areas where there is intense malaria transmission.

2) **People who are or will be exposed to mosquitoes in malarious areas** should know the four principles—the **ABCD**— of malaria protection:

a) Be **A**ware of the risk, the incubation period, the possibility of delayed onset, and the main symptoms.

b) Avoid being **B**itten by mosquitoes, especially between dusk and dawn.

c) Take antimalarial drugs (**C**hemoprophylaxis) when appropriate, to prevent infection developing into clinical disease.

d) Immediately seek **D**iagnosis and treatment if a fever develops one week or more after entering an area where there is a malaria risk and up to 3 months (or, rarely, later) after departure from a risk area.

The risk of malaria infection varies among countries and between different areas of each country. For more information, see the country list in WHO's annually updated publication *International Travel and Health*, which can be found at:

<http://www.who.int/ith>

Depending on the malaria risk in the area visited, the recommended prevention method may be mosquito bite prevention only, or mosquito bite prevention in combination with chemoprophylaxis. Alternatively, in rural areas with multidrug-resistant malaria and only a very low risk of *P. falciparum* infection, mosquito bite prevention can be combined with standby emergency treatment.

3A) **Pregnant travelers** must be advised of the following:

a) Malaria during pregnancy increases the risk of maternal death, miscarriage, stillbirth, low birthweight and neonatal death.

b) Pregnant travelers should not visit malarious areas unless this is absolutely necessary.

c) Pregnant women have been shown to be particularly susceptible to mosquito bites. Extra diligence is needed in using measures to protect against mosquito bites.

d) There is very limited information on the safety and efficacy of most antimalarials in pregnancy, particularly during the first trimester. There is no prophylactic or treatment regimen that is effective and safe for pregnant women in areas of multidrug-resistant malaria.

e) Prophylaxis with chloroquine (with or without proguanil) can be safely prescribed, including during the first 3 months of pregnancy, but its use is now very limited. Mefloquine prophylaxis may be given during the second and third trimesters, but there is limited information on its safety during the first trimester. Doxycycline is contraindicated during pregnancy. Atovaquone–proguanil has not been sufficiently investigated to be prescribed in pregnancy. In light of the danger of malaria to mother and fetus, experts increasingly agree that travel of pregnant women to a chloroquine-resistant *P. falciparum* area during the first trimester of pregnancy should be avoided or delayed at all costs; if this is truly impossible, good preventive measures should be taken, including prophylaxis with mefloquine where this is indicated.

f) Medical help should be sought immediately if malaria is suspected; standby emergency treatment should be taken only if no medical help is immediately available. Medical help must be sought as soon as possible after standby treatment (see 9AII5 and 9AII6).

g) Women of childbearing age should preferably avoid pregnancy until 3 months after they have stopped mefloquine prophylaxis, and for 1 week after doxycycline, and 3 weeks after atovaquone-proguanil. If pregnancy occurs during antimalarial prophylaxis, this is not considered to be an indication for pregnancy termination.

3B) **Parents of young children** must be advised of the following:

   a) *Falciparum* malaria in a young child may be rapidly fatal. Early symptoms are atypical and difficult to recognize, and life-threatening complications can occur within hours of the initial symptoms. In infants, fever may be absent.

   b) Babies and young children should not be taken to areas with risk of *falciparum* malaria. If travel cannot be avoided, children must be very carefully protected with preventive measures.

   c) Chemoprophylaxis dosage schedules for children should be based on body weight. Long-term travelers and expatriates should adjust the chemoprophylaxis dosage according to the increasing weight of the growing child.

   d) Chloroquine (5 mg base/kg/week in one dose; or 10 mg base/kg/week divided into 6 daily doses) and proguanil (3 mg/kg/day) are safe, but their use is now very limited. Mefloquine (5 mg/kg/week) may be given to infants of more than 5 kg body weight. Atovaquone–proguanil (in pediatric tablets) is generally not recommended for prophylaxis in children who weigh less than 11 kg, because of limited data; in the USA and Belgium it is given for prophylaxis in infants of more than 5 kg body weight. Doxycycline cannot be used in children less than eight years of age.

   e) All antimalarial drugs should be kept out of the reach of children and stored in childproof containers: chloroquine is particularly toxic in case of overdose.

4) **Chemoprophylaxis:** Before travel, the most appropriate chemoprophylactic antimalarial drug(s) (if any) for the destination(s) should be prescribed in the correct dosages.

   a) In areas with only very limited risk of malaria transmission, chemoprophylaxis may not be indicated, as the risk of side effects associated with antimalarials may outweigh the potential benefits. Travelers should, however, always be aware of the possibility of malaria if they develop a febrile disease.

   b) In areas where only *P. vivax* malaria occurs, and those rare places where *P. falciparum* remains fully sensitive to chloroquine, chemoprophylaxis with chloroquine (5 mg base/kg/week in one dose; or 10 mg base/kg/week divided into 6 daily doses) on its own can be used.

   c) In areas with risk of *P. vivax* and *P. falciparum* malaria transmission, and emerging chloroquine resistance, chloroquine chemoprophylaxis should be combined with proguanil (3 mg/kg/day).

d) In areas with high risk of *P. falciparum* malaria and reported antimalarial drug resistance, the chemoprophylaxis choices are atovaquone–proguanil (adult dose: 250 mg atovaquone plus 100 mg proguanil daily), doxycycline (1.5 mg/kg/day), or mefloquine (5 mg/kg/week). This choice also applies to areas with moderate/low *P. falciparum* risk and reported high levels of drug resistance. The selection depends on the reported resistance pattern in the area to be visited, the contraindications of the various drugs, and personal preferences. Annually updated information on recommended prophylaxis options is available from WHO at:

<http://www.who.int/ith/>

e) Antimalarials that have to be taken daily (atovaquone-proguanil, chloroquine, doxycycline, proguanil) should be started the day before arrival in the risk area. Weekly chloroquine should be started 1 week before arrival. Mefloquine should preferably be started 2-3 weeks before departure, to achieve higher pre-travel blood levels and to allow side effects to be detected before travel so that possible alternatives can be considered.

f) All prophylactic drugs should be taken with unfailing regularity for the duration of the stay in the malaria risk area, and should be continued for 4 weeks after the last possible exposure to infection, since parasites may still emerge from the liver during this period. The single exception is atovaquone–proguanil, which can be stopped 1 week after return because of its effect on early liver-stage parasites. Premature interruption of the daily atovaquone-proguanil prophylaxis regimen may lead to loss of this causal prophylactic effect, in which case atovaquone-proguanil prophylaxis should also be continued for 4 weeks upon return.

g) All antimalarial drugs have specific contraindications and possible side effects. Serious adverse events— defined as constituting an apparent threat to life, requiring or prolonging hospitalization, or resulting in persistent or significant disability or incapacity—are rare, and normally only identified in post-marketing surveillance once a drug has been in use for some time. Severe neuropsychiatric disturbances (seizures, psychosis, encephalopathy) occur in approximately 1 in 10 000 travelers receiving mefloquine prophylaxis, and have also been reported for chloroquine at a similar rate. The risk of serious adverse reactions can be reduced by carefully observing the contraindications for each drug. A traveler who develops severe side-effects to an antimalarial should stop taking the drug and seek immediate medical attention.

5) **Standby emergency treatment (SBET):** The most important factors that determine the survival of patients with *falciparum* malaria are early diagnosis and immediate treatment. Non-immune individuals exposed to or infected with malaria should obtain prompt medical attention when malaria is suspected. A minority will be exposed to a high risk of infection while at least 12–24 hours away from competent medical attention. WHO recommends that prescribers issue antimalarial medicines to be carried for self-administration by persons who may be in such exposed situations. Also, in light of the spread of counterfeit medicines, some travelers may opt to buy a reserve antimalarial treatment before departure, so that they can be confident of drug quality should they become ill.

Persons prescribed standby treatment must receive precise instructions on recognition of symptoms, when and how to take treatment, the complete treatment regimen to be taken, possible side-effects, and action to be taken in the event of drug failure. They must be made aware that self-treatment is a temporary measure and medical advice is to be sought as soon as possible. If several people travel together, the individual dosages for SBET should be specified. Weight-based dosages for children need to be clearly indicated.

6) **Treatment upon return:**

The following antimalarials are suitable for treatment of **uncomplicated *falciparum* malaria** in travelers returning to non-endemic countries:

- Artemether–lumefantrine (adult dose, 4 tablets twice a day for 3 days).
- Atovaquone–proguanil (15/6 mg/kg, usual adult dose, 4 tablets once a day for 3 days).
- Quinine (10 mg salt/kg bw every 8 h) plus doxycycline (3.5 mg/kg bw once a day) or clindamycin (10 mg/kg bw twice a day); all drugs to be given for 7 days. Doxycycline cannot be used during pregnancy and in children less than eight years of age.

The treatment for ***vivax* and *ovale* malaria** in travelers is with chloroquine (25 mg base/kg bw divided over 3 days), combined with primaquine (usual dose 0.25 mg base/kg bw, taken with food once daily for 14 days). For travelers returning from Oceania and southeast Asia the dose of primaquine should be 0.5 mg/kg bw. In moderate G6PD deficiency, primaquine 0.75 mg base/kg bw should be given once a week for 8 weeks. In severe G6PD deficiency, primaquine should not be given. Primaquine is contraindicated during pregnancy and in young infants. Late onset *vivax* or *ovale* malaria may occur from the development of intrahepatic parasites after chemoprophylaxis is discontinued. *Malariae* malaria in travelers can be treated with chloroquine (25 mg base/kg bw divided over 3 days).

Returning travelers with **severe *falciparum* malaria** should be managed in an intensive care unit. Parenteral antimalarial treatment should be started without delay with whichever effective antimalarial is first available:

- Artesunate[1] (first choice) (2.4 mg/kg bw i.v. or i.m. given on admission (time = 0), then at 12 h and 24 h, then once a day).
- Artemether (3.2 mg/kg bw i.m. given on admission then 1.6 mg/kg bw per day).
- Quinine (20 mg salt/kg bw on admission (i.v. infusion or divided i.m. injection), then 10 mg/kg bw every 8 h; infusion rate should not exceed 5 mg salt/kg bw per hour).

If these medicines are not available, use parenteral quinidine with careful clinical and electrocardiographic monitoring.

B. *Control of patient, contacts and the immediate environment:*

1) In non-endemic areas, report to local health authority: Obligatory case report as a Disease under Surveillance by WHO, Class 1 (see *Reporting*), preferably limited to smear confirmed cases; Class 3 (reporting of probable and confirmed cases) is the more practical procedure in endemic areas.

2) Isolation: For hospitalized patients, blood precautions. In non-endemic areas where malaria transmission is possible, patients should be in mosquito-proof areas from dusk to dawn, until microscopy shows that they have no gametocytes in the blood.

---

[1]Artesunate is not yet FDA-approved in the United States, but is available from the CDC on an emergency compassionate use basis. More information can be found at <http://www.cdc.gov/malaria>

Blood donations

In non-endemic areas, blood donors should be questioned for a history of malaria or a history of travel to, or residence in, a malarious area. In many non-endemic areas, travelers who have not taken antimalarial drugs and who have been free of symptoms may donate blood 6 months after return from an endemic area. In some others, travelers to an area with malaria are deferred from donating blood for 1 year after their return; former residents of malaria-risk areas are deferred for 3 years; and persons diagnosed with malaria cannot donate blood for 3 years after treatment, during which time they must have remained free of symptoms of malaria. Immigrants or visitors from areas where *P. malariae* malaria is or has been endemic may be a source of trans-fusion-induced infection for many years. Such areas in-clude malaria endemic countries of the Americas, tropical Africa, the southwestern Pacific, and south and southeast Asia.

3) Concurrent disinfection: Not applicable.
4) Quarantine: Not applicable.
5) Immunization of contacts: Not applicable.
6) Investigation of contacts and source of infection: Determine history of previous infection or of possible exposure. If a history of sharing needles is obtained from the patient, investigate and treat all persons who shared the equipment. In transfusion-induced malaria, all donors must be located and their blood examined for malaria parasites and for antimalarial antibodies; parasite-positive donors must receive treatment. Malaria cases in non-endemic areas are usually imported, but some cases with no travel history have been reported in recent years: some of these events are believed to have been caused by infected mosquitoes air-transported from an endemic area; in other situations, infected migrants from endemic areas to non-malarious areas have been the source for outbreaks of local transmission where competent vectors are present. If the area is receptive to malaria (competent vectors present), persons living in the same community as well as health services should be advised about the risk of malaria; people developing malaria-like symptoms must be examined by microscopic examination of blood smears or rapid diagnostic tests. The flight range of anopheline mosquitoes may reach 2 km, but in most cases it is only a few hundred meters. Vector control should only be considered if several cases occur in a small area. Malaria outbreaks in receptive areas can also be triggered by a heavy influx of seasonal laborers and/or immigrants from nearby

endemic countries. In the USA, several cases of locally-acquired malaria have occurred since the mid-1980s after importation of infection in humans or mosquitoes.

7) Specific treatment for all forms of malaria:

a) *P. falciparum* in almost all endemic areas of the world is resistant to chloroquine, and in most areas to sulfadoxine-pyrimethamine (which was initially used to replace chloroquine). Identifying suitable antimalarial drug policies poses a major challenge to national programs in endemic countries. WHO now recommends that *P. falciparum* endemic countries with chloroquine resistance adopt artemisinin-based combination therapy (ACT). ACTs are highly effective, providing a greater than 90% cure rate in almost all situations. There are four ACT regimens currently recommended for use and the choice of the ACT depends on the efficacy of the non-artemisinin partner medicine in that particular area or country:

- Artemether-lumefantrine (adult dose, 4 tablets twice a day for 3 days).
- Artesunate plus mefloquine (4 mg/kg bw of artesunate given once a day for 3 days and 25 mg base/kg bw of mefloquine usually split over 2 or 3 days).
- Artesunate plus amodiaquine (4 mg/kg bw of artesunate and 10 mg base/kg bw of amodiaquine, given once a day for 3 days).
- Artesunate plus sulfadoxine-pyrimethamine (4 mg/kg bw of artesunate given once a day for 3 days and a single administration of sulfadoxine-pyrimethamine (25/1.25 mg base/kg bw) on day 1.

In addition to improving efficacy, the use of combination therapy will help delay the emergence of drug resistance to the non-artemisinin partner medicine in the combination.

Alternatives to ACTs for the treatment of uncomplicated *P. falciparum* malaria would be a combination of oral quinine (30 mg salt/kg/day in 3 divided doses for 7 days) together with either oral doxycycline (2 mg/kg once a day, maximal 100 mg/dose) or tetracycline (5 mg/kg/dose, maximal 250 mg/dose, 4 times a day for 7 days) or clindamycin (10 mg/kg bw twice a day). If the patient is pregnant or under 8 years of age, doxycycline and tetracycline are contraindicated, and quinine should be given with clindamycin.

b) For *P. falciparum* infections acquired in areas of multi-drug resistance (southeast Asia, Amazon Basin), ACT treatment with artesunate+mefloquine or artemether-lumefantrine is recommended. Artemether-lumefantrine tablets contain 20mg artemether and 120 mg of lumefantrine. Adult dosage: 6 doses given over 3 days (4 tablets each at 0 hours, 8 hours, 24 hours, 36 hours, 48 hours, and 60 hours). Pediatric dosage by weight: 5–14 kg 1 tablet at same time intervals, 15–24 kg 2 tablets at same time intervals, 25–34 kg 3 tablets at same time intervals, >34 kg adult regimen). Artemether-lumefantrine is not yet available in the United States.

c) Severe *falciparum* malaria is a medical emergency. After rapid clinical assessment and confirmation of the diagnosis, full doses of parenteral antimalarial treatment should be started without delay with whichever effective antimalarial is first available. In low transmission areas or outside malaria endemic areas the recommended choice is artesunate 2.4 mg/kg bw i.v. or i.m. given on admission (time = 0), then at 12 h and 24 h, then once a day. For children in high transmission areas, any of the following antimalarial medicines can be used:

- Artesunate (2.4 mg/kg bw i.v. or i.m. given on admission (time = 0), then at 12 h and 24 h, then once a day).
- Artemether (3.2 mg/kg bw i.m. given on admission then 1.6 mg/kg bw per day).
- Quinine (20 mg salt/kg bw on admission (i.v. infusion or divided i.m. injection), then 10 mg/kg bw every 8 h; infusion rate should not exceed 5 mg salt/kg bw per hour).

Details on the management of severe malaria can be found in: *Management of severe malaria—a practical handbook* (WHO, Geneva, 2000), available at: <http://www.who.int/malaria/docs/hbsm_toc.htm>

d) For *P. vivax* infections the recommended treatment is chloroquine (25 mg base/kg divided over 3 days) combined with primaquine to prevent relapses that occur as a result of the late development of intrahepatic stages. Primaquine can produce hemolysis, especially in those with G6PD deficiency; patients should be tested for G6PD deficiency before primaquine is given. In areas where re-infection is very frequent, the risks of widespread use of primaquine may exceed the benefits. The decision to administer primaquine is made on an individual basis, after consideration of the potential risk of adverse reactions. A dose of 0.25 mg base/kg/day taken with food for 14 days (15 mg base or 26.3 mg of primaquine phosphate for the average adult) is often effective. Larger daily doses (30 mg base) are generally required for use in the southwestern Pacific and for some strains from southeast Asia and South America. In moderate G6PD deficiency, primaquine, 0.75 mg base/kg, may be given once weekly for 8 doses (45 mg base or 79 mg primaquine phosphate for the average adult). Primaquine should not be administered during pregnancy, in young infants, and in severe G6PD deficiency. In areas where confirmed chloroquine-resistant *P. vivax* infections have been reported, any of the recommended ACTs can be given, with the exception of artesunate plus sulfadoxine-pyrimethamine; quinine and artemether-lumefantrine are possible alternatives.

e) For prevention of relapses in mosquito-acquired *P. vivax* and *P. ovale* infections, administer primaquine, as described above, after testing for G6PD deficiency to prevent drug-induced hemolysis. Primaquine is not required in the treatment of induced malaria (e.g. transfusion), since no liver phase occurs.

f) *P. malariae* infections can be treated with chloroquine (25 mg base/kg bw divided over 3 days).

WHO recommendations, products and drug policies can be found online at:

<http://www.who.int/malaria/>

US guidelines may differ and can be found at:

<http://www.cdc.gov/malaria/>

C. *Epidemic measures:* Determine the nature and extent of the epidemic situation. Malaria epidemics must be controlled through rapid and vigorous action and effective treatment of all cases; in confirmed *P. falciparum* epidemics where a large part of the population is infected, mass fever treatment, based only on clinical grounds (fever) without laboratory confirmation of diagnosis, may be necessary to cope with the patient load. In *falciparum* malaria epidemics the inclusion of an anti-gametocyte drug like primaquine in a single adult dose of 30–45 mg may be considered, but possible benefits must be weighed against possible side-effects in G6PD-deficient persons. As soon as possible, full coverage vector control measures should be instituted. Usually, indoor residual spraying is preferred because of its rapid effect; this may be followed by the use of ITNs or LLINs and anti-larval measures.

D. Disaster implications: Disasters in endemic areas may lead to malaria epidemics, often as a result of population movements, ecological changes favoring vector breeding, breakdown of health services, crowding of people in poorly-constructed housing or the existence of a large number of people without adequate housing, creating high-risk, high-exposure situations. In complex emergencies in Africa, malaria has presented with an epidemic pattern, taking an extraordinarily high toll among children, and often adults. At such times the drug resistance situation often turns out to be worse than had been assumed from national data, and therefore artemether-lumefantrine, to which parasites from most parts of the world are still sensitive, is recommended for use as the first-line medicine. Control priorities are early effective treatment and vector control; the latter is usually only possible after the acute emergency is over, and focuses on personal protection with ITNs or LLINs for high risk groups, combined with indoor residual spraying where feasible. In densely populated refugee camps, space spraying may be effective in the emergency phase; environmental measures may be relevant later. In areas of intense transmission in Africa, intermittent preventive treatment in pregnancy should be provided as soon as antenatal care services have been established or re-established. Health education on a continuous basis, as in any context, is required to support these interventions and promote better malaria control.

More information can be found at:

<http://www.who.int/malaria/interagencyfieldhandbook.html>
<http://www.who.int/malaria/docs/dip_mal0508.pdf>

E. International measures:

1) Important international measures include the following:

   a) Disinsectization of aircraft before boarding passengers or in transit, using a residual spray application of an effective insecticide.

   b) Disinsectization of aircraft, ships and other vehicles on arrival if the health authority at the place of arrival has reason to suspect importation of malaria vectors.

   c) Enforcing and maintaining rigid anti-mosquito sanitation within the mosquito flight range of all ports and airports.

2) In special circumstances, screen and treat potentially infected migrants, refugees, seasonal workers and persons taking part in periodic mass movement before their arrival in an area or country where malaria has been eliminated. Arrange housing of such populations as much as possible in non-receptive areas, and/or in well-constructed, screened

housing that prevents mosquito entry. Primaquine, 30–45 mg base (0.5–0.75 mg/kg), given as a single dose, renders the gametocytes of *P. falciparum* non-infectious, but possible benefits must be weighed against possible side-effects in G6PD-deficient persons.

3) As one of the world's major global public health problems, malaria is a disease under surveillance by WHO. It is addressed by the global Roll Back Malaria Initiative, the United Nations' Millennium Development Goals, the Global Fund to fight AIDS, Tuberculosis and Malaria, UNICEF, the US President's Malaria Initiative, the World Bank Booster Program, and other partners. National health administrations in endemic countries are expected to notify WHO annually of the following:

a) Recorded malaria cases/deaths, epidemics, coverage of major interventions—for further guidance, see *Framework for Monitoring Progress & Evaluating Outcomes and Impact* (WHO/CDS/RBM, 2000.25), or:
<http://whqlibdoc.who.int/hq/2000/WHO_CDS_RBM_2000.25.pdf>

b) The situation of antimalarial drug resistance.

c) Those international ports and airports free of malaria. Further information can be found at:
<http://www.rbm.who.int>
- and:
<http://www.who.int/malaria>

MALIGNANT NEOPLASMS ASSOCIATED WITH INFECTIOUS AGENTS
[CCDM19: Editorial Board]

Infectious agents are risk factors for several malignancies. Among the agents implicated in the pathogenesis of various human malignancies, either directly or indirectly, are parasites, viruses and the bacterium *Helicobacter pylori*. The infectious agent is not a sufficient cause for all cases of agent-related malignancy; other causes are involved; cofactors, both external (environmental) and internal (genetic and physiological at immunological and molecular levels), play important roles in each of these malignancies, which usually represent the late outcome of the infection. With the exception of cervical cancer, for which infection with human papillomavirus is involved in essentially all cases, cancers with similar or identical histology occur independent of infection, so infection is not required for carcinogenesis.

Most of the infectious agents implicated in the etiology of tumors are viruses. A common feature of most virus-related cancers is the persistence of the virus following infection early in life or the presence of immuno-suppression: this often leads to integration and development of cancer, usually in a single cell clone (monoclonal tumor). Both DNA and RNA viruses are involved.

The 4 strongest viruses directly or indirectly involved in the pathogenesis of human malignancies are:

1) Hepatitis B virus (HBV) and hepatitis C virus (HCV).
2) Epstein-Barr virus (EBV).
3) Human papillomaviruses (HPV, mainly types 16 and 18).
4) Human herpesvirus-8 (HHV-8), also called Kaposi sarcoma-associated herpesvirus (KSHV).

The first 3 occur worldwide and produce many more unapparent than apparent infections; most result in a latent virus state that is subject to reactivation. Monoclonality of the tumor cells and integration of the virus into the tumor cell strongly support a causal association further strengthened by epidemiologic studies. The associated malignancies occur in special host and geographic settings. Retroviruses—including human T-cell lymphotropic virus (HTLV-1)—are associated with human T-cell leukemia/lymphoma.

I. HEPATOCELLULAR
CARCINOMA   ICD-9 155.0; ICD-10 C22.0
(HCC, Primary liver cancer, Primary hepatocellular carcinoma)
[CCDM19: S. D. Holmberg]
[CCDM18: E. K. Yeoh]

Hepatocellular carcinoma is the 5th most common cancer in men and the 8th most common in women worldwide, with an estimated one-half to one million new cases per year. It is estimated that 50–55% of these cancers are attributable to chronic hepatitis C virus (HCV) infection, and another 25–30% to chronic hepatitis B virus (HBV) infection.

Periodic screening of carriers of HBV for alpha-fetoprotein—a serologic marker associated with hepatocellular cancer—and ultrasound screening can, in some cases, detect the tumor at an early, resectable stage. Newer technologies, such as CT or MRI scanning, are being evaluated as screening strategies for hepatocellular carcinoma, but are currently too expensive for most populations.

Hepatocellular cancer is one of the most common malignant neoplasms in many parts of Asia and Africa, and its occurrence correlates with rates of chronic HBV and HCV infection in the population. Thus, it occurs with high frequency in areas with high prevalence of HBV carriers, including most of Asia, Africa, the South Pacific and part of the Middle East. Rates are intermediate on the Indian subcontinent and relatively low in North America and western Europe. In developed countries, including Japan, and other countries such as Pakistan, Egypt and Mongolia, HCV infection is considered the dominant viral etiology of hepatocellular cancer.

See *Viral hepatitis B* and *C* for methods of control. The administration of hepatitis B vaccine to all newborns may help prevent development of hepatocellular cancer, because immunization interrupts mother-to-infant transmission. WHO recommends that all countries integrate hepatitis B vaccine into routine childhood immunization schedules. Almost all countries are now implementing this recommendation, which should eventually lead to elimination of HBV transmission and control of hepatocellular cancer caused by HBV. No vaccine is available for HCV infection, but testing the blood supply for HCV antibody will prevent its transmission by transfusion. Hepatocellular cancer cases should be reported to a tumor registry according to standard cancer registration procedures.

II. BURKITT LYMPHOMA   ICD-9 200.2; ICD-10 C83.7
(BL, African Burkitt lymphoma, Endemic Burkitt lymphoma, Burkitt tumor)
[CCDM18 & 19: E. K. Yeoh]

Burkitt lymphoma (BL) is a monoclonal tumor of B cells occurring worldwide, which is hyperendemic in highly malarious areas of altitudes below 1 000 meters/3 000 feet with heavy rainfall (above 1 000 millimeters/40 inches a year), such as tropical Africa and lowland Papua New Guinea. African children commonly show jaw involvement. The tumor may also develop as a rare event in immunosuppressed patients (patients with organ transplant or familial X-linked immunodeficiency, and more commonly in AIDS). The tumors may be monoclonal, polyclonal or mixed; not all are Burkitt-type, but all are acute lymphoblastic sarcomas.

Epstein-Barr virus (EBV), a herpesvirus responsible for infectious mononucleosis, plays an important pathogenic role in about 97% of cases in Africa and Papua New Guinea, where EBV infection occurs in infancy and where malaria, an apparent cofactor, is holoendemic. EBV is also associated with Burkitt lymphoma in about 30% of cases in non-malarious areas and areas of low endemicity for Burkitt lymphoma (American form). Regardless of the presence of EBV, there is a specific chromosomal translocation t(8;14) involving the proto-oncogene *c-myc* locus on the long arm of chromosome 8 and the immunoglobulin heavy chain locus on chromosome 14. Variant translocations t(2;8) and (8;22) involve the *c-myc* gene and the immunoglobulin kappa and lambda chain loci, located, respectively on chromosomes 2 and 22. The subsequent activation of the *c-myc* gene plays an important role in malignant transformation. Recent studies suggest that the chromosomal breakpoint locations in African cases differ from those in American cases, suggesting a molecular heterogeneity in Burkitt lymphoma in general. Other genetic alterations include the inactivation of tumor suppressor gene p53. The estimated time range of tumor development is 2–12 years from primary EBV infection, but is much shorter in AIDS patients in whom an EBV-related lymphoma (often CNS) develops. Evidence from serology, virology and epidemiology points to a strong role of EBV infection in the causation of the African form of the disease.

Burkitt lymphoma is a highly aggressive tumor, but can nevertheless be cured in 90% of cases with intensive multiple chemotherapy. Prevention of EBV infection early in life and control of malaria (see *Malaria*, section 9) might reduce tumor incidence in Africa and Papua New Guinea. Subunit vaccines against EBV are in the trial stage. Chemotherapy is usually effective after the tumor develops. Cases should be reported to a tumor registry.

III. NASOPHARYNGEAL
CARCINOMA   ICD-9 147.9; ICD-10 C11
[CCDM18 & 19: B. Sylla]

Nasopharyngeal carcinoma (NPC) is a malignant tumor of the epithelial cells of the nasopharynx that usually occurs in adults aged 20–40 years. Incidence is particularly high (about 10-fold when compared with the general population) among groups from China (Taiwan and southern China), even in those who have moved elsewhere. This risk decreases in subsequent generations after emigration from Asia.

IgA antibody to the EBV viral capsid antigen in both serum and nasopharyngeal secretions is characteristic of the disease and has been used in China as a screening test for the tumor. Its appearance may precede the clinical appearance of nasopharyngeal carcinoma by several years and its reappearance after treatment heralds recurrence.

The serological and virological evidence relating EBV to NPC is similar to that for African Burkitt lymphoma (high EBV antibody titers, genome in tumor cells); this relationship has been found without respect to the geographical origin of the patient. The tumor occurs worldwide, but is highest in southern China, southeastern Asia, northern and eastern Africa and the Arctic. Male cases outnumber female cases by about 2:1. Chinese with HLA-2 and SIN-2 antigen profiles have a particularly high risk.

EBV infection occurs early in life in settings where nasopharyngeal carcinoma is most common, yet the tumor does not appear until age 20–40 years, which suggests the occurrence of some secondary reactivating factor, with epithelial invasion later in life. Repeated respiratory infections or chemical irritants, such as nitrosamines in dried foods, may play a role. The higher frequency of the tumor in persons of southern Chinese origin without respect to later residence, and the association with certain HLA haplotypes, suggest a genetic susceptibility. A lower incidence among those who have migrated to the USA and elsewhere suggests that one or more environmental factor(s), such as the nitrosamines present in smoked fish and other foods, may be associated cofactors.

Early detection in highly endemic areas (screening for EBV IgA antibodies to viral capsid antigen) permits early treatment. A subunit vaccine against EBV infection is under study. Chemotherapy after early recognition is the only specific therapy. Cases should be reported to a tumor registry.

IV. MALIGNANCIES POSSIBLY RELATED TO EBV   ICD-9 201; ICD-10 C81
[CCDM18 & 19: B. Sylla]

A. HODGKIN DISEASE

Hodgkin disease (HD) is a tumor of the lymphatic system occurring in 4 histological subtypes: nodular sclerosis, lymphocyte predominance, mixed cellularity and lymphocyte depletion. The histology shows the presence of a highly specific but non-pathognomonic cell, the Reed-Sternberg cell, also seen in cases of infectious mononucleosis. The cause of Hodgkin disease is not certain, but laboratory and epidemiological evidence implicates EBV in at least half the cases. The disease is more common in industrialized countries, but age-adjusted incidence is relatively low. It is more common in higher socioeconomic settings, in smaller families, and in Caucasians compared with Americans of African origin.

Cases that develop after infectious mononucleosis occur some 10 years later; cases in older adults, if EBV-related, are probably the result of virus reactivation in the presence of a deteriorating immune system. The high frequency of EBV found in cases of Hodgkin disease diagnosed among HIV-infected patients and the relatively short incubation period appear related to the severe immunodeficiency of HIV infection; whether the presence of EBV in the tumor cell is cause or effect is not known. Among HIV-infected patients, particularly those infected through IV drug use, a higher proportion of Hodgkin disease cases are EBV-associated. Cases should be reported to a tumor registry.

B. NON-HODGKIN LYMPHOMAS   ICD-10 B21.2, C83.0, C83.8, C83.9, C85

The incidence of lymphomas in AIDS patients is about 50–100 times that in the general population. While these cases may be related to EBV, the virus most associated with non-Hodgkin lymphoma (NHL) tumors such as high grade and CNS lymphomas is HIV. Since 1980, NHL has shown a dramatic increase among young, single white men with AIDS in the USA. About 4% of AIDS patients present with lymphoma, and perhaps 30% will eventually develop one if survival is sufficiently long. Whether EBV is a causal factor in EBV-associated lymphomas in HIV-infected patients or simply enters the tumor cell after it has been formed is not clear, but accumulating evidence points to the former possibility.

A marked increase in NHL not explained by the increase in AIDS patients has been noted in recent years. The disease commonly occurs in the presence of other forms of immunodeficiency, such as those in post-transplant patients, people given immunosuppressive drugs, and people with inherited forms of immunodeficiency. There are few epidemiological clues as to the risk factors responsible. Altered antibody patterns to EBV characteristic of those seen in immunodeficiency states occur in many cases of NHL; these changes have been shown to precede the development of NHL. Molecular techniques have evidenced the EBV genome in 10%–15% of tumor cells of the spontaneous form of NHL. Cases should be reported to a tumor registry.

V. KAPOSI SARCOMA   ICD-9 173.0-173.9; ICD-10 C46.0-C46.9

(Idiopathic multiple pigmented hemorrhagic sarcoma)
[CCDM18 & 19: D. Parkin]

Kaposi sarcoma (KS) is a vascular neoplastic disorder that involves spindle cell proliferation, characterized by red-purple or blue-brown macules, plaques, and nodules of the skin and other organs. Skin lesions may be firm or compressible, solitary or multiple. First described in 1872, it was considered a rare tumor of unknown etiology before its frequent diagnosis in HIV-infected patients.

There are 4 epidemiological forms of KS. The classical form occurs in older males of mainly Mediterranean or eastern European Jewish backgrounds. An endemic form occurs in all age groups in parts of equatorial Africa; neither has a known precipitating environmental factor nor is associated with immune deficiency. The remaining types—in recipients of organ transplants who undergo immunosuppressive treatment or in HIV-infected persons—are accompanied by immune impairment. Overall, males are predominantly afflicted. The epidemic form presents the most aggressive clinical course and is seen almost exclusively in HIV-infected individuals. Despite differences in clinical manifestations and serostatus, it is appropriate to consider all forms of Kaposi sarcoma as one entity, given the identical immunohistochemical features of the characteristic spindle cell of the tumor.

Kaposi sarcoma-associated herpesvirus (KSHV), or human herpesvirus 8 (HHV-8), is believed to be the causal agent of Kaposi sarcoma. Discovered in 1994, it is a new human *Gammaherpesvirus* related to an oncogenic herpesvirus of monkeys, *Herpesvirus saimiri*. Evidence of viral infection is found in virtually all cases, and several lines of evidence point to a key etiologic role in this disease. KSHV infection precedes clinical sarcoma, is highly associated with increased risk in all populations studied thus far, and affects the endothelial (spindle) cell thought to be the prime determinant of tumorigenesis. KSHV has also been shown to induce transformation of primary endothelial cells.

Sero-epidemiological analysis suggests that KSHV has a more limited distribution than any of the other 7 human herpesviruses. In North America, seroprevalence ranges from 0%–1% in blood donors to about 35% in HIV-infected individuals and up to 100% in Kaposi sarcoma patients with AIDS. In Milan, Italy, blood donors have a 4% seropositivity rate. Data suggest even higher KSHV rates in central Africa, where 58% of persons aged 14–84 were KSHV positive in one study and seroprevalence (similar in men and women) increased linearly with age.

Serological analyses also suggest that infection occurs primarily in sexually active people, particularly men who have sex with men. Differences in risk of Kaposi sarcoma for AIDS patients who acquired HIV via sexual transmission and those whose HIV infections derived from blood product exposure support the role of sexual transmission: only 1% to 3% of hemophilia- and transfusion-related AIDS patients develop Kaposi. Transplacental transmission of anti-KSHV antibody is almost certain and the virus may also be transmitted transplacentally since children of KSHV-positive mothers are at increased risk of infection after the neonatal period. In Africa, the high seroprevalence among adolescents and the relatively linear increase in prevalence with age suggest that nonsexual modes of transmission for KSHV may also be important.

There is no known cure for Kaposi sarcoma, but partial and complete remissions have been noted. Cases should be reported to a tumor registry.

VI. LYMPHATIC TISSUE MALIGNANCY

ICD-9 202;
ICD-10 C84.1, C84.5, C91.4, C91.5
(Adult T-cell leukemia [ATL], T-cell lymphosarcoma [TLCL], peripheral T-cell lymphoma [Sézary disease], Hairy cell leukemia) [CCDM18 & 19: E. K. Yeoh]

Adult T-cell leukemia (ATL), a leukemia/lymphoma of T-cell origin commonly seen in Japan, is identical to T-cell lymphoma sarcoma-cell leukemia (TLCL), seen less commonly in the Caribbean, the Pacific coast of South America, equatorial Africa, and southern USA. These malignancies primarily involve adults, and are associated with human T-cell lymphotrophic virus (HTLV-1), a member of the family of retroviruses. The latent period between infection and the emergence of ATL is 20–30 years. Infection early in life, primarily through breast milk, leads to tumor development in the adult, peaking at about age 50. This suggests the risk of ATL is lower should infection occur later in life through transfer of blood or blood products, IV drug use, or sexual activity. The same virus causes tropical spastic paraparesis (also called HTLV-1-associated myelopathy in Japan). Adult Japanese and Afro-Caribbeans are at highest risk.

Serological, virological and epidemiological evidence strongly implicate HTLV-1 in the causation of full leukemia/lymphoma. Control measures are similar to those for prevention of AIDS (see *Acquired immunodeficiency syndrome*, section 9). The effectiveness of screening donor blood for antibodies against HTLV-1 and 2 has yet to be demonstrated. In the USA, although the low overall virus prevalence renders transmission from blood donors a rare event, screening donor units for the virus is now a standard procedure. Cases should be reported to a tumor registry.

VII. CERVICAL CANCER   ICD-9 180; ICD-10 C53
(Carcinoma of the uterine cervix)
[CCDM19: E. Unger]
[CCDM18: S. Francheschi]

Cervical cancer is the second most common cancer in women worldwide, and the most common among women in Latin America, India and sub-Saharan Africa. Cervical cancer risk is associated with lower socioeconomic status, early start of sexual activity, and multiple sexual partners. Of all deaths from cervical cancer, 80% occur in developing countries.

Human papillomavirus (HPV) infection is now considered the cause of cervical cancer. These double-stranded DNA viruses are a large family of over 100 closely related viruses, called types, numbered in the order of their discovery. About 40 types infect mucosal surfaces and are those most commonly found in the genital tract. The so-called "low-risk" mucosal types of HPV cause benign warts (see *Warts, viral*) and low-grade cervical lesion; "high-risk" types, most notably HPV types 16, 18, 31, 33, and 45, have been found in tumor tissues of about 90% of cervical cancer cases worldwide. HPV is an extremely common sexually acquired infection. In most instances the virus clears within 1-2 years and is not associated with symptoms. The prevalence of HPV in populations peaks around the age of sexual debut and gradually decreases with age, with a second peak at older ages being observed in some populations. Invasive cervical disease is preceded by a long pre-invasive phase of growth, recognized histologically as cervical intraepithelial neoplasia (CIN) of increased severity or grades (CIN 1-3). The histologic precursors are detectable with exfoliated cervical cytology, the basis of the Papanicolaou test (Pap test). Detection and treatment of pre-cancers based on organized Pap test screening programs dramatically reduce cervical cancer incidence and mortality, when fully implemented and maintained. However, those countries with the greatest burden of disease do not have sufficient trained personnel and infrastructure for this complex approach to prevention.

The strong etiologic association of cervical cancer with certain types of HPV suggests that prevention of HPV infection would prevent cervical cancer. At time of writing in early 2008, two vaccine formulations had recently completed phase 3 trials and were under review or approved by many national regulatory agencies. Both vaccines target HPV 16 and 18, and one also includes HPV 6 and 11. As HPV 16 and 18 account for approximately 70% of cancers worldwide, either vaccine has the potential to reduce cervical cancer substantially. Cost-effective strategies for vaccine implementation and monitoring are being developed, but there will be a delay between initiation of vaccine programs and an impact on disease. In countries without well-developed cervical cancer screening programs, cervical cancer control strategies may use a combined approach of screening and vaccination. In these settings, low cost, rapid approaches to screening, such as visual inspection of the cervix with a colposcope and possible use of acetic acid, as commonly used in developing countries ("see and treat"), or a simplified HPV test, are being evaluated. Cases should be reported to a tumor registry.

VIII. MALIGNANCY RELATED TO LIVER FLUKES CHOLANGIOCARCINOMA
[CCDM19: Y. Wattanagoon]

ICD–10 C22.1

Cholangiocarcinoma is malignancy of the biliary duct system. Incidence is low in western countries, but notably high in Asia, where the prevalence of liver fluke infections (*Opisthorchis viverrini and Clonorchis sinensis*) is high. Cholangiocarcinoma can be divided into 2 types: the intrahepatic or peripheral type, which involves the intrahepatic bile ducts, and the extrahepatic type, which involves the extrahepatic bile ducts.

The incidence of Cholangiocarcinoma in the northeastern part of Thailand is the highest in the world—135.4/100 000 population in males and 43/100 000 population in females—and has been associated with high prevalence of *O. viverrini* infection, which is acquired from consumption of raw freshwater cyprinoid fish. Consumption of fermented food containing high levels of N-nitrosocompound and nitrosamines also accelerates carcinomatous changes of the epithelial cells in the bile duct.

Cholangiocarcinoma related to liver fluke infection may appear early in the fourth decade of life. Persons infected with liver flukes may have been carrying infection from as early as one year old. Cholangiocarcinoma can manifest as malignant obstructive jaundice or as a non-jaundice type with liver mass. Cholangitis is a common complication. Alkaline phosphatase level is very high in both types. Tumor marker levels (e.g. CA 19-9, CA 125 and CEA) are high, but AFP is normal. Ultrasonography of the liver may show single or multiple masses with localized dilatation of bile ducts in peripheral type, or diffuse intrahepatic/extrahepatic bile duct dilatation. CT scan or MRI is useful for staging of the disease or for planning surgical intervention. Surgical resection of the tumor mass can cure the disease in the early stages only. In late cases, palliative biliary bypass with stent using endoscopy or surgery can relieve the symptoms, but does not affect survival. Results of chemotherapy are not good.

Mass treatment of liver fluke infection with antihelminthic drugs has reduced the prevalence of liver fluke infection in endemic areas; however, the most important preventive measure for liver fluke infection is through health education aimed at changing eating habits, avoiding consumption of raw freshwater fish.

Early markers for the detection of cholangiocarcinoma in high-risk groups (i.e. people with history of liver fluke infection) may include alkaline phosphatase levels. High levels may be an indication of cholangiocarcinoma, which should be checked by ultrasonography of the liver. After confirming diagnosis, cases should be reported to a tumor registry.

MEASLES   ICD-9 055; ICD-10 B05
(Rubeola, Hard measles, Red measles, Morbilli)
[CCDM19: P. Strebel]
[CCDM18: B. Hersh]

1. Identification—An acute, highly communicable viral disease with prodromal fever, conjunctivitis, coryza, cough, and small spots with white or bluish-white centers on an erythematous base on the buccal mucosa (Koplik spots). A characteristic red blotchy rash appears on the third to seventh day; the rash begins on the face, then becomes generalized, lasts 4–7 days, and sometimes ends in brawny desquamation. Leukopenia is common. The disease is more severe in infants and adults than in children. Complications may result from viral replication or bacterial superinfection, and include otitis media, pneumonia, laryngotracheobronchitis (croup), diarrhea, and encephalitis.

The case-fatality rate in developing countries is estimated to be 3%–5%, but may reach 10%–30% in some localities. Both acute and delayed mortality in infants and children have been documented. Measles is a more severe disease in the very young and in malnourished children, in whom it may be associated with hemorrhagic rash, protein-losing enteropathy, otitis media, oral sores, dehydration, diarrhea, blindness, and severe skin infections. Children with clinical or subclinical vitamin A deficiency are at particularly high risk of severe disease. In children whose nutrition status is borderline, measles often precipitates acute kwashiorkor and exacerbates vitamin A deficiency that may lead to blindness. Very rarely (in about 1/100 000 cases), subacute sclerosing panencephalitis (SSPE) develops several years after infection; over 50% of SSPE cases had measles diagnosed in the first 2 years of life. The WHO clinical case-definition for measles reads "any person with fever and maculopapular rash and cough/coryza/conjunctivitis."

Diagnosis is usually on clinical and epidemiological grounds, although laboratory confirmation is preferred. The detection of measles-specific IgM antibodies, present 3–4 days after rash onset, or a significant rise in antibody concentrations between acute and convalescent sera, confirms the diagnosis. Less commonly used techniques include identification of viral antigen in nasopharyngeal mucosal swabs by FA techniques, or virus isolation in cell culture from blood or nasopharyngeal swabs collected before day 4 of rash, or from urine specimens before day 8 of rash. RT-PCR can be used to identify measles RNA in urine, blood, and nasopharyngeal mucus.

2. Infectious agent—Measles virus, a member of the genus *Morbillivirus* of the family Paramyxoviridae.

3. Occurrence—Prior to widespread immunization, measles was common in childhood, so that more than 90% of people had been infected by age 20; few went through life without becoming infected. In the pre-vaccine era, there were an estimated 100 million cases and 6 million measles deaths a year. Measles, endemic in large metropolitan communities, attained epidemic proportions about every second or third year. In smaller communities and areas, outbreaks tended to be more widely spaced and somewhat more severe. With longer intervals between outbreaks, as in some Sahelian populations, in the Arctic and some islands, measles outbreaks often involved a large proportion of the population, with a high case-fatality rate. In temperate climates, measles occurs primarily in the late winter and early spring. In tropical climates, measles occurs primarily in the dry season.

With effective childhood immunization programs, measles cases in many industrialized countries have dropped by 99%, and generally occur in young un-immunized children or older children, adolescents or young adults who received only one dose of vaccine.

In 1994, the countries of the western hemisphere established a regional target of elimination of indigenous measles transmission by the end of the year 2000, through a comprehensive measles immunization strategy. This included the provision of measles vaccine to at least 95% of children aged 12–15 months, through routine immunization services, with another opportunity for measles immunization to all children, and careful measles surveillance. The second opportunity for measles immunization provides immunity to children who escaped routine immunization and those who failed to respond immunologically to the first vaccine, and is usually provided through Supplementary Immunization Activities (SIAs). One-off "catch-up" campaigns target all children aged 9 months to 14 years regardless of disease history or previous vaccination status, and "follow-up" campaigns are conducted every 3–4 years, targeting all children 9 months to 4 years. In Canada and the USA, the second opportunity for measles immunization is provided through routine immunization services, generally at school entry.

At time of writing in early 2008, strong country and regional measles surveillance systems indicate that the western hemisphere has been free of endemic measles since November 2002, thereby achieving the goal of measles elimination—although importations continue to occur, requiring maintenance of very high population immunity through vaccination. Also at time of writing, WHO is discussing the possibility of adding the goal of global measles elimination, rather than control.

Despite the existence of a safe, effective and inexpensive measles vaccine for 40 years, measles remains a leading vaccine-preventable killer of children worldwide. WHO estimates that there were approximately 17 million cases and 242 000 measles deaths worldwide in 2006. Over 95% of measles deaths occur in countries with per capita gross national products lower than $1 000, with over 85% in children aged under 5 years, and over 80% in southeast Asia and Africa. After achieving the global goal to halve measles mortality by 2005, the World Health Assembly adopted the new target of reducing global measles deaths by 90% from the 2000 level of 757 000 before the end of 2010; it recommended that all countries fully implement the WHO/UNICEF comprehensive immunization strategy for sustainable measles mortality reduction.

4. **Reservoir**—Humans.

5. **Mode of transmission**—Airborne by droplet spread, direct contact with nasal or throat secretions of infected persons; less commonly by articles freshly soiled with nose and throat secretions. Measles is one of the most highly communicable infectious diseases.

6. **Incubation period**—About 10 days, but may be 7 to 18 days from exposure to onset of fever, usually 14 days until rash appears; rarely, as long as 19–21 days. Immune globulin given for passive protection early in the incubation period may extend this period.

7. **Period of communicability**—From 1 day before the beginning of the prodromal period (usually about 4 days before rash onset) to 4 days after rash appearance; minimal after the second day of rash. The vaccine virus has not been shown to be communicable.

8. **Susceptibility**—All persons who have not had the disease or been successfully immunized are susceptible. Acquired immunity after illness is permanent. Infants born to mothers who have had the disease are protected against disease for the first 6–9 months or more, depending on the amount of residual maternal antibody at the time of pregnancy and the rate of antibody degradation. Maternal antibody interferes with response to vaccine. Immunization at 12–15 months induces immunity in 94%–98% of recipients; re-immunization increases immunity levels to about 99%. Children born to mothers with vaccine-induced immunity receive less passive antibody; they may become susceptible to measles and require measles immunization at an earlier age than is usually recommended.

9. **Methods of control—**

  A. Preventive measures:

  1) Public education by health departments and private physicians should encourage measles immunization for all susceptible infants, children, adolescents and young adults. Those for whom vaccine is contraindicated, and un-immunized persons identified more than 72 hours after exposure to measles in families or institutions, may be partially or completely protected by IG given soon after exposure.

  2) Immunization: Live attenuated measles vaccine is the vaccine of choice, indicated for all persons not immune to measles, unless specifically contraindicated (see 9A2c, below). A single injection of live measles vaccine, often combined with other live vaccines (mumps, rubella), can be administered concurrently with other inactivated vaccines or toxoids; it should induce active immunity in 94%–98% of susceptible individuals, probably for life, by producing a mild or inapparent noncommunicable infection. Another dose of measles vaccine may increase immunity levels up to 99%.

  About 5%–15% of non-immune vaccinees may develop malaise and fever to 39.5°C (103°F) within 5–12 days after immunization; this lasts 1–2 days, with little disability. Rash, coryza, mild cough and Koplik spots may occasionally occur. Febrile seizures occur infrequently and without sequelae; the highest incidence is in children with a previous history or a close family (parents or siblings) history of seizures. Encephalitis and encephalopathy have been reported (at the rate of less than one case per million doses distributed) following measles immunization—this is lower than the background rate and consequently may not be caused by the vaccine.

  Current recommendations in the USA and other industrialized countries advise a routine 2-dose measles vaccination schedule. The initial dose is at 12–15 months or as soon as possible thereafter; the following dose, usually at school entry (4–6 years), can be administered as early as 4 weeks after the initial dose where the risk of exposure to measles is high. Both doses are generally given as combined measles, mumps and rubella vaccine (MMR).

  Routine immunization with MMR at 12 months is particularly important in areas where measles cases occur. During community outbreaks, the recommended age for immunization using monovalent vaccine can be lowered to 6–11 months. A second dose of measles vaccine is then given at 12–15 months, and a third dose at school entry.

  The optimal age for immunization in developing countries

depends on the persistence of maternal antibodies in the infant and the increased risk of exposure to measles at a younger age. In most developing country settings, WHO recommends measles immunization of all children at 9 months, with another opportunity for measles immunization, generally through SIAs. In Latin America, due to the markedly decreased risk of an infant being exposed to measles virus, PAHO recommends routine immunization at 12–15 months for all children, with another opportunity for measles immunization through periodic SIAs.

a) Vaccine shipment and storage: Immunization may not produce protection if the vaccine has been improperly handled or stored. Prior to reconstitution, freeze-dried measles vaccine is relatively stable and can be stored with safety for a year or more in a freezer or at refrigerator temperatures (2°–8°C/35.6°–46.4°F). Reconstituted vaccine must be kept at refrigerator temperatures and discarded after 8 hours; both freeze-dried and reconstituted vaccine must be protected from prolonged exposure to ultraviolet light, which may inactivate the virus.

b) Re-immunizations: In the USA and other industrialized countries, in addition to routine re-immunization of children entering school, measles re-immunization is offered at entry to high school and colleges, and to international travelers and health care workers, unless they have a documented history of measles disease or immunization with 2 doses of vaccine, or serological evidence of measles immunity. In those who have received only inactivated vaccine, re-immunization may produce reactions such as local edema and induration, lymphadenopathy and fever, but will protect against the atypical measles syndrome. Use of inactivated measles vaccine was discontinued more than 30 years ago.

c) Contraindications to the use of live virus vaccines:

i) Patients with primary immune deficiency diseases affecting T-cell function or acquired immune deficiency due to leukemia, lymphoma or generalized malignancy, or those undergoing therapy with corticosteroids, irradiation, alkylating drugs or antimetabolites, should not receive live virus vaccines. Infection with HIV is not an absolute contraindication: unless severely immunocompromised, WHO recommends measles immunization of HIV-infected infants at 6 months of age followed by an additional dose at 9 months. The USA and other industrialized countries recommend measles vaccination only in asymptomatic HIV-positive individuals; low CD4 counts are a contraindication to measles vaccine because of the risk of viral pneumonia.

ii) In patients with severe acute illness with or without fever, immunization should be deferred until recovery from the acute phase; minor febrile illnesses such as diarrhea or upper respiratory infections are not a contraindication.

iii) Persons with anaphylactic hypersensitivity to a previous dose of measles vaccine, gelatin or neomycin should not receive measles vaccine. Egg allergy, even if anaphylactic, is no longer considered a contraindication.

iv) Purely on theoretical grounds, vaccine should not be given to pregnant women; mothers should be advised of the theoretical risk of fetal damage if they become pregnant within 1 month after receipt of measles-containing vaccine.

v) Vaccine should be given at least 14 days before IG or blood transfusion. IG or blood products can interfere with the response to measles vaccine for varying periods depending on the dose of IG. The usual dose administered for hepatitis A prevention can interfere for 3 months; very large doses of intravenous IG can interfere for up to 11 months.

B. Control of patient, contacts and the immediate environment:

1) Report to local health authority: Obligatory case report in most countries, Class 2 (see *Reporting*). Early reporting (within 24 hours) provides opportunity for better outbreak control.
2) Isolation: Impractical in the community at large; if practicable, children with measles should be kept out of school for 4 days after appearance of the rash. In hospitals, respiratory isolation from onset of catarrhal stage of the prodromal period up to and including the fourth day of rash reduces the exposure of other patients at high risk.
3) Concurrent disinfection: Not applicable.
4) Quarantine: Usually impractical. Quarantine of institutions, wards or dormitories can sometimes be of value; strict segregation of infants if measles occurs in an institution.
5) Immunization of contacts: Live virus vaccine should be administered within 72 hours of exposure. Alternatively, IG may be given (0.25 ml/kg or 0.11 ml/lb; for immunocompromised persons, 0.5 ml/kg or 0.22ml/lb up to a maximum of 15 ml within 72 hours of exposure, for maximal protection). IG should be used within 6 days of exposure for susceptible household or other contacts with high risk of complications (contacts under 1 year of age, pregnant women or immuno-

compromised persons), or where measles vaccine is contraindicated. Live measles vaccine should be given 5–6 months later to those for whom vaccine is not contraindicated.

6) Investigation of contacts and source of infection: Search and immunize exposed susceptible contacts to limit the spread of disease. Healthy carrier state does not occur.

7) Specific treatment: None. During measles infection, vitamin A reserves fall rapidly (especially in malnourished children), which further weakens immunity. Vitamin A supplementation at the time of measles diagnosis replaces body reserves, prevents blindness due to corneal ulceration and keratomalacia, and significantly reduces measles fatality. The following Vitamin A schedule is recommended:

Age	Immediately	Next day
<6 months	50 000 IU	50 000 IU
6–11 months	100 000 IU	100 000 IU
12 months	200 000 IU	200 000 IU

A third dose of vitamin A should be given 2–4 weeks later if there are signs of vitamin A deficiency on diagnosis (night blindness, Bitot spots, conjunctival or corneal dryness, corneal clouding or ulceration).

C. Epidemic measures:

1) Prompt reporting (within 24 hours) of suspected cases, and comprehensive immunization programs for all susceptibles, are needed to limit spread. In day care, school and college outbreaks, all persons without documentation of 2 doses of live virus vaccine at least 1 month apart on or after the first birthday should be immunized unless they have documentation of prior physician-diagnosed measles, or laboratory evidence of immunity.

2) In institutional outbreaks, new admissions should receive vaccine or IG.

3) In many developing countries, measles has a relatively high case-fatality rate. If vaccine is available, prompt use at the beginning of an epidemic is essential to limit spread; if vaccine supply is limited, priority should be given to young children for whom the risk is greatest.

D. Disaster implications:
Introduction of measles into refugee populations with a high proportion of susceptibles can result in devastating epidemics with high fatality rates. Providing measles vaccine to displaced persons living in camp settings within a week of entry is a public health priority.

E. International measures:
Persons traveling to measles-endemic areas should ensure that they are immune to measles.

MELIOIDOSIS
(Whitmore disease)
[CCDM19: K. Glynn]
[CCDM18: A. Plant]

ICD-9 025; ICD-10 A24.1–A24.4

1. **Identification**—An uncommon bacterial infection; clinical manifestations range from none or asymptomatic pulmonary consolidation to localized cutaneous or visceral abscesses, necrotizing pneumonia and/or a rapidly fatal septicemia. Melioidosis may simulate typhoid fever or tuberculosis, with pulmonary cavitation, empyema, chronic abscesses and osteomyelitis. Overwhelming infection can occur, resulting in death from septic shock within 48 hours of generalized symptoms. A specific syndrome of meningoencephalitis with flaccid paraparesis or peripheral motor weakness occurs in 5% of cases in northern Australia. Cerebral abscess is occasionally reported. Mortality ranges from 40 to 75% despite rational use of antimicrobial therapy. Fatality rate of melioidosis is greater in persons with underlying disease such as diabetes mellitus, renal dysfunction and chronic pulmonary disease, and in immunosuppressed individuals.

Diagnosis depends on isolation of the causative agent from clinical specimens (blood, urine, sputum, skin lesions and throat swab); a rising antibody titer in serological tests is confirmatory. Direct immunofluorescent microscopy is 98% specific but only about 70% sensitive compared with culture. The possibility of melioidosis must be kept in mind in any unexplained suppurative disease, especially cavitating pulmonary disease, in patients living in or returned from endemic areas; disease may become manifest as long as 25 years after exposure.

2. **Infectious agent**—*Burkholderia pseudomallei*, the Whitmore bacillus, is a saprophytic gram-negative motile rod.

3. **Occurrence**—Clinical disease is uncommon, generally occurring in individuals with impaired immunocompetence whose non-intact skin had intimate contact with contaminated soil or surface water. It may appear as a complication of overt wounds or follow aspiration of water. Melioidosis is emerging as a significant cause of community-acquired sepsis in the tropics with a variety of clinical presentations. Cases have been recorded in many tropical and subtropical areas of Africa, America, Asia, Australia/ Pacific Islands, India, and the Middle East. In certain areas, 5%–20% of agricultural workers have demonstrable antibodies but no history of overt disease; in Thailand it is considered to be a disease of rice farmers. The disease is reported to be highly seasonal, with 75%–85% of cases presenting during the rainy season when exposure to the organism is believed to be greatest. Worldwide, fatal pulmonary melioidosis has been increasing among travelers returning from areas of endemicity, and it has been a pathogen commonly isolated from troops of all nationalities who have served in areas with endemic disease. Following the Tsunami of 2004, an

increase in the number of melioidosis cases was observed, mainly among repatriated tourists. Highest risk for melioidosis exists for servicemen, adventure travelers, eco-tourists, construction and resource extraction workers and persons whose contact to contaminated soil or water may expose them.

4. Reservoir—The organism is saprophytic in certain soils and waters. Various animals, including sheep, goats, horses, swine, monkeys and rodents (plus various animals in zoological gardens) can become infected, without evidence that they are important reservoirs, except in the transfer of the agent to new foci.

5. Mode of transmission—Usually, contact with contaminated soil or water through overt or inapparent skin wounds, inhalation of soil dust, and—rarely—aspiration or ingestion of contaminated water. Transmission can also occur through contact with rodents. Person-to-person transmission is possible through direct or sexual contact, or through use of injection needles. Transmission may also occur *in utero* or through breastfeeding.

6. Incubation period—May range from 1 to 21 days, and can be as short as a few hours with high inoculum. However, years may elapse between presumed exposure and appearance of clinical disease.

7. Period of communicability—Person-to-person transmission can occur via contact with blood and body fluids of an infected person, but this is rare. Laboratory-acquired infections may rarely occur, especially if procedures produce aerosols.

8. Susceptibility—Disease in humans is more common than previously thought, especially among people in endemic areas who have close contact with soil or water containing the infectious agent. Melioidosis is considered to be under-diagnosed in most endemic areas. Approximately two-thirds of adult cases have a predisposing medical condition such as diabetes, cirrhosis, alcoholism or renal failure, which may precipitate disease or recrudescence in asymptomatic infected individuals.

9. Methods of control—

    A. Preventive measures:

        1) Persons with debilitating disease, including diabetes, and those with traumatic wounds should avoid exposure to soil or water in endemic areas.

        2) In endemic areas, skin lacerations, abrasions or burns that have been contaminated with soil or surface water should be immediately and thoroughly cleaned.

3) Use of boots and gloves is recommended for occupations that involve contact with soil and water, such as work in rice fields.

B. Control of patient, contacts and the immediate environment:

1) Report to local health authority: No official report, Class 5 (see *Reporting*).
2) Isolation: Respiratory and sinus drainage precautions. Common blood and body fluid precautions should be taken. Patients or health care workers with known immunocompromised conditions should not have direct contact with cases.
3) Concurrent disinfection: Safe disposal of sputum and wound discharges.
4) Quarantine: Not applicable.
5) Immunization of contacts: Not applicable.
6) Investigation of contacts and source of infection: Human carriers are not known.
7) Specific treatment: Melioidosis requires long courses of antimicrobial therapy. Initial treatment consists of supportive measures and 10 days of intensive-phase therapy with intravenous ceftazidime, imipenem, or meropenem. Following intensive-phase therapy, treatment is ambulatory eradication-phase therapy with 20–24 weeks of oral trimethoprim-sulfamethoxazole with or without doxycycline (NB: doxycycline cannot be used in children less than eight years of age). The infection may be slow to respond to treatment, and even with 20 weeks of treatment, 10% of cases relapse. Treatment for an inadequate length of time leads to a high probability of relapse. Abscesses should be drained if possible.

C. Epidemic measures: Usually a sporadic disease. Outbreaks should be investigated to determine if there is a point source.

D. Disaster implications: None, except as in C, above.

E. International measures: None except as in C, above. Risk of introduction should be considered when animals are moved to areas where the disease is unknown.

F. Measures in the case of deliberate use: B. pseudomallei is a potential agent for deliberate use that is moderately easy to disseminate and has low morbidity rates, although the case fatality rate among overt cases is high. Control measures include rapid identification (and control) of the point source. In the unlikely event of the spread of *B. pseudomallei*, the value of prophylactic medication is unproven but may be efficacious. Post-exposure prophylaxis with trimethoprim-sulfamethoxazole (co-trimoxazole) is recommended. There is no vaccine available for human melioidosis.

For more information on the deliberate use of infectious agents to cause harm, see the section on *Deliberate use*.

GLANDERS   ICD-9 024; ICD-10 A24.0

Glanders is a highly communicable disease of horses, mules and donkeys; it has disappeared from most areas of the world, although enzootic foci are believed to exist in Asia and some eastern Mediterranean countries. Clinical glanders no longer occurs in the western hemisphere. Rare and sporadic human infections are reported almost exclusively in those whose occupations involve contact with animals or work in laboratories (e.g. veterinarians, equine butchers and pathologists). Infection with *Burkholderia mallei*, the glanders bacillus, cannot be differentiated serologically from infection with *B. pseudomallei*; characterization of the isolated organism alone can lead to specific diagnosis. Prevention depends on control of glanders in equine species and care in handling causative organisms. Treatment: see Melioidosis. *B. mallei*, like *B. pseudomallei*, is a potential agent for deliberate use. For more information on the deliberate use of infectious agents to cause harm, see the section on *Deliberate use*.

MENINGITIS
I. VIRAL MENINGITIS   ICD-9 047.9; ICD-10 A87
(Aseptic meningitis, Serous meningitis, Nonbacterial or Abacterial meningitis)
(Nonpyogenic meningitis: ICD-9 322.0; ICD-10 G03.0)
[CCDM19: Editorial Board]
[CCDM18: D. Lavanchy]

1. **Identification**—A relatively common but rarely serious clinical syndrome with multiple viral etiologies, characterized by sudden onset of febrile illness with signs and symptoms of meningeal involvement. CSF findings are pleocytosis (usually mononuclear, occasionally polymorphonuclear in early stages), increased protein, normal sugar and absence of bacteria. A rubella-like rash characterizes certain types caused by echoviruses and coxsackieviruses; vesicular and petechial rashes may also occur. Active illness seldom exceeds 10 days. Transient paresis and encephalitic manifestations may occur; paralysis is unusual. Residual signs lasting a year or more may include weakness, muscle spasm, insomnia and personality changes. Recovery is usually complete. GI and respiratory symptoms may be associated with enterovirus infection.

Various diseases caused by non-viral infectious agents may mimic aseptic meningitis: these include inadequately treated pyogenic meningitis, tuberculous and cryptococcal meningitis, meningitis caused by other fungi, cerebrovascular syphilis, and lymphogranuloma venereum. Post-infectious and post-vaccinal reactions require differentiation from sequelae to measles, mumps, varicella and immunization against rabies and smallpox; these syndromes are usually encephalitic in type. Leptospirosis, listeriosis, syphilis, lymphocytic choriomeningitis, viral hepatitis, infectious mononucleosis, influenza and other diseases may produce the same clinical syndrome, as discussed in the chapters dealing with those diseases.

Infection by enteroviruses transmitted from the mother is a frequent cause of neonatal fever with neurological signs. In countries that are polio-free, the most prevalent infectious agent causing paralysis is enterovirus 71, responsible for outbreaks of meningitis and paralysis in many countries. Children and adults with B cell deficiencies are subject to chronic relapsing meningitis, usually caused by enteroviruses.

Under optimal conditions, specific identification is possible in about half of all cases, through serological and isolation techniques. Viral agents may be isolated in early stages from throat washings and stool, occasionally from CSF and blood, and through cell culture techniques and animal inoculation. PCR identification in CSF (and stool for enteroviruses) yields a more rapid diagnosis and probes are available for the identification of most viruses.

2. **Infectious agents**—A wide variety of infectious agents exist, many associated with other specific diseases. Several viruses can produce meningeal features. At least half of cases have no obvious cause. In epidemic periods, mumps may be responsible for more than 25% of cases of established etiology in non-immunized populations. In the USA, enteroviruses (picornaviruses) cause most cases of known etiology, followed by coxsackievirus. These include coxsackievirus group B types 1-6 and echovirus types 2, 5, 6, 7, 9 (most), 10, 11, 14, 18 and 30, and enterovirus 71. Coxsackievirus group A (types 2, 3, 4, 7, 9 and 10), arboviruses, measles, herpes simplex and varicella viruses, lymphocytic choriomeningitis virus, adenovirus and others provide sporadic cases. Incidence of specific types varies with geographic location and time. *Leptospira* may cause up to 20% of cases of aseptic meningitis in various areas (see *Leptospirosis*).

3. **Occurrence**—Worldwide, as epidemics and sporadic cases; true incidence unknown. Seasonal increases in late summer and early autumn are due mainly to arboviruses and enteroviruses, while late winter outbreaks may be due primarily to mumps.

4., 5., 6., 7., and 8. **Reservoir, Mode of transmission, Incubation period, Period of communicability** and **Susceptibility**—Vary according to the specific infectious agent (please see specific disease chapters).

9. **Methods of control—**

A. **Preventive measures:** Depend on causes (please see specific disease chapters).

B. **Control of patient, contacts and the immediate environment:**

1) Report to local health authority: In selected endemic areas; in many countries not a reportable disease, Class 3 (see *Reporting*). If laboratory-confirmed, specify infectious agent; otherwise, report as "cause undetermined."

2) Isolation: Specific diagnosis depends on laboratory data not usually available until after recovery. Therefore, enteric precautions are indicated for 7 days after onset of illness, unless a non-enteroviral diagnosis is established.

3) Concurrent disinfection: No special precautions needed beyond routine sanitary practices.

4) Quarantine: Not applicable.

5) Immunization of contacts: See specific infectious agent.

6) Investigation of contacts and source of infection: Not usually indicated.

7) Specific treatment: Acyclovir may be given for herpes simplex meningitis. Pleconaril is available experimentally for enteroviral infections in many industrialized countries. In the rare event of agammaglobulinemia with chronic enteroviral meningitis, patients should receive IG.

C. **Epidemic measures:** See specific infectious agent.

D. **Disaster implications:** None.

E. **International measures:** WHO Collaborating Centres provide support as required. More information can be found at:

<http://www.who.int/collaboratingcentres/database/en/>

II. BACTERIAL MENINGITIS   ICD-9 320; ICD-10 G00

Neisseria meningitidis, *Streptococcus pneumoniae* and *Haemophilus influenzae* type b (Hib) cause more than 75% of all cases of bacterial meningitis in most studies, and 90% of bacterial meningitis in children. Meningitis due to Hib, previously the most common cause of bacterial meningitis, has largely been eliminated in many industrialized countries through immunization programs. Meningococcal disease is unique among the major causes of bacterial meningitis in that it causes both endemic disease and also large epidemics. The less common bacterial causes of meningitis, such as staphylococci, enteric bacteria, group B streptococci and *Listeria*, occur in persons with specific susceptibilities (such as neonates and patients with impaired immunity) or as the consequence of head trauma.

II. A. MENINGOCOCCAL
   INFECTION   ICD-9 036; ICD-10 A39
(Meningococcemia, not meningitis: ICD-10 A39.2-A39.4)
MENINGOCOCCAL
   MENINGITIS   ICD-9 036.0; ICD-10 A39.0
(Cerebrospinal fever)

1. Identification—An acute bacterial disease, characterized by sudden onset of fever, intense headache, nausea and often vomiting, stiff neck and photophobia. A petechial rash with pink macules or occasionally vesicles may be observed in Europe and North America, but rarely in Africa. Case fatality rates formerly exceeded 50%. Antibiotics, intensive care units and improved supportive measures have decreased this, but case fatality remains high at 8%–15%. In addition, 10%–20% of survivors will suffer long-term sequelae, including mental retardation, hearing loss, and loss of limb use. Invasive disease is characterized by one or more clinical syndromes including bacteremia, sepsis, or meningitis, the latter being the most common presentation. Meningococcemia, or meningococcal sepsis, is the most severe form of infection, with petechial rash, hypotension, disseminated intravascular coagulation and multi-organ failure. Other forms of meningococcal disease, such as pneumonia, purulent arthritis, and pericarditis, are less common.

The gold standard for diagnosis is recovery of meningococci from a sterile site, primarily cerebrospinal fluid (CSF) or blood; however, the sensitivity of culture, especially in patients who have received antibiotics, is low. In culture-negative cases, identification of group-specific meningococcal polysaccharides in CSF by latex agglutination is of help but false-negative results are common, especially for serogroup B. Polymerase chain reaction offers the advantage of detecting meningococcal DNA in CSF or plasma and not requiring live organisms; it is not yet widely available in many countries. Microscopic examination of Gram-stained smears from petechiae may show *Neisseria*.

2. Infectious agent—*Neisseria meningitidis*, the meningococcus, is a Gram-negative, aerobic diplococcus. *Neisseria* are divided into serogroups according to the immunological reactivity of their capsular polysaccharide. Group A, B, and C organisms account for at least 90% of cases, although the proportion of groups Y and W135 is increasing in several regions. In most European and many Latin American countries, serogroups B and C cause the majority of disease, while serogroup A causes the majority of disease in Africa and Asia. Serogroups A, B, C, Y, W-135 and X are all capable of causing outbreaks—most characteristically serogroup A, which is responsible for major epidemics, particularly in the so-called African meningitis belt (see Occurrence). Outbreaks of *N. meningitidis* are usually caused by closely related strains. Molecular subtyping of isolates (multi-locus enzyme electrophoresis or pulsed-field gel electrophoresis of enzyme-restricted DNA fragments) may allow identification of an "outbreak strain" and assist in better differentiation of outbreaks from endemic disease.

3. Occurrence—In Europe and North America the incidence of meningococcal disease is higher during winter and spring; in Sub-Saharan Africa the disease classically peaks during the dry season. Infants have the highest risk of meningococcal disease. Rates of disease decrease after infancy and then increase in adolescence and young adulthood. In addition to age, other individual risk factors for meningococcal disease include underlying immune deficiencies, such as asplenia, properdin deficiency, and a deficiency of terminal complement components. Crowding, low socioeconomic status, active or passive exposure to tobacco smoke and concurrent upper respiratory tract infections increase the risk of meningococcal disease. In some countries males are at higher risk than females. New military recruits have also been consistently found to have higher risk of disease; it may be similar reasons that cause increased risk among university students living in dormitories.

The highest burden of the disease undoubtedly lies in the African meningitis belt, a large area that stretches from Senegal to Ethiopia and affects all or part of 21 countries. In this region, high rates of sporadic infections (1–20 cases per 100 000 population) occur in annual cycles, with periodical superimposition of large-scale epidemics (usually caused by serogroup A, occasionally serogroup C, and more recently by serogroup W-135). In the countries of the African meningitis belt, epidemics with incidence rates as high as 1 000 cases per 100 000 population have occurred every 8–12 years over at least the past 50 years. In addition, major epidemics have occurred in adjacent countries not usually considered part of the African meningitis belt (such as Kenya and the United Republic of Tanzania).

In 2000, an epidemic of serogroup W-135 meningococcal disease associated with the Hajj occurred in Saudi Arabia; in 2000 and 2001, in several countries, cases of serogroup W-135 occurred among returning pilgrims and their close contacts. In 2002, the first major serogroup W-135 epidemic occurred in Burkina Faso, with over 13 000 cases and 1 400 deaths reported.

During the 1980s and 1990s, serogroup B has emerged as the most common cause of disease in Europe and most of the Americas. Epidemics characterized by a 5- to 10-fold increase in incidence for 10–20 years have been reported from many countries in Europe, Central and South America, and most recently in New Zealand and the US Pacific northwest. Community outbreaks of group C disease have occurred with increasing frequency in Canada and the USA since 1990. During the late 1990s, group Y disease has become as common as groups B and C in parts of the USA.

4. **Reservoir**—Humans.

5. **Mode of transmission**—Direct contact, including respiratory droplets from noses and throats of infected people; infection usually causes only a subclinical mucosal infection. Up to 5%–10% of people may be asymptomatic carriers with nasopharyngeal colonization by *N. meningitidis*. Less than 1% of those colonized will progress to invasive disease. Carrier rates of 25% have been documented in some populations in the absence of any cases of meningococcal disease. In contrast, during some meningococcal outbreaks in industrialized countries, no carriers of the "outbreak stain" have been identified. Fomite transmission is insignificant.

6. **Incubation period**—2 to 10 days, commonly 3 to 4 days.

7. **Period of communicability**—Until live meningococci are no longer present in discharges from nose and mouth. Meningococci usually disappear from the nasopharynx within 24 hours after institution of antimicrobial treatment to which the organisms are sensitive, and with substantial concentrations in oronasopharyngeal secretions. Penicillin will temporarily suppress the organisms, but does not usually eradicate them from the oronasopharynx.

8. **Susceptibility**—Susceptibility to the clinical disease is low and decreases with age; this induces a high ratio of carriers to cases. Persons deficient in certain complement components are especially prone to recurrent disease; splenectomized persons are susceptible to bacteremic illness. Group-specific immunity of unknown duration follows even subclinical infections.

9. **Methods of control**—

  A. *Preventive measures:*

  1) Educate the public on the need to reduce direct contact and exposure to droplet infection.
  2) Reduce overcrowding in living quarters and workplaces, such as barracks, schools, camps and ships.
  3) Vaccines containing groups A, C, Y and W-135 meningococcal polysaccharides are available; two polysaccharide vaccines are currently available on the market (quadrivalent ACYW-135 vaccine, and bivalent AC). Bivalent polysaccharide meningococcal vaccines against serogroups A and C are safe and effective in adults and children over 2, but do not elicit long-term protection, particularly in children under 5. The serogroup A polysaccharide can induce antibodies in children as young as 3 months, but the C polysaccharide is poorly immunogenic and ineffective in children under 2. Serogroup Y and W135 polysaccharides are also immunogenic in adults and children over 2, but immunogenicity and

clinical protection have not been fully documented. Meningococcal polysaccharide vaccines are effective for outbreak control and for prevention among high-risk groups, such as travelers to countries where disease is epidemic, Hajj pilgrims, military groups, and individuals with underlying immune dysfunctions. Because these vaccines are often poorly immunogenic in young children and have limited duration of efficacy, they are not generally used in routine childhood immunization programs. Re-immunization may be considered within 3–5 years if indications still exist. No vaccine effective against group B meningococci is currently licensed, although several have been developed and show some efficacy in older children and adults.

B. Control of patient, contacts and the immediate environment:

1) Report to local health authority: Obligatory case report in most countries, Class 2 (see *Reporting*).
2) Isolation: Respiratory isolation for 24 hours after start of chemotreatment.
3) Concurrent disinfection: Of discharges from the nose and throat and articles soiled therewith. Terminal cleaning.
4) Quarantine: Not applicable.
5) Protection of contacts: Close surveillance of household, day care, and other intimate contacts for early signs of illness, especially fever, to initiate appropriate therapy without delay; prophylactic administration of an effective chemotherapeutic agent to intimate contacts (household contacts, military personnel sharing the same sleeping space and people socially close enough to have shared eating utensils, e.g. close friends at school but not the whole class). Younger children in day care centers, even if not close friends, should all be given prophylaxis after an index case is identified. Rifampicin, ceftriaxone and ciprofloxacin are equally effective prophylactic agents. Rifampicin is administered twice daily for 2 days: adults 600 mg per dose; children over 1 month old, 10 mg/kg; under 1 month, 5 mg/kg. Rifampicin should not be given to pregnant women and may reduce the effectiveness of oral contraceptives.

For adults, ceftriaxone, 250 mg IM, given in a single dose, is effective; 125 mg IM for children under 15. Ciprofloxacin, 500 mg PO, may be given as a single dose to adults. Because in most countries 50% of *N. meningitidis* isolates are resistant to sulfadiazine, the latter is rarely used for prophylaxis. If the organisms have been shown to be sensitive to sulfadiazine, it may be given to adults and older children at a dosage of 1 gram every 12 hours for 4 doses; for infants and children, the dosage is 125–150 mg/kg/day divided into 4 equal doses, on each of 2 consecutive days. Health care personnel are rarely at risk even when caring for infected patients; only intimate exposure to nasopharyngeal secretions (e.g. as in mouth-to-mouth resuscitation) warrants prophylaxis. Because of the efficacy of prophylaxis, immunization is generally not recommended.

6) Investigation of contacts and source of infection: Throat or nasopharyngeal cultures are of no value in deciding who should receive prophylaxis, since carriage is variable, and there is no consistent relationship between that found in the normal population and that found in an epidemic.

7) Specific treatment: Penicillin given parenterally in adequate doses is the drug of choice for proven meningococcal disease; ampicillin and chloramphenicol are also effective. Penicillin-resistant strains have been reported in many countries, including Spain, the UK and the USA; strains resistant to chloramphenicol have been reported in France and in Viet Nam. Treatment should start as soon as the presumptive clinical diagnosis is made, even before meningococci have been identified. In children, until the specific agent has been identified, the drug chosen must be effective against *Haemophilus influenzae* type b (Hib) as well as *Streptococcus pneumoniae*. While ampicillin is the drug of choice for both as long as the organisms are ampicillin-sensitive, it should be combined with a third-generation cephalosporin, or chloramphenicol or vancomycin should be substituted in the many places where ampicillin-resistant *H. influenzae* b or penicillin-resistant *S. pneumoniae* strains are known to occur. Patients with meningococcal or Hib disease should receive rifampicin prior to discharge if neither a third-generation cephalosporin nor ciprofloxacin was given as treatment, to ensure elimination of the organism.

C. Epidemic measures:

1) When an outbreak occurs, major emphasis must be placed on careful surveillance, early diagnosis, and immediate treatment of suspected cases. A high index of suspicion is necessary. A threshold approach tailored to the epidemiology of the country is used in many developing countries to differentiate endemic disease from outbreaks. Thresholds (alert and epidemic) from a country with high rates of endemic disease (African meningitis belt) are given here as an example. When thresholds are passed, immunization campaigns must be implemented.

Alert threshold: 5 cases/100 000 population **or** increase in relation to previous non-epidemic years. Once alert threshold is reached: mandatory investigation, confirmation of agent, reinforcing of surveillance, enhancing of preparedness, and treatment of patients.

Epidemic threshold: 10 cases/100 000 population and alert threshold crossed early in meningitis season **or** weekly doubling of cases each week during a three week period or 15 cases/100 000 population or 2 cases at a mass gathering among refugees or displaced persons. Once epidemic threshold is reached: mass vaccination, provision of drugs to health units, treatment of cases and public education.

In some industrialized countries, the following steps are used to decide whether to declare an outbreak and initiate vaccination:

a) Determine whether it is an organization-based outbreak (e.g. school, university, prison) or a community-based outbreak (town, city, county)
b) Investigate links between cases, because secondary or co-primary cases are excluded from calculations
c) Calculate attack rates with the outbreak strain among the population at risk
d) Subtype *N. meningitidis* isolates, if available, from cases of disease, using molecular typing methods.

   If at least 3 cases have occurred during a 3 month period, the attack rate exceeds 10 cases per 100 000 in the population at risk, and the strain is vaccine-preventable (serogroup A, C, Y or W-135), immunization of those in the group at risk should be considered.

2) Reduce overcrowding and ventilate living and sleeping quarters for all people exposed to infection because of living conditions (e.g. soldiers, miners and prisoners).
3) Mass chemoprophylaxis is usually not effective in controlling outbreaks; in outbreaks involving small populations (e.g. a single school), chemoprophylaxis to all members of the community may be considered, especially if the outbreak is caused by a serogroup not included in the available vaccine. If undertaken, chemoprophylaxis should be administered to all members at the same time. Intimate contacts should all be considered for prophylaxis, regardless of whether the entire small population is treated (see 9B5).
4) The use of vaccine in all age groups affected is strongly recommended if an outbreak occurs in a large institutional or community setting in which the cases are due to groups A, C, W-135 or Y (see 9A3). Meningococcal vaccine has been very effective in halting epidemics due to A and C serogroups.

In countries where large-scale epidemics occur, mass vaccination of the entire population in affected areas should be considered when vaccine supply and administrative facilities allow. Geographical distribution of cases, age-specific attack rates and available resources all must be considered in estimating the target population. Decisions about vaccination should consider where the intervention is likely to have the largest impact in preventing disease and death.

D. Disaster implications: Epidemics may develop in situations of forced crowding.

E. International measures: WHO Collaborating Centres provide support as required. More information can be found at:
<http://www.who.int/collaboratingcentres/database/en/>

Although the disease is not covered by *International Health Regulations*, some countries may require a valid certificate of immunization against meningococcal meningitis as a condition of entry, e.g. Saudi Arabia for Hajj pilgrims. For further information, please see:

<http://www.who.int/topics/meningitis/en/>

II. B. HEMOPHILUS MENINGITIS ICD-9 320.0; ICD-10 G00.0
(Meningitis due to *Haemophilus influenzae*)

1. Identification—Before widespread use of *Haemophilus* b (Hib) conjugate vaccines, in industrialized countries Hib most commonly presented as meningitis. Epiglottitis and bacteremia without focus were the next most common presentations. In developing countries, the primary manifestation of Hib disease is lower respiratory tract infection. Hib may account for 5–8% of all pneumonia in children in these areas, and causes an estimated 480 000 pneumonia deaths each year among children under 5.

Infection is usually associated with bacteremia. Onset can be subacute but is usually sudden, including fever, vomiting, lethargy and meningeal irritation, with bulging fontanelle in infants or stiff neck and back in older children. Progressive stupor or coma is common. Occasionally, there is a low-grade fever for several days, with more subtle CNS symptoms. Overall mortality rate for Hib meningitis is 5%; 6% of the survivors have permanent sensorineural hearing loss; 25% have significant handicap of some type.

Diagnosis may be made through isolation of organisms from blood or CSF. Specific capsular polysaccharide may be identified by CIE or LA techniques.

2. Infectious agent—*H. influenzae* are Gram-negative coccobacilli that are divided into unencapsulated (nontypeable) and encapsulated strains. The encapsulated strains are further classified into serotypes a through f, based on the antigenic characteristics of their polysaccharide capsules. *H. influenzae* serotype b (Hib) is the most pathogenic.

3. Occurrence—Worldwide; most prevalent among children aged 2 months to 3 years; unusual over the age of 5. In developing countries, peak incidence is in children below 6 months; in industrialized countries, generally in children 6–12 months. As of the late 1990s, with widespread vaccine use in early childhood, Hib meningitis has virtually disappeared in industrialized countries. Secondary cases in families and day care centers are rare.

4. Reservoir—Humans.

5. Mode of transmission—Droplet infection and discharges from nose and throat during the infectious period. The portal of entry is most commonly the nasopharynx.

6. Incubation period—Unknown; probably short, 2–4 days.

7. Period of communicability—As long as organisms are present, which may be for a prolonged period even without nasal discharge. Non-communicable within 24–48 hours of starting effective antibiotherapy.

8. Susceptibility—Susceptibility assumed to be universal. Immunity associated with the presence of circulating bactericidal and/or anticapsular antibody, acquired trans-placentally, from prior infection, or through immunization.

9. Methods of control

    A. Preventive measures:

        1) Routine childhood immunization. Several protein polysaccharide conjugate vaccines have been shown to prevent meningitis in children more than 2 months of age, and are licensed in many countries, both individually and combined with other vaccines. Immunization is recommended, starting at 2 months of age, followed by additional doses after an interval of 2 months; dosages vary with the vaccine in use. All vaccines require boosters at 12–15 months of age. Immunization is not routinely recommended for children over 5.

           Despite the availability of Hib conjugate vaccines since the 1980s, and despite its virtual elimination in most industrialized countries, Hib disease remains common in many developing countries, where cost and the non-recognition of Hib disease burden constitute major obstacles to the introduction of Hib conjugate vaccine. Efforts to introduce Hib conjugate vaccine are, however, increasing worldwide.

        2) Monitor for cases occurring in susceptible population settings, such as day care centers and large foster homes.

3) Educate parents about the risk of secondary cases in siblings under 4 and the need for prompt evaluation and treatment if fever or stiff neck develops.

B. Control of patient, contacts and the immediate environment:

1) Report to local health authority: In selected endemic areas, Class 3 (see *Reporting*).
2) Isolation: Respiratory isolation for 24 hours after start of chemotherapy.
3) Concurrent disinfection: Not applicable.
4) Quarantine: Not applicable.
5) Protection of contacts: Recommended for Hib but not other serotypes of *H. influenzae*. Rifampicin prophylaxis (orally once daily for 4 days in a 20 mg/kg dose, maximal dose 600 mg/day) for all household contacts (including adults) in households with one or more children under 1 (other than the index case) or with a child of 1–3 who is inadequately immunized. When 2 or more cases of invasive disease have occurred within 60 days and unimmunized or incompletely immunized children attend the childcare facility, administration of rifampicin to all attenders and supervisory personnel is indicated. When a single case has occurred, the use of rifampicin prophylaxis is controversial.
6) Investigation of contacts and source of infection: Observe contacts under 6 years old, especially infants, for signs of illness, such as fever.
7) Specific treatment: Ampicillin has been the drug of choice (parenteral 200–400 mg/kg/day). However, about 30% of strains are now resistant due to beta-lactamase production: ceftriaxone, cefotaxime or chloramphenicol is thus recommended concurrently or singly until antimicrobial susceptibility has been ascertained. The patient should be given rifampicin prior to discharge from hospital, to ensure elimination of the organism.

C. Epidemic measures: Not applicable.

D. Disaster implications: None.

E. International measures: None.

II. C. PNEUMOCOCCAL MENINGITIS ICD-9 320.1; ICD-10 G00.1

1. Identification—Pneumococcal meningitis has a high case-fatality rate. It can be fulminant and occurs with bacteremia but not necessarily with any other focus, although there may be otitis media or mastoiditis.

Onset is usually sudden with high fever, lethargy or coma, and signs of meningeal irritation. It is a sporadic disease in young infants, the elderly and other high-risk groups, including asplenic and hypogammaglobulinemic patients. Receipt of a cochlear implant and basilar fracture causing persistent communication with the nasopharynx are predisposing factors (see *Pneumonia, pneumococcal*). Diagnosis may be made by isolation of organisms from blood or CSF. Pneumococcal capsular polysaccharide may be identified by CIE or LA techniques.

2. **Infectious agent**—*Streptococcus pneumoniae* is a Gram-positive diplococcus. Nearly all strains causing meningitis and other severe forms of pneumococcal disease are encapsulated; there are 90 known capsular serotypes. The distribution of serotypes varies regionally and with age. In North America the 7 serotypes in pneumococcal conjugate vaccine are those that cause 80% of pneumococcal meningitis in children, and the majority of pneumococcal meningitis in adults.

3. **Occurrence**—Worldwide; most prevalent among children 2 months to 3 years; in developing countries infants are at highest risk; in North America, peaks at 6–18 months. The elderly, and adults who are immunocompromised or have certain chronic illness, are also at higher risk.

4. **Reservoir**—Humans. Pneumococci are often found in the upper respiratory tract of healthy persons. Carriage is more common in children than in adults.

5. **Mode of transmission**—Droplet spread and contact with respiratory secretions; direct contract with a person with pneumococcal disease generally results in nasopharyngeal carriage of the organism rather than in disease.

6. **Incubation period**—Unknown; probably short, 1–4 days.

7. **Period of communicability**—As long as organisms are present, which may be for a prolonged period, especially in immunocompromised hosts.

8. **Susceptibility**—Assumed to be universal. Immunity is associated with the presence of circulating bactericidal and/or anticapsular antibody, acquired trans-placentally, from prior infection or from immunization.

9. **Methods of control**

   A. *Preventive measures:* Vaccination is the mainstay of prevention. In many industrialized countries, pneumococcal conjugate vaccine is recommended for children under 2 and those aged 2–4 years with certain high-risk conditions, such as immunocompromising conditions, sickle cell disease, asplenia, heart or lung disease, or cochlear implantation. The vaccine covers the 7 serotypes most often causing pneumococcal meningitis in industrialized countries. Other countries are currently using conjugate vaccine in selected high-risk populations. A polysaccharide vaccine containing 23 of the most common serotypes has been available since 1983, and is recommended in several countries for use in persons 65 and older and those aged 2–64 with immunocompromising conditions or certain chronic illnesses.

B. *Control of patient, contacts and the immediate environment:*

1) Report to local health authority: In selected areas, Class 3 (see *Reporting*).
2) Isolation: Standard precautions for hospitalized patients.
3) Concurrent disinfection: Of nasal and throat secretions.
4) Quarantine: Not applicable.
5) Protection of contacts: Not applicable, except in an outbreak setting (see *Epidemic measures*).
6) Investigation of contacts and source of infection: Generally not useful.
7) Specific treatment: Penicillin, ceftriaxone, or cefotaxime are the drugs of choice. Because resistance is common in many areas, blood and CSF culture should be performed for all patients with suspected bacterial meningitis, and susceptibility testing performed on pneumococci. Where resistance is widespread, ceftriaxone or cefotaxime given along with vancomycin are recommended for empirical therapy until susceptibility results are known. Intravenous dexamethasone early in the course of the illness along with antibiotics has been shown to reduce the long-term complications of pneumococcal meningitis.

C. *Epidemic measures:* Pneumococcal meningitis can occur as part of a cluster of pneumococcal disease in institutional settings. Immunization using either the 23-valent polysaccharide vaccine or the 7-valent conjugate vaccine, depending on the setting, should be used to control outbreaks. Targeted antimicrobial prophylaxis (e.g. penicillin) may be useful in some outbreaks, especially those caused by non-vaccine type strains and when the outbreak strain is not resistant to antimicrobial agents. Widespread antimicrobial prophylaxis is not always effective and can induce resistance.

D. *Disaster implications:* None.

E. *International measures:* None.

II. D. NEONATAL MENINGITIS

ICD-9 320.8, 771.8;
ICD-10 P37.8,
P35-P37, G00, G03

[CCDM18: W. Perea]

Infants with neonatal meningitis develop lethargy, seizures, apneic episodes, poor feeding, hypo- or hyperthermia, and sometimes respiratory distress, usually in their first week of life. The WBC count may be elevated or depressed. CSF culture yields group B streptococci, *Listeria monocytogenes* (see *Listeriosis*), *E. coli* K-1 or other organisms acquired from the birth canal. Infants aged 2 weeks to 2 months may develop similar symptoms, with recovery from the CSF of group B streptococci or organisms of the Klebsiella-Enterobacter-Serratia group, acquired from the nursery environment. Meningitis in both groups is associated with septicemia. Treatment is with ampicillin, plus a third-generation cephalosporin or aminoglycoside, until the causal organism has been identified and its antimicrobial susceptibilities determined.

MOLLUSCUM CONTAGIOSUM

ICD-9 078.0;
ICD-10 B08.1

[CCDM18 & 19: F. Ndowa]

1. Identification—A viral disease of the skin resulting in smooth-surfaced, firm and spherical papules with umbilication of the vertex. The lesions may be flesh-colored, white, translucent or yellow. Most papules are 2-5 mm in diameter; giant-cell papules (above 15 mm diameter) are occasionally seen. Lesions in adults are most often on the lower abdominal wall, pubis, genitalia or inner thighs; on children, they are most often on the face, trunk and proximal extremities. Immunocompetent hosts usually have 15-35 lesions; immunocompromised hosts (e.g. patients with HIV infection) may develop hundreds of disseminated lesions of the body and face. Occasionally the lesions itch and show a linear orientation, which suggests autoinoculation by scratching. In some patients, 50-100 lesions may become confluent and form a single plaque.

Without treatment, molluscum contagiosum persists for 6 months to 2 years. Any one lesion has a life span of 2-3 months. Lesions may resolve spontaneously or as a result of inflammatory response following trauma or secondary bacterial infection. Treatment (mechanical removal of the lesions) may shorten the course of illness.

Diagnosis can be clinical when multiple lesions are present. For confirmation, the core can be expressed onto a glass slide and examined by ordinary light microscopy for classic basophilic, Feulgen-positive, intra-cytoplasmic inclusions, the "molluscum" or "Henderson-Paterson bodies." Histology can confirm the diagnosis.

2. Infectious agent—Member of Poxviridae family, genus *Mollusci-poxvirus*; the genus comprises at least two species differentiated by DNA endonuclease cleavage maps. The virus has not been grown in cell culture.

3. Occurrence—Worldwide. Serological tests are not well standard-ized and skin inspection is the only screening technique available; epidemiological studies of the disease have therefore been limited. Population surveys have been conducted only in Fiji and Papua New Guinea, where the peak disease incidence occurs in childhood.

4. Reservoir—Humans.

5. Mode of transmission—Usually through direct contact. Transmis-sion can be sexual or non-sexual, the latter includes spread via fomites. Autoinoculation is also suspected.

6. Incubation period—For experimental inoculation, 19–50 days; clinical reports give 7 days to 6 months.

7. Period of communicability—Unknown, probably as long as le-sions persist.

8. Susceptibility—All ages may be affected; more often seen in children. Disease is more common in HIV-infected patients, in whom lesions may disseminate.

9. Methods of control—

> **A. Preventive measures:** Avoid contact, or sharing bathtubs, bath towels or sponges, with affected patients.
>
> **B. Control of patient, contacts and the immediate environment:**
>
> 1) Report to local health authority: Official report not ordinarily justifiable, Class 5 (see *Reporting*).
> 2) Isolation: Generally not indicated. Infected children with visible lesions should be excluded from close contact sports.
> 3) Concurrent disinfection: None.
> 4) Quarantine: None.
> 5) Immunization of contacts: None.
> 6) Investigation of contacts and source of infection: Examine sexual partners where applicable.
> 7) Specific treatment: Indicated to minimize risk of transmis-sion. Curettage with local anesthesia or topical application of

428 / MONONUCLEOSIS

cantharidin or peeling agents (salicylic or lactic acid). Freezing with liquid nitrogen has some advocates. Self-applied 0.5% podophyllotoxin cream has been effective. No therapy is effective in immunocompromised patients, because of the rapid occurrence of new lesions—as shown by the futility of both systemic and intralesional interferon.

C. Epidemic measures: Suspend direct contact activities.

D. Disaster implications: None.

E. International measures: None.

MONONUCLEOSIS, INFECTIOUS   ICD-9 075; ICD-10 B27
(Gammaherpesviral mononucleosis, Mononucleosis due to Epstein-Barr virus, Glandular fever, Monocytic angina)
[CCDM19: Editorial Board]

1. Identification—An acute viral syndrome characterized clinically by fever, sore throat (often with exudative pharyngotonsillitis), lymphadenopathy (especially posterior cervical) and splenomegaly; characterized hematologically by mononucleosis and lymphocytosis of 50% or greater, including 10% or more atypical cells; and characterized serologically by the presence of heterophiles and Epstein-Barr virus (EBV) antibodies. Recovery usually occurs in a few weeks, but a very small proportion of individuals can take months to regain their former level of energy. There is no evidence that this is due to abnormal persistence of the infection in a chronic form.

In young children the disease is generally mild and more difficult to recognize. Jaundice occurs in about 4% of infected young adults, although 95% have abnormal liver function tests; splenomegaly occurs in 50%. Duration is from 1 to several weeks; the disease is rarely fatal, and is more severe in older adults.

The causal agent, EBV, is also closely associated with the pathogenesis of several lymphomas and nasopharyngeal cancer (see *Malignant neoplasms associated with infectious agents*). Fatal immunoproliferative disorders involving a polyclonal expansion of EBV infected B-lymphocytes may occur in persons with an X-linked recessive immunoproliferative disorder; they can also occur in persons with acquired immune defects, including patients infected with HIV, transplant recipients, and persons with other conditions requiring long-term immunosuppressive therapy.

About 10%–15% of those with classical infectious mononucleosis cases are heterophile-negative. A heterophile-negative form of a syndrome resembling infectious mononucleosis is due to cytomegalovirus, and accounts for 5% to 7% of the "mono syndrome" (see *Cytomegalovirus infections*); other rare causes are toxoplasmosis and herpesvirus type 6 (see *Exanthema subitum*, following rubella). A mononucleosis-like illness may occur early in HIV-infected patients. Differentiation depends on laboratory results that include the EBV IgM test; only EBV elicits the "true" heterophile antibody. EBV accounts for over 80% of both heterophile positive and heterophile negative cases of the mononucleosis syndrome.

Laboratory diagnosis is based on the finding of a lymphocytosis exceeding 50% (including 10% or more abnormal forms), abnormalities in liver function tests (AST), or an elevated heterophile antibody titer after adsorption of the serum on guinea pig kidney. The most sensitive and commercially available test is the absorbed horse-RBC test; the most specific of the common tests is the beef-cell hemolysin test; and the most frequently used procedure is a commercial, qualitative slide agglutination assay. Very young children may not show an elevation of the heterophile titer, and heterophile-negative and clinically atypical forms rarely occur in the elderly. If available, the IFA test for IgM and IgA antibody, specific for viral capsid antigen (VCA) or antibody against "early antigen" of the causal virus, is helpful in diagnosis of heterophile-negative cases; antibody specific for the EBV nuclear antigen (EBNA) is usually absent during the acute phase of illness. Therefore, a positive anti-VCA titer and a negative anti-EBNA titer are diagnostic responses of an early primary EBV infection.

2. **Infectious agent**—Epstein-Barr virus, human (gamma) herpesvirus 4, closely related to other herpesviruses morphologically, but distinct serologically; it infects and transforms B-lymphocytes.

3. **Occurrence**—Worldwide. Infection is common and widespread in early childhood in developing countries and in socio-economically depressed population groups, where it is usually mild or asymptomatic. Typical infectious mononucleosis occurs primarily in industrialized countries, where age of infection is delayed until older childhood and young adulthood, so that it is most commonly recognized in high school and college students. About 50% of those infected develop clinical infectious mononucleosis; the others are mostly asymptomatic.

4. **Reservoir**—Humans.

5. **Mode of transmission**—Person-to-person spread by the oropharyngeal route, via saliva. Young children may be infected by saliva on the hands of nurses and other attendants and on toys, or by pre-chewing of baby food by the mother, a practice in some countries. Kissing facilitates spread among young adults. Spread may also occur via blood

transfusion to susceptible recipients, but ensuing clinical disease is uncommon. Reactivated EBV may play a role in the interstitial pneumonia of HIV infected infants and in hairy leukoplakia and B-cell tumors in HIV-infected adults.

6. Incubation period—From 4 to 6 weeks.

7. Period of communicability—Prolonged; pharyngeal excretion may persist in cell-free form for a year or more after infection; 15%–20% or more of EBV antibody-positive healthy adults are long-term oropharyngeal carriers.

8. Susceptibility—Susceptibility is general. Infection confers a high degree of resistance; immunity from unrecognized childhood infection may account for low rates of clinical disease in lower socioeconomic groups. Reactivation of EBV may occur in immunodeficient individuals and may result in elevated antibody titers to EBV (but not heterophile antibody), and possibly in the development of lymphomas.

9. Methods of control—

A. *Preventive measures:* Undetermined. Use hygienic measures, including handwashing, to avoid salivary contamination from infected individuals; avoid drinking beverages from a common container, in order to minimize contact with saliva.

B. *Control of patient, contacts and the immediate environment:*

1) Report to local health authority: Official report not ordinarily justifiable, Class 5 (see *Reporting*).
2) Isolation: Not applicable.
3) Concurrent disinfection: Of articles soiled with nose and throat discharges.
4) Quarantine: Not applicable.
5) Immunization of contacts: Not applicable.
6) Investigation of contacts and source of infection: For the individual case, of little value.
7) Specific treatment: None. Non-steroidal anti-inflammatory drugs, or steroids given in small doses in decreasing amounts over about a week, are of value in severe toxic cases, and in patients with severe oropharyngeal involvement and airway encroachment.

C. *Epidemic measures:* None.

D. *Disaster implications:* None.

E. *International measures:* None.

MUMPS
(Infectious parotitis)
[CCDM19: J. Seward, P. Strebel]
[CCDM18: S. Robertson]

ICD-9 072; ICD-10 B26

1. Identification—An acute viral disease characterized by fever, swelling and tenderness of one or more salivary glands— usually the parotid and sometimes the sublingual or submaxillary glands. Not all cases of parotitis are caused by mumps infection, but other parotitis-causing agents do not produce parotitis on an epidemic scale. Orchitis, most commonly unilateral, occurs in 20%–30% of affected post-pubertal males, but sterility is extremely rare. Mumps orchitis has been reported to be a risk factor for testicular cancer. As many as 40%–50% of mumps infections have been associated with respiratory symptoms, particularly in children aged under five years. Mumps can cause sensorineural hearing loss in both children and adults. Pancreatitis, usually mild, occurs in 4% of cases; a suggested association with diabetes remains unproven.

Symptomatic aseptic meningitis occurs in up to 10% of mumps cases; patients usually recover without complications, though many require hospitalization. Mumps encephalitis is rare (1–2/10 000 cases), but can result in permanent sequelae, such as paralysis, seizures and hydrocephalus; the case-fatality rate for mumps encephalitis is about 1%. Mumps infection during the first trimester of pregnancy has been associated with spontaneous abortion, but there is no firm evidence that mumps during pregnancy causes congenital malformations.

Acute mumps infection can be confirmed through: a positive serological test for mumps-specific IgM antibodies; seroconversion; a significant (at least 4-fold) rise in serum mumps IgG titer as determined by standard serological assay; detection of virus by reverse transcription polymerase chain reaction (RT-PCR); or isolation of mumps virus from an appropriate clinical specimen (throat swab, urine, CSF). In research settings, typing methods can distinguish wild-type mumps virus from vaccine virus. Diagnosis may be more challenging in vaccinated populations where the IgM response may be absent or short-lived and viral load may be lower.

2. Infectious agent—Mumps virus, a member of the family Paramyxoviridae, genus *Rubulavirus*.

3. Occurrence—In unvaccinated populations, about one-third of exposed susceptible people have unapparent or sub-clinical infections, especially young children. In temperate climates, winter and spring are peak seasons. In the absence of immunization mumps is endemic, with an annual incidence usually 100–1 000 per 100 000 population and epidemic peaks every 2–5 years. In many industrialized countries, mumps was a major cause of viral encephalitis. Serosurveys conducted prior to mumps vaccine introduction found that in some countries 90% of persons were immune by age 15 years, while in other countries a large proportion of the adult population remained susceptible. In countries where mumps vaccine has not been introduced, the incidence of mumps remains high, mostly affecting children aged five to nine.

By the end of 2006, 112 of 193 WHO Member States included mumps vaccine in their national immunization schedules. In countries where mumps vaccine coverage has been sustained at high levels, the incidence of the disease has dropped markedly.

4. **Reservoir**—Humans.

5. **Mode of transmission**—Airborne transmission or droplet spread; also direct contact with the saliva of an infected person.

6. **Incubation period**—About 16–18 days (range 12–25).

7. **Period of communicability**—Virus has been isolated from saliva (from seven days before the onset of parotitis to nine days afterwards) and from urine (six days before to 15 days after). Maximum infectiousness occurs between two days before onset of illness and four days afterwards. Unapparent infections can be communicable.

8. **Susceptibility**—Immunity is generally lifelong, and develops after either unapparent or clinical infections.

9. **Methods of control**—

   A. *Preventive measures:*

      Public education should encourage mumps immunization for susceptible individuals. Routine mumps vaccination is recommended in countries with an efficient childhood vaccination program and sufficient resources to maintain high levels of vaccine coverage. Mumps vaccination is recommended at age 12–18 months, as part of the measles/mumps/rubella (MMR) vaccine, though most countries have a two-dose schedule, with the 2nd dose given at least 1 month after the first dose. More than 90% of recipients develop immunity that is long-lasting and may be lifelong.

      Live attenuated mumps virus vaccines are available as monovalent vaccines or trivalent MMR vaccines. Hydrolyzed gelatin and/or sorbitol are used as stabilizers in mumps vaccine, along with neomycin as a preservative. Mumps vaccines are cold-chain dependent and should be protected from light.

      Different strains of live attenuated mumps vaccine have been developed in Japan, Russia, Switzerland and the USA. All licensed strains are judged acceptable by WHO for public health programs, except the Rubini strain, which is not recommended because of demonstrated low efficacy; persons who received this strain should be re-vaccinated with another strain. In most industrialized countries, only the Jeryl-Lynn strain or strains derived from it are accepted, because they show no confirmed association with aseptic meningitis.

The reported incidence of adverse events depends on the strain of mumps vaccine. The most common adverse reactions are fever and parotitis. Rare adverse reactions include orchitis, sensorineural deafness, and thrombocytopenia. Aseptic meningitis, resolving spontaneously in less than one week without sequelae, has been reported at frequencies ranging from 0.1 to 100 cases per 100 000 vaccine doses. This reflects differences in vaccine strains and their preparation, as well as variations in study design and case ascertainment. Better data are needed to establish more precise estimates of aseptic meningitis incidence in recipients of different strains of mumps vaccine. The rates of aseptic meningitis due to mumps vaccine are at least 100-fold lower than rates of aseptic meningitis due to infection with wild mumps virus.

Accumulated global experience in industrialized countries shows that 2 doses of vaccine are needed for protection against mumps. The first dose is usually given as MMR vaccine at the age of 12–18 months. The age of administration of the second dose may range from the 2nd year of life to age at school-entry, depending on programmatic considerations aimed at optimizing vaccination coverage. Less commonly, the second vaccination may be delivered through supplementary campaigns in developing countries.

Countries intending to use mumps or MMR vaccine during mass campaigns should give special attention to planning. The mumps vaccine strain should be carefully selected, and health workers should receive training on expected rates of adverse events following immunization, and on community advocacy and health education activities.

Vaccine is contraindicated in the immunosuppressed; however, treatment with a low dose of steroids (less than 2 mg/kg/day) on alternate days, topical steroid use, and aerosolized steroid preparations are not contraindications to administration of mumps vaccine. For theoretical reasons, pregnant women or women planning a pregnancy in the next month (28 days in the USA) should not receive mumps vaccine, although no evidence exists that mumps vaccine causes fetal damage.

B. Control of patient, contacts and the immediate environment:

1) Report to local health authority: WHO recommends making mumps a notifiable disease in all countries, Class 3 (see *Reporting*).

2) Isolation: Respiratory isolation for five days from onset of parotitis. Exclusion from school or workplace until five days after onset of parotitis if susceptible contacts (those not immunized) are present.

3) Concurrent disinfection: Of articles soiled with nose and throat secretions.

4) Quarantine: Exclusion of susceptibles from school or the workplace from the 12th until the 25th day after exposure if other susceptibles are present.

5) Immunization of contacts: Immunization after exposure may not always prevent infection. IG is not effective and not recommended.

6) Investigation of contacts and source of infection: Immunization of susceptible contacts.

7) Specific treatment: None.

C. Epidemic measures: Immunize susceptibles, especially those at risk of exposure. Serological screening to identify susceptibles is impractical and unnecessary, since there is no risk in immunizing those who are already immune.

D. Disaster implications: None.

E. International measures: None.

MYALGIA, EPIDEMIC ICD-9 074.1; ICD-10 B33.0
(Epidemic pleurodynia, Bornholm disease, Devil's grippe)
[CCDM18 & 19: D. Lavanchy]

1. Identification—An acute viral disease characterized by paroxysmal spasmodic pain in the chest or abdomen, which may be intensified by movement, usually accompanied by fever and headache. The pain tends to be more abdominal than thoracic in infants and young children, while the reverse applies to older children and adults. Most patients recover within 1 week of onset, but relapses occur; no fatalities have been reported. Localized epidemics are characteristic. It is important to differentiate from more serious medical or surgical conditions.

Complications occur infrequently and include orchitis, pericarditis, pneumonia and aseptic meningitis. During outbreaks of epidemic myalgia, cases of group B coxsackievirus myocarditis of the newborn have been reported. While myocarditis in adults is a rare complication, the possibility should always be considered.

Diagnosis is suggested by the appearance of similar symptoms among multiple family members. It is confirmed by a significant rise in antibody titer against specific etiologic agents in acute and convalescent sera, or by isolation of the virus in cell culture or neonatal mice from throat secretions or patient feces.

2. Infectious agents—Group B coxsackievirus types 1–3, 5 and 6 and echoviruses 1 and 6 are associated with the illness. Many group A and B coxsackieviruses and echoviruses have been reported in sporadic cases.

3. Occurrence—An uncommon disease, occurring in summer and early autumn; usually in children and young adults aged 5–15, but all ages may be affected. Multiple cases in a household can occur frequently. Outbreaks have been reported in Europe, Australia, New Zealand and North America.

4. Reservoir—Humans.

5. Mode of transmission—Directly by fecal-oral or respiratory droplet contact with an infected person, or indirectly by contact with articles freshly soiled with feces or throat discharges of an infected person who may or may not have symptoms. Group B coxsackieviruses have been found in sewage and flies, though the relationship to transmission of human infection is not clear.

6. Incubation period—Usually 3–5 days.

7. Period of communicability—Apparently during the acute stage of disease; stools may contain virus for several weeks.

8. Susceptibility—Probably general; type-specific immunity presumably results from infection.

9. Methods of control—

   A. **Preventive measures:** Avoid fecal-oral contact and/or respiratory droplet contact with infected persons and/or associated materials.

   B. **Control of patient, contacts and the immediate environment:**

   1) Report to local health authority: Obligatory report of epidemics, Class 4 (see *Reporting*).
   2) Isolation: Ordinarily limited to enteric precautions. Because of possible serious illness in the newborn, if a patient in a maternity unit or nursery develops an illness suggestive of enterovirus infection, precautions should be instituted at once. Individuals with suspected enterovirus infections (including health personnel) should be excluded from visiting maternity and nursery units and from contact with infants and women near term.

3) Concurrent disinfection: Prompt and safe disposal of respiratory discharges and feces; wash or dispose of articles soiled therewith. Careful attention must be given to prompt, thorough handwashing when handling discharges, feces and articles soiled therewith.

4) Quarantine: Not applicable.

5) Immunization of contacts: Not applicable.

6) Investigation of contacts and source of infection: Of no practical value.

7) Specific treatment: None.

C. Epidemic measures: General notice to physicians of the presence of an epidemic and the necessity for differentiation of cases from more serious medical or surgical emergencies.

D. Disaster implications: None.

E. International measures: None.

MYCETOMA	ICD-9 039; ICD-10 B47

ACTINOMYCETOMA	ICD-9 039; ICD-10 B47.1
EUMYCETOMA	ICD-9 117.4; ICD-10 B47.0

(Maduromycosis, Madura foot)
[CCDM18: L. Severo]
[CCDM19: M. Brandt, K. Glynn]

1. Identification—A clinical syndrome caused by a variety of aerobic actinomycetes (bacteria) and eumycetes (fungi), characterized by swelling and suppuration of subcutaneous tissues and formation of sinus tracts with visible granules in the pus draining from the sinus tracts. Lesions are usually on the foot or lower leg, sometimes on the hand, shoulders and back, and rarely at other sites.

Mycetoma may be difficult to distinguish from chronic osteomyelitis and botryomycosis (a clinically and pathologically similar entity caused by a variety of bacteria, including staphylococci and Gram-negative bacteria). Specific diagnosis depends on visualizing the granules in fresh preparations or histopathological slides, and isolation of the causative actinomycete or fungus in culture.

2. Infectious agents—Eumycetoma is caused by: *Madurella mycetomatis*; *M. grisea*; *Scedosporium apiospermum* (with a teleomorph, *Pseudallescheria boydii*); *Exophiala jeanselmei*; *Acremonium recifei*; *A. falciforme*; *Leptosphaeria senegalensis*; *Neotestudina rosatii*; *Pyre-*

nochaeta romeroi; and several other species. Actinomycetoma is caused by: *Nocardia brasiliensis*; *N. asteroids*; *N. otitidiscaviarum*; *Actinomadura madurae*; *A. pelletieri*; *Nocardiopsis dassonvillei*; *Streptomyces somaliensis;* and *S. sudanensis* sp. *Nov.*

3. Occurrence—Common in Mexico, Africa, southern Asia and other tropical and subtropical areas, especially where people go barefoot.

4. Reservoir—Soil and decaying vegetation.

5. Mode of transmission—Subcutaneous implantation of conidia or hyphal elements from a saprophytic source by penetrating wounds (thorns, splinters).

6. Incubation period—Usually months.

7. Period of communicability—No person-to-person transmission.

8. Susceptibility—Causal agents are widespread in nature, but clinical infection is rare, which suggests intrinsic resistance.

9. Methods of control—

   A. Preventive measures: Protect against puncture wounds by wearing shoes and protective clothing.

   B. Control of patient, contacts and the immediate environment:

   1) Report to local health authority: Official report not ordinarily justifiable, Class 5 (see *Reporting*).
   2) Isolation: Not applicable.
   3) Concurrent disinfection: Not applicable. Ordinary cleanliness.
   4) Quarantine: Not applicable.
   5) Immunization of contacts: Not applicable.
   6) Investigation of contacts and source of infection: Not indicated.
   7) Specific treatment: Some patients with eumycetoma may benefit from itraconazole or ketoconazole. Treatment with voriconazole or posaconazole has been helpful in eumycetoma caused by *S. apiospermum*. Terbinafine has also been helpful in some cases of eumycetoma. Some cases of actinomycetoma may benefit from clindamycin, trimethoprim-sulfamethoxazole, long-acting sulfonamides, or imipenem. Penicillin alone is usually not useful (unlike for actinomycosis), but amoxicillin-clavulanic acid has been used successfully. Resection of small lesions may be helpful; amputation may be required for an extremity with advanced lesions.

   C. Epidemic measures: Not applicable, a sporadic disease.

D. Disaster implications: None.

E. International measures: WHO Collaborating Centres provide support as required. More information can be found at:

http://www.who.int/collaboratingcentres/database/en/

NAEGLERIASIS, ACANTHAMEBIASIS, AND BALAMUTHIASIS ICD-9 136.2; ICD-10 B60.2, B60.1
(Primary amebic meningoencephalitis, PAM; Granulomatous amebic encephalitis, GAE)
[CCDM19: M. Eberhard, A. Gabrielli, L. Savioli, G. Visvesvara]
[CCDM18: L. Savioli]

1. Identification—In naegleriasis, *Naegleria fowleri*, a free-living ameboflagellate, invades the brain and meninges via the nasal mucosa and olfactory nerve; it causes a typical syndrome of fulminating pyogenic meningoencephalitis (primary amebic meningoencephalitis, or PAM) with sore throat, severe frontal headache, occasional olfactory hallucinations, nausea, vomiting, high fever, nuchal rigidity and somnolence, and death within 10 days, usually on the fifth or sixth day. The disease occurs mainly in active immunocompetent children, young men and women, who have had recent contact with warm, freshwater.

In acanthamebiasis, several species of *Acanthameba* can invade the brain and meninges of immunocompromised individuals, probably after entry through a skin lesion and without involvement of the nasal and olfactory tissues; this causes a granulomatous disease (granulomatous amebic encephalitis, or GAE) of insidious onset and lasting from weeks to several months; *Balamuthia mandrillaris* (leptomyxid amebae) is also responsible for GAE. CFR may be high in *Acanthameba* infections.

In addition to causing GAE, several species of *Acanthameba* (*A. polyphaga*, *A. castellanii*, *A. hatchetti*) have been associated with chronic granulomatous lesions of the skin, with or without secondary invasion of the CNS. Infections of the eye (Conjunctivitis due to *Acanthameba*, ICD-10 H13.1) and of the cornea (Keratoconjunctivitis due to *Acanthameba*, ICD-10 H19.2) have resulted in blindness.

Diagnosis of suspected PAM or GAE is made through microscopic examination of wet mount preparations of fresh CSF showing motile amebae, and of stained smears. In suspected *Acanthameba* infections, diagnosis is made by microscopic examination of scrapings, swabs or aspirates of the eye and skin lesions; or by culture on non-nutrient agar seeded with *Escherichia coli*, *Klebsiella aerogenes* or other suitable *Enterobacter* species. *Balamuthia* require mammalian cell cultures for isolation. The trophozoites of *Naegleria* may become flagellated after a few hours in water. Pathogenic *N. fowleri*, *Acanthameba* species and *Balamuthia* can be differentiated morphologically and through immunological testing. Amebae have been misidentified as macrophages and have been mistaken for *Entameba histolytica* when microscopic diagnoses are made under low magnification.

2. Infectious agents—*Naegleria fowleri*, several species of *Acanthameba* (*A. culbertsoni*, *A. polyphaga*, *A. castellanii*, *A. astronyxis*, *A. hatchetti*, *A. rhysodes*), and *Balamuthia mandrillaris*.

3. Occurrence—The organisms are distributed globally in the environment. Cases have been diagnosed in many countries on all continents, including more than 160 cases of PAM in healthy people, over 100 cases of GAE in immunodeficient patients (including several with AIDS), and over 1 000 cases of keratitis, primarily in wearers of contact lenses.

4. Reservoir—*Acanthameba* and *Naegleria* are free-living in aquatic and soil habitats. Little is known about the reservoir of *Balamuthia*, although it has recently been isolated from soil.

5. Mode of transmission—*Naegleria fowleri* infection occurs through exposure of the nasal passages to contaminated water, most commonly by diving or swimming in freshwater, especially stagnant ponds or lakes in warm climate areas or during late summer; in thermal springs or bodies of water warmed by the effluent of industrial plants; or in hot tubs, spas or inadequately maintained public swimming pools. *Naegleria* trophozoites colonize the nasal tissues, then invade brain and meninges by extension along the olfactory nerves.

Acanthameba and *Balamuthia* trophozoites reach the CNS through hematogenous spread, probably from a skin lesion or other site of primary colonization, frequently in chronically ill or immunosuppressed patients with no history of swimming or known source of infection. Eye infections have occurred primarily in soft contact lens wearers; homemade saline used as a cleaning or wetting solution and exposure to spas or hot tubs have been implicated as sources of corneal infection.

6. Incubation period—From 3 to 15 days in documented cases of *Naegleria* infection; usually longer in infections with *Acanthameba* and *Balamuthia*.

7. Period of communicability—No person-to-person transmission observed.

8. Susceptibility—Unknown. Apparently healthy individuals develop *Naegleria fowleri* infection; immunodeficient individuals have increased susceptibility to infection with *Acanthameba* and probably *Balamuthia*. *Naegleria* and *Balamuthia* have not been found in asymptomatic individuals; *Acanthameba* has been found in the respiratory tract of healthy people.

9. **Methods of control—**

A. *Preventive measures:*

1) Educate the public to the dangers of swimming in lakes and ponds where infection is known or presumed to have been acquired, and of allowing such water to be forced into the nose through diving or underwater swimming.

2) Protect nasopharynx from exposure to water likely to contain *N. fowleri*. In practice, this is difficult, since the amebae may occur in a wide variety of aquatic bodies, including swimming pools.

3) Swimming pools containing residual free chlorine of 1–2 ppm are considered safe. No infection is known to have been acquired in a standard chlorinated swimming pool.

4) Soft contact lens wearers should not wear lenses while swimming or in hot tubs, and should follow strictly the wear and care procedures recommended by lens manufacturers and health care professionals.

B. *Control of patient, contacts and the immediate environment:*

1) Report to local health authority: Not reportable in most countries, Class 3 (see *Reporting*).

2) Isolation: Not applicable.

3) Concurrent disinfection: Not applicable.

4) Quarantine: Not applicable.

5) Immunization of contacts: Not applicable.

6) Investigation of contacts and source of infection: A history of swimming or introducing water into the nose within the week prior to onset of symptoms may suggest the source of infection.

7) Specific treatment: *N. fowleri* is sensitive to amphotericin B; recovery has followed intravenous or intrathecal administration of amphotericin B at various dosages, alone or in conjunction with intravenous administration of miconazole, oral rifampicin or ketoconazole. Despite the sensitivity of the organisms to antibiotics in laboratory studies, recoveries have been rare. For eye infections due to *Acanthameba*, the most effective drugs are the diamidines propamidine and dibromopropamidine, and polyhexamethylene biguanide (PHMB) biocide has also proven effective; treatment of choice, however, is topical polyhexamethylene biguanide (PHMB).

C. **Epidemic measures:** Multiple cases may occur following exposure to an apparent source of infection. Any grouping of cases warrants prompt epidemiological investigation and the prohibition of swimming in implicated waters.

D. **Disaster implications:** None.

E. **International measures:** None.

F. **Measures in case of deliberate use:** *N. fowleri* can in principle be used as a biological agent against humans. Primary hazards are droplet or aerosol exposure of mucous membranes (eye, nose, or mouth) to trophozoites and tissue homogenates. Containment requirements correspond to biosafety level 2.

For more information on the deliberate use of infectious agents to cause harm, see the section on *Deliberate use*.

NOCARDIOSIS
ICD-9 039.9; ICD-10 A43
[CCDM19: K. Glynn]
[CCDM18: J. Iredell]

1. Identification—A chronic bacterial disease of animals and humans that may be localized or disseminated. Any of the *Nocardia* species may cause respiratory and disseminated infections, with high associated mortality, and a particular propensity to cause brain abscess. Nocardiae (especially *N. brasiliensis*) may also cause cutaneous and/or lymphocutaneous disease of the extremities, or actinomycotic mycetomas, predominantly in tropical and subtropical regions such as central and South America (see *Mycetoma, Actinomycetoma and Eumycetoma*).

Microscopic examination of stained smears of sputum, pus, CSF, bronchial washings or tissue may reveal beaded gram-positive, weakly acid-fast, branched filaments; culture confirmation is desirable but often difficult, and any suspicion of nocardial infection should be passed on to the microbiology laboratory to enhance diagnosis. Biopsy or autopsy usually clearly establishes involvement, although histopathology may be non-specific.

2. Infectious agents—*Nocardia asteroides sensu stricto*, *N. farcinica*, *N. nova*, *N. brasiliensis*, *N. transvalensis*, *N. otitidiscaviarum*, *N. cyriaciageorgica* and *N. abscessus*; aerobic actinomycetes.

3. Occurrence—An occasional sporadic disease in people and animals in all parts of the world. No evidence of age, gender, or racial differences.

4. Reservoir—Found worldwide as a soil saprophyte.

5. Mode of transmission—Typically acquired through inhalation or skin inoculation.

6. Incubation period—Uncertain; probably a few days to a few weeks.

7. Period of communicability—Not directly transmitted from humans or from animals to humans.

8. Susceptibility—Organism-specific virulence variation and host exposure are important determinants. Immunocompromised status (e.g. due to alcoholism, diabetes or steroid use) is a risk factor in more than 60% of infections, but the incidence in those with AIDS is lower than expected, even accounting for sulfamethoxazole prophylaxis.

9. Methods of control—

    A. Preventive measures: None.

    B. Control of patient, contacts and the immediate environment:

        1) Report to local health authority: Official report not ordinarily justifiable, Class 5 (see *Reporting*).
        2) Isolation: Not applicable.
        3) Concurrent disinfection: Of discharges and contaminated dressings.
        4) Quarantine: Not applicable.
        5) Immunization of contacts: Not applicable.
        6) Investigation of contacts and source of infection: Most disease is sporadic. Occasional outbreaks may occur from environmental sources, and transmission through health care workers is probably rare.
        7) Specific treatment: Successful treatment usually involves both surgical drainage and antimicrobial therapy. Trimethoprim-sulfamethoxazole (TMP-SMX), sulfisoxazole and sulfadiazine may not be effective due to the development of resistance in some species. A combination of agents, such as TMP-SMX, amikacin and a β-lactam, has been found to be effective. Minocycline or linezolid may be tried in patients allergic to sulfonamides who do not have a brain abscess.

    C. Epidemic measures: Not applicable, a sporadic disease.

    D. Disaster implications: None.

    E. International measures: None.

ONCHOCERCIASIS
ICD-9 125.3; ICD-10 B73
(River blindness)

[CCDM19: M. Eberhard, H. Remme, F. Richards]
[CCDM18: M. Behrend]

1. Identification—A chronic nonfatal filarial disease with fibrous nodules in subcutaneous tissues, particularly of the head and shoulders (America) or pelvic girdle and lower extremities (Africa). Adult worms are found in these nodules, which occur superficially, and also in deep-seated bundles lying against the periosteum of bones or near joints. The female worm discharges microfilariae that migrate through the skin, often causing an intense pruritic rash when they die, with disfiguring skin lesions including chronic papular and lychenified dermatitis, altered pigmentation, edema, and atrophy of the skin.

Pigment changes, particularly of the lower limbs, give the condition known as "leopard skin," while loss of skin elasticity and lymphadenitis may result in "hanging groin." Microfilariae frequently reach the eye, where their invasion and subsequent death causes visual impairment and blindness, with the predominant inflammatory response being due to endosymbiotic *Wolbachia* bacteria. The greater the body load of microfilaria, the greater the risk of developing skin and eye disease. Microfilariae may be found in organs and tissues other than skin and eye, but the clinical significance of this is not yet clear; in heavy infections they may also be found in blood, tears, sputum and urine. Onchocerciasis is a risk factor for epilepsy and hyposexual dwarfism.

Disease manifestations vary between geographical zones, probably as a result of differences in parasite strains, with onchocercal blindness most prevalent in African savanna while skin manifestations predominate in forest areas. In Yemen and central Sudan, the major disease manifestation is Sowda, a pruritic skin condition usually affecting one limb.

Laboratory diagnosis is made through microscopic examination of fresh superficial skin biopsy incubated in water or saline with observation of one or more emerging microfilariae, or through the finding of adult worms in excised nodules. Differentiation of the microfilariae from those of other filarial diseases is required where the latter are also endemic. Other diagnostic clues include evidence of ocular manifestations and slit-lamp observations of microfilariae in the cornea, anterior chamber or vitreous body. The Mazzotti reaction (characteristic pruritus after oral administration of 25 mg of diethylcarbamazine citrate or topical application of the drug as a skin test) may be used, but oral DEC administration even in small doses has been generally abandoned as this test may be dangerous in heavily infected individuals. Serum antibody testing (using recombinant antigens) may be used for diagnosis, and a new skin patch test involving transdermal delivery of a low dose of diethylcarbamazine citrate was shown to be safe and sensitive in clinical trials and is undergoing large-scale field testing. PCR on material obtained from skin scratches can be used to detect parasite DNA, and is used in some research labs.

2. Infectious agent—*Onchocerca volvulus*, a filarial worm belonging to the class Nematoda.

3. Occurrence—Worldwide some 37 million people are thought to be infected with *O. volvulus;* over 99% of cases occur in sub-Saharan Africa, where the disease is transmitted in an extensive area extending from Senegal to Ethiopia down to Angola in the west and Malawi in the east. It also occurs focally in Yemen, and in six countries in the Americas: Guatemala (principally on the western slope of the continental divide near Lake Atitlan); southern Mexico (states of Chiapas and Oaxaca); Venezuela, with foci in the north and south; and small areas in Brazil (states of Amazonas and Roraima), Colombia (Cauca) and Ecuador (Esmeraldas). Regional control programs in both Africa and the Americas have had a major impact on the prevalence of disease, and in some areas it has been virtually eliminated.

4. Reservoir—Humans. The disease can be transmitted experimentally to chimpanzees and has been found rarely in nature in gorillas. Different species cannot be distinguished morphologically, but species-specific DNA probes exist that are routinely used for their differentiation in control programs.

5. Mode of transmission—Human onchocerciasis can only be acquired through the bite of infected female blackflies of the genus *Simulium*: the most important vectors in Africa and Yemen are the *Simulium damnosum* complex and the *S. neavei* complexes, as well as *S. albivirgulatum* in Democratic Republic of Congo. In Central America, mainly *S. ochraceum*; in South America, *S. metallicum* complex, *S. sanguineum/amazonicum* complex, *S. quadrivittatum* and other species. Microfilariae, ingested by a blackfly feeding on an infected person, penetrate thoracic muscles of the fly, develop into infective larvae, migrate to the cephalic capsule, are liberated on the skin, and enter the bite wound during a subsequent blood-meal.

6. Incubation period—Microfilariae are found in the skin usually only after 1 year or more from the time of the infective bite, though they have been found in children as young as 6 months. In Africa, vectors could be infective 7 days after a blood-meal; in Guatemala the extrinsic incubation period is measurably longer (up to 14 days) because of lower temperatures.

7. Period of communicability—Adult worms live as long as 10–14 years and people can infect flies as long as living microfilariae occur in their skin, i.e. up to for 10–14 years after last exposure to *Simulium* bites if untreated. No direct person-to-person transmission occurs.

8. Susceptibility—Susceptibility is probably universal. Re-infection of infected people is common; severity of disease depends on cumulative effects of the repeated infections.

9. **Methods of control—**

A. *Preventive measures:*

1) Avoid bites of *Simulium* flies by wearing protective clothing and headgear as much as possible, or by use of an insect repellent such as diethyltoluamide (DEET).

2) The Onchocerciasis Control Program (OCP), a coordinated program in western Africa sponsored by the World Bank, UNDP, FAO and WHO, covered the area in 11 countries where primarily the savanna ("blinding") form of the infection was endemic. Control has been based mainly on anti-blackfly measures, with insecticides applied systematically to breeding sites in the rivers of the area. When OCP was phased out in 2002, following the achievement of its objective to eliminate onchocerciasis as a disease of public health importance in the savanna areas of 10 West African countries (Sierra Leone being the exception), the use of insecticides to control onchocerciasis largely ceased, and was replaced by mass treatment programs using the microfilaricide ivermectin, which is being donated for this purpose by the manufacturers. The African Program for Onchocerciasis Control (APOC) was established in 1996 to implement effective and sustainable annual ivermectin community treatment throughout Africa to prevent disease from onchocerciasis. APOC ensured treatment of over 46 million people in 2007 and aims to establish sustainable treatment in all remaining endemic areas in Africa by 2015. The Onchocerciasis Elimination Program for the Americas (OEPA) uses semiannual mass distribution of ivermectin to prevent disease and interrupt onchocerciasis transmission.

3) Provide annual or 6-monthly ivermectin treatment to the eligible population of all endemic communities in an onchocerciasis focus in order to prevent onchocercal morbidity and reduce—and, where possible, interrupt—transmission and prevent new infections.

4) Provide facilities for diagnosis and treatment of individual patients.

B. *Control of patient, contacts and the immediate environment:*

1) Report to local health authority: Official report not ordinarily justifiable, Class 5 (see *Reporting*).
2) Isolation: Not applicable.
3) Concurrent disinfection: Not applicable.
4) Quarantine: Not applicable.
5) Immunization of contacts: Not applicable.

6) Investigation of contacts and source of infection: A community problem.

7) Specific treatment: Ivermectin, given as a single oral dose of 150 micrograms/kg annually or semiannually, kills microfilaria and blocks release of new microfilariae from the uterus of the adult female worm, effectively reducing the number of microfilariae in the skin and eyes over a period of 6–12 months. The duration of the effect of such treatment is not well defined. In endemic communities, ivermectin treatment for whole eligible population at least once yearly is recommended.

Research is under way to identify or develop safe and effective drugs that would sterilize or kill the adult worm; some of these (such as moxydectin and doxycycline) are undergoing clinical trials. Some authorities recommend a 3–4 week course of doxycycline treatment in individuals not exposed to re-infection (though doxycycline cannot be used in children less than eight years of age). Diethylcarbamazine citrate (DEC) is effective against microfilariae, but it may cause severe adverse reactions and is no longer recommended for treatment of onchocerciasis. Suramin kills the adult worms, but because of the risk of severe adverse events, including nephrotoxicity, it is rarely used to treat onchocerciasis.

If onchocercal subcutaneous nodules are detected and can be safely removed, they are often excised under local anesthesia.

C. Epidemic measures: In areas of high prevalence, concerted efforts to provide community mass drug administration, as described in 9A.

D. Disaster implications: None.

E. International measures: Please see section 9A.

ORF VIRUS DISEASE   ICD-9 051.2; ICD-10 B08.0
(Contagious pustular dermatitis, Human Orf, Ecthyma contagiosum)
[CCDM19: Editorial Board]

1. Identification—A proliferative cutaneous viral disease transmissible to humans through contact with infected sheep and goats, and, occasionally, wild ungulates (deer, reindeer). The lesion in humans, usually solitary and located on hands, arms or face, is a red to violet vesiculonodule, maculopapule or pustule, progressing to a weeping nodule with central umbilication. There may be several lesions, each up to 3 cm in diameter and lasting 3–6 weeks. With secondary bacterial infection, lesions may become pustular. Regional adenitis occurs in a few cases. A maculopapular rash may occur on the trunk. Erythema multiforme and erythema multiforme bullosum are rare complications. Disseminated disease and serious ocular damage have been reported. The disease has been confused with cutaneous anthrax and malignancy.

Diagnosis is through a history of contact with sheep, goats or wild ungulates, in particular their young; in the presence of negative results of conventional bacteriology, through electron microscopy demonstration of ovoid parapoxvirions in the lesion or by growth of the virus in ovine, bovine or primate cell cultures; or through positive serological tests.

2. Infectious agent—Orf virus, a DNA virus belonging to the genus *Parapoxvirus* of Poxviruses (family *Poxviridae*). The agent is closely related to other parapoxviruses that can be transmitted to humans as occupational diseases, such as milkers' nodule virus of dairy cattle and bovine papular stomatitis virus of beef cattle. Contagious ecthyma parapoxvirus of domesticated camels may infect people on rare occasions.

3. Occurrence—Probably worldwide among farm workers; a common infection among shepherds, veterinarians and abattoir workers in areas producing sheep and goats, and an important occupational disease in New Zealand.

4. Reservoir—Probably in various ungulates (sheep, goats, reindeer, musk oxen). The virus is very resistant to physical factors, except UV light, and may persist for months in soil and on animal skin and hair.

5. Mode of transmission—Direct contact with the mucous membranes of infected animals, with lesions on udders of nursing dams, or through intermediate passive transfer from apparently normal animals contaminated by contact, knives, shears, stalls mangers and sides, trucks, and clothing. Person-to-person transmission is rare. Human infection may follow production and administration of vaccines to animals.

6. Incubation period—Generally 3–6 days.

7. Period of communicability—Unknown. Human lesions show a decrease in the number of virus particles as the disease progresses.

8. Susceptibility—Susceptibility is probably universal; recovery produces variable levels of immunity.

9. Methods of control—

   A. *Preventive measures:* Good personal hygiene and use of gloves. Washing of hands and exposed areas with soap and water. Domestic and wild ungulates should be considered a potential source of infection. Ensure general cleanliness of animal housing areas. The efficacy and safety of Parapoxvirus vaccines in animals has not been fully determined.

B. Control of patient, contacts and the immediate environment:

1) Report to local health authority: Not required, but desirable when a human case occurs in areas not previously known to have the infection, Class 5 (see *Reporting*).
2) Isolation: Not applicable.
3) Concurrent disinfection: Boil, autoclave or incinerate dressings.
4) Quarantine: Not applicable.
5) Immunization of contacts: Not applicable.
6) Investigation of contacts and source of infection: Secure history of contact.
7) Specific treatment: None.

C. Epidemic measures: None.

D. Disaster implications: None.

E. International measures: None for humans.

PARACOCCIDIOIDOMYCOSIS

ICD-9 116.1;
ICD-10 B41

(South American blastomycosis, Paracoccidioidal granuloma)
[CCDM19: M. Brandt]
[CCDM18: L. Severo]

1. Identification—Paracoccidioidomycosis is a polymorphic disease, often severe and progressive, although some self-limited cases have been reported. In younger patients, the disorder is subacute and carries a severe prognosis; in adults, the course is chronic and the outcome better if appropriate therapy is given. The lungs are the site of primary infection but the patient's symptoms may not reflect this. The acute or subacute form (less common) usually afflicts children, adolescents and young adults, who present clinical manifestations compatible with involvement of the reticuloendothelial system, i.e. lymph node hypertrophy, hepatomegaly, and/or splenomegaly. In this clinical form mucosal and pulmonary involvement is infrequent. In the adult form, most patients present respiratory problems, and seek medical advice as a result of the following symptoms, in order of decreasing frequency:

a) Mucosal ulcerations occurring in the upper respiratory and digestive tracts, mostly in the mouth and nose.
b) Difficulties in swallowing and changes in voice.
c) Cutaneous lesions, often located on the face or limbs.
d) Enlarged lymph nodes, especially in the cervical area.
e) Respiratory problems, such as shortness of breath, persistent cough, purulent or blood-tinged sputum, and chest pain.

These symptoms are accompanied by weakness, malaise, fever and weight loss.

Keloidal blastomycosis (Lobo disease), a disease involving only the skin and formerly confused with paracoccidioidomycosis, is caused by *Lacazia loboi*, a fungus known only in tissue form and not yet grown in culture. Histology and culture distinguish the two diseases. Serological techniques are useful in diagnosis.

2. Infectious agent—*Paracoccidioides brasiliensis*, a dimorphic fungus.

3. Occurrence—Endemic in tropical and subtropical regions of Latin America, from Mexico to Argentina. Some countries are not affected (e.g. some Caribbean Islands and Chile). Brazil is the heart of the area of endemicity, with considerably fewer cases reported from Colombia, Venezuela, Ecuador and Argentina. Occupational distribution reveals a predilection for agricultural workers. Highest incidence is in adults aged 30–50, and paracoccidioidomycosis is more common in males than in females, with a mean ratio of 15:1.

4. Reservoir—Presumably soil or fungus-laden dust.

5. Mode of transmission—The route of infection is still a matter of debate. At present, the inhalation theory is accepted by most investigators.

6. Incubation period—Highly variable, from 1 month to many years. There is an indication that the fungus can remain dormant in residual lymph node lesions. Dormancy may be the reason why outbreaks have not been reported.

7. Period of communicability—Not transmitted from person to person.

8. Susceptibility—Unknown.

9. Methods of control—

  A. Preventive measures: None.

  B. Control of patient, contacts and the immediate environment:

   1) Report to local health authority: Official report not ordinarily justifiable, Class 5 (see *Reporting*).

2) Isolation: Not applicable.
3) Concurrent disinfection: Of discharges and contaminated articles. Terminal cleaning.
4) Quarantine: Not applicable.
5) Immunization of contacts: Not applicable.
6) Investigation of contacts and source of infection: Not indicated.
7) Specific treatment: Presently, itraconazole is considered the best choice, as it is effective in 95% of cases, with low relapse rates. Amphotericin B is usually reserved for severely disseminated or critically ill patients such as those with juvenile-form presentations or those who are immunosuppressed. Oral support therapy with itraconazole is also given to these patients for prolonged periods of time. Sulfonamides are cheaper, but much less effective than azoles requiring long-term treatment periods.

C. Epidemic measures: Not applicable, a sporadic disease.

D. Disaster implications: None.

E. International measures: None.

PARAGONIMIASIS   ICD-9 121.2; ICD-10 B66.4
(Pulmonary distomiasis, Lung fluke disease)
[CCDM19: M. Eberhard]
[CCDM18: D. Engels]

1. Identification—A trematode disease most frequently involving the lungs. Symptoms include cough, hemoptysis and pleuritic chest pain. Chest X-ray findings may include diffuse and/or segmental infiltrates, nodules, cavities, ring cysts and/or pleural effusions. Extrapulmonary disease is not uncommon, with flukes found in such sites as the CNS, subcutaneous tissues, intestinal wall, peritoneal cavity, liver, lymph nodes and genitourinary tract. Infection usually lasts for years, and the infected person may appear well. The disease may be mistaken for tuberculosis, clinically and on chest X-rays.

Sputum generally contains orange-brown flecks, sometimes diffusely distributed, in which masses of eggs are seen microscopically and establish the diagnosis. However, acid-fast staining for tuberculosis destroys the eggs and precludes diagnosis. Eggs are also swallowed, especially by children, and may be found in feces by some concentration techniques.

2. Infectious agents—*Paragonimus westermani*, *P. skrjabini* and other species in Asia; *P. africanus* and *P. uterobilateralis* in Africa; *P. mexi-*

canus (*P. peruvianus*) and other species in the Americas; *P. kellicotti* in North America.

3. Occurrence—The disease has been reported in eastern, southwestern and southeast Asia, India, Africa and the Americas. China, where an estimated 20 million people are infected, is now the major endemic area, followed by India (Manipur province), Lao People's Democratic Republic, and Myanmar. The disease has been almost eliminated from Japan, while fewer than 1 000 people are infected in the Republic of Korea. Of the Latin American countries, Ecuador is the most affected, with an estimated prevalence of 500 000 infections; cases have also occurred in Brazil, Colombia, Costa Rica, Mexico, Peru and Venezuela. The disease is rare in Canada and the USA.

4. Reservoir—Humans, dogs, cats, pigs and wild carnivores are definitive hosts and act as reservoirs.

5. Mode of transmission—Infection occurs through consumption of raw, salted, marinated or partially cooked flesh of freshwater crabs—such as *Eriocheir* and *Potamon*— or crayfish—such as *Cambaroides*— containing infective larvae (metacercariae). Larvae excyst in the duodenum, penetrate the intestinal wall, migrate through the tissues, become encapsulated (usually in the lungs), and develop into egg-producing adults. Eggs are expectorated in sputum and, when this is swallowed, are passed in the feces, gain access to freshwater, and embryonate in 2-4 weeks. Larvae (miracidia) hatch, penetrate suitable freshwater snails (*Semisulcospira, Thiara, Aroapyrgus* or other genera), and undergo a cycle of development of approximately 2 months. Larvae (cercariae) emerge from the snails to encyst in freshwater crabs and crayfish. Pickling of these crustaceans in wine, brine or vinegar, a common practice in Asia, does not kill encysted larvae. Infections often occur in tourists sampling "native" or exotic foods.

6. Incubation period—Flukes mature and begin to lay eggs approximately 6-10 weeks after ingestion of the infective larvae. The long, variable, poorly defined interval until symptoms appear depends on the organ invaded and the number of worms involved.

7. Period of communicability—Eggs may be discharged by those infected for up to 20 years; duration of infection in mollusk and crustacean hosts is not well defined. Not directly transmitted from person to person.

8. Susceptibility—Susceptibility is general.

9. Methods of control—

  A. Preventive measures:

   1) Educate the public in endemic areas about the life cycle of the parasite.
   2) Stress thorough cooking of crustaceans.

    3) Dispose of sputum and feces in a sanitary manner.
    4) Control snails through molluskicides where feasible.

B. *Control of patient, contacts and the immediate environment:*

    1) Report to local health authority: Official report not ordinarily justifiable, Class 5 (see *Reporting*).
    2) Isolation: Not applicable.
    3) Concurrent disinfection: Of sputum and feces.
    4) Quarantine: Not applicable.
    5) Immunization of contacts: Not applicable.
    6) Investigation of contacts and source of infection: None.
    7) Specific treatment: Praziquantel and triclabendazole.

C. *Epidemic measures:* In an endemic area, the occurrence of small clusters of cases, or even sporadic infections, is an important signal for examination of local waters for infected snails, crabs and crayfish, and determination of reservoir mammalian hosts, to establish appropriate controls.

D. *Disaster implications:* None.

E. *International measures:* WHO Collaborating Centres provide support as required. More information can be found at:

http://www.who.int/collaboratingcentres/database/en/

PEDICULOSIS AND PHTHIRIASIS

ICD-9 132;
ICD-10 B85

[CCDM19: M. Eberhard, J. Watson]
[CCDM18: P. Guillet]

    1. Identification—Infestation by head lice (*Pediculus capitis*) occurs on hair, eyebrows and eyelashes; infestation by body lice (*P. corporis*) is of the clothing, especially along the seams of inner surfaces. Crab lice (*Phthirus pubis*) usually infest the pubic area, and—more rarely—facial hair (including eyelashes in heavy infestations), axillae, and body surfaces. Infestation may result in severe itching and excoriation of the scalp or body. Secondary infection may lead to regional lymphadenitis (especially cervical).

    2. Infesting agents—The ectoparasites *Pediculus capitis* (head louse), *P. corporis* (body louse), and *Phthirus pubis* (crab louse); adult lice, nymphs and nits (egg cases) infest people. Lice are host-specific, and those of lower animals do not infest humans, although they may be present transiently. Both sexes feed on blood.

The body louse is the species involved in outbreaks of epidemic typhus caused by *Rickettsia prowazekii*, trench fever caused by *Bartonella quintana*, and epidemic relapsing fever caused by *Borrelia recurrentis*.

3. Occurrence—Worldwide. Outbreaks of head lice are common among children in schools and institutions everywhere. Body lice are prevalent among populations with poor personal hygiene, especially in cold climates where heavy clothing is worn and bathing is infrequent, or when people cannot change clothes (e.g. in the case of refugees).

4. Reservoir—Humans.

5. Mode of transmission—For head and body lice, direct contact with infested persons and objects used by them; for body lice, indirect contact with the personal belongings of infested persons, especially shared clothing and headgear. Crab lice are most frequently transmitted through sexual contact. Lice leave a febrile host; fever and overcrowding increase transfer from person to person.

6. Incubation period—Life cycle of 3 stages: eggs, nymphs and adults. The most suitable temperature range for egg production and hatching is 29°C to 32°C (84.2°F to 89.6°F). Eggs of human lice do not hatch at temperatures under 22°C (71.6°F). Under optimal conditions, lice eggs hatch in 7–10 days. The nymphal stages last about 9–12 days for head and body lice, and 13–17 days for crab lice. The egg-to-egg cycle averages about 3 weeks. The life cycle of the adult louse is about one month.

7. Period of communicability—As long as lice or eggs remain viable on the infested person or on fomites. The adult's life span on the host is approximately one month. Nits remain viable on clothing for 1 month. Body lice can survive for up to a week off the host without feeding; head lice and crab lice only about 2 days. Nymphs can survive 24 hours without feeding. Under suitable environmental conditions, head and crab lice eggs can remain viable away from the host for up to 7–10 days; body lice eggs remain viable for up to a month.

8. Susceptibility—Any person may become infested under suitable conditions of exposure. Repeated infestations may result in dermal hypersensitivity.

9. Methods of control—

A. *Preventive measures:*

1) Educate the public about diagnosis, treatment, and prevention, including the value of destroying eggs and lice through early detection; safe and thorough treatment of the hair; laundering clothing and bedding in hot water (55°C or 131°F for 20 min); and dry cleaning and/or the use of dryers set on "hot cycle."

2) For head lice, avoid head-to-head contact with an infested person, and avoid contact with items that have been in contact with hair from an infested person (e.g. hats, scarves, combs, brushes, pillowcases, towels, etc.). For body and pubic lice, avoid direct physical contact with infested individuals and their belongings, especially clothing and bedding.

3) Perform direct inspection of body and clothing for evidence of body lice when indicated. Evidence does not support the efficacy and cost-effectiveness of regular screening of children in classroom or school-wide settings for head lice and nits. In the USA, the American Academy of Pediatrics discourages such screening.

4) Individuals may protect themselves by wearing silk or plastic clothing tightly fastened around wrists, ankles and neck, and by impregnating their clothes, hair and skin with repellents or permethrin.

B. Control of patient, contacts and the immediate environment:

1) Report to local health authority: Official report not ordinarily justifiable; school authorities should be informed, Class 5 (see *Reporting*).

2) Isolation: For body lice, contact isolation if possible, until 24 hours after application of an effective insecticide.

3) Concurrent disinfection: Clothing, bedding and fomites should be treated by laundering in hot water, drying in a hot dryer, dry cleaning, or applying an effective chemical insecticide (see 9B7).

4) Quarantine: Not applicable.

5) Immunization of contacts: Not applicable.

6) Investigation of contacts and source of infestation: Examine household and close personal contacts; treat those infested.

7) Specific treatment: For head and pubic lice: 1% permethrin (a synthetic pyrethroid) cream rinse with 10 minutes' exposure; pyrethrins synergized with piperonyl butoxide (10 minutes); and malathion 0.5%, an organophosphate (8–12 hours). None of these treatments is 100% effective; retreatment may be necessary after an interval of 9–10 days for permethrin and pyrethrins, and 7–9 days for malathion. Carbaryl and Benzyl benzoate are not recommended in some countries for treatment of lice. Resistance to permethrin and pyrethrins is widespread. Malathion resistance has been detected so far in France and the UK. Carbaryl resistance is emerging in the UK. Lindane is approved as a second-line drug for lice, but because of toxicity, side effects and low efficacy, its use should be limited to patients who cannot

tolerate or have failed treatment with other products that pose less risk.

For body lice: Clothing and bedding should be washed using the hot water cycle of an automatic washing machine or dusted with pediculicides using power dusters, hand dusters or 2-ounce sifter cans. Recommended dusts include 1% malathion and 0.5% permethrin.

C. *Epidemic measures:* Mass treatment as recommended in 9B7 above, using insecticides clearly known to be effective against prevalent strains of lice. In typhus epidemics, individuals may protect themselves by wearing silk or plastic clothing tightly fastened around wrists, ankles and neck, and by impregnating their clothes with repellents or permethrin.

D. *Disaster implications:* Diseases for which body and head lice are vectors are particularly prone to occur at times of social upheaval (see *Typhus fever*, section I, Epidemic louse-borne).

E. *International measures:* None.

PERTUSSIS   ICD-9 033.0, 033.9; ICD-10 A37.0, A37.9

PARAPERTUSSIS   ICD-9 033.1; ICD-10 A37.1
(Whooping Cough)
[CCDM19: P. Duclos, S. Halperin]
[CCDM18: P. Duclos]

1. Identification—An acute bacterial infection of the respiratory tract caused by *Bordetella pertussis*. The initial catarrhal stage has an insidious onset with an irritating cough that gradually becomes paroxysmal, usually within 1–2 weeks, and lasts for 1–2 months or longer. Paroxysms are characterized by repeated violent coughing; each series of paroxysms has many coughs without intervening inhalation and can be followed by a characteristic crowing or high-pitched inspiratory whoop. Paroxysms frequently end with the expulsion of clear, tenacious mucus, often followed by vomiting. Infants under 6 months, partially vaccinated children, adolescents and adults often do not have the typical whoop or cough paroxysm.

The number of fatalities in vaccinated populations is low. Most deaths occur in infants under 6 months, often in those too young to have completed primary immunization. In recent years, all deaths from pertussis in most industrialized countries occurred in infants under 6 months. In non-immunized populations, especially those with underlying malnutrition and multiple enteric and respiratory infections, pertussis is among the most lethal diseases of infants and young children. Complications include pneumonia, atelectasis, seizures, encephalopathy, weight loss, hernias and death. Pneumonia is the most common cause of death; fatal encephalopathy, probably hypoxic, and inanition from repeated vomiting occasionally occur. Case-fatality rates in unprotected children are less than 1 per thousand in industrialized countries; in developing countries they are estimated at 3.7% for children under 1 and 1% for children 1 to 4 years. In several industrialized countries with high rates of infant immunization for many years an increasing proportion of cases has been reported in adolescents and adults, whose symptoms vary from a mild, atypical respiratory illness to the full whooping syndrome. Many such cases occur in previously immunized persons and suggest waning immunity following immunization.

Parapertussis is a similar but occasional and milder disease due to *Bordetella parapertussis*. Diagnosis is based on the recovery of the causal organism from nasopharyngeal specimens obtained during the catarrhal and early paroxysmal stages on Bordet-Gengou or Regan-Lowe culture media both supplemented with 15% defibrinated sheep or horse blood. WHO considers culture as the "gold standard" of laboratory confirmation; it is the most specific diagnosis, but it is not highly sensitive (60%). Polymerase chain reaction (PCR) is more sensitive, and can be performed on the same biological samples as cultures. It requires more technical skills to perform, however, and requires more expensive equipment. Direct fluorescent antibody staining of nasopharyngeal secretions is not recommended because of frequent false-positive and false-negative results. Indirect diagnosis by evaluating the immune response to the infection rather than directly detecting the organism (serology) consists of detecting specific IgG antibodies directed against the pertussis toxin in the serum of the infected individual, collected at the beginning of cough (acute serum); and in serum collected one month later (convalescent serum). Criteria for diagnosing pertussis using a single serum specimen have been proposed. The presence of antibodies in excess of population based threshold levels in the serum of a non-vaccinated individual indicates infection. Serology cannot be used for diagnosis during the year following vaccination, since it does not differentiate between antibodies due to the vaccine and those due to natural infection.

Differentiation between *B. parapertussis* and *B. pertussis* is based on culture and genetic, biochemical and immunological differences.

2. **Infectious agents**—*B. pertussis*, the bacillus of pertussis *stricto sensu*; *B. parapertussis* causes parapertussis. The *Bordetella* are Gram-negative aerobic bacteria; *B. pertussis* and *B. parapertussis* are similar species but the latter lacks the expression of the gene coding for pertussis toxin.

3. **Occurrence**—An endemic disease common to children (especially young children) everywhere, regardless of ethnicity, climate or geo-

graphic location. Outbreaks occur typically every 3 to 4 years. A marked decline has occurred in incidence and mortality rates over the past 40 years, chiefly in communities with active immunization programs and where good nutrition and medical care are available. In 2003, despite an estimated global vaccination coverage of around 75% with 3 doses of pertussis-containing vaccines, there were still an estimated 17.6 million pertussis cases, with an estimated 279 000 deaths. A substantial proportion of those deaths are occurring in Africa, where vaccine coverage is lowest. Altogether, in 2006 an estimated 26.3 million children had not received full immunization with three doses of DTP. Incidence rates have increased in countries where pertussis immunization rates fell in the past (e.g. Japan in the early 1980s, Sweden and the United Kingdom), and dropped again when immunization programs were reestablished. In countries with high vaccination coverage, the incidence rate in children under 15 is less than 1 per 100 000.

4. **Reservoir**—Humans are believed to be the only host for pertussis. *B. parapertussis* can also be isolated from ovines.

5. **Mode of transmission**—Direct contact with discharges from respiratory mucous membranes of infected persons by the airborne route, probably via large droplets. In vaccinated populations, bacteria are frequently brought home by an older sibling, and sometimes by a parent. Indirect spread through the air or contaminated objects occurs rarely if at all.

6. **Incubation period**—Average 9–10 days (range 6–20 days).

7. **Period of communicability**—Highly communicable in the early catarrhal stage and at the beginning of the paroxysmal cough stage (first 2 weeks). Thereafter, communicability gradually decreases and becomes negligible in about 3 weeks, despite persisting spasmodic cough with whoop. When treated with erythromycin, clarithromycin or azithromycin, patients are no longer contagious after 5 days of treatment.

8. **Susceptibility**—Susceptibility of non-immunized individuals is universal. The highest incidence of pertussis is in infants, and school-aged children are often the source of infection for younger siblings at home, but infection also occurs in adolescents and adults. Incidence, morbidity and mortality are higher in females than males. Secondary attack rates of up to 90% have been observed in non-immune household contacts. Although antibodies cross the placenta, transplacental immunity in infants has not been demonstrated.

Incidence is highest in children aged less than 5 years, except where infant vaccination programs have been very effective, and a shift has occurred toward adolescents. Milder and missed atypical cases occur in all age groups. One attack usually confers prolonged immunity, although subsequent attacks (some of which may be attributable to *B. parapertussis*) can occur. Cases in previously immunized adolescents and adults in countries with long-standing and successful immunization programs occur because of waning immunity, and are a source of infection for non-immunized young children.

9. **Methods of control—**

A. *Preventive measures:*

1) Educate the public, particularly parents of infants, about the dangers of whooping cough and the advantages of initiating immunization on time (between 6 weeks and 3 months depending on the country), and of adhering to the immunization schedule. This continues to be important because of the wide negative publicity given to adverse immunization reactions.

2) Immunization is the most rational approach to pertussis control: whole-cell vaccine against pertussis (wP) has been effective in preventing pertussis for more than 40 years. Active primary immunization against *B. pertussis* infection is done by administering 3 doses of a vaccine consisting of either a suspension of killed bacteria (wP) or acellular preparations (aP) that contain 1–5 different components of *B. pertussis*. These are usually given in combination with diphtheria and tetanus toxoids adsorbed on aluminum salts (Diphtheria and Tetanus Toxoids and Pertussis Vaccine Adsorbed, DTwP or DTaP). In terms of severe adverse effects aP and wP vaccines appear to have the same high level of safety; local and transient systemic reactions are less commonly associated with aP vaccines. Similar high efficacy levels (more than 80%) occur with the best aP and wP vaccines, although the level of efficacy may vary within each group. Protection is greater against severe disease, and begins to wane after about 5 years. Acellular pertussis vaccines do not protect against infection by *B. parapertussis*.

Although the use of aP vaccines is less commonly associated with local and systemic reactions such as fever, price considerations affect their use, and wP vaccines are the vaccines of choice for most developing countries. Japan, USA and many other industrialized countries have completely replaced wP vaccines with aP vaccines. Schedules vary: North America vaccinates at 2, 4, 6 months; France and the United Kingdom at 2, 3, 4 months; and Sweden at 3, 5, 12 months. Many developing countries vaccinate at 6, 10 and 14 weeks of age, according to the initially proposed schedule of the expended program on immunization. In all countries and particularly where pertussis is still endemic and poses a serious health problem, the priority should be to reach at least 90% coverage with a primary series of 3 doses of DTP in infants in all areas. In countries where immunization programs have considerably reduced pertussis incidence, a booster dose approximately one to six years after the primary series is recommended. The optimal timing of the booster dose of DTP—as well as the possible need and timing for additional booster doses—depends on the epidemiological situation, and should be assessed by national programs. Some other countries recommend booster doses at 15–18 months of age and at school entry. As of 2006, 67 of 193 WHO member states had a recommended schedule including one booster dose in addition to the initial series, and 57 countries recommended 2 or more booster doses. Vaccines containing wP are not recommended after the seventh birthday, since local reactions may be increased in older children and adults. Formulations of acellular pertussis vaccine for use in adolescents and adults have been licensed and are available in several countries. As of 2006, 10 countries were reporting the introduction of adolescent or adult booster doses in the routine immunization scheme.

DTaP/DTwP can be given simultaneously with oral poliovirus vaccine (OPV), inactivated poliovirus vaccine (IPV), *Hemophilus influenzae* type b (Hib), hepatitis B (HepB) vaccine, pneumococcal and meningococcal conjugate vaccines and measles, mumps and rubella vaccine (MMR) at different sites. Combination vaccines with Hib, IPV and HepB are available and are widely used in Europe and North America.

Minor adverse reactions such as local redness and swelling, fever and agitation often occur after immunization with wP vaccine (1 in 2–10). Prolonged crying and febrile seizures are less common (<1 in 100); hypotonic-hyporesponsive episodes are rare (<1 in 2 000). Although febrile seizures and hypotonic-hyporesponsive episodes may follow DTwP and are disturbing to parents and physicians alike, there is no scientific evidence that these reactions have any permanent consequences. Recent detailed reviews of all available studies conclude that there is no demonstrable causal relationship between DTwP and chronic nervous system dysfunction in children. The only true contraindication to immunization with aP or wP is an anaphylactic reaction to a previous dose or to any constituent of the vaccine. In young infants with suspected evolving and progressive neurological disease, immunization may be delayed for some months to permit diagnosis, in order to avoid possible confusion about the cause of symptoms.

3) When an outbreak occurs, consider protection of health workers who have been exposed to pertussis cases, using a 7-day course of erythromycin. Clarithromycin and azithromy-

cin are expensive but better-tolerated alternatives. Use of aP can be considered for health workers where ongoing transmission is a concern.

B. Control of patient, contacts and the immediate environment:

1) Report to local health authority: Case report of suspected and confirmed cases obligatory in most countries, Class 2 (see *Reporting*); early reporting permits better outbreak control. The WHO-recommended clinical case definition is "a case diagnosed as pertussis by a physician or a person with a cough lasting at least 2 weeks and at least one of the following symptoms: paroxysms (fits) of coughing, inspiratory 'whooping,' post-tussive vomiting (vomiting immediately after coughing) without other apparent cause."

2) Isolation: Respiratory isolation for known cases. Suspected cases should be removed from the presence of young children and infants, especially non-immunized infants, until the patients have received at least 5 days of antibiotics. Suspected cases who do not receive antibiotics should be isolated for 3 weeks after onset of paroxysmal cough or until the end of cough, whichever comes first.

3) Concurrent disinfection: Disinfection measures are of little impact.

4) Quarantine: Inadequately immunized household contacts under 7 may be excluded from schools, day care centers and public gatherings for 21 days after last exposure or until the cases and contacts have received 5 days of appropriate antibiotics.

5) Protection of contacts: All contacts must have their immunization status verified and brought up-to-date. Passive immunization has not been demonstrated to be effective, and there is no such product currently commercially available. The initiation of active immunization following recent exposure is not effective against infection but should be undertaken to protect the child against further exposure in case he or she has not been infected. Close contacts under 7 who have not received 4 DTP doses or have not received a DTP dose within 3 years should be given a dose as soon after exposure as possible. A 7-day course of erythromycin or clarithromycin, or a 5-day course of azithromycin, for household and other close contacts—regardless of immunization status and age— is recommended for households where there is a child under 1. Prophylactic antibiotic therapy in the early incubation period may prevent disease, but difficulties of early diagnosis, the costs involved and concerns related to the occurrence of drug resistance all limit prophylactic treatment to the following selected individual conditions:

- Children under 1 year and pregnant women in the last 3 weeks of pregnancy (because of the risk of transmission to the newborn)
- Stopping infection among household members, particularly if the household contains children aged less than 1 and pregnant women in the last 3 weeks of pregnancy.

6) Investigation of contacts and source of infection: A search for early, missed and atypical cases is indicated where a non-immune infant or young child is or might be at risk.

7) Specific treatment: Erythromycin, clarithromycin and azithromycin shorten the period of communicability, but do not reduce symptoms except when given during the incubation period, in the catarrhal stage or early in the paroxysmal stage.

C. Epidemic measures: A search for unrecognized and unreported cases may be indicated to protect preschool children from exposure and to ensure adequate preventive measures for exposed children under 7. Accelerated immunization, with the first dose at 4 – 6 weeks of age and the second and third doses at 4-week intervals, may be indicated; more important is to make sure that immunization is completed for those whose schedule is incomplete, and that the vaccines are given on time according to the national schedule.

D. Disaster implications: Pertussis is a potential problem if introduced into crowded refugee camps containing many non-immunized children.

E. International measures: Ensure completion of primary immunization of infants and young children before they travel to other countries; review need for a booster dose.

PINTA   ICD-9 103; ICD-10 A67
(Carate)
[CCDM18 & 19: G. Antal]

1. Identification—An acute and chronic nonvenereal treponemal skin infection. A scaling painless papule with satellite lymphadenopathy appears 1–8 weeks after infection, usually on the hands, legs or dorsum of the feet. Within 3–12 months a maculopapular, erythematous secondary rash appears, and may evolve into tertiary splotches of altered (dyschromic) skin pigmentation of variable size. These treponema-containing macules pass through stages of blue to violet to brown pigmentation, finally becoming treponema-free depigmented (achromic) scars. Lesions coexist at different stages of evolution and are most common on the face and extremities. Organ systems are not involved; physical disability and death do not occur.

Spirochetes are demonstrable in dyschromic (but not achromic) lesions through darkfield or direct FA microscopic examination. Serological tests for syphilis usually become reactive before or during the secondary rash, and thereafter behave as in venereal syphilis.

2. Infectious agent—*Treponema carateum*, a spirochete.

3. Occurrence—Found only among isolated rural populations living under crowded unhygienic conditions in the American tropics. Predominantly a disease of older children and adults. Surveys carried out during the mid-1990s by PAHO/WHO in targeted Amazonian populations in Brazil, Peru and Venezuela found few cases, mostly inactive. WHO concludes that pinta is a residual problem, and that the infection is on its way to elimination and eradication, as sanitation improves and access to antibiotics increases. Isolated foci may still exist in Central America and Cuba.

4. Reservoir—Humans.

5. Mode of transmission—Presumably person-to-person through direct and prolonged contact with initial and early dyschromic skin lesions. The location of primary lesions suggests that trauma provides a portal of entry; lesions in children occur in those body areas most scratched. Various biting and sucking arthropods, especially blackflies, are suspected, but not proven, biological vectors.

6. Incubation period—Usually 2–3 weeks.

7. Period of communicability—Unknown; potentially communicable while dyschromic skin lesions are active, sometimes for many years. Not highly contagious; several years of intimate contact may be necessary for transmission.

8. Susceptibility—Undefined; presumably as in other treponematoses.

9. Methods of control—

    *A. **Preventive measures:*** Those applicable to other nonvenereal treponematoses apply to pinta; see *Yaws*, 9A.

    *B. **Control of patient, contacts and the immediate environment:***

        1) Report to local health authority: In selected endemic areas; in most countries, not a reportable disease, Class 3 (see *Reporting*).

        2), 3), 4), 5), 6) and 7) Isolation, Concurrent disinfection, Quarantine, Immunization of contacts, Investigation of contacts and source of infection and Specific treatment: See *Yaws*, 9B2 through 9B7.

C, D. and ***E. Epidemic measures, Disaster implications*** and ***International measures:*** See *Yaws*, C, D and E.

PLAGUE
(Pestis)
[CCDM19: E. Bertherat, K. Gage]
[CCDM18: E. Bertherat]

ICD-9 020; ICD-10 A20

1. Identification—An acute bacterial zoonosis of rodents, caused by *Yersinia pestis*. Plague is typically transmitted by fleas or through direct contact with infected animals, although human cases are occasionally acquired through inhalation of infectious respiratory droplets or other materials. Initial signs and symptoms may be nonspecific, with fever, chills, malaise, myalgia, nausea, prostration, sore throat and headache. Lymphadenitis often develops in those lymph nodes that drain the site of inoculation. This is bubonic plague, and the location of buboes can vary depending on the circumstances of exposure, with flea bites on the legs typically resulting in the appearance of buboes in the inguinal area. Axillary buboes can be associated with flea bites as well as with handling of infected animals. Cervical buboes are rare in the USA and certain other countries, but are relatively common in many developing countries, where people sleep on the dirt floors of flea-infested huts. Regardless of the location, the involved nodes become swollen, inflamed and tender, and may suppurate. The septicemic form of plague can occur subsequent to bubonic plague (secondary septicemic plague) or without prior lymphadenopathy (primary septicemic plague), and involves bloodstream dissemination to diverse parts of the body, including, in some instances, the meninges. Septicemic cases also can experience endotoxic shock and disseminated intravascular coagulation (DIC), in some instances without localizing signs of infection. Secondary involvement of the lungs results in pneumonia; mediastinitis or pleural effusion may develop. Secondary pneumonic plague is of special significance, since respiratory droplets may serve as the source of person-to-person transfer with resultant primary pneumonic or pharyngeal plague; this can lead to localized outbreaks or devastating epidemics. Though naturally acquired plague usually presents as bubonic plague, purposeful aerosol dissemination as a result of deliberate use would be manifest primarily as pneumonic plague

Untreated bubonic plague has a case-fatality rate of about 50%–60%. Untreated primary septicemic plague and pneumonic plague are almost invariably fatal. Modern therapy markedly reduces fatalities from bubonic plague; pneumonic and septicemic plague also responds if recognized and treated early (within about 2 days). Plague is a medical and a public health emergency.

The main laboratory approaches to diagnosing plague are as follows. Visualization of characteristic bipolar staining, "safety pin" ovoid, gram-negative organisms in direct microscopic examination of material aspirated from a bubo, sputum or CSF is suggestive, but not conclusive, evidence of plague infection. Examination by FA test, antigen capture by ELISA or dipstick formats, or PCR are more specific and particularly useful in some instances. In the USA, cases are considered confirmed following isolation of *Yersinia pestis* by culture of bubo aspirates, blood, CSF or sputum samples, or demonstration of a 4-fold or greater rise or fall in antibody titer. Recently, the World Health Organization has proposed the use of dipstick assays designed to detect *Y. pestis* antigen as a means for case confirmation. Slow growth of the organism at normal incubation temperatures may lead to misidentification by automated systems. The passive hemagglutination test (PHA) using *Yersinia pestis* Fraction-1 antigen is most frequently used for serodiagnosis. Rapid diagnostic tests for detecting F1 antigen have been developed, produced and evaluated. They are used routinely in endemic African countries. Medical personnel should be aware of areas where the disease is endemic, and should entertain the diagnosis of plague early on; unfortunately, plague is often misdiagnosed, especially in travelers who develop illness after returning from an endemic area.

2. Infectious agent—*Yersinia pestis*, the plague bacillus.

3. Occurrence—Plague continues to be a threat because of vast areas of persistent wild rodent infection; contact of wild rodents with domestic rats occurs frequently in some enzootic areas. Wild rodent plague exists in the Americas, with foci in northeastern Brazil, the Andean region near the border of Ecuador and Peru, and the western half of the USA, causing sporadic cases and occasional outbreaks, including an outbreak of pneumonic plague in Ecuador in 1998; scattered locations in east-central and southern Africa, as well as the interior of Algeria and perhaps other African countries bordering the Mediterranean Sea; central, southwestern and southeastern Asia; and extreme southeastern Europe, near the Caspian Sea. While urban plague has been controlled in most of the world, since 1990 the disease has occurred in several African countries, including Botswana, the Democratic Republic of Congo (DRC), Kenya, Madagascar, Malawi, Mozambique, the United Republic of Tanzania, Uganda, Zambia and Zimbabwe and Algeria. Plague is endemic in China, India, Lao People's Democratic Republic, Mongolia, Myanmar, Viet Nam and Indonesia. Outbreaks occasionally appear in areas that have been free of the disease for many decades, as was demonstrated in Algeria in 2003. Since the beginning of the 90s, there has been an increase in the annual incidence of human cases of plague; moreover, the disease has reappeared in countries where it had not been reported for decades. Today the distribution of plague coincides with the geographical distribution of its natural foci. In 2007, 7 countries reported 2 021 cases with 156 deaths. Among these, 99.6% of cases were reported from Africa. DRC has the most active foci of plague worldwide, with more than 1 000 suspected cases a year; following the eruption of several severe outbreaks of pneumonic plague in DRC, the diagnosis is now systematically evoked when a deadly outbreak with hemorrhagic signs is reported in Central Africa.

Human plague in the western USA is sporadic (typically 5–15 cases per year since 1970), with only single cases or small common source clusters in an area, usually following exposure to wild rodents or their fleas—although cases have also been acquired by persons handling infected rabbits, wild carnivores or domestic cats. No person-to-person transmission has occurred in the USA since 1924, although secondary plague pneumonia occurred in about 20% of bubonic cases in one reported series. Five instances of primary plague pneumonia through cat-to-human transmission have been recorded.

4. **Reservoir**—Wild rodents are the natural vertebrate hosts of plague, and play a key role in maintaining natural plague cycles by serving as sources of infection (amplifying hosts) for the flea vectors of the disease, some species of which can survive for weeks to months in the burrows of their hosts and appear to represent a significant reservoir of infection. In North America, the most important rodents include species of ground squirrels, prairie dogs, chipmunks, wood rats, deer mice and voles. Certain other mammals, including lagomorphs (rabbits and hares), wild carnivores and domestic cats may also become infected, and act as sources of infection to people. In many developing countries, commensal rats play epidemiologically important roles by moving infected fleas into human dwellings from wild lands or agricultural fields.

5. **Mode of transmission**—Two main patterns of transmission for naturally acquired human plague can be distinguished:

a) Human intrusion into the zoonotic (sylvatic) cycle during or following an epizootic. A sub-population of the community, involved in specific activities— e.g. hunting, trapping, trekking, farming—is at risk: USA, central Asia, China.

Human cases have been linked to domestic pets, particularly house cats and dogs, carrying plague-infected wild rodent fleas into homes. Cats may occasionally transmit infection through bites or respiratory droplets; cats develop plague abscesses that have been a source of infection to veterinary personnel.

b) Infection in commensal rodents and their fleas, themselves infected by contact with peri-domestic mammals, leads to an entry of the bacteria into human habitat. In that case, the disease is the manifestation of poverty and insufficient conditions of hygiene. In such conditions person-to-person transmission by *Pulex irritans* fleas ("human" flea) can also occur. Risk of exposure concerns the community as a whole: Africa, India, and South America.

On a worldwide basis the most frequent source of exposure for human cases are the bites of infectious infected rat fleas, especially the oriental rat flea (*Xenopsylla cheopis*). In some countries, wild rodent fleas can also be an important source of infection. The primary vector in North America is the ground squirrel flea *Oropsylla montana*.

Other important sources of human infection include the handling of infected animals, especially rodents and rabbits, but also wild carnivores and domestic cats; rarely, airborne droplets from human patients or household cats with plague pharyngitis or pneumonia; and careless manipulation of laboratory cultures. Human cases acquired by inhalation (primary pneumonic plague) have been reported in the past couple of decades in developing countries, such as India. Person-to-person transmission by *Pulex irritans* fleas (the "human" flea) is presumed to be important in the Andean region of South America and in other places where plague occurs and this flea is abundant in homes or on domestic animals. Poor rodent sanitation practices and certain activities, including hunting, trapping, cat ownership and rural residence, carry increased risk of exposure. In the case of deliberate use plague bacilli would possibly be transmitted as an aerosol. For more information on the deliberate use of infectious agents to cause harm, see the section on *Deliberate use*.

6. Incubation period—From 1 to 7 days; may be a few days longer in immunized persons who develop illness. For primary plague pneumonia, incubation period can be less than one day, up to four days, and is usually short.

7. Period of communicability—Fleas may remain infective for months under suitable conditions of temperature and humidity. Bubonic plague is not usually transmitted directly unless there is contact with pus from suppurating buboes. Pneumonic plague may be highly communicable under appropriate climatic conditions; overcrowding and cool temperatures facilitate transmission.

8. Susceptibility—Susceptibility among humans is general. Immunity after recovery is relative; it may not protect against a future large inoculum.

9. Methods of control—

A. *Preventive measures:* The basic objective is to reduce the likelihood of people being bitten by infectious fleas, having direct contact with infective tissues and exudates, or of being exposed to patients with pneumonic plague.

1) Educate the public in enzootic areas on the modes of human and domestic animal exposure; on rat-proofing buildings and preventing access to food and shelter by peri-domestic or wild rodents through appropriate storage and disposal of food, garbage and refuse; and on the importance of avoiding flea bites by use of insecticides and repellents. In sylvatic or rural plague areas, the public should be advised to use insect repellents when walking or working in suspect areas, and be warned not to camp near rodent burrows and to avoid handling of rodents—but to report dead or sick animals to health authorities or other appropriate persons. Dogs and cats in such areas should be protected periodically with appropriate insecticides to reduce the risk that infectious fleas will be transported into human environs, and should not be allowed to roam freely in plague-affect areas. Any animal carcasses brought home by these animals should be disposed of safely.

2) Survey rodent populations periodically to determine whether epizootics are in progress or conditions indicate that one is likely. The effectiveness of rodent sanitation measures in homes and public areas also should be evaluated. Although flea control is the primary means for controlling plague, rat suppression by poisoning (see 9B6) may be necessary to augment basic environmental sanitation measures; rat control should always be preceded by measures to control fleas. Areas of plague activity can be identified by surveillance of natural foci by testing fleas collected from rodents and their burrows or nests; bacteriologic testing of sick or dead wild rodents; and serological analyses of samples from wild carnivores and outdoor ranging dogs and cats. Regular testing should take place to ensure the effectiveness of insecticides on target flea populations.

3) Control rats on ships and docks and in warehouses by rat-proofing or periodic fumigation, combined when necessary with destruction of rats and their fleas in vessels and in cargoes, especially containerized cargoes, before shipment and on arrival from locations endemic for plague.

4) Wear gloves when hunting and handling wildlife. Veterinarians and their staff should wear gloves and masks when examining sick cats.

5) Plague vaccine should not be relied upon as the sole preventive measure, and immunized persons should take other appropriate prevention precautions as indicated elsewhere in this section. Live attenuated vaccines are used in some countries, but can produce adverse reactions, and their efficacy has not been proven. Different vaccination strategies have been used in the past involving both a killed and a live

attenuated vaccine, but these strategies have only conferred protection against bubonic plague and not against primary pneumonic plague. Currently, the next generation of plague vaccines is being researched—and, in some cases, vaccines are in clinical trials. Both new, live attenuated vaccines and recombinant F1-V vaccines are being examined.

B. Control of patient, contacts and the immediate environment:

1) Report to local health authority any suspected case. Case reports of suspected and confirmed cases from plague-endemic areas are no longer required by the *International Health Regulations,* but cases that occur outside plague-endemic areas or are likely to pose a threat for spread of the disease to other areas are still reportable. In the USA, because of the rarity of naturally acquired primary plague pneumonia, even a single case should initiate prompt investigation, and in the unlikely circumstance that a natural source of infection cannot be identified, public health and law enforcement authorities might be reasonably suspicious of deliberate use. For more information on the deliberate use of infectious agents to cause harm, see the section on *Deliberate use.*

2) Isolation: Rid patients living in rat- and flea-infested dwellings of fleas and treat their clothing and baggage with an appropriate insecticide; hospitalize if practical. Strict isolation is only required for patients with pneumonic plague, for whom precautions against airborne spread are required until 48 hours of appropriate antibiotherapy have been completed and there has been a favorable clinical response (see 9B7). For patients with bubonic plague (if there is no cough and the chest X-ray is negative), drainage and secretion precautions are indicated for 48 hours after start of effective treatment.

3) Concurrent disinfection: Disinfect articles and surfaces contaminated with potentially infectious sputum and purulent discharges. Human cadavers and animal carcasses should be handled with strict aseptic precautions.

4) Quarantine: Quarantine measures have been shown to be ineffective in controlling plague outbreaks, and can trigger panic in the population. Those who have been in household or face-to-face contact with patients with pneumonic plague should be provided chemoprophylaxis (see 9B5) and placed under surveillance for 7 days; those who refuse chemoprophylaxis should be maintained in strict isolation with careful surveillance for 7 days.

5) Protection of contacts: In epidemic situations where human dwellings are invaded by flea-infested rats or harbor human

fleas (*Pulex irritans*) that also might act as vectors, consideration should be given to dis-insecting family members and other close contacts with an appropriate insecticide. All close contacts should be evaluated for chemoprophylaxis. Close contacts of confirmed or suspected plague pneumonia cases (including medical personnel) should be provided with chemoprophylaxis for a period of 7 days using tetracycline (2 g/day in two or four equal doses for adults; 25–50 mg/kg/day in two or four equal doses for children over eight years of age), doxycycline (100 mg twice daily for persons >45 kg; 2.2 mg/kg for those over eight years of age <45 kg) or chloramphenicol (30 mg/kg daily in 4 divided doses). Tetracycline and doxycyline cannot be used in children less than eight years of age. Contacts also should be advised about appropriate measures they can take to protect themselves and their families from plague, and should be placed under surveillance.

6) Investigation of contacts and source of infection: Search for sick or dead rodents and their fleas and, if possible, submit these for laboratory analysis. Identify household members and others likely to have had potential similar plague exposures to the cases under investigation. If pneumonic plague is involved, identify household members and others who are likely to have had face-to-face contact with pneumonic plague patients. Determine whether case contacts show evidence of plague and provide medical care, treatment and chemoprophylaxis as needed.

7) Specific treatment: Rapid diagnosis and treatment are essential to reduce complications and fatality. The laboratory confirmation is of first importance but must not delay the set up of the treatment. Although streptomycin (adults—2 g/day in two equal doses; children—30 mg/kg/day in two equal doses) is the drug of choice, gentamicin (adults—3 mg/kg/day in 3 equal doses; children— 6.0-7.5 mg/kg/day in 3 equal doses) can be used when the former is not readily available; tetracyclines (adults—2 g/day in 4 equal doses; children over eight years of age—25–50 mg/day in 4 equal doses) and chloramphenicol (50 mg/kg/day in 4 equal doses for children and adults) are alternative choices. Chloramphenicol is required for treatment of plague meningitis. All are highly effective if used early. After a satisfactory response to drug treatment, reappearance of fever may result from a secondary infection or a suppurative bubo that may require incision and drainage.

C. Epidemic measures:

1) Investigate all suspected plague deaths with autopsy and laboratory examinations when indicated. Develop and carry

out case-finding. Establish the best possible facilities for diagnosis and treatment. Alert existing medical facilities to report cases immediately, and to use full diagnostic and therapeutic services.

2) Attempt to prevent or mitigate public hysteria by appropriate informational and educational releases through the press and news media.

3) Institute intensive flea control in affected areas and during epidemics. Apply flea control measures in expanding circles from known outbreak sites. Flea control should precede anti-rodent measures, and the latter should not be executed until the efficacy of the flea control measures has been demonstrated. To control fleas, apply insecticidal dusts to rodent runs, harborages, nests and burrows in and around known or suspected plague areas. All insecticides used for such control should be safe for human residents, labeled for flea control, and known to be effective against local fleas. If non-burrowing rodents are involved, insecticide bait stations can be used. If urban rats are involved, dis-insect houses and other structures with insecticidal dusts; dust the bodies and clothing of all residents in the immediate vicinity. After appropriate flea control measures have been taken, rat populations can be suppressed by environmental modifications intended to reduce rodent food and harborage, and applications of appropriate rodent poisons can be considered.

4) Implement tracing of contacts and medical surveillance/chemoprophylaxis.

5) Protect field workers against fleas; dust clothing with insecticide powder and use insect repellents daily. Antibiotic prophylaxis should be provided for those with documented close exposure (see 9B5).

D. Disaster implications: Plague could become a significant problem in or near endemic areas when there are social upheavals, crowding and unhygienic conditions. See preceding and following paragraphs for appropriate actions.

E. International measures:

1) According to the new *International Health Regulations* (June 2007), any event of potential international concern is subject to a notification to WHO. Plague cases will be notified only if the assessment done by the country shows that the public health impact can be considered as serious with at least one of the following characteristics: unusual or unexpected event; risk of international spread; significant risk of international travel; or trade restriction. Thus, the occurrence of a pneumonic plague case in a well-known focus should not be systematically notified. Conversely, the appearance of a

bubonic case in a non-endemic region is typically an event to be notified.

2) Measures applicable to ships, aircraft and land transport arriving from plague areas are specified in *International Health Regulations*.

3) All ships should be free of rodents or periodically de-ratted.

4) Rat-proof buildings at seaports and airports; apply appropriate insecticides; eliminate rats with effective rodenticides.

5) WHO Collaborating Centres provide support as required. More information can be found at: <http://www.who.int/collaboratingcentres/database/en/>.

F. Measures in the case of deliberate use: *Y. pestis* is distributed worldwide; techniques for mass production and aerosol dissemination are thought to exist. The fatality rate of primary pneumonic plague is high, and there is a real potential for secondary spread, particularly in those circumstances where cases are treated in home environments without modern medical care. For these reasons, the risk of a biological attack with plague is considered to be of serious public health concern. In some countries, a few sporadic cases may be missed or not attributed to a deliberate act, particularly in those with natural foci listed. Any suspect case of pneumonic plague should be reported immediately to the local health department. The sudden appearance of many patients presenting with fever, cough, a fulminant course and high case-fatality rate should provide a suspect alert for plague; if cough is primarily accompanied by hemoptysis, this presentation favors the tentative diagnosis of pneumonic plague. For a suspected or confirmed outbreak of pneumonic plague, follow the treatment and containment measures outlined in 9B. Depending on the extent of dissemination, mass prophylaxis of potentially exposed populations may be considered. For more information on the deliberate use of infectious agents to cause harm, see the section on *Deliberate use*.

PNEUMONIA

I. PNEUMOCOCCAL PNEUMONIA
[CCDM19: M. Moore, S. Qazi]
[CCDM18: N. Shindo]

ICD-9 481; ICD-10 J13

1. Identification—*Streptococcus pneumoniae* (pneumococcus) is the most common bacterial etiology of community-acquired pneumonia among all ages. In Europe and North America, estimates of the rate of pneumococcal pneumonia vary widely, from approximately 30 cases per 100 000 to nearly 100 per 100 000 adults each year, depending on the population studied and the diagnostic tests used. Clinical manifestations include sudden onset, high fever, rigors, pleuritic chest pain, dyspnea, tachypnea, and cough productive of "rusty" sputum. Onset may be less abrupt, especially among the elderly; fever, shortness of breath, or altered mental status may provide the first evidence of pneumonia. In infants and young children, fever, vomiting and convulsions may be the initial manifestations. Laboratory findings include leukocytosis (neutrophilia) and elevated C-reactive protein. Typical chest radiograph findings show lobar or segmental consolidation; consolidation may be bronchopneumonic, especially in children and the elderly. Pneumococcal pneumonia is an important cause of death in infants and the elderly. Persons suffering from chronic conditions and immune deficiencies are at increased risk. Infection can be complicated by empyema, acute respiratory distress syndrome, septic shock, and purpura fulminans. The case-fatality rate also varies widely, from 5–35%, depending on the setting (e.g., outpatients vs. inpatients) and the population (e.g., healthy adults vs. persons with alcoholism). In developing countries, case-fatality rates among children are often over 10%, and as high as 60% among infants under 6 months of age. Pneumococcal pneumonia among previously healthy individuals with other respiratory infections (e.g., influenza) is well-described.

Pneumonia is generally treated empirically with antimicrobial agents that have good activity against pneumococcus. A microbiologic diagnosis of pneumococcal pneumonia can further guide antibiotic therapy. The presence in sputum of many Gram-positive diplococci together with polymorphonuclear leukocytes suggests pneumococcal pneumonia; however, Gram stain and culture of respiratory secretions are performed less frequently than previously, largely due to technical aspects of obtaining good quality specimens and the difficulty of distinguishing infection from respiratory tract colonization. Definitive diagnosis of pneumococcal pneumonia is established by isolation of pneumococci from blood or, less commonly, pleural fluid. Among adults, the diagnosis can also be established by identification of pneumococcal polysaccharide in urine. For children, urine antigen testing is not useful because nasopharyngeal colonization can cause excretion of pneumococcal antigen in urine. Most pediatric cases are diagnosed by isolation of pneumococci from blood. Patients suspected of having pneumococcal pneumonia should be treated promptly, preferably after collection of appropriate diagnostic specimens, according to established guidelines. If pneumococcus is isolated, susceptibility testing should be performed, and antimicrobial therapy tailored to susceptibility results.

2. **Infectious agent**—*Streptococcus pneumoniae* (pneumococcus) is a Gram-positive, lancet-shaped, encapsulated diplococcus that often

asymptomatically colonizes the human nasopharynx. Children are colonized with *S. pneumoniae* more often than adults. Current data suggest that a hypothetical vaccine including six serotypes (1, 5, 6B, 14, 19F, 23F, assuming 6A cross-protection from 6B) could cover 70% of invasive disease worldwide, ranging from 66% in North America to 76% in Africa.

3. Occurrence—Pneumococcal pneumonia is an endemic disease among the elderly and those with underlying medical conditions. Infection is more frequent among malnourished populations and lower socioeconomic groups, especially in developing countries. It occurs in all climates and seasons, peaking in winter in temperate zones. Certain serotypes may cause epidemics, especially among institutionalized populations, the homeless, and in developing countries. Incidence is high in certain geographic areas (e.g., Papua New Guinea) and in certain ethnic groups, such as Alaska Natives and Australian Aboriginals. An increased incidence often accompanies epidemics of influenza.

4. Reservoir—Humans. Pneumococci are commonly found in the upper respiratory tract of healthy people worldwide.

5. Mode of transmission—Droplet spread. Person-to-person transmission of the organisms is common, but illness among casual contacts and attendants is infrequent.

6. Incubation period—Not well determined; may be as short as 1–3 days. Infection is thought to be preceded by asymptomatic colonization.

7. Period of communicability—Presumably until discharges of mouth and nose no longer contain sufficient numbers of pneumococci, which usually occurs within 24 hours of initiation of effective antibiotic therapy.

8. Susceptibility—Susceptibility is increased among certain populations, including infants, the elderly, and persons with underlying illnesses such as anatomical or functional asplenia, sickle cell disease, cardiovascular disease, diabetes mellitus, cirrhosis, Hodgkin's disease, lymphoma, multiple myeloma, chronic renal failure, nephrotic syndrome, HIV infection, and recent organ transplantation. Malnutrition and low birthweight are important risk factors for infection among infants and young children in developing countries. Susceptibility to infection is also increased by processes affecting the integrity of the lower respiratory tract, including influenza, pulmonary edema, aspiration following alcoholic intoxication or other causes, chronic lung disease, or exposure to irritants (e.g., cigarettes, cooking fire smoke). Previously healthy persons can develop pneumococcal pneumonia. Serotype-specific immunity usually follows infection and may last for years.

9. **Methods of control—**

A. *Preventive measures:*

1) Avoid crowding in living quarters whenever practical, particularly in institutions. Prevent malnutrition and encourage physical activity. Bedridden patients should lie in an upright position, at a 30- to 45-degree incline.

2) A protein-polysaccharide conjugate vaccine including seven of the commonest serotypes was introduced in 2000 and subsequently included in the routine infant immunization schedules in many countries. The vaccine has been shown to be highly effective at preventing invasive pneumococcal disease and pneumococcal pneumonia, with important reductions in disease incidence demonstrated in the target age population (direct effects) as well as those too old or too young to receive the vaccine (indirect, or herd, effects). It should be noted that the evidence for this is mostly from developed countries, and at time of writing in early 2008 there is little information about the effectiveness of the vaccine in developing countries.

   WHO considers that it should be a priority to include pneumococcal conjugate vaccine in all national immunization programs—though countries, and particularly developing countries, should consider switching to newer vaccines with more serotypes once these are available and affordable.

3) A 23-valent polysaccharide vaccine (PPV23) is available for persons aged more than two years. In some countries it is recommended for high-risk persons (individuals 65 years of age and older and those with anatomic or functional asplenia, sickle cell disease, HIV infection and a variety of chronic systemic illnesses, including heart and lung disease, cirrhosis of the liver, renal insufficiency and diabetes mellitus). The role of PPV23 in preventing pneumococcal disease among HIV-infected persons in sub-Saharan Africa is unclear. WHO has recently convened a working group to prepare a revised position statement on the use of this vaccine. More information can be found at:

   <http://www.who.int/immunization/sage/ppv_member ship/en/index.html>

   PPV23 is not effective in children under two years of age and has no impact on pneumococcal carriage. For most eligible patients, vaccine need be given only once; however, re-immunization is generally safe, and vaccine should be offered to eligible patients whose immunization status cannot be determined. Re-immunization is recommended once for persons over 2 years of age who are at highest risk for serious pneumococcal infection (e.g., asplenic patients), and those likely to have a rapid decline in pneumococcal antibody levels, provided that 5 years or more have elapsed since receipt of the 1st dose of vaccine. Re-immunization after 3 years should also be considered for children with functional or anatomic asplenia, and those who present conditions associated with rapid antibody decline after initial immunization (e.g., nephrotic syndrome, renal failure, renal transplantation) who would be 10 years or younger at re-immunization. In addition, persons aged 65 years and older should be given another dose of vaccine if they received the vaccine more than 5 years previously and were under 65 at the time of primary immunization.

B. *Control of patient, contacts and the immediate environment:*

1) Report to local health authority: Obligatory report of epidemics in some countries; no individual case report, Class 4 (see *Reporting*).
2) Isolation: Respiratory isolation may be warranted for hospitalized patients with highly antibiotic resistant infection, who may transmit it to patients at high risk of pneumococcal disease.
3) Concurrent disinfection: Hand hygiene and cough etiquette.
4) Quarantine: Not applicable.
5) Immunization of contacts: Not applicable (See 9C).
6) Investigation of contacts and source of infection: Of no practical value.
7) Specific treatment: Antibiotic treatment of infants and young children with pneumonia should start presumptively based on a clinical diagnosis. If tachypnea and chest indrawing are present, infants aged less than 2 months should be transferred to hospital care without delay; if pneumococcal pneumonia is identified, parenteral penicillin G or ampicillin are preferred treatments (or erythromycin for those hypersensitive to penicillin). Based on a recent clinical trial in Pakistan, immediate treatment of children aged 3–59 months with severe pneumonia with oral amoxicillin may result in equivalent outcome compared to hospitalization and intravenous ampicillin. Because pneumococci resistant to penicillin and other antimicrobials are increasingly recognized, sensitivities of strains isolated from normally sterile sites, including blood or CSF, should be determined. Caution should be exercised in interpreting susceptibility results, as the same isolate may be considered susceptible or resistant to certain antibiotics (e.g., penicillin, third generation cephalosporins)

depending on the site of infection (e.g., blood vs. meninges). In developing countries, WHO guidelines recommend trimethoprim-sulfamethazole, ampicillin or amoxicillin for home-treatment of non-severe pneumonia for children under 5 years of age (NB: recommended duration of treatment in non-severe pneumonia, based on findings from RCTs, is 3 days, instead of the standard 5 days). WHO guidelines are not intended for industrialized countries, most of which have no unified guidelines for the treatment of pneumococcal disease, although professional societies have published recommendations for the treatment of community-acquired pneumonia and pneumonia in children.

C. *Epidemic measures:* In outbreaks in institutions or in other closed groups, immunization may be carried out unless it is known that the type causing disease is not included in the vaccine. Based on experience with *Haemophilus influenzae* type b vaccine, there is a theoretical concern that immunization with PPV23 may be followed by a period of a few days of increased susceptibility to infection. If PPV23 is used, or if the outbreak is particularly explosive, antibiotic prophylaxis may need to be considered.

D. *Disaster implications:* Crowding of populations in temporary shelters bears a risk of disease, especially for the very young and the elderly.

E. *International measures:* None.

II. MYCOPLASMA PNEUMONIA ICD-9 483; ICD-10 J15.7

1. **Identification**—Predominantly a febrile lower respiratory infection causing about 20% of pneumonias; less often, a pharyngitis that sometimes progresses to tracheobronchitis or pneumonia. Onset is gradual with headache, malaise, cough (often paroxysmal), sore throat and sometimes chest discomfort that may be pleuritic. Sputum, scant at first, may increase later. Early patchy infiltration of the lungs is often more extensive on X-rays than clinical findings suggest. In severe cases, the pneumonia may progress from one lobe to another and become bilateral. Leukocytosis occurs after the first week in approximately one-third of cases. Duration varies from a few days to a month or more. Complications such as CNS involvement (e.g., encephalitis, acute disseminated encephalomyelitis) and Stevens-Johnson syndrome are infrequent; fatalities are rare.

Differentiation is required from atypical pneumonia due to many other agents: other bacteria; adenoviruses; influenza; respiratory syncytial virus;

parainfluenza; measles; Q fever; psittacosis; certain mycoses; severe acute respiratory syndrome (SARS); and tuberculosis.

Diagnosis is based on a rise in antibody titers between acute and convalescent sera collected 3-6 weeks apart. Diagnosis by PCR using throat swabs/sputum is possible in some countries. The infectious agent may be cultured on special media.

2. Infectious agent—*Mycoplasma pneumoniae* belongs to the Mycoplasmas (Molicutes), placed between bacteria and viruses. Because Mycoplasmas lack cell walls, cell wall synthesis inhibitors such as the penicillins and cephalosporins are not effective in treatment. Along with *Streptococcus pneumoniae* and *Haemophilus influenzae*, *Mycoplasma pneumoniae* is one of the most common agents of community-acquired pneumonia.

3. Occurrence—Worldwide; sporadic, endemic and occasionally epidemic, especially in institutions and military populations. Outbreaks often occur in schools and households. Attack rates vary from 5 to more than 50/1 000/year in military populations and 1 to 3/1 000/year in civilians. Epidemics occur more often in late summer and autumn; endemic disease is not seasonal, but there can be variation from year to year and among different geographic areas. Men and women of all ages are equally affected. Infection is most frequent among school-age children and young adults.

4. Reservoir—Humans.

5. Mode of transmission—Probably droplet inhalation, direct contact with an infected person (probably including those with sub-clinical infections). Secondary cases of pneumonia among contacts, family members and attendants are frequent.

6. Incubation period—6 to 32 days.

7. Period of communicability—Probably less than 20 days. Treatment reduces carriage but does not reliably eradicate the organism from the respiratory tract, where it may persist for weeks.

8. Susceptibility—Clinical pneumonia occurs in about 3-30% of infections with *M. pneumoniae*. Disease varies from mild afebrile pharyngitis to febrile illness of the upper or lower respiratory tract. Duration of immunity is uncertain. Second attacks of pneumonia may occur. Protection against repeat infection has been correlated with humoral antibodies that persist up to 1 year.

9. Methods of control—

    A. Preventive measures: Avoid crowded living and sleeping quarters whenever possible, especially in institutions, barracks and ships.

B. Control of patient, contacts and the immediate environment:

1) Report to local health authority: Obligatory report of epidemics in some countries; no individual case report, Class 4 (see *Reporting*).
2) Isolation: Not applicable. Respiratory secretions may be infectious.
3) Concurrent disinfection: Hand hygiene and cough etiquette.
4) Quarantine: Not applicable.
5) Immunization of contacts: Not applicable.
6) Investigation of contacts and source of infection allows for treatment of clinical disease among family members.
7) Specific treatment: Azolides (e.g., azithromycin, clarithromycin) or erythromycin or a tetracycline. Azolides or macrolides are preferred for children under 8 years of age, in whom tetracycline cannot be used.

C. Epidemic measures: No reliably effective measures for control are available, although antimicrobial prophylaxis has been used in some institutional outbreak settings.

D. Disaster implications: None.

E. International measures: WHO Collaborating Centres provide support as required. More information can be found at:

<http://www.who.int/collaboratingcentres/database/en/>

III. PNEUMOCYSTIS PNEUMONIA   ICD-9 136.3; ICD-10 B59
(Interstitial plasma-cell pneumonia, PCP)

1. Identification—An acute to sub-acute, often fatal, pulmonary disease, especially in persons with HIV/AIDS or other causes of immunosuppression, and in malnourished, premature infants. Clinically, patients present with dyspnea on exertion, dry, non-productive cough, and fever. Auscultatory signs are usually minimal or absent. Chest radiographs typically show bilateral diffuse interstitial infiltrates.

Demonstration of the causative agent in material from induced sputum, bronchoalveolar lavage, or transbronchial or open lung biopsy establishes the diagnosis. Staining with methenamine silver or Giemsa can identify the organism. There is no satisfactory routine culture method or serological test at present.

2. Infectious agent—*Pneumocystis jiroveci* (previously known as *Pneumocystis carinii* and classified as a protozoa). Currently, it is considered a fungus, based on nucleic acid and biochemical analysis.

3. Occurrence—Worldwide; may be endemic and epidemic in debilitated, malnourished or immunosuppressed infants. It affected approximately 60% of patients with HIV infection in the USA, Europe and Australia before the routine use of prophylactic medication and HAART. It is a common cause of pneumonia in HIV-infected young infants in developing countries with high HIV prevalence, particularly in sub-Saharan Africa.

4. Reservoir—Humans. Organisms have been demonstrated in rodents, cattle, dogs and other animals, but the ubiquitous presence of the organism and its sub-clinical persistence in man renders these potential animal sources of human infection of little public health significance.

5. Mode of transmission—Airborne animal-to-animal transmission has occurred in rats. The mode of transmission in people is not known. In one USA study, approximately 75% of healthy individuals were reported to have humoral antibody to *P. jiroveci* by the age of 4 years, suggesting that sub-clinical infection is common. Pneumonitis in the compromised host may result from either a reactivation of latent infection or a newly acquired infection.

6. Incubation period—Unknown. Analysis of data from institutional outbreaks and animal studies indicates that the onset of disease often occurs 1–2 months after establishment of the immunosuppressed state.

7. Period of communicability—Unknown.

8. Susceptibility—Susceptibility is enhanced by prematurity, chronic debilitating illness and disease or treatments that impair immune mechanisms. Infection with HIV is a predominant risk factor.

9. Methods of control—

  A. *Preventive measures:* Among immunosuppressed patients— especially those with HIV infection, those treated for lymphatic leukemia and those with organ transplants—prophylaxis with either oral trimethoprim-sulfamethoxazole, dapsone, or atovaquone is effective in preventing endogenous re-activation for as long as the patient receives the drug.

  B. *Control of patient, contacts and the immediate environment:*

  1) Report to local health authority: Official report not ordinarily justifiable, Class 5; when cases occur in people with evidence of HIV infection, case report may be required in some countries, Class 2 (see *Reporting*).
  2) Isolation: Not applicable.
  3) Concurrent disinfection: Insufficient knowledge.
  4) Quarantine: Not applicable.
  5) Immunization of contacts: Not applicable.

6) Investigation of contacts and source of infection: Not applicable.
7) Specific treatment: Trimethoprim-sulfamethoxazole is the drug of choice. Alternate drugs are pentamidine (IM or IV), dapsone-trimethoprim, atovaquone, and clindamycin-primaquine.

C. *Epidemic measures:* Knowledge of the source and mode of transmission is so incomplete that there are no generally accepted measures.

D. *Disaster implications:* None.

E. *International measures:* None.

IV. CHLAMYDIAL PNEUMONIAS
IV.A. PNEUMONIA DUE TO *CHLAMYDIA TRACHOMATIS*   ICD-9 482.8; ICD-10 P23.1
(Neonatal eosinophilic pneumonia, Congenital pneumonia due to *Chlamydia*)

1. Identification—A sub-acute chlamydial pulmonary disease typically occurring between 4 and 11 weeks of age among infants whose mothers have chlamydial infection of the uterine cervix. Clinically, the disease is characterized by insidious onset, cough (characteristically staccato), lack of fever, patchy infiltrates on chest radiograph with hyperinflation, eosinophilia, and elevated IgM and IgG. About half of infant cases show prodromal rhinitis and conjunctivitis. Duration of illness is commonly 1–3, weeks but may extend as long as 2 months. The illness is usually moderate, but can progress to severe pneumonia. One study suggests that infants with *C. trachoma* pneumonia are at increased risk of chronic cough and abnormal lung function.

A wide variety of diagnostic tests are available, including direct fluorescent antibody tests, enzyme immunoassays, DNA probes, and nucleic acid amplification systems. Although elevated serum IgM suggests recent infection, microimmunofluorescent assays, considered optimal for detection of antibody, are not widely available.

2. Infectious agent—*Chlamydia trachomatis* of immunotypes D to K.

3. Occurrence—Probably coincides with the worldwide distribution of genital chlamydial infection. The disease has been recognized in many countries. Epidemics have not been recognized.

4. Reservoir—Humans. Experimental infection with *C. trachomatis* has been induced in nonhuman primates and mice; animal infections are not known to occur in nature.

5. Mode of transmission—From the infected cervix to an infant during birth, with resultant nasopharyngeal infection (and occasionally chlamydial conjunctivitis). Respiratory transmission has not been established.

6. Incubation period—Pneumonia may occur in infants from 1 to 18 weeks of age (more commonly between 4 and 11 weeks). Nasopharyngeal infection is usually not recognized before 2 weeks of age.

7. Period of communicability—Unknown.

8. Susceptibility—Unknown. Maternal antibody does not protect the infant from infection.

9. Methods of control—

   A. Preventive measures: See *chlamydial conjunctivitis (Conjunctivitis,* section IV).

   B. Control of patient, contacts and the immediate environment:

   1) Report to local health authority: Official report not ordinarily justifiable, Class 5 (see *Reporting*).
   2) Isolation: Universal precautions in hospitals and nurseries.
   3) Concurrent disinfection: Of discharges from nose and throat.
   4) Quarantine: Not applicable.
   5) Immunization of contacts: Not applicable.
   6) Investigation of contacts and source of infection: Examine parents for infection and treat if positive.
   7) Specific treatment: Oral erythromycin (50 mg/kg/day) is the drug of choice for infants. Sulfisoxazole is a possible alternative.

   C. Epidemic measures: No epidemic occurrence recognized.

   D. Disaster implications: None.

   E. International measures: None.

IV.B. PNEUMONIA DUE TO CHLAMYDIA PNEUMONIAE ICD-9 482.8; ICD-10 J16.0

1. Identification—An acute chlamydial respiratory disease with cough, frequently a sore throat and hoarseness, and fever at the onset; sputum is scanty and chest pain is rare. Inflammatory signs are sometimes subtle. Pulmonary rales are usually present. The clinical picture is similar to pneumonia caused by *Mycoplasma*. Radiographic abnormalities include bilateral infiltrates, sometimes with pleural effusions. Age distribution has 2 peaks: one among children of 5–15 years of age and one in persons aged 60 and older. Outbreaks in communities, households, day care centers, and schools are often reported. Illness is usually mild, but recovery is slow, with cough persisting for 2–6 weeks. Death is rare in uncomplicated cases.

Laboratory diagnosis is primarily serological. Microimmunofluorescence testing of paired sera collected 4–8 weeks apart is the recommended approach. The organism can be isolated from throat swab specimens in special cell lines.

2. Infectious agent—*Chlamydia pneumoniae*, biovar TWAR, is the species name for the human-specific organism with distinct morphological and serological differences from *C. psittaci* and *C. trachomatis.*

3. Occurrence—Presumably worldwide. Antibodies are rare in children under 5 years of age; seroprevalence increases among teenagers and young adults to a plateau of about 50% by age 20–30, which persists into old age. While clinical disease is encountered most frequently in young adults, disease has occurred in all age groups. No seasonality has been noted.

4. Reservoir—Presumably humans. No avian association has been found; no isolations or antibodies were found in pigeons and other birds captured at the site of an outbreak, nor in dogs or cats.

5. Mode of transmission—Not defined, although droplet transmission is most likely.

6. Incubation period—Unknown; may be 3–4 weeks.

7. Period of communicability—Not defined but presumably long; some military outbreaks have lasted as long as 8 months.

8. Susceptibility—Presumably universal with increased likelihood of clinical disease in the presence of pre-existing chronic disease. Serological evidence of recall type immune response suggests immunity after infection; second episodes of pneumonia have been observed in military recruits, with a secondary type of serological response to the second attack.

9. Methods of control—

    A. Preventive measures:

        1) Avoid crowding in living and sleeping quarters.
        2) Apply personal hygiene measures: cover mouth when coughing and sneezing and wash hands frequently.

B. Control of patient, contacts and the immediate environment:

1) Report to local health authority: Obligatory report of epidemics; no individual case report, Class 4 (see *Reporting*).
2) Isolation: Not applicable. Universal precautions should be practiced.
3) Concurrent disinfection: Of discharges from nose and throat.
4) Quarantine: Not applicable.
5) Immunization of contacts: Not applicable.
6) Investigation of contacts and source of infection: Examine all members of the family for infection and treat if positive.
7) Specific treatment: A definite diagnosis is difficult at the early stages of illness. Current recommendations for empiric treatment of community-acquired pneumonia in adults include regimens effective against *C. pneumoniae*, including, in adults, macrolides, azolides and tetracyclines. In children macrolides are the drug of choice—tetracyclines cannot be used in children less than eight years of age. Fluoroquinolones are alternative agents. Treatment may have to be as long as 6 weeks for *C. pneumoniae* pneumonia.

C. Epidemic measures: Case-finding and appropriate treatment.

D. Disaster implications: None.

E. International measures: None.

OTHER PNEUMONIAS   ICD-9 480, 482; ICD-10 J12, J13, J15, J16.8, J18

Among the known viruses, a pneumonitis may be produced by: adenoviruses; respiratory syncytial virus: parainfluenza viruses; human bocavirus; and probably others as yet unidentified. Because these agents cause upper respiratory disease more often than pneumonia, they are presented under Respiratory Disease, Acute Viral. Viral pneumonia occurs in measles, influenza and chickenpox. Infection by *Chlamydia psittaci* is presented as Psittacosis (q.v.). Pneumonia is also caused by infection with rickettsiae (see *Q fever*) and *Legionella* (see *Legionellosis*). It can be associated with the invasive phase of nematode infections, such as ascariasis, and with mycoses such as aspergillosis, histoplasmosis and coccidioidomycosis.

Various pathogenic bacteria commonly found in the mouth, nose and throat, such as *Haemophilus influenzae* (see Meningitis), *Staphylococcus aureus*, *Klebsiella pneumoniae*, *Streptococcus pyogenes* (group A hemolytic streptococci), *Neisseria meningitidis*, *Bacteroides* species, *Moraxella catarrhalis* and anaerobic cocci, can cause pneumonia, either as a primary pathogen or as a complication of chronic pulmonary disease, or after aspiration of gastric contents or tracheostomy. With increased use of antimicrobial and immunosuppressive treatment, pneumonias caused by enteric Gram-negative bacilli have become more common, especially those caused by *Escherichia coli, Pseudomonas aeruginosa* and *Proteus* species. Management depends on the organism involved.

POLIOMYELITIS, ACUTE   ICD-9 045; ICD-10 A80
(Polioviral fever, Infantile paralysis)
[CCDM18 & 19: R. B. Aylward]

1. Identification—A viral infection recognized by acute onset of flaccid paralysis. Infection occurs in the GI tract with spread to regional lymph nodes and, in a minority of cases, to the CNS. Flaccid paralysis occurs in less than 1% of infections; over 90% are unapparent or result in non-specific fever. Aseptic meningitis occurs in about 1% of infections. Fever, malaise, headache, nausea and vomiting are recognized in 10% of infections. If disease progresses to major illness, severe muscle pain and stiffness of the neck and back with flaccid paralysis may occur. Paralysis of poliomyelitis is usually asymmetric, with fever present at onset. Maximum extent of paralysis is usually reached within 3–4 days. The site of paralysis depends on the location of nerve cell destruction in the spinal cord or brain stem; legs are affected more often than the arms. Paralysis of the respiration and/or swallowing muscles can be life-threatening. Some improvement in paralysis may occur during convalescence, but paralysis still present after 60 days is likely to be permanent. Infrequently, recurrence of muscle weakness following recovery may occur many years after the original infection has resolved ("postpolio syndrome"); this is not believed to be related to persistence of the virus itself. With progress made towards global eradication, poliomyelitis must now be distinguished from other paralytic conditions by isolation of virus from stool. Other enteroviruses (notably types 70 and 71), echoviruses and coxsackieviruses have been reported to cause an illness simulating paralytic poliomyelitis.

The most frequent cause of acute flaccid paralysis (AFP) that must be distinguished from poliomyelitis is Guillain-Barré syndrome (GBS). Paralysis in GBS is typically symmetrical, and may progress for periods as long as 10 days. Fever, headache, nausea, vomiting and pleocytosis characteristic of poliomyelitis are usually absent in GBS; high protein and low cell counts in CSF and sensory changes are seen in the majority of GBS cases. Acute motor axonal neuropathy ("China paralytic syndrome") is an important cause of AFP in northern China, and is probably present elsewhere; it is seasonally epidemic and closely resembles poliomyelitis. Fever and CSF pleocytosis are usually absent, but paralysis may persist for several months. Other causes of AFP include transverse myelitis, traumatic neuritis, infectious and toxic neuropathies, tick paralysis, myasthenia gravis, porphyria, botulism, insecticide poisoning, polymyositis, trichinosis, and periodic paralysis.

Differential diagnosis of acute non-paralytic poliomyelitis includes other forms of acute nonbacterial meningitis, purulent meningitis, brain abscess, tuberculous meningitis, leptospirosis, lymphocytic choriomeningitis, infectious mononucleosis, the encephalitides, neurosyphilis and toxic encephalopathies.

Definitive laboratory diagnosis requires isolation of the wild poliovirus from stool samples, CSF or oropharyngeal secretions. Specialized laboratories can differentiate "wild" from vaccine virus strains. Rises in antibody levels (4-fold or greater) are less helpful in the diagnosis of wild poliomyelitis infection, since type-specific neutralizing antibodies may already be present when paralysis develops, and significant titer rises may not be demonstrable in paired sera. Antibody response following immunization mimics the response after infection with wild type viruses, and the widespread use of live polio vaccines makes interpretation of antibody levels difficult, except to rule out polio in cases where no antibody has developed in immunocompetent children.

2. Infectious agent—Poliovirus (genus *Enterovirus*) types 1, 2 and 3; all types cause paralysis. Wild poliovirus type 1 is isolated from paralytic cases most often, and type 3 less so. Circulating wild type 2 poliovirus has not been detected since October 1999. Type 1 most frequently causes epidemics. Paralytic polio cases have also been reported, rarely, due to outbreaks caused by circulating vaccine-derived polioviruses (cVDPVs) types 1, 2 and 3. Most vaccine-associated cases are due to type 2 or 3 Sabin-like polioviruses.

3. Occurrence—Historically, poliomyelitis occurred worldwide sporadically and as epidemics, with an increase during the late summer and autumn in temperate countries. In tropical countries, a less pronounced seasonal peak occurred in the hot and rainy season. With improved immunization and the global initiative to eradicate poliomyelitis, by the end of 2007 polioviruses were limited to only four countries that had not succeeded in interrupting transmission (Afghanistan, India, Nigeria and Pakistan). The greatest risks of polio are now in south Asia (70% of cases in 2007) and in West/Central Africa (30% of cases in 2007). Poliomyelitis remains primarily a disease of infants and young children. In the four countries that have not yet succeeded in interrupting transmission, 80%–90% of cases are in children aged less than three, and virtually all cases are in those under five. Clusters of susceptible persons—including groups that refuse immunization, minority populations, migrants and other unregistered children, nomads, refugees and the urban poor—are at high risk.

Although wild poliovirus transmission has ceased in most countries, importation remains a threat. A large outbreak of poliomyelitis occurred in 1992–1993 in the Netherlands among members of a religious group that refuse immunization, and virus was also found among members of a related religious group in Canada, although no cases occurred. Between 2003 and 2007, imported wild poliovirus caused paralytic cases in 27 countries, primarily in Africa, Asia and the Middle East. Until recent changes in immunization policy, and with the exception of rare imported cases, the few cases of poliomyelitis recognized in industrialized countries were caused by vaccine virus strains. About half of vaccine-associated paralytic poliomyelitis (VAPP) cases occurred among adult contacts of vaccinees.

Since 2000, 10 polio outbreaks due to cVDPVs have been reported from 9 countries, all of which continue to use OPV for routine immunization. These outbreaks have been associated with areas of low OPV coverage, and the cases were clinically indistinguishable from polio caused by wild poliovirus.

4. Reservoir—Humans, most frequently people with inapparent infections, especially children. No long-term carriers of wild type poliovirus have been detected.

5. Mode of transmission—Primarily person-to-person spread, principally through the fecal-oral route; virus is detectable more easily and for a longer period in feces than in throat secretions. Where sanitation levels are high, pharyngeal spread may be relatively more important. In rare instances, milk, foodstuffs and other materials contaminated with feces have been incriminated as vehicles. No reliable evidence of spread by insects exists.

6. Incubation period—Commonly 7-14 days for paralytic cases; reported range of 3 to possibly 35 days.

7. Period of communicability—Not precisely defined, but transmission is possible as long as the virus is excreted. Poliovirus is demonstrable in throat secretions as early as 36 hours, and in feces 72 hours, after exposure to infection in both clinical and inapparent cases. Virus typically persists in the throat for approximately 1 week, and in feces for 3-6 weeks. Cases are most infectious during the days before and after onset of symptoms.

8. Susceptibility—Susceptibility to infection is universal; paralysis occurs in only about 1% of infections. Residual paralysis is observed in 0.1% to 1% of cases, depending primarily on the virulence of the strain. The rate of paralysis among infected non-immune adults is higher than that among non-immunized infants and young children. Type-specific immunity, apparently of lifelong duration, follows both clinically recognizable and inapparent infections. Second attacks are rare and result from infection with a poliovirus of a different type. Infants born of immune mothers have transient passive immunity.

Intramuscular injections, trauma or surgery during the incubation period or prodromal illness may provoke paralysis in the affected extremity. Tonsillectomy increases the risk of bulbar involvement. Excessive muscular activity in the prodromal period may predispose to paralysis.

9. **Methods of control—**

A. *Preventive measures:*

1) Educate the public on the advantages of immunization in early childhood.
2) Both a trivalent live, attenuated oral poliovirus vaccine (OPV) and an injectable, inactivated poliovirus vaccine (IPV) are commercially available for routine immunization. Since 2005, monovalent oral poliovirus vaccines (mOPV) types 1 and 3 have been developed and licensed for use in mass campaigns to provide higher, type-specific seroconversion rates in areas where one or both of these serotypes are circulating.

   OPV simulates natural infection by inducing both circulating antibody and resistance to infection of the pharynx and intestine, and also immunizes some susceptible contacts through secondary spread. In developing countries, lower rates of seroconversion and reduced vaccine efficacy for OPV have been reported; this can be overcome by administration of numerous extra doses in immunization programs and/or supplemental campaigns. Breastfeeding does not cause a significant reduction in the protection provided by OPV. WHO recommends the use of OPV alone for immunization programs in developing countries because of the capacity to induce mucosal immunity, low cost, ease of administration, and superior capacity to provide population immunity through community spread.

   IPV, like OPV, provides excellent individual protection by inducing circulating antibody that blocks the spread of virus to the CNS, and also protects against pharyngeal infection, but does not induce intestinal immunity comparable to OPV. Many middle-income countries and most industrialized countries have switched to IPV alone for routine immunization, because wild type polioviruses have been eliminated, ongoing global eradication efforts have reduced the risk of importations, and the risk of paralysis from OPV in these countries is considered greater than that from wild poliovirus.

   A few individuals with underlying primary immune deficiency disorders have been identified who chronically excreted an OPV-derived poliovirus, and the significance of these chronic excreters as a risk to polio eradication is under review. No secondary cases have been associated with or attributed to long-term excreters of vaccine-derived polioviruses.

More troublesome are outbreaks of poliomyelitis caused by circulating vaccine-derived polioviruses (cVDPVs). These are capable of spreading through populations and becoming manifest in non-vaccinated or incompletely vaccinated individuals. The extent of this problem is being evaluated, with on average one such outbreak being detected each year, arising primarily in areas of low OPV coverage

3) Recommendations for routine and supplementary immunization:

In developing countries, WHO recommends 4 doses of OPV at 6, 10 and 14 weeks of age, with an additional dose at birth or at the measles contact (usually 9 months of age), depending on the endemicity and/or risk of polio in the country. In endemic countries, WHO recommends the use of national supplemental immunization campaigns administering two or more doses of OPV one month apart to all children under five regardless of prior immunization status. These campaigns should be conducted during the cool, dry season to achieve maximum effect. On the attainment of a high level of control in a country, targeted house-to-house mop-up immunization campaigns in high-risk areas are recommended to interrupt the final chains of transmission.

Where polio is still endemic or at high risk of importation and spread, WHO recommends the use of OPV for all infants, including those who may be infected with HIV in whom it has been shown to be safe. Diarrhea is not a contraindication to OPV. In industrialized countries, contraindications to OPV frequently include congenital immunodeficiency (B-lymphocyte deficiency, thymic dysplasia), current immunosuppressive treatment, disease states associated with immunosuppression (e.g. lymphoma, leukemia, and generalized malignancy), and the presence of immunodeficient individuals in the households of potential vaccine recipients. IPV should be used in such people. OPV causes paralytic poliomyelitis in vaccine recipients or their healthy contacts at a rate of approximately one in every 2.5 million doses administered, or 1 in 800 000 first vaccinations. In Romania, multiple injections of antibiotics at the time of vaccination were associated with an increased risk of vaccine-associated poliomyelitis (VAPP).

With progress towards eradication, the risk profile of paralytic poliomyelitis is changing, particularly in industrialized and high/middle income countries. Many of these have decided that the risks of paralytic poliomyelitis due to adverse events associated with continued use of OPV in routine immunization are greater than those due to the handling or circulation of wild poliovirus, and have adopted one of two approaches to prevent or minimize immunization-related adverse events:

a) Replacement of OPV by inactivated poliovirus vaccine (IPV) for routine immunization.
b) Introduction of mixed OPV/IPV use—for example, effective January 2000, all children in the USA were to receive 4 doses of IPV at ages 2, 4 and 6–18 months and 4–6 years. In these countries, OPV is now reserved for special circumstances, such as mass campaigns to control possible outbreaks.

Immunization of adults: Routine immunization for adults is not considered necessary. Primary immunization is advised for previously non-immunized adults traveling to endemic countries, members of communities or population groups in which poliovirus disease is present, laboratory workers handling specimens containing poliovirus, and health care workers who may be exposed to patients excreting wild type polioviruses. In most industrialized countries, IPV is recommended for adult primary immunization, e.g. 2 doses at a 1–2 month interval and a third dose 6–12 months later. Those having previously completed a course of immunization and currently at increased risk of exposure are often given an additional dose of IPV. A single, lifetime booster is recommended for previously immunized adults traveling to polio-infected areas.

Some countries have established special immunization requirements for travelers from polio-endemic and re-infected countries, and travelers should check immunization requirements prior to departure.

B. Control of patient, contacts and the immediate environment:

1) Report to local health authority: Obligatory case report of paralytic cases as a Disease under surveillance by WHO, Class 1. In countries undertaking poliomyelitis eradication and/or certification, each case of acute flaccid paralysis (AFP), including Guillain-Barré syndrome, in children aged under 15 years must be reported and fully investigated. Non-paralytic cases are also reported to the local health authority, Class 2 (see *Reporting*).
2) Isolation: Enteric precautions in the hospital for wild virus disease; of little value under home conditions because many household contacts are infected before poliomyelitis has been diagnosed.

3) Concurrent disinfection: Throat discharges, feces and articles soiled therewith. In communities with modern and adequate sewage disposal systems, feces and urine can be discharged directly into sewers without preliminary disinfection. Terminal cleaning.

4) Quarantine: Of no community value.

5) Protection of contacts: Immunization of familial and other close contacts is recommended but may not contribute to immediate control; the virus has often infected susceptible close contacts by the time the initial case is recognized.

6) Investigation of contacts and source of infection: Occurrence of a single case of poliomyelitis due to wild poliovirus in a country that has interrupted transmission is a public health emergency prompting immediate investigation and planning for a large-scale response. A thorough search for additional cases of AFP in the area around the case assures early detection, facilitates control, and permits appropriate treatment of unrecognized and unreported cases.

7) Specific treatment: None; attention during acute illness to complications of paralysis requires expert knowledge and equipment, especially for patients in need of respiratory assistance. Physical therapy is used to attain maximum function after paralytic poliomyelitis and can prevent many deformities that are late manifestations of the illness.

C. *Epidemic measures:* In any country that has previously interrupted transmission of wild poliovirus, a single case of poliomyelitis must now be considered a public health emergency, requiring an extensive supplementary immunization response over a large geographic area. Responses should be initiated within 4 weeks of confirmation of the index case, and should consist of a minimum of 3 mass immunization rounds spaced 4–6 weeks apart (with at least 2 rounds after the last detected case), using the appropriate type-specific monovalent OPV, covering a minimum of 2–5 million children, and achieving at least 95% coverage in each administrative area.

D. *Disaster implications:* Overcrowding of non-immune groups and collapse of the sanitary infrastructure pose an epidemic threat.

E. *International measures:*

1) Poliomyelitis is a Disease under surveillance by WHO and targeted for eradication. Since 2007, countries party to the International Health Regulations (2005) are required to inform WHO immediately of individual cases of paralytic

polio due to wild poliovirus, and to report details and extent of virus transmission. Countries should also report wild poliovirus isolated from other sources (e.g. environmental sampling), and polio cases due to circulating vaccine-derived poliovirus. Planning of a large-scale immunization response must begin immediately and be completed within 72 hours, and if appropriate, be coordinated with bordering countries. Primary isolation of the virus is best accomplished in a designated Global Polio Eradication Laboratory. Once a wild poliovirus is isolated, molecular epidemiology can help trace the source. At-risk countries should submit weekly reports on cases of poliomyelitis, AFP cases and AFP surveillance performance to their respective WHO offices until the world has been certified polio-free.

2) International travelers visiting polio-infected areas should be adequately immunized. For more information see the WHO publication *International travel and health*.

3) WHO Collaborating Centres provide support as required. More information can be found at:

http://www.who.int/collaboratingcentres/database/en/

Further information can be found at:

http://www.who.int/gpv/

PSITTACOSIS ICD-9 073; ICD-10 A70
(*Chlamydia* [or *Chlamydophila*] *psittaci* infection, Ornithosis, Parrot fever, Avian chlamydiosis)
[CCDM19: L. Hicks]

1. Identification—An acute generalized chlamydial disease with variable clinical presentations, caused by infection with the bacterium *Chlamydia psittaci*. It is primarily an infection of birds, but can cause pneumonia and other severe health problems in humans. Fever, headache, rash, myalgia, chills and upper or lower respiratory tract disease are common. Respiratory symptoms are often mild when compared with the extensive pneumonia demonstrable by X-ray examination. Cough is initially absent or nonproductive; when present, sputum is mucopurulent and scant. Pleuritic chest pain and splenomegaly occur infrequently; pulse may be slow in relation to temperature. Encephalitis, myocarditis and thrombophlebitis are occasional complications; relapses may occur. Although usually mild or moderate, human disease can be severe, especially in untreated elderly persons.

Diagnosis may be suspected in patients with appropriate symptoms, a history of exposure to birds, and a 4-fold increase in antibody titers to chlamydial antigens in sera collected at least 2–3 weeks apart. Isolation of the infectious agent from sputum, blood or postmortem tissues in mice, eggs or cell culture, under safe laboratory conditions only, confirms the diagnosis. Recovery of the infectious agent may be difficult, especially if the patient has received broad-spectrum antibiotics.

2. **Infectious agent**—*Chlamydia* (or *Chlamydophila*) *psittaci*.

3. **Occurrence**—Worldwide. May be associated with a pet bird, whether obviously sick or apparently healthy. Outbreaks occasionally occur in households, pet shops, aviaries, avian exhibits and pigeon lofts. Most human cases are sporadic; many infections are probably not diagnosed.

4. **Reservoir**—Mainly in birds of the parrot family (a.k.a. psittacine birds—including parakeets, parrots and love birds); less often in poultry, pigeons, canaries and sea birds. Apparently healthy birds can be carriers and shed the infectious agent, particularly when subjected to stress through crowding and shipping.

5. **Mode of transmission**—By inhaling the agent from desiccated droppings, secretions and dust from feathers of infected birds. Imported psittacine birds are the most frequent source of exposure, followed by turkey and duck farms; processing and rendering plants have also been sources of occupational disease. Geese and pigeons are occasionally responsible for human disease. Laboratory infections can occur. Rarely, person-to-person transmission may occur during acute illness with paroxysmal coughing. Due to a lack of specific laboratory testing, there is a possibility that such reported cases may have been caused by the recently described *C. pneumoniae* rather than *C. psittaci*.

6. **Incubation period**—From 1 to 4 weeks.

7. **Period of communicability**—Birds (diseased or seemingly healthy) may shed the agent intermittently, and sometimes continuously, for weeks or months.

8. **Susceptibility**—Susceptibility is general, post-infection immunity incomplete and transitory. Older adults may be more severely affected. There is no evidence that persons with antibodies are protected.

9. **Methods of control**—

   A. *Preventive measures:*

      1) Educate the public to the danger of exposure to infected pet birds. Medical personnel responsible for occupational health

in processing plants should be aware that febrile respiratory illness with headache or myalgia among employees exposed to birds may be psittacosis.

2) Regulate the importation, raising and trafficking of birds of the parrot family. Prevent or eliminate avian infections through quarantine and appropriate antibiotics.

3) Psittacine birds offered for sale should be raised under psittacosis-free conditions and handled in such a manner as to prevent infection. Tetracyclines can be effective in controlling disease in psittacines and other companion birds if properly administered to ensure adequate intake for at least 30 and preferably 45 days.

4) Conduct surveillance at pet shops and aviaries where psittacosis has occurred or where birds epidemiologically linked to cases were obtained, and of farms or processing plants to which human psittacosis was traced. Infected birds must be treated or destroyed, and the area where they were housed thoroughly cleaned and disinfected with a phenolic compound.

B. *Control of patient, contacts and the immediate environment:*

1) Report to local health authority: Obligatory case report in many countries, Class 2 (see *Reporting*).

2) Isolation: Not applicable. Coughing patients should be instructed to cough into paper tissue or upper arm.

3) Concurrent disinfection: Of all discharges.

4) Quarantine: Of infected farms (or premises with infected birds) until the buildings have been disinfected and diseased birds destroyed or adequately treated with tetracycline.

5) Immunization of contacts: Not applicable.

6) Investigation of contacts and source of infection: Trace origin of suspected birds. If they cannot be killed, ship swab-cultures of their cloacae or droppings to the laboratory in appropriate transport media and shipping containers, in compliance with postal regulations; after the cultures are taken, the birds should be treated with a tetracycline drug. If they can be killed, immerse bodies after slaughter in 2% phenolic or equivalent disinfectant. Place in plastic bags, close securely and ship frozen (on dry ice) to nearest laboratory capable of isolating *Chlamydia*.

7) Specific treatment: Antibiotics of the tetracycline group, given to those over eight years of age, until 10-14 days after temperature returns to normal. Erythromycin is an alternative when tetracycline is contraindicated (in pregnancy and in children under eight).

C. *Epidemic measures:* Cases are usually sporadic or confined to family outbreaks, but epidemics related to infected aviaries or bird suppliers may be extensive. Report outbreaks of avian psittacosis to agricultural and public health authorities. In poultry flocks, large doses of tetracycline can suppress, but not eliminate, infection, and thus may complicate investigations.

D. *Disaster implications:* None.

E. *International measures:* Compliance with national regulations to control importation of psittacine birds.

Q FEVER
(Query fever)
[CCDM19: R. Massung]
[CCDM18: D. Raoult]

ICD-9 083.0; ICD-10 A78

1. **Identification**—An acute febrile disease; onset may be sudden with chills, retrobulbar headache, weakness, malaise and severe sweats. There is considerable variation in severity and duration; infections may be inapparent or present as a nonspecific fever of unknown origin. A pneumonitis may be found on X-ray examination, but cough, expectoration, chest pain and physical findings in the lungs are not prominent. Abnormal liver function tests are common. Acute and chronic granulomatous hepatitis, which can be confused with tuberculous hepatitis, has been reported. Chronic Q fever manifests primarily as endocarditis and this form of the disease can occur in up to half the people with antecedent valvular disease. Q fever endocarditis can occur on prosthetic or abnormal native cardiac valves; these infections may have an indolent course, extending over years, and can present up to 2 years after initial infection. Other rare clinical syndromes, including neurological syndromes, have been described. The case-fatality rate in untreated acute cases is usually less than 1%; it is negligible in treated cases, except for individuals who develop endocarditis, in whom protracted antibiotic courses are the rule. A post-Q fever fatigue syndrome has been described.

Laboratory diagnosis is made by demonstration of a rise in specific antibodies between acute and convalescent stages by IF or CF, or by IgM detection through IF or ELISA. Diagnosis is facilitated by use of 2 antigen preparations: phase I, which represents the infectious agent, and phase II, which is a laboratory-generated attenuated form with truncated LPS. Antibodies to phase II antigens are found at higher levels than Phase I antibodies in the acute period, and the reverse is true in chronic disease; high antibody titers to phase I may indicate chronic infection, such as endocarditis. Recovery of the infectious agent from blood is diagnostic, but requires BSL-3 containment facilities, as the procedure poses a hazard to laboratory workers. Bacteria may be identified in tissues (liver biopsy or heart valve) by immunohistochemistry and EM. PCR has also been used.

2. Infectious agent—*Coxiella burnetii*. The organism can be found in high concentrations in tissues of infected animals, particularly placenta tissues, and is highly resistant to many disinfectants and environmental conditions.

3. Occurrence—Reported from all continents; the real incidence is greater than that reported, because of the mildness of many cases, limited clinical suspicion, and lack of availability of diagnostic assays and laboratories. It is endemic in areas where reservoir animals are present, and affects veterinarians, meat workers, sheep (and occasionally dairy) workers, and farmers. Epidemics have occurred among workers in stockyards, meatpacking and rendering plants, and laboratories, and in medical and veterinary centers that use sheep (especially pregnant ewes) in research. Individual cases may occur where no direct animal contact can be demonstrated. Evidence of previous infection is common among researchers working with *C. burnetii*, and cases have occurred among casual visitors to such facilities.

4. Reservoir—Sheep, cattle, goats, cats, dogs, some wild mammals (bandicoots and many species of feral rodents), birds and ticks are natural reservoirs. Trans-ovarial and trans-stadial transmission are common in ticks that participate in wildlife cycles in rodents, larger animals and birds. Infected animals are often asymptomatic, but shed massive numbers of organisms in placental tissues at parturition; abortions may occur in sheep and goats, particularly in naive populations where the agent has recently been introduced.

5. Mode of transmission—Commonly through airborne dissemination of *Coxiellae* in dust from premises contaminated by placental tissues, birth fluids and excreta of infected animals; in establishments processing infected animals or their byproducts; and in necropsy rooms. Airborne particles containing organisms may be carried downwind for a distance of one kilometer or more; contamination also occurs through direct contact with infected animals and other contaminated materials, such as wool, straw, fertilizer and laundry. Raw milk from infected cattle or goats contains organisms and may be responsible for some cases. Direct transmission by blood or marrow transfusion has been reported. Tick-to-human transmission occurs rarely, if ever. There have also been rare cases of person-to-person transmission, e.g. following delivery of an infant from an infected woman, or autopsy of an infected cadaver.

6. Incubation period—Dependent on the size of the infecting dose; typically 2–3 weeks; range: 3–30 days.

7. Period of communicability—Direct person-to-person transmission occurs rarely, if ever. However, contaminated clothing may be a source of infection.

8. Susceptibility—Susceptibility is general. Immunity following recovery from clinical illness may be life-long, with cell-mediated immunity lasting longer than humoral immunity. Antibodies detected by CF persist for 3–5 years: antibodies detected by IF may persist as long as 10–15 years.

9. Methods of control—

A. Preventive measures:

1) Educate persons in high-risk occupations (sheep, goat and dairy farmers, veterinary researchers, abattoir workers, etc.) on sources of infection and the necessity for adequate disinfection and disposal of animal products of conception; restrict access to sheds, barns and laboratories with potentially infected animals; and stress the value of inactivation procedures such as pasteurization of milk.

2) Pasteurizing milk from cows, goats and sheep at 62.7°C (145°F) for 30 minutes or at 71.6°C (161°F) for 15 seconds, or boiling, inactivates Q fever *Coxiellae*.

3) The only commercially available vaccine is in Australia. Immunization with inactivated vaccines prepared from *C. burnetii* phase I-infected yolk sac is useful in protecting laboratory workers and is strongly recommended for those working with live *C. burnetii*. It should also be considered for abattoir workers and others in hazardous occupations, including those carrying out medical research with pregnant sheep. To avoid severe local reactions, vaccine administration should be preceded by a skin sensitivity test with a small dose of diluted vaccine; vaccine should not be given to individuals with a positive skin or antibody test or a documented history of Q fever.

4) Research workers using pregnant sheep should be identified and enrolled in a health education and surveillance program. This should include a baseline serum evaluation, followed by periodic (yearly) evaluations. Persons at risk (i.e. those with valvular heart disease, pregnant women, and persons who are immunosuppressed) should be advised of the risk of serious illness that may result from Q fever. Animals used in research can also be assessed for Q fever infection through serology. Laboratory clothes must be appropriately bagged and washed to prevent infection of laundry personnel. Sheep-holding facilities should be away from populated areas, and measures should be implemented in order to

prevent airflow to other occupied areas; no casual visitors should be permitted.

B. *Control of patient, contacts and the immediate environment:*

1) Report to local health authority. Q fever is a notifiable disease in the USA, but not in many countries; Class 3 (see *Reporting*).
2) Isolation: Not applicable.
3) Disinfection: Autoclaving is recommended to sterilize research materials, veterinary byproducts, and contaminated clothing. Gamma irradiation is effective for inactivation of live bacteria, but typically limited to small volumes such as antigen preparations. Quaternary ammonium compounds combined with detergents (MicroChem, Enviro-Chem), or 70% ethanol, may be used for surface disinfection. Universal precautions should be used during postmortem examination of suspected cases in humans or animals.
4) Quarantine: Not applicable.
5) Immunization of contacts: Unnecessary.
6) Investigation of contacts and source of infection: Search for history of: contact with sheep, cattle or goats on farms or in research facilities, or parturient cats; consumption of raw milk; or direct or indirect association with a laboratory that handles *C. burnetii*.
7) Specific treatment: Acute disease: Tetracyclines (particularly doxycycline) administered orally for 14–21 days; doxycycline and hydroxychloroquine may prevent the development of endocarditis in patients with acute Q fever and valvulopathy. Quinolones are also used to treat Q fever (NB tetracyclines cannot be used in children less than eight years of age). In cases of pregnancy: cotrimoxazole throughout the pregnancy. Chronic disease (endocarditis): doxycycline in combination with hydroxychloroquine for 18 to 36 months or doxycycline plus rifampin for 3 years; doxycycline plus quinolone is also used. Surgical replacement of the infected valve may be necessary in some patients for hemodynamic reasons.

C. *Epidemic measures:* Outbreaks are generally of short duration; control measures are limited essentially to elimination of sources of infection, observation of exposed people, and provision of antibiotics to those becoming ill. Detection is particularly important in pregnant women, the immunosuppressed, and patients with cardiac valve lesions.

D. *Disaster implications:* None.

E. **International measures:** Measures to ensure the safe importation of goats, sheep and cattle, and their products (e.g. wool, hides). WHO Collaborating Centres provide support as required. More information can be found at:

http://www.who.int/collaboratingcentres/database/en/

F. **Measures in case of deliberate use:** *C. burnetii* is easy to produce in animals, can be desiccated and transmitted through aerosol. It is thought that scientists have worked on its possible use as a bioterrorism weapon. Immunocompromised patients, people with valvular diseases, and pregnant women should be actively diagnosed and treated.

For more information on the deliberate use of infectious agents to cause harm, see the section on *Deliberate use*.

RABIES   ICD-9 071; ICD-10 A82
(Hydrophobia)
(Post-exposure prophylaxis [PEP] Guide follows at end of chapter)
[CCDM19: T. Hemachuda, F. Meslin, C. Rupprecht, H. Wilde]
[CCDM18: F. Meslin]

1. **Identification**—Rabies is an acute viral infection, causing progressive viral encephalomyelitis that is nearly always fatal. Transmission is usually through saliva via the bite of an infected animal, with dogs being the main transmitter of rabies to humans. Onset is generally heralded by a sense of apprehension, headache, fever, malaise and sensory changes (paresthesia) at the site of an animal bite. Excitability, aero- and/or hydrophobia, often with spasms of swallowing muscles, are frequent symptoms. Delirium with occasional convulsions follows. Such classic symptoms of furious rabies are noted in two-thirds of the cases, whereas the remaining present as paralysis of limbs and respiratory muscles with sparing of consciousness. Phobic spasms may be absent in this paralytic form. Coma and death ensue within 1–2 weeks, mainly due to cardiac failure. Diagnosis is made through specific FA staining of brain tissue or virus isolation in mouse or cell cultures. Antemortem diagnosis can be made by specific FA staining of viral antigens in frozen skin sections taken from the back of the neck at the hairline, detection of viral antibodies in serum and CSF, and specific amplification of viral nucleic acids in saliva or skin biopsies by RT-PCR. Serological diagnosis is based on neutralization tests in cell culture or in mice. Viral shedding in body secretions is intermittent and molecular studies need to be repeated if initially found negative.

2. Infectious agents—Lyssaviruses, such as rabies virus, are in the family *Rhabdoviridae* in the genus *Lyssavirus*. All members of the genus are antigenically related, but use of monoclonal antibodies and nucleotide sequencing demonstrates differences according to animal species or geographical origin. Lyssaviruses in Africa (Mokola and Duvenhage) and Eurasia (European bat lyssaviruses) have been associated with fatal encephalitis. A lyssavirus, first identified in 1996 in several species of flying foxes and bats in Australia, has been associated with 2 human deaths from rabies. These viruses, named Australian bat lyssaviruses, are closely related, but not identical, to classical rabies virus. Illnesses suspected due to rabies by other lyssaviruses may be diagnosed by the standard FA test on brain tissue or by suggested antemortem tests. Several other lyssaviruses (e.g. Aravan virus, Irkut virus, Khujand virus, Lagos bat virus, West Caucasian bat virus) have been characterized as etiological agents of rabies in mammals, but have not so far been identified in human infections.

3. Occurrence—Worldwide, more than 10 million human exposures are estimated, and an estimated 55 000 rabies deaths occur each year, almost all in developing countries, particularly in Asia (31 000 deaths) and Africa (24 000 deaths). Most human deaths follow dog bites for which adequate post-exposure prophylaxis was not or could not be provided. In Latin America, a regional dog rabies control program coordinated by PAHO since 1983 has led to a reduction of almost 95% in the number of human deaths, with only 26 cases reported in 2007, 46% of which followed contacts with hematophagous bats. During the past 12 years, although reduction of the numbers of human cases have been reported in several Asian countries (particularly Thailand), drastic increases have occurred in China—where since 1996 the number of notified human rabies deaths has continuously increased, reaching 3 300 in 2006—and Viet Nam. Western, central and eastern Europe, including Russia, report less than 50 human rabies deaths annually. In the USA between 2000 and 2007, 20 of 25 human deaths from rabies were acquired domestically. Of those infected within the USA, almost all were bat-associated rabies (as identified by viral variant analysis). Rabies can present in atypical forms, and medical personnel unfamiliar with the disease may misdiagnose it. This is one factor in underreporting of this disease worldwide.

Rabies is a zoonotic disease, primarily associated with the bite of infected mammals. Given the global distribution of bat rabies, few areas are truly free of autochthonous rabies in the animal population. Some sites include insular locations in the western Pacific and parts of the Caribbean. Dogs transmit rabies in most developing countries, whereas in many developed countries, rabies is a disease of wild carnivores, with sporadic spillover infection to domestic animals. In Canada, and the USA, oral immunization of free-ranging wild carnivores has controlled rabies over large areas, via the distribution of vaccine-laden baits. By 2000, many western European countries had likewise successfully eliminated fox rabies by oral immunization.

4. Reservoirs—All mammals are susceptible. Reservoirs and important vectors include wild and domestic Canidae, such as dogs, foxes, coyotes, wolves and jackals; also, skunks, raccoons, raccoon dogs, mongooses and other common carnivores, such as cats in North America. In developing countries, dogs remain the principal reservoir. Infected populations of vampire, frugivorous and insectivorous bats occur in Mexico and Central and South America, and infected insectivorous bats are present throughout Canada, the USA and Eurasia. In Africa and Australia, infected frugivorous and insectivorous bat species are involved in transmission. Many other mammals, such as rabbits, squirrels, chipmunks, rats, mice and opossums are very rarely infected.

5. Modes of transmission—The most common form of exposure is virus-laden saliva from a rabid animal introduced though a bite or scratch (and very rarely into a fresh break in the skin or through intact mucous membranes). Person-to-person transmission is theoretically possible, but is rare and not well documented. Several cases of rabies transmission by transplant of cornea, solid organs and blood vessels from persons dying of undiagnosed CNS disease have been reported from Asia, Europe and North America. Airborne spread has been suggested in a cave where heavy infestations of bats were roosting, and demonstrated in laboratory settings, but this occurs very rarely. Transmission from infected vampire bats feeding on domestic animals is common in Latin America. Rabid insectivorous or frugivorous bats can transmit rabies to terrestrial animals, wild or domestic.

6. Incubation period—The period is highly variable, but usually 3–8 weeks, and very rarely as short as a few days, or as long as several years. The length of the incubation period depends in part on wound severity, wound location in relation to nerve supply, and relative distance from the brain; the amount and variant of virus; the degree of protection provided by clothing; and other factors.

7. Period of communicability—Defined periods of communicability of animal hosts are only known with reliability in domestic dogs, cats, and ferrets, and are usually for 3–7 days before onset of clinical signs (rarely over 4 days) and throughout the course of the disease. Longer periods of excretion before onset of clinical signs (14 days) have been observed with certain canine rabies virus variants in experimental infections, but these are the exception. Excretion in other animals is highly variable: for example, in one study bats shed virus for 12 days before evidence of illness, while in another, skunks shed virus for at least 8 days before onset of clinical signs.

8. Susceptibility—All mammals are susceptible to varying degrees; the degree of susceptibility may be influenced by the virus variant as well as by certain host parameters (age, health, nutrition, etc.). Humans may be more resistant to infection than several other animal species; for example, a study in the Islamic Republic of Iran showed that, of those bitten by proven rabid animals and not treated, about 40% developed the disease.

9. **Methods of control—**

   A. *Preventive measures:* Many preventive measures are possible at the level of the primary animal host(s) and transmitter(s) of rabies to humans. Such measures are part of a comprehensive rabies control program.

   1) Register, license and vaccinate all owned dogs, and other pets when feasible, in enzootic countries; control ownerless animals and strays. Educate pet owners and the public on the importance of local community responsibilities (e.g. pets should be leashed in congested areas when not confined on the owner's premises; strange-acting or sick animals of any species— domestic or wild—should be avoided and not handled; animals that have bitten a person or another animal should be reported to relevant authorities, such as the police/local health departments; if possible, such animals should be confined and observed as a preventive measure; and wildlife should be appreciated in nature and not be kept as pets). Where animal population reduction is impractical, animal contraception and repetitive vaccination campaigns may prove effective.

   2) Maintain active surveillance for animal rabies. Laboratory capacity should be developed to perform FA diagnosis on all wild mammals involved in human or domestic animal exposures, and all domestic animals clinically suspected of having rabies.

   3) Detain and observe for 10 days any healthy-appearing dog or cat known to have bitten a person (stray or ownerless dogs and cats may be euthanized and examined for rabies by fluorescent microscopy); dogs and cats showing suspicious clinical signs of rabies should be euthanized and tested for rabies. If the biting animal was infective at the time of the bite, it usually develops signs of rabies within 4-7 days, such as change in behavior, excitability or paralysis, followed by acute death. All wild mammals that have bitten a person should be euthanized and the brain examined for evidence of rabies.

   4) In a timely manner, submit to a qualified laboratory the intact head of suspect animals, packed in ice (not frozen), for viral diagnosis.

5) Euthanize unvaccinated domestic animals bitten by known rabid animals; if detention is elected, hold the animal in a secure facility for at least 6 months under veterinary supervision, and vaccinate against rabies 30 days before release. If previously vaccinated, booster immediately with rabies vaccine, and detain for at least 45 days.

6) Immunize wild carnivore reservoirs and free-ranging domestic dogs, using vaccine-laden baits containing attenuated or recombinant rabies viral vectors, as utilized in Europe and North America.

7) Cooperate with wildlife conservation authorities in programs to reduce the carrying capacity of wildlife hosts of sylvatic rabies, and to reduce exposures to domestic animals and human populations—such as in circumscribed enzootic areas near campsites, and in areas of dense human habitation.

8) Vaccinate individuals at high risk of exposure (e.g. veterinarians and veterinary technicians, animal control staff, wildlife researchers, cavers, staff of quarantine kennels, laboratory and field personnel working with rabies virus, and long-term travelers to rabies-endemic areas). Such persons should receive pre-exposure immunization, using potent and safe cell-culture vaccines (CCVs). Vaccine can be administered in doses of 1.0 ml or 0.5 ml intramuscularly (IM) on days 0, 7 and 21 or 28. Post-immunization serological testing is advisable every 6 months to 2 years, depending upon the defined level of exposure, as long as the risk remains. Results with intradermal (ID) immunization (using WHO recommended schedules) for Human Diploid Cell rabies Vaccine (HDCV), Purified Chick Embryo (PCECV) and Purified Vero Cell Vaccines (PVRVP) have been equivalent to what is expected from the intramuscular schedule. Antibody response to ID immunization has been less than ideal in some groups receiving chloroquine for antimalarial chemoprophylaxis. Although the comparative immune response has not been evaluated for antimalarials structurally related to chloroquine (e.g. mefloquine, hydroxychloroquine), similar precautions for individuals receiving these drugs should be followed. The human diploid cell vaccine (HDCV) was the original gold standard for modern human rabies prophylaxis, but is too expensive for developing countries. Other cell-culture vaccines fulfilling basic WHO requirements for the ID route, such as purified vero cell and chick embryo cell vaccines, are widely and successfully used in canine rabies-endemic countries.

If a risk of exposure continues, single booster doses are

given, or—preferably—serum is tested at regular intervals for neutralizing antibody detection, dependent upon relative risk of exposure, and booster doses are given only when indicated.

9) Prevention of rabies after animal bites ("post-exposure prophylaxis" or PEP) consists of the following:

a) *First aid:* Clean and flush the wound immediately with soap or detergent and water (or water alone), then apply either 70% ethanol, tincture of aqueous solution of iodine or povidone iodine, or Dakins solution (household bleach: 3 tablespoons of bleach plus ½ teaspoon baking soda in 1 liter of boiled water). The wound should not be sutured unless unavoidable. Sutures, if required, should be placed after local infiltration of antiserum (see 9b); they should be loose, and should not interfere with free bleeding and drainage.

b) *Specific treatment (serum and vaccine):* Specific passive prophylaxis in humans is provided by administration of human (HRIG) or equine (ERIG) rabies immune globulin at the site of the bite as soon as possible after exposure, to neutralize the virus; and is followed by vaccine at a different site to elicit active immunity. Animal studies suggest that human disease caused by the Australian bat lyssavirus may be prevented by rabies vaccine and RIG, and such PEP is recommended for persons bitten or scratched by any bat in Australia. Although PEP may not always be effective for the prevention of bat lyssaviruses throughout the world, it should always be performed.

Passive immunization: HRIG should be used in a single dose of 20 IU/kg, and ERIG in a single dose of 40 IU/kg. All or as much as possible of this should be infiltrated into and around the bite wound; the remainder, if any, should be given IM. Where serum of animal origin (ERIG) is used, an intradermal or subcutaneous test dose has been used preceding administration to detect potential allergic sensitivity, but the utility of this testing for predictive risk has been questionable.

WHO-approved cell-culture vaccines should be applied according to the WHO and USA-CDC approved "Essen Regimen," in 5 IM doses of 0.5 or 1.0 ml on days 0, 3, 7, 14 and 28 (see manufacturer's instructions), in the deltoid region or lateral thigh muscles. This is to start as soon as possible after exposure. In Europe, Asia, Africa, South and Central America, a second WHO-approved regimen is widely used and found to be safe and effective; this is referred to as the "2-1-1" or "Zagreb" Regimen, and consists of two full intramuscular doses at two sites on day 0, and one injection each on days 7 and 21. It saves one vaccine dose and one clinic visit.

Reduced-dose, WHO-approved, multi-site intradermal post-exposure schedules have been approved by local authorities in several rabies-endemic countries of Asia and Africa where the cost of vaccine is a significant deterrent to proper post-exposure prophylaxis. WHO recommends 2 ID multi-site regimens with cell-culture vaccines known to be safe and immunogenic: i) the 2-site Thai Red Cross regimen (2-2-2-2); and ii) the 8-site Oxford regimen (8-0-4-0-1-1). If properly applied using potent modern vaccines, these schedules result in an antibody response equivalent to that seen with the two WHO-approved intramuscular regimens.

It has been well documented that subjects with severe immunodeficiency (very low CD4 counts) will not respond well to rabies vaccination. Some may not develop neutralizing antibody at all. Careful wound cleansing and the use of immunoglobulin is thus of great importance in such patients. Vaccination must be administered in the usual dose. A serum specimen should be collected at the time when the last dose of vaccine is administered and tested for rabies antibodies. If sensitization reactions appear in the course of immunization, consult the health department or infectious disease consultants for guidance. If the person has had a previous full course of pre- or post-exposure rabies immunization with an approved vaccine (see 9A8), only 2 doses of vaccine need to be given—one immediately, and one 3 days later. In the previously vaccinated person, RIG and ERIG are not used.

c) The combination of local wound treatment, passive immunization with RIG and active vaccination is recommended for all severe exposures (category III, see end of this item), virtually guaranteeing complete protection. Pregnancy and infancy are never contraindications to post-exposure prophylaxis (PEP). Persons presenting even months after the bite must be dealt with in the same way as recent exposures. Factors to be considered in the initiation of PEP are nature of the contact; rabies endemicity at site of encounter or origin of animal; animal species involved; vaccination/clinical status; availability of animal for observation; type of vaccine used; and laboratory results of animal for rabies, if available.

d) Modern cell-culture vaccines (CCVs) are considered to be safe and well tolerated, although reported reaction rates to primary immunization have varied with the monitoring system. Following IM immunization with the human diploid cell vaccine, mild and self-limited local reactions, such as pain at the site of injection, redness, and swelling, occur in 21%–74% of cases. Mild systemic reactions, such as fever, headache, dizziness, and gastrointestinal symptoms, occur in 5%–40% of cases, and systemic hypersensitivity following booster injections occurs in 6% of vaccines, but is less common following primary immunization. When further purification steps are added, systemic hypersensitivity reactions become very rare. With chick embryo and Vero cell-based vaccines, the rates of local and mild systemic reactions are similar to those of the human diploid cell vaccine, but no systemic hypersensitivity reactions have been reported. Compared with IM vaccination, the ID application is at least as safe and well tolerated, although local irritation may be more frequent. No significant adverse reactions have been attributed to HRIG; however, antiserum from a nonhuman source produces serum sickness in 5%–40% of recipients. Newer, commercially produced purified animal globulins, in particular purified equine globulin, have only a 1–6% risk of serum sickness reactions. The commonly used skin test for ERIG will not predict serum sickness. Serious anaphylaxis is extremely rare with purified ERIG products (2 in over 150 000 cases in one series). The risk of contracting fatal rabies outweighs the risks for allergic reactions.

B. Control of patient, contacts and the immediate environment:

1) Report to local health authority: Obligatory case report required in most countries, Class 2 (see *Reporting*).
2) Isolation: Contact with salivary secretions of a rabid patient should be avoided during the illness.
3) Concurrent disinfection: Of saliva and articles soiled therewith. Although transmission from a patient to attending personnel has not been documented, immediate attendants should be warned of the potential hazard of infection from saliva, and should wear gloves, protective gowns, and other appropriate personal protection equipment to avoid exposure from a coughing patient.
4) Quarantine: Not applicable.
5) Immunization of contacts: Contacts who receive a bite or have an open wound or mucous membrane exposure

to the patient's saliva should receive specific PEP (see 9A9b).

6) Investigation of contacts and source of infection: Search for rabid animals and for people and other animals bitten.

7) Specific treatment: For clinical rabies, intensive supportive medical care.

C. Epidemic (epizootic) measures: Applicable only to animals; a sporadic disease in humans.

1) Establish control area under authority of laws, regulations and ordinances, in cooperation with appropriate human, agricultural and wildlife conservation authorities.

2) Immunize dogs and cats through officially sponsored, intensified mass programs that provide immunizations at temporary and emergency stations. For protection of other domestic animals, use approved vaccines appropriate for each animal species.

3) In urban areas of industrialized countries, strict enforcement of regulations requiring collection, detention and euthanasia of ownerless and stray dogs, and of non-immunized dogs found off owners' premises; control of the dog population by castration, spaying or drugs have been effective in breaking transmission cycles.

4) Immunization of wildlife through baits containing vaccine has contained red fox rabies in western Europe and southern Canada, and coyote, gray fox, and raccoon rabies in the USA.

D. Disaster implications: A potential problem exists if the disease is freshly introduced or enzootic in an area where there are many stray dogs or wild reservoir animals. Similarly, in disaster areas—for example after hurricanes or tsunamis—many stray animals may occur after human evacuations, with subsequent bites to animal control or humane society personnel taking part in future rescue attempts.

E. International measures:

1) Strict compliance by common carriers and travelers with national laws and regulations (see *International travel and Health*, WHO 2007, chapter 5, p 73). Immunization of animals, certificates of health and origin, and microchip identification of animals may be required.

2) WHO Collaborating Centres and other international organizations and institutions prepared to collaborate with national

services on request. See WHO Expert Consultation on Rabies, first report, TRS 931, WHO, Geneva, 2005, annex 3, pp 76–80. More information on Collaborating Centres can be found at <http://www.who.int/collaboratingcentres/data base/en/>.

POST-EXPOSURE PROPHYLAXIS GUIDE

In addition to prophylaxis as described under 9A, B, Consult regional, provincial, local, state, or national health officials if questions arise about the need for rabies prophylaxis.

WHO recommendations for PEP rabies management follow:

Category of exposure	Type of contact with a suspect or confirmed rabid domestic or wild[a] animal or if the animal is unavailable for observation	WHO Recommendations
Category I (no exposure)	Touching or feeding of animal; licks on intact skin	None, if reliable case history available
Category II	Nibbling of uncovered skin Minor scratches or abrasion without bleeding	Administer vaccine immediately[b] Stop prophylaxis if animal remains healthy throughout observation (10 days) or is euthanized and found to be negative for viral antigens by appropriate laboratory techniques[c]
Category III	Single or multiple transdermal bites or scratches; contamination of mucous membranes with saliva (licks); licks on broken skin	Administer HRIG or ERIG followed by vaccine immediately[b] Stop prophylaxis if animal remains healthy throughout observation (10 days), or is euthanized and found to be negative for viral antigens by appropriate laboratory techniques

[a]Exposure to most small mammals, such as insectivores (e.g. shrews), rodents (e.g. mice, rats, squirrels, etc.), and lagomorphs (e.g. rabbits and hares) seldom if ever requires specific rabies prophylaxis.

[b]The placing of an apparently healthy dog or cat in or from a low-risk area under careful supervision may warrant delaying prophylaxis.

[c]Applicable only to dogs and cats. Except for threatened or endangered species, other animals suspected of rabies should be euthanized and their tissues examined using appropriate laboratory techniques.

508 / RABIES

USA recommendations for post-exposure management follow (ACIP: Human Rabies Prevention–United States, 1999: Recommendations of Advisory Committee on Immunization Practices (ACIP). *MMWR*, **48**: (RR) 1–21, 1999):

Vaccination Status	Regimen[a]
Not previously vaccinated	**Wound cleansing** All PEP to begin with immediate and thorough cleansing of all wounds with soap and water. If available, a virucidal agent such as a povidone-iodine solution should be used to irrigate the wounds. **HRIG** Administer 20 IU/kg body weight. If anatomically feasible, *the full dose* should be infiltrated around the wound(s); any remaining volume should be administered intramuscularly (IM) at an anatomic site distant from that of vaccine administration (such as the anterior-lateral aspect of the thigh). RIG should not be administered in the same syringe or location as the vaccine. Because HRIG may partially suppress active production of antibody, no more than the recommended dose should be given. **Vaccine** HDCV or PCECV, 1.0 ml, IM (deltoid area[b]); one each on days 0[c], 3, 7, 14, and 28.
Previously vaccinated[d]	**Wound cleansing** All post-exposure prophylaxis to begin with immediate and thorough cleansing of all wounds with soap and water. If available, a virucidal agent such as a povidone-iodine solution should be used to irrigate wounds. **RIG** RIG should *not* be administered. **Vaccine** HDCV or PCEV, 1.0 mL, IM (deltoid area[b]); one each on days 0[c] and 3.

[a]Regimens are applicable for all age groups, including children.

[b]The deltoid area is the only acceptable site of vaccination for adults and older children. For younger children, the outer aspect of the thigh may be used. Never administer vaccine in the gluteal area.

[c]Day 0 is the day the 1st dose of vaccine is administered.

[d]History of pre-exposure vaccination with HDCV, RVA (rabies vaccine, adsorbed), or PCECV; prior post-exposure prophylaxis with HDCV, RVA, or PCECV; or previous vaccination with any other type of rabies vaccine and a documented history of antibody response to the prior vaccination.

RAT-BITE FEVER
[CCDM19: K. Glynn]

ICD-9 026; ICD-10 A25

The general term "rat-bite fever" refers to two rare bacterial zoonoses: streptobacillosis (also known as streptobacillary fever or Haverhill fever) is caused by *Streptobacillus moniliformis*; and Sodoku (or spirillary fever) is caused by *Spirillum minus*. Because of their clinical and epidemiological similarities, only streptobacillosis is presented in detail below; variations manifested by *S. minus* infection are noted in a brief summary.

I. STREPTOBACILLOSIS   ICD-9 026.1; ICD-10 A25.1
(Streptobacillary fever, Haverhill fever, Epidemic arthritic erythema)

1. Identification—An abrupt onset of chills, fever, headache and muscle pain is followed within 1–3 days by a maculopapular rash most marked on the extremities. The rash may also be petechial, purpuric or pustular. A non-suppurative polyarthritis may develop in over half of cases. There is usually a history of a rat bite, which healed normally, within the previous 10 days. Relapses are common in untreated patients, with an approximate case-fatality rate of 7%–10%. Bacterial endocarditis, pericarditis, parotitis, tenosynovitis and focal abscesses of soft tissues or the brain may occur late in untreated cases. Laboratory confirmation is through isolation of the organism by inoculating material from the primary lesion, lymph node, blood, joint fluid or pus into the appropriate bacteriological medium enriched with 20% blood, serum, or ascitic fluid, or into laboratory animals (guinea pigs or mice that are not naturally infected). *S. moniliformis* is a fastidious, slow-growing organism; therefore, cultures should be maintained for at least three weeks. Serological testing is currently not reliable.

2. Infectious agent—*Streptobacillus moniliformis*.

3. Occurrence—Worldwide, but uncommon in North and South America and most European countries.

4. Reservoir—Infected rats, rarely other rodents (squirrels, mice, gerbils), and cats, dogs, ferrets, and weasels, which may become infected when hunting rodents.

5. Mode of transmission—*S. moniliformis* and *S. minus* are commensal organisms of rats, and can be found in the oral, nasal and conjunctival secretions and urine of an infected animal. Transmission most frequently occurs through biting, but sporadic cases may occur without history of a bite. Blood from an experimental laboratory animal has infected humans. Direct contact with rats is not necessary; infection has occurred in people working or living in rat-infested buildings. In outbreaks of Haverhill fever, milk or water contaminated by rat urine or feces has usually been suspected as the vehicle of infection.

6. Incubation period—Usually from 3 to 10 days; can range from 2 days to 3 weeks.

7. Period of communicability—No direct person-to-person transmission has been reported.

8. Susceptibility—No information.

9. Methods of control—

A. *Preventive measures:* Rat-proof dwellings and reduce rat populations. Prevent contamination of food and water sources by rodents. Use appropriate restraining techniques and protective equipment when handling rodents. Penicillin or doxycycline may be used as prophylaxis following a rat bite, since up to 10% of rat bites may result in rat-bite fever. Doxycycline cannot be used in children less than eight years of age.

B. *Control of patient, contacts and the immediate environment:*

1) Report to local health authority: Obligatory report of epidemics in most countries; no case report required, Class 4 (see *Reporting*).
2) Isolation: Standard precautions are recommended.
3) Concurrent disinfection: Not applicable.
4) Quarantine: Not applicable.
5) Immunization of contacts: Not applicable.
6) Investigation of contacts and source of infection: To establish whether there are additional unrecognized cases.
7) Specific treatment: Penicillin, tetracyclines or erythromycin, for 7–10 days. Treatment may shorten clinical course and reduce occurrence of complications. Tetracyclines cannot be used in children less than eight years of age.

C. *Epidemic measures:* A cluster of cases requires search for a common source, possibly contaminated food and water.

D. *Disaster implications:* None.

E. *International measures:* None.

II. SPIRILLOSIS   ICD-9 026.0; ICD-10 A25.0
(Spirillary fever, Sodoku, Rat-bite fever due to *Spirillum minus*)

Rat bite fever caused by *Spirillum minus* is the common form of sporadic rat-bite fever in Asia and Africa. Clinically, *Spirillum minus* disease differs from streptobacillary fever in the presence of an indurated or ulcerated lesion at the site of the bite when fever develops, the rarity of arthritic symptoms, and the presence of a distinctive rash of reddish or purplish plaques. The incubation period is usually between 14 and 18 days, with a range of 1 day to 6 weeks. Complications may resemble those of streptobacillary fever. Untreated, the case-fatality rate is approximately 10%. Laboratory methods are essential for differentiation; animal inoculation is used for isolation of *S. minus,* since it has not been successfully cultured on artificial media.

RELAPSING FEVER   ICD-9 087; ICD-10 A68
(Borrelia burgdorferi, Lyme borreliosis, Lyme disease)
(Borrelia recurrentis, Louse-borne relapsing fever)
[CCDM19: B. Chomel]
[CCDM18: D. Hulínská]

1. Identification—Relapsing fever is a zoonotic disease caused by several species of the spirochete *Borrelia*. It can be transmitted by lice or ticks depending on the species and the part of the world in which it occurs. It is a systemic louse-borne epidemic or tick-borne sporadic spirochetal disease in which periods of fever lasting 2–7 days alternate with afebrile periods of 7 days (range: 4–14 days); the number of relapses varies from 1 to 10 or more. Incubation period lasts on average 7 days (range: 2–18 days). Total duration of the louse-borne disease averages 13–16 days; this is usually longer (report of up to 10 years) for the tick-borne disease. Transitory petechial rashes are common during the initial febrile period. Symptoms vary with host immunity, the strain of *Borrelia* involved, and phase of the epidemic. Hematuria is rare, but epistaxis has been reported. Gastrointestinal involvement is common; respiratory and neurological symptoms are frequently observed in the USA, southern Europe and western Mediterranean countries; and meningeal symptoms are seen in Spain. Neuropsychiatric symptoms are more common in tick-borne than in louse-borne epidemics. Predisposing factors (thiamine and vitamin B deficiency) may lead to neuritis or encephalitis. Severity varies according to individual susceptibility (e.g. in Africa infections are severe for Europeans, but milder for the local population) and to geography (e.g. tick-borne infections may be severe in Egypt and Pakistan, and mild in Poland and Romania). The overall case-fatality rate in untreated cases is between 2% and 10%.

Diagnosis is made by the demonstration of the infectious agent in dark field preparations of fresh blood or stained thick or thin blood films taken during a febrile period, by intraperitoneal inoculation of immature laboratory mice with blood taken during the febrile period, or by blood culture in special media (BSK). *Borreliae* are usually absent from the blood between relapses.

2. Infectious agents—For louse-borne disease, *Borrelia recurrentis*, a gram-negative spirochete. In tick-borne borreliosis, different strains have been distinguished by area of first isolation and/or vector rather than by inherent biological differences. Strains isolated during a relapse often show antigenic differences from those obtained during the paroxysm immediately preceding it. In North America, most human cases are caused by *B. hermsii* transmitted by *Ornithodoros hermsii*. The classical agent of relapsing fever in Europe is *B. hispanica*. A "Spain strain" has recently been implicated in severe human disease. New relapsing fever-like spirochetes transmitted by hard ticks (*Ixodes, Amblyomma*) cause a tick-associated rash (Master disease) different from that transmitted by soft ticks (*Ornithodoros*).

3. Occurrence—Typically, the epidemic form is spread by lice, whereas the endemic or sporadic forms are spread by ticks. Louse-borne relapsing fever occurs in limited areas in Asia, eastern Africa (Burundi, Ethiopia and Sudan), highlands of central Africa, and South America. Tick-borne disease is endemic throughout tropical Africa, with other foci in India, the Islamic Republic of Iran, Portugal, Saudi Arabia, Spain, northern Africa, central Asia, and North and South America. Sporadic human cases and occasional outbreaks of tick-borne disease occur in limited areas of western Canada, the USA, and Europe. Relapsing fever has been observed in all parts of the world except Australia and New Zealand.

4. Reservoir—For *B. recurrentis*, humans; for tick-borne relapsing fever, *Borreliae*, wild rodents and argasid (soft) ticks.

5. Mode of transmission—Vector-borne; no direct person-to-person transmission. Louse-borne relapsing fever is acquired by crushing an infective louse, *Pediculus humanus*: this results in contamination of the bite wound or an abrasion of the skin. In tick-borne disease, people are infected by the bite or coxal fluid of an argasid tick, principally *Ornithodoros moubata* and *O. hispanica* in Africa, *O. rudis* and *O. talaje* in Central and South America, *O. tholozani* in the Near and Middle East, and *O. hermsii* and *O. turicata* in the USA. These ticks usually feed several times at night, engorge rapidly, and leave the host; they live 2–5 years (up to 10 years) and remain infective throughout their life span.

6. Incubation period—Louse-borne relapsing fever: usually 8 days (range 5–15 days). A short 2–4 day incubation has been observed in North Africa. Tick-borne relapsing fever: about 7 days (range 2–18 days).

7. Period of communicability—Lice become infective 4-5 days after ingestion of blood from an infected person, and remain so for life (20-30 days). Infected ticks can live and remain infective for several years without feeding; they pass the infection trans-ovarially to their progeny.

8. Susceptibility—Susceptibility is general. Duration and degree of immunity after clinical symptoms are unknown; repeated infections may occur.

9. Methods of control—

A. *Preventive measures:*

1) Control lice using measures prescribed for louse-borne typhus fever (see *Typhus fever*, Epidemic louse-borne, 9A).
2) Control ticks by measures prescribed for *Rocky Mountain spotted fever*, 9A. Soft tick-infested human habitations may present a major problem, and eradication of the ticks may be difficult. Closing crevasses in wall structures and installing rodent proofing to prevent future colonization by rodents and their soft ticks are the mainstay of prevention and control. Spraying with approved acaricides, such as diazinon, chlorpyrifos, propoxur, pyrethrum or permethrin, may be tried.
3) Use personal protective measures, including repellents and permethrin on clothing and bedding, for people with exposure in endemic foci. Dimethyl phthalate (5%) and 10% carbolic soap are effective.
4) Antibiotic chemoprophylaxis with tetracyclines may be taken after exposure (arthropod bites) when the risk of acquiring the infection is high. Tetracyclines cannot be used in children less than eight years of age. No vaccines against *Borreliae* are available yet for human use.

B. *Control of patient, contacts and the immediate environment:*

1) Report to local health authority: Report of louse-borne relapsing fever required as a Disease under Surveillance by WHO, Class 1; tick-borne disease, in selected areas, Class 3 (see *Reporting*).
2) Isolation: Blood/body fluid precautions. Patients, clothing, household contacts and immediate environment must be deloused or freed of ticks.
3) Concurrent disinfection: Not applicable, if disinfection of environment has been carried out properly.
4) Quarantine: Not applicable.
5) Immunization of contacts: Not applicable.

6) Investigation of contacts and source of infection: For individual tick-borne cases, search for additional associated cases and sources of infection; for louse-borne disease, application of appropriate lousicidal preparation to infested contacts (see *Pediculosis*, 9B6 and 9B7).

7) Specific treatment: Erythromycin, tetracycline, chloramphenicol (500 mg every 6 hours) or doxycycline (100 mg every 12 hours), for 7 days. Tetracycline and doxycyline cannot be used in children less than eight years of age.

C. *Epidemic measures:* For louse-borne relapsing fever, when case reporting has been properly done and cases are localized, dust or spray contacts and their clothing with 1% permethrin (residual effect insecticide), and apply permethrin spray at 0.03–0.3 kg/hectare (2.47 acres) to the immediate environment of all reported cases. Provide facilities for washing clothes and for bathing to affected populations; establish active surveillance, especially in refugee camps. Where infection is known to be widespread, apply permethrin systematically to all people in the community. For tick-borne relapsing fever, apply permethrin or other acaricides to target areas where vector ticks are thought to be present; for sustained control, a treatment cycle of 1 month is recommended during the transmission season. Since animals (horses, camels, cows, sheep, pigs, and dogs) can also play a role in tick-borne relapsing fever, persons entering tick-infested areas (hunters, soldiers, vacationers and others) should be educated regarding tick-borne relapsing fever.

D. *Disaster implications:* A serious potential hazard among louse-infested populations. Epidemics are common in wars, famines and other situations with increased prevalence of pediculosis (e.g. overcrowded, malnourished populations with poor personal hygiene), especially with important population movements and in refugee camps.

E. *International measures:*

1) Prompt notification by governments to WHO and adjacent countries of an outbreak of louse-borne relapsing fever in any areas of their territories, with further information on the source and type of the disease and the number of cases and deaths.

2) Louse-borne relapsing fever is not a disease subject to the International Health Regulations, but WHO considers it a Disease under Surveillance, and the measures outlined under 9E1 should be followed.

RESPIRATORY DISEASE, ACUTE VIRAL
(Excluding influenza)
(Acute viral rhinitis, Pharyngitis, Laryngitis)
[CCDM19: S. Qazi]
[CCDM18: O. Fontaine]

Numerous acute respiratory illnesses of known and presumed viral etiology are grouped here. Clinically, infections of the upper respiratory tract (above the epiglottis) can be designated as acute viral rhinitis or acute viral pharyngitis (common cold, upper respiratory infections), and infections involving the lower respiratory tract (below the epiglottis) can be designated as croup (laryngotracheitis), acute viral tracheobronchitis, bronchitis, bronchiolitis or acute viral pneumonia. These respiratory syndromes are associated with a large number of viruses, each of which can produce a wide spectrum of acute respiratory illness and differ in etiology between children and adults.

The illnesses caused by known agents have important common epidemiological attributes, such as reservoir and mode of transmission. Many of the viruses invade any part of the respiratory tract; others show a predilection for certain anatomical sites. Some predispose to bacterial complications. Morbidity and mortality from acute respiratory diseases are especially significant in children. In adults, relatively high incidence and resulting disability, with consequent economic loss, make acute respiratory diseases a major health problem worldwide. As a group, acute respiratory diseases are one of the leading causes of death from any infectious disease.

Several other infections of the respiratory tract are presented as separate chapters because they are sufficiently distinctive in their manifestations and occur in regular association with a single infectious agent: examples include influenza, psittacosis, hantavirus pulmonary syndrome, chlamydial pneumonia, vesicular pharyngitis (herpangina), epidemic myalgia (pleurodynia), and severe acute respiratory syndrome (SARS). Particularly in pediatric practice, influenza must be considered in cases of acute respiratory tract disease.

Symptoms of upper respiratory tract infection, mainly pharyngotonsillitis, can be produced by bacterial agents, among which A streptococcus is the most common. Viral infections should be differentiated from bacterial or other infections for which specific antimicrobial measures are available. For instance, although viral pharyngotonsillitis is more common, group A streptococcal infection should be ruled out by rapid streptococcal antigen test and culture, particularly in children aged more than two. In non-streptococcal outbreaks, it is important to identify the cause in a representative sample of cases through appropriate clinical and laboratory methods, in order to rule out other diseases (e.g. mycoplasmal pneumonia, chlamydial pneumonia, legionellosis and Q fever), for which specific treatments may be effective.

I. ACUTE VIRAL
RHINITIS—COMMON COLD ICD-9 460; ICD-10 J00
(Rhinitis, Coryza [acute])

1. Identification—An acute catarrhal infection of the upper respiratory tract characterized by coryza, sneezing, lacrimation, irritation of the nasopharynx, chilliness and malaise lasting 2–7 days. Fever is uncommon in children over three, and rare in adults. No fatalities have been reported, but disability is important because it affects work performance and industrial and school absenteeism; illness may be accompanied by laryngitis, tracheitis or bronchitis, and may predispose to more serious complications, such as sinusitis and otitis media. WBC counts are usually normal, and bacterial flora of the respiratory tract are within normal limits in the absence of complications.

Cell or organ culture studies of nasal secretions may show a known virus. Specific clinical, epidemiological and other manifestations aid differentiation from similar diseases due to toxic, allergic, physical or psychological stimuli.

2. Infectious agents—Rhinoviruses, of which there are more than 100 recognized serotypes, are the major known causal agents of the common cold in adults; they account for 20%–40% of infections, especially in the autumn. Coronaviruses, such as 229E, OC43 and B814, are responsible for about 10%–15% common colds in adults, and influenza for another 10%–15%; they appear especially important in the winter and early spring, when the prevalence of rhinoviruses is low. Other known respiratory viruses account for a small proportion of common colds in adults. In infants and children, parainfluenza viruses, respiratory syncytial viruses (RSV), influenza, adenoviruses, certain enteroviruses, and coronaviruses all cause illnesses similar to the common cold. The cause of about half of common colds has not been identified.

3. Occurrence—Worldwide, both endemic and epidemic. In temperate zones, incidence rises in autumn, winter and spring; in tropical settings, incidence is highest in the rainy season. Many people, except in small isolated communities, have 1–6 colds yearly. Incidence is highest in children under five, and gradually declines with increasing age.

4. Reservoir—Humans.

5. Mode of transmission—Presumably direct contact or inhalation of airborne droplets; more importantly, indirect transmission through hands and articles freshly soiled by nose and throat discharges of an infected person. Contaminated hands carry rhinovirus, RSV and probably other similar viruses to the mucous membranes of the eye or nose.

6. Incubation period—Between 12 hours and 5 days, usually 48 hours, varying with the agent.

7. Period of communicability—Nasal washings taken 24 hours before onset and for 5 days after onset have produced symptoms in experimentally infected volunteers.

8. Susceptibility—Susceptibility is universal. Inapparent and abortive infections occur; frequency of healthy carriers is undetermined but known to be rare with some viral agents, notably rhinoviruses. Frequently repeated attacks are most likely due to the multiplicity of agents, but may be due to the short duration of homologous immunity against different serotypes of the same virus or to other causes.

9. Methods of control—

A. Preventive measures:

1) Educate the public in personal hygiene, such as covering the mouth when coughing and sneezing, safe disposal of oral and nasal discharges, and frequent handwashing.
2) When possible, avoid crowding in living and sleeping quarters, especially in institutions, in barracks and onboard ships. Provide adequate ventilation.
3) Oral live adenovirus vaccines have proven effective against adenovirus 4, 7 and 21 infections in military recruits, but are not indicated in civilian populations because of the low incidence of specific disease.
4) Do not smoke in households with children, whose risk of pneumonia increases when exposed to passive smoke.

B. Control of patient, contacts and the immediate environment:

1) Report to local health authority: Official report not ordinarily justifiable, Class 5 (see *Reporting*).
2), 3), 4), 5), 6), and 7): Isolation, Concurrent disinfection, Quarantine, Immunization of contacts, Investigation of contacts and source of infection, and Specific treatment: See section II, 9B2 through 9B7.

C., D,. and E. Epidemic measures, Disaster implications, and *International measures:* See section II, 9C, 9D and 9E.

II. ACUTE FEBRILE RESPIRATORY
DISEASE ICD-9 461–466; 480; ICD-10 J01-J06; J12
(Excluding Streptococcal pharyngitis, q.v., J02.0)

1. Identification—Viral diseases of the respiratory tract may be characterized by fever, cough, increased respiratory rate and one or more systemic reactions, such as chills or chilliness, headache, general aching, malaise and anorexia; occasionally in infants by GI disturbances. Localizing signs also occur at various sites in the respiratory tract, either alone or in combination, such as rhinitis, pharyngitis or tonsillitis, laryngitis, laryngo-tracheitis, bronchitis, bronchiolitis, pneumonitis or pneumonia. There may be associated conjunctivitis. Symptoms and signs usually subside in 2–5 days without complications; infection may, however, be complicated by bacterial sinusitis, otitis media, or—more rarely—bacterial pneumonia. WBC counts and respiratory bacterial flora are within normal limits unless modified by complications.

In very young infants, it may be difficult to distinguish between pneumonia, sepsis and meningitis. Specific diagnosis depends on isolation of the causal agent from respiratory secretions in appropriate cell or organ cultures, identification of viral antigen in nasopharyngeal cells by FA, ELISA and RIA tests, and/or antibody studies of paired sera.

2. Infectious agents—Viruses considered etiologic agents of acute febrile respiratory illnesses are: parainfluenza virus, types 1, 2, 3 and rarely type 4; respiratory syncytial virus (RSV); adenovirus, especially types 1–5, 7, 14 and 21; rhinoviruses; certain coronaviruses; certain types of coxsackievirus groups A and B; and echoviruses. Influenza virus (see *Influenza*) can produce the same clinical picture, especially in children. Some of these agents tend to cause more severe illnesses; others have a predilection for certain age groups and populations. RSV, the major viral respiratory tract pathogen of early infancy, produces illness with greatest frequency during the first 2 years of life; it is the major known causal agent of bronchiolitis and is a cause of pneumonia, croup, bronchitis, otitis media, and febrile upper respiratory illness. The parainfluenza viruses are the major known causal agents of croup and also cause bronchitis, pneumonia, bronchiolitis and febrile upper respiratory illness in pediatric populations. RSV and the parain-fluenza viruses may cause symptomatic disease in adults, particularly the debilitated elderly. Adenoviruses are associated with several forms of respiratory disease; types 4, 7 and 21 are common causes of acute respiratory disease in non-immunized military recruits; in young in-fants, adenoviruses are the most aggressive viral agents to cause significant mortality.

3. Occurrence—Worldwide. Seasonal in temperate zones, with great-est incidence during autumn and winter, and occasionally spring. In tropical zones, respiratory infections tend to be more frequent in wet and in colder weather. In large communities, some viral illnesses are constantly present, usually with little seasonal pattern (e.g. adenovirus type 1); others tend to occur in sharp outbreaks (e.g. RSV).

Annual incidence is high, particularly in infants and children, with 2–6 episodes per child per year, and depends on the number of susceptibles and the virulence of the agent. During the season where incidence is high, attack rates for preschool children may average 2% per week, as compared to 1% per week for school-age children and 0.5% per week for adults. Under special host and environmental conditions, certain viral infections may disable more than half a closed community within a few weeks (e.g. outbreaks of adenovirus type 4 or 7 in military recruits).

4. Reservoir—Humans. Many known viruses produce inapparent infections; adenoviruses may remain latent in tonsils and adenoids. Viruses of the same group cause similar infections in many animal species, but are of minor importance as sources of human infections.

5. Mode of transmission—Directly by oral contact or droplet spread; indirectly by hands, handkerchiefs, eating utensils or other articles freshly soiled by respiratory discharges of an infected person. Viruses discharged in the feces, including enteroviruses and adenoviruses, may be transmitted by the fecal-oral route. Outbreaks of illness due to adenovirus types 3, 4 and 7 have been related to swimming pools.

6. Incubation period—From 1 to 10 days.

7. Period of communicability—Shortly prior to and for the duration of active disease; little is known about subclinical or latent infections. Especially in infants, RSV shedding may very rarely persist several weeks after clinical symptoms subside.

8. Susceptibility—Susceptibility is universal. Illness is more frequent and more severe in infants, children and the elderly. Infection induces specific antibodies that are usually short-lived. Reinfection with RSV and parainfluenza viruses is common, but illness is generally milder. Individuals with compromised cardiac, pulmonary or immune systems, including those with HIV infection, are at increased risk of severe illness.

9. Methods of control—

    A. Preventive measures: See section I, 9A. Those at high risk of RSV-related complications include infants, children aged under two with chronic lung disease who have required medical treatment for lung disease within 6 months of the RSV season, and premature infants of <35 weeks gestation at birth. These high-risk infants may benefit from intravenous Palivizumab. Palivizumab, an RSV monoclonal antibody preparation that is given monthly (IM) during the course of the RSV-season, has reduced RSV-related hospitalization by about half in such infants. HIV-infected children have a 2.5 fold greater risk of hospitalization for RSV-associated LRTI and have a higher case fatality rate. The increase in RSV-associated morbidity and mortality in HIV infected children may however be related to heightened susceptibility to co-infection with other pathogens, including bacteria and *Pneumocystis jiroveci.*

B. **Control of patient, contacts and the immediate environment:**

1) Report to local health authority: Obligatory report of epidemics in some countries; no individual case report, Class 4 (see *Reporting*).
2) Isolation: Contact isolation is desirable in children's hospital wards. Outside hospitals, ill people should avoid direct and indirect exposure of young children, debilitated or aged people, or patients with other illnesses.
3) Concurrent disinfection: Of eating and drinking utensils. Sanitary disposal of oral and nasal discharges.
4) Quarantine: Not applicable.
5) Immunization of contacts: Not applicable.
6) Investigation of contacts and source of infection: Not generally indicated.
7) Specific treatment: None. Indiscriminate use of antibiotics is to be discouraged; they should be reserved for patients with group A streptococcal pharyngitis and patients with identified bacterial complications such as otitis media, pneumonia or sinusitis. There is a lack of consensus regarding appropriate management of infants with RSV infection, specifically with respect to the use of aerosolized ribavirin. Despite studies in the USA and Canada, no clear improvement in clinical outcomes attributed to the use of aerosolized ribavirin is consistent across all studies. Cough medicines, decongestants and antihistaminics are of questionable effectiveness, and may be hazardous, especially in children.

C. **Epidemic measures:** No effective measures known. Some nosocomial transmission can be prevented by good infection control procedures, including handwashing; procedures such as ultraviolet irradiation, aerosols and dust control have not proven useful. Avoid crowding (see section I, 9A2).

D. **Disaster implications:** None.

E. **International measures:** WHO Collaborating Centres provide support as required. More information can be found at: <http://www.who.int/collaboratingcentres/database/en/>

RICKETTSIOSES, TICK- and MITE-BORNE (or ACARI-BORNE)   ICD-9 082; ICD-10 A77
(Spotted fever group)
[CCDM19: M. Eremeeva, G. Dasch]
[CCDM18: D. Raoult]

Rickettsioses, or Rickettsial infections, are a closely related group of bacterial infections causing clinically similar diseases characterized by fever, rash, and vasculitis which can be associated with multi-organ involvement such as hepatosplenomegaly, heart failure, renal failure, bleeding, and neurological complications. They are transmitted by ixodid (hard) ticks or mites, which are widely distributed throughout the world; tick species differ markedly according to geographical area. For all of these diseases, control measures are similar, and doxycycline is the reference treatment—though this cannot be used in children less than eight years of age. IFA tests become positive generally in the second week of illness. The Weil-Felix tests using Proteus OX-19 and Proteus OX-2 antigens are less sensitive and less specific, and should be confirmed by more agent-specific serologic tests.

I. ROCKY MOUNTAIN SPOTTED FEVER   ICD-9 082.0; ICD-10 A77.0
(Febre Maculosa)

1. Identification—This prototypic disease of the spotted fever group of *Rickettsiae* is characterized by the sudden onset of moderate to high fever, which ordinarily persists for 2–3 weeks in untreated cases; significant malaise; deep muscle pain; severe headache; chills; and conjunctival injection. A maculopapular rash generally appears on the extremities on the 3rd to 5th day; this soon includes the palms and soles, and spreads rapidly to the body trunk. A petechial exanthem occurs in 40% to 60% of patients, generally on or after the 6th day. The case-fatality rate ranges between 20% and 80% in different regions in the absence of specific treatment; with prompt recognition and treatment, death is uncommon, yet 3%–5% of cases reported in the USA during recent years have been fatal. Risk factors associated with more severe disease and death include delayed antibiotic therapy and patient age of over 40. Absence or delayed appearance of the typical rash, or failure to recognize it, especially in dark-skinned individuals, contribute to delay in diagnosis and thence to increased fatality.

The early stages of Rocky Mountain spotted fever (RMSF) may be confused with ehrlichiosis, meningococcemia (see *Meningitis*) and enteroviral infection.

The serological response to specific antigens confirms the diagnosis. During the early stages, *Rickettsiae* may sometimes be detected in blood by PCR, and more frequently in skin biopsies using immunostains or PCR.

Culturing blood or buffy coats on cell culture monolayers permits isolation of the organisms and facilitates precise confirmatory diagnosis. Identification is based on DNA sequencing of OmpA, OmpB, GltA and/or Sca4 gene fragments.

2. Infectious agent—*Rickettsia rickettsii*.

3. Occurrence—Throughout the USA, primarily from April through September, mainly in the southeast and south central regions; highest incidence rates are seen in North Carolina and Oklahoma. Few cases are reported from the Rocky Mountain region. In the western USA, adult males are infected most frequently, while in the east, incidence is higher in children; the difference relates to conditions of exposure to infected ticks. Infection has also been documented in Argentina, Brazil, Canada, Colombia, Costa Rica, western and central Mexico, and Panama.

4. Reservoir—Maintained in nature among ticks by trans-ovarial and trans-stadial passage. The *Rickettsiae* can be transmitted to dogs, various rodents and other animals; animal infections are usually subclinical, but persistent infections in rodents and disease in dogs have been observed. Dogs are useful sentinels for spotted fever group *rickettsiae*. Clustered cases of RMSF in humans and dogs may occur at the same time.

5. Mode of transmission—Typically through the bite of an infected tick. At least 4–6 hours of attachment and feeding on blood by the tick are required before the *Rickettsiae* become infectious for people. Contamination of breaks in the skin or mucous membranes with crushed tissues or feces of the tick may also lead to infection. In eastern and southern USA, the common vector is the American dog tick, *Dermacentor variabilis*, and in northwestern USA, the Rocky Mountain wood tick, *D. andersoni*. The principal vector in Latin America is *Amblyomma cajennense*. The brown dog tick, *Rhipicephalus sanguineus,* may also transmit *R. rickettsii*.

6. Incubation period—From 3 to about 14 days.

7. Period of communicability—Not directly transmitted from person to person. The tick remains infective for life, commonly as long as 18 months.

8. Susceptibility—Susceptibility is general. One attack probably confers lasting immunity.

9. Methods of control—

    A. Preventive measures:

        1) See also *Lyme disease*, 9A. Remove attached or crawling ticks immediately after exposure to tick-infested habitats.

2) Removing ticks from dogs, and using acaridal collars or treatments on them, minimizes the tick population near residences.

3) Vaccine is not available. Antibiotic prophylaxis following a tick bite is not recommended.

B. Control of patient, contacts and the immediate environment:

1) Report to the local health authority: Case reporting is obligatory in most countries, Class 2 (see *Reporting*).

2) Isolation: Not applicable.

3) Concurrent disinfection: Carefully remove all ticks from patients.

4) Quarantine: Not applicable.

5) Immunization of contacts: Unnecessary.

6) Investigation of contacts and source of infection: Not beneficial except as a community measure. See Lyme disease, 9C.

7) Specific treatment: Tetracyclines (usually doxycylin e) in daily oral or intravenous doses for 5–7 days, and for at least 48 hours once the patient is afebrile. Tetracyclines cannot be used in children less than eight years of age. Chloramphenicol may also be used, but only when there is an absolute contraindication for using tetracyclines. Treatment should be initiated on clinical and epidemiological considerations without waiting for laboratory confirmation of the diagnosis.

C. Epidemic measures: See *Lyme disease*, 9C.

D. Disaster implications: None.

E. International measures: WHO Collaborating Centres provide support as required. More information can be found at http://www.who.int/collaboratingcentres/database/en/.

II. BOUTONNEUSE FEVER   ICD-9 082.1; ICD-10 A77.1
(Mediterranean tick fever, Mediterranean spotted fever, Marseilles fever, Kenya tick typhus, India tick typhus, Israeli tick typhus, Astrakhan fever)

1. Identification—A mild to severe febrile illness of a few days to 2 weeks; there may be a primary lesion or eschar at the site of a tick bite. This eschar (tache noire), often evident at the onset of fever, is a small ulcer 2–5 mm in diameter with a black center and red areola; regional lymph nodes are often enlarged. In some areas, such as the Negev in Israel and Astrakhan, Russia, primary lesions are rarely seen. A generalized maculopapular erythematous rash usually involving palms and soles appears about the 4th to 5th day and persists for 6–7 days; with antibiotic therapy, fever lasts no more than 2 days. The case-fatality rate is low (less than 3%), even without specific treatment.

Diagnosis is confirmed by serological tests or PCR or immunostains of biopsied tissues. Culturing blood on human fibroblast monolayers permits demonstration of the organisms by DFA testing.

2. Infectious agent—*Rickettsia conorii* and closely related organisms.

3. Occurrence—Widely distributed throughout the African continent, in India and in those parts of Europe and the Middle East adjacent to the Mediterranean and the Black and Caspian seas. Expansion of the European endemic zone to the north occurs when tourists take their dogs with them; the dogs acquire infected ticks, which establish colonies when the dogs return home, with subsequent transmission. In more temperate areas, the highest incidence is during warmer months when ticks are numerous; in tropical areas, disease occurs throughout the year.

4. Reservoir—As in *RMSF* (see section I, 4).

5. Mode of transmission—In the Mediterranean area, bite of infected *Rhipicephalus sanguineus*, the brown dog tick.

6. Incubation period—Usually 5-7 days.

7., 8., and **9. Period of communicability, Susceptibility and Methods of control**—As in *RMSF*, above (see section I, 7, 8 and 9).

III. AFRICAN TICK BITE FEVER   ICD-9 082.8; ICD-10 A77.8

1. Identification—The disease is milder than other rickettsioses. Clinically similar to Boutonneuse fever (see above), but fever is less common, and rash is noticed in only half the cases and may be vesicular. Aphthous stomatitis is common. Multiple eschars, lymphangitis, lymphadenopathy, and edema localized to the eschar site are seen more commonly than with Boutonneuse fever. Outbreaks of disease may occur when groups of travelers (such as people on safari in Africa) are bitten by ticks. Cases are occasionally imported into the USA and Europe.

2. Infectious agent—*Rickettsia africae*.

3. Occurrence—Sub-Saharan Africa, including Botswana, South Africa, Swaziland and Zimbabwe; and the Lesser Antilles.

4. Reservoir—As in *RMSF*, above (see section I, 4).

5. Mode of transmission—As in *RMSF*, above (see section I, 5). *Amblyomma hebraeum* and *A. variegatum* are the major vectors.

6. Incubation period—5 to 10 days (mean 6.6 ± 3.0 days after tick bite).

7., 8., and **9. Period of communicability, Susceptibility and Methods of control**—As in *RMSF*, above (see section I, 7, 8 and 9).

IV. QUEENSLAND TICK TYPHUS   ICD-9 082.3; ICD-10 A77.3

1. Identification—Clinically similar to Boutonneuse fever (see section II); the rash can be vesicular.

2. Infectious agent—*Rickettsia australis*.

3. Occurrence—Queensland, New South Wales, Tasmania and coastal areas of eastern Victoria, Australia.

4. Reservoir—As in *RMSF*, above (see section I, 4).

5. Mode of transmission—As in *RMSF*, above (see section I, 5). *Ixodes holocyclus*, which infests small marsupials and wild rodents, is probably the major vector.

6. Incubation period—About 7-10 days.

7., 8., and **9. Period of communicability, Susceptibility and Methods of control**—As in *RMSF*, above (see section I, 7, 8 and 9).

V. NORTH ASIAN TICK FEVER   ICD-9 082.2; ICD-10 A77.2
(Siberian tick typhus)

1. Identification—Clinically similar to Boutonneuse fever (see section II); lymphadenitis is common.

2. Infectious agent—*Rickettsia sibirica*.

3. Occurrence—North China, Mongolia and Asiatic areas of Russia.

4. Reservoir—As in *RMSF*, above (see section I, 4).

5. Mode of transmission—Through the bite of ticks in the genera *Dermacentor* and *Haemaphysalis*, which infest certain wild rodents.

6. Incubation period—3 to 7 days.

7., 8., and **9. Period of communicability, Susceptibility and Methods of control**—As in *RMSF*, above (see section I, 7, 8 and 9).

VI. TICK-BORNE LYMPHADENOPATHY (TIBOLA)   ICD-9 082x; ICD-10 A77.x
(*Dermacentor*-borne necrosis and lymphadenopathy [DEBONEL])

1. Identification—Mild rickettsiosis; main symptoms include necrosis and erythema, often found on the head; cervical lymphadenopathy and enlarged lymph nodes; and, rarely, maculopapular rash.

2. Infectious agent—*Rickettsia slovaca*.

3. Occurrence— Europe and Asia.

4. Reservoir—Lagomorphs and rodents.

5. Mode of transmission—Through the bite of *Dermacentor marginatus*, which infests certain wild rodents.

6. Incubation period—2 to 7 days.

7., 8., and 9. Period of communicability, Susceptibility and Methods of control—As in *RMSF*, above (see section I, 7, 8 and 9).

VII. FLINDERS ISLAND SPOTTED FEVER   ICD-9 082.x, ICD-10 A77.x
(Thai tick typhus)

1. Identification—Mild spotted fever, maculopapular rash; eschar and adenopathy are rare.

2. Infectious agent—*Rickettsia honei*.

3. Occurrence—Australia, Thailand, Flinders Island, Tasmania.

4. Reservoir—Not well determined; however, reptiles, migratory birds and rodents are suspected.

5. Mode of transmission—Through the bite of ticks *Aponomma hydrosauri, Ixodes tasmanii, I. granulatus*.

6. Incubation period—3 to 7 days.

7, 8, and 9. Period of communicability, Susceptibility and Methods of control—As in *RMSF*, above (see section I, 7, 8 and 9).

VIII. AUSTRALIAN SPOTTED FEVER   ICD-9 082.x, ICD-10 A77.x

1. Identification—Fever, eschar, maculopapular or vesicular rash, adenopathy; fatalities have been reported.

2. Infectious agent—*Rickettsia marmionii*

3. Occurrence—Australia.

4. Reservoir—Rodents, reptiles.

5. Mode of transmission—Through the bite of ticks, *I. holocyclus* and *H. novaeguineae*.

6. Incubation period—3 to 7 days.

7., 8., and 9. Period of communicability, Susceptibility and Methods of control—As in *RMSF*, above (see section I, 7, 8 and 9).

IX. FAR-EASTERN TICK-BORNE RICKETTSIOSIS ICD-9 082.x, ICD-10 A77.x

1. Identification—Fever, eschar, faint macular or maculopapular rash, lymphadenopathy, enlarged lymph nodes, lymphangitis.

2. Infectious agent—*Rickettsia heilongjiangensis.*

3. Occurrence—Far east of Russia, northern China.

4. Reservoir—Rodents, lagomorphs.

5. Mode of transmission—Through the bite of ticks *D. silvarum*, *Haemaphysalis concinna* and *H. japonica douglasii.*

6. Incubation period—3 to 7 days.

7., 8., and 9. Period of communicability, Susceptibility and Methods of control—As in *RMSF*, above (see section I, 7, 8 and 9).

X. ORIENTAL SPOTTED FEVER ICD-9 082.x, ICD-10 A77.x

1. Identification—Fever, eschar, macular or maculopapular rash, lymphadenopathy, enlarged lymph nodes; fatalities have been described.

2. Infectious agent—*Rickettsia japonica.*

3. Occurrence—Japan.

4. Reservoir—Rodents, reptiles.

5. Mode of transmission—Through the bite of ticks *H. flava*, *H. longicornis, D. taiwanensis*, and *I. ovatus.*

6. Incubation period—3 to 7 days.

7., 8., and 9. Period of communicability, Susceptibility and Methods of control—As in *RMSF*, above (see section I, 7, 8 and 9).

XI. MACULATUM
INFECTION   ICD-9 082.x, ICD-10 A77.x

1. Identification—A mild febrile illness with eschar, maculopapular to vesicular rash.

2. Infectious agent—*Rickettsia parkeri*.

3. Occurrence—Coastal regions of southeastern USA; southern South America, including Argentina, Uruguay and parts of Brazil.

4. Reservoir—Rodents.

5. Mode of transmission—Through the bite of ticks *Amblyomma maculatum* and *A. triste*.

6. Incubation period—2–10 days (median, 5 days).

7., 8., and **9. Period of communicability, Susceptibility and Methods of control**—As in *RMSF*, above (see section I, 7, 8 and 9).

XII. RICKETTSIALPOX   ICD-9 083.2; ICD-10 A79.1
(Vesicular rickettsiosis)

1. Identification—An acute febrile illness transmitted by mites. An initial skin lesion at the site of a mite bite, often associated with lymphadenopathy, is followed by fever; a disseminated vesicular skin rash appears, which generally does not involve the palms and soles, and lasts only a few days. It may be confused with chickenpox. Death is uncommon, and the infection is responsive to tetracyclines—though these cannot be used in children less than eight years of age. Acute hepatitis may be one of the leading symptoms before development of specific vesicular rash. Diagnosis is made by serology or by PCR, or by immunostains of biopsied tissues.

2. Infectious agent—*Rickettsia akari*.

3. Occurrence—Urban areas of the eastern USA; most cases have been described from New York City and in Russia and neighboring countries. *R. akari* has also been detected in Africa and the Republic of Korea.

4. Reservoir—Mice (*Mus musculus*) in urban sites in the USA. Commensal rats are reported to be the reservoir in Russia, and *Apodemus* in the Republic of Korea.

5. Mode of transmission—Through the bite of a mite (*Liponyssoides sanguineus*).

6. Incubation period—6 to 15 days.

7., 8., and **9. Period of communicability, Susceptibility and Methods of control**—Incidence has been markedly reduced by changes in management of garbage in tenement housing, so that few cases have been diagnosed in recent years. Prevention includes rodent elimination and mite control.

RUBELLA   ICD-9 056; ICD-10 B06
(German measles)

CONGENITAL RUBELLA   ICD-9 771.0; ICD-10 P35.0
(Congenital rubella syndrome)
[CCDM19: P. Duclos, S. Reef]
[CCDM18: S. Robertson]

1. Identification—For most people, rubella is a mild febrile viral disease with a diffuse punctate and maculopapular rash. Clinically, rubella is indistinguishable from febrile rash illness due to measles, dengue, parvovirus B19, human herpesvirus 6, Coxsackie virus, Echovirus, adenovirus or scarlet fever. Children usually present few or no constitutional symptoms, but adults may experience a 1–5 day prodrome of low-grade fever, headache, malaise, mild coryza and conjunctivitis. Post-auricular, occipital and posterior cervical lymphadenopathy is the most characteristic clinical feature, and precedes the rash by 5–10 days. Leukopenia is common and thrombocytopenia can occur, but hemorrhagic manifestations are rare. Arthralgia and, less commonly, arthritis complicate a substantial proportion of infections, particularly among adult females. Encephalitis is seen in 1:6 000 cases, and occurs with a higher frequency in adults. Up to 50% of rubella infections are subclinical.

For surveillance purposes, the WHO-recommended case definition of a suspected rubella case is any person with fever, non-vesicular (maculopapular) rash and adenopathy (cervical, sub-occipital or post-auricular). Laboratory diagnosis of rubella is required, since clinical diagnosis is often inaccurate. Laboratory confirmation is usually based on a positive rubella-specific IgM ELISA test on a blood specimen obtained within 28 days after the rash onset. An epidemiologically confirmed rubella case is a patient with suspected rubella with an epidemiological link to a laboratory-confirmed case. Other methods for rubella diagnosis include paired serum specimens that show seroconversion, or at least a 4-fold rise in rubella-specific IgG antibody titer, positive rubella PCR test, and virus isolation; PCR and virus isolation may be only available in higher-level reference laboratories.

Rubella is important because of its ability to produce anomalies in the developing fetus. Congenital rubella syndrome (CRS) occurs in up to 90% of infants born to women who are infected with rubella during the first 10 weeks of pregnancy; defects are rare when maternal infection occurs after the 20th week of gestation. Congenital malformations and fetal death may occur following inapparent maternal rubella.

Fetuses infected early are at greatest risk of intrauterine death, spontaneous abortion and congenital malformations of major organ systems. These include single or combined defects such as hearing impairment, cataracts, microphthalmia, congenital glaucoma, microcephaly, meningoencephalitis, developmental delay, patent ductus arteriosus, atrial or ventricular septal defects, purpura, hepatosplenomegaly, jaundice, and radiolucent bone disease. Moderate and severe CRS is usually recognizable at birth; mild CRS with only slight cardiac involvement or hearing impairment may not be detected for months or even years after birth. Insulin-dependent diabetes mellitus is recognized as a frequent late manifestation of CRS.

Laboratory confirmation of CRS in an infant is based on a positive rubella-specific IgM ELISA test on a blood specimen; the persistence of a rubella-specific IgG antibody titer in a blood specimen beyond the time expected from passive transfer of maternal IgG antibody; isolation of the virus from a throat swab or urine specimen; or detection of rubella virus by PCR. Almost all infants with CRS have a positive rubella IgM test in the first 3 months of life, and >30% remain positive during the second 6 months of life. Rubella virus has been isolated from throat and urine specimens of infants with CRS, and from cataract surgery aspirates in children up to 3.

2. Infectious agent—Rubella virus (family Togaviridae; genus *Rubivirus*).

3. Occurrence—In the absence of generalized immunization, rubella occurred worldwide at endemic levels with epidemics every 5-9 years. Large rubella epidemics resulted in very high levels of morbidity: for example, the USA epidemic in 1964-1965 led to an estimated 12.5 million cases of rubella, over 20 000 cases of CRS, and 11 000 fetal deaths; the incidence of CRS during endemic periods was 0.1-0.2 per 1 000 live births, and 1-4 per 1 000 live births during epidemics. In countries where rubella vaccine has not been introduced, rubella remains endemic. In 1999, an estimated minimum of 100 000 CRS cases occurred each year in developing countries.

As of end-2006, 123 countries/territories (64% of the world total) regularly use rubella vaccine in their national immunization programs, with the highest coverage in the Americas (97% of countries), Europe (96%), the Eastern Mediterranean region (71%), and the Western Pacific (67%). Of these 123 countries, 107 include 2 doses in the routine schedule, and nine provide a 3rd dose during adolescence. In many countries, sustained high levels of rubella immunization have drastically reduced or practically eliminated rubella and CRS.

4. Reservoir—Humans.

5. Mode of transmission—Contact with nasopharyngeal secretions of infected people. Infection is by droplet spread or direct contact with patients. Infants with CRS shed large quantities of virus in their pharyngeal secretions and urine, and serve as a source of infection to their contacts.

6. Incubation period—From 14–17 days with a range of 14–21 days.

7. Period of communicability—For about 1 week before and at least 4 days after onset of rash; highly communicable. Infants with CRS may shed virus for months after birth.

8. Susceptibility—Immunity is usually permanent after natural infection, and thought to be long-term, probably lifelong, after immunization; but persistent immunity may require contact with endemic cases. Infants born to immune mothers are ordinarily protected for 6–9 months, depending on the amount of maternal antibodies acquired transplacentally.

9. Methods of control—Rubella control is needed primarily to prevent defects in the offspring of women who acquire the disease during pregnancy.

A. Preventive measures:

1) Educate the general public on modes of transmission, and stress the need for rubella immunization. Health care providers must be aware of the risks caused by rubella in pregnancy.
2) WHO recommends use of the vaccine in all countries where control or elimination of CRS is considered a public health priority. The primary purpose of rubella vaccination is to prevent the occurrence of congenital rubella infection, including CRS. This can be done using combined vaccines (MR or MMR), and current efforts in global measles control should be used as an opportunity to pursue control of rubella. Two approaches are recommended to prevent the occurrence of CRS:

   a) Prevention of CRS only, through immunization of adolescent girls or women of childbearing age.
   b) Elimination of rubella as well as CRS, through universal immunization of infants and ensuring immunity in women of childbearing age. For increased impact men should also be vaccinated.

   To achieve rubella and CRS elimination rapidly, countries may wish to conduct mass campaigns in adults, both male and female. Decisions on which approach is taken should be based on level of susceptibility in women of childbearing age, burden of disease due to CRS, strength of the basic immunization program as indicated by routine measles vaccine coverage, infrastructure, and resources for child and adult immunization programs. Following well-designed and well-implemented programs, rubella and CRS have almost disappeared from many countries. Two regions—the Americas and Europe—have adopted a goal of rubella elimination.

A policy of rubella vaccination of adults is unlikely to alter rubella transmission dynamics, and in practice is difficult to implement with high coverage rates. Inadequately implemented childhood vaccination may run the risk of increasing the number of susceptibles among women—and the possibility of increased numbers of cases of CRS—until immunized child cohorts become adults. Consequently, it is essential that childhood rubella vaccination programs achieve and maintain high levels of coverage (estimated at above 80% to be effective) to decrease the incidence of rubella on a long-term basis.

A single dose of live, attenuated rubella virus vaccine elicits a significant and long-lasting antibody response in about 95%–100% of susceptible individuals aged 9 months or older. Rubella vaccines are cold-chain dependent, and should be protected from light. Several rubella vaccines are available as single antigen, measles-rubella (MR), measles-mumps-rubella (MMR), or measles-mumps-rubella-varicella (MMRV) vaccines. Most of the currently licensed vaccines are based on the live attenuated RA27/3 strain of rubella virus; other live attenuated rubella virus strains are used in China and Japan.

Following the introduction of large-scale rubella vaccination, coverage should be measured periodically by age and locality. In addition, surveillance is needed for rubella and CRS. If resources permit, longitudinal serological surveillance can be used to monitor the impact of the immunization program, especially through assessing rubella IgG antibody in serum samples from women attending antenatal clinics.

Rubella vaccine should be avoided in pregnancy because of the theoretical—but never demonstrated—teratogenic risk. No CRS occurred in more than 2 000 susceptible pregnant women who were unknowingly pregnant and received RA 27/3 rubella vaccine in early pregnancy. If pregnancy is being planned, however, an interval of one month should be observed after rubella immunization. Receipt of rubella vaccine during pregnancy is not an indication for abortion.

Rubella vaccine should not be given to anyone with an immunodeficiency or who receives immunosuppressive therapy. Asymptomatic HIV-infected persons can be immunized.

3) In case of infection with wild rubella virus early in pregnancy, culturally appropriate counseling should be provided. Abortion may be considered in those countries where this is an option.

4) Intramuscular Immune Globulin (IG) given in a dose of 20 mL within 72 hours of rubella exposure may decrease clinical disease, viral shedding and the rate of viremia in exposed susceptible persons. IG may be considered for a susceptible pregnant woman exposed to the disease who would not be in a position to consider abortion. The absence of clinical signs in a pregnant woman who has received IG does not guarantee that fetal infection has been prevented. Infants with congenital rubella have been born to mothers who were given IG shortly after exposure.

B. Control of patient, contacts and the immediate environment:

1) Report to local health authority: In countries where rubella eradication is a goal, all cases of rubella and of CRS should be reported. In many countries, reporting is obligatory, Class 3 (see *Reporting*). Early reporting of suspected cases permits early establishment of control measures.

2) Isolation: In hospitals, patients suspected of having rubella should be managed under contact isolation precautions; attempts should be made to prevent exposure of non-immune pregnant women. Exclude children from school and adults from work for 7 days after onset of rash. Infants with CRS may shed virus for prolonged periods of time. All persons having contact with infants with CRS should be immune to rubella (naturally or through immunization); contact between these infants and pregnant women should be avoided. In hospitals, contact isolation precautions should be applied to infants under 12 months with CRS, unless urine and pharyngeal virus cultures are negative for rubella virus.

3) Concurrent disinfection: Not applicable.

4) Quarantine: Not applicable.

5) Immunization of contacts: Immunization of contacts will not necessarily prevent infection or illness. Passive immunization with IG is not indicated (except possibly as in 9A4).

6) Investigation of contacts and source of infection: Identify pregnant female contacts, especially those in the first trimester. Such contacts should be tested serologically for suscep-

tibility or early infection (IgM antibody), and advised accordingly.

7) Specific treatment: None.

C. Epidemic measures:

1) Prompt reporting of all confirmed and suspected cases; the country's established goal for rubella control/elimination will dictate the level of investigation required. During an outbreak, a limited number (5–10) of suspect cases (see definition earlier) should be investigated with laboratory tests to confirm that disease is due to rubella.

2) The medical community and general public should be informed about rubella epidemics in order to identify and protect susceptible pregnant women. Active surveillance for infants with CRS should be carried out until 9 months after the last reported rubella case.

D. Disaster implications: None.

E. International measures: None.

SALMONELLOSIS   ICD-9 003; ICD-10 A02
[CCDM19: C. B. Behravesh, M. Lynch, J. Schlundt]
[CCDM18: P. Braam]

1. Identification—A bacterial disease commonly manifested by acute enterocolitis, with sudden onset of headache, abdominal pain, diarrhea, nausea and sometimes vomiting. Dehydration, especially among infants or in the elderly, may be severe. Fever is almost always present. Anorexia and diarrhea often persist for several days. Infection may begin as acute enterocolitis and develop into septicemia or focal infection. Occasionally, the infectious agent may localize in any tissue of the body, produce abscesses, and cause septic arthritis, cholecystitis, endocarditis, meningitis, pericarditis, pneumonia, pyoderma, or pyelonephritis. Investigations suggest that up to 2% of all cases of salmonellosis cause extra-intestinal infections. Deaths are uncommon, except in the very young, the very old, the debilitated and the immunosuppressed. However, morbidity and associated costs of salmonellosis may be high.

In cases of septicemia, *Salmonella* may be isolated on enteric media from feces and blood during acute stages of illness. In cases of enterocolitis, fecal excretion usually persists for several days or weeks beyond the acute phase; administration of antibiotics may not decrease this duration. For detection of asymptomatic infections, 3–10 grams of fecal material is preferred to rectal swabs; this should be inoculated into an appropriate enrichment medium. Specimens should be collected over several days, since excretion of the organisms may be intermittent. Serological tests are not useful in diagnosis.

2. Infectious agents—Nearly all *Salmonella* isolated from ill persons are serotypes of *S. enterica* subsp. *enterica*. Approximately 2 500 serotypes of *Salmonella* have been identified. Numerous serotypes of *Salmonella* are pathogenic for both animals and people. *S. enterica* subsp. *enterica* serovar Typhi and serovar Paratyphi occur primarily in developing areas, such as Southeast Asia, Africa and South America, and cause systemic illness that leads to an estimated 20 million cases and 200 000 deaths worldwide each year. These strains are of human origin and cause typhoid and paratyphoid fevers—which are presented in a separate chapter.

Numerous serotypes of *Salmonella* are pathogenic for both animals and humans, or are spread from animal reservoirs. There is much variation in the relative prevalence of different serotypes from country to country; in most countries that maintain *Salmonella* surveillance, *Salmonella enterica* subsp. *enterica* serovar Typhimurium (commonly *S.* Typhimurium) and *Salmonella enterica* subsp. *enterica* serovar Enteritidis (*S.* Enteritidis) are the most commonly reported. In most areas, a small number of serotypes account for the majority of confirmed cases.

S. Enteritidis emerged as a major concern for food safety in Europe and the Americas in the 1980s. By 1993 this serovar, typically transmitted through poultry, was the most frequently reported serovar in humans in both USA and Europe. The serovar thereafter spread to chicken production systems in the rest of the world (apart from Australia).

3. Occurrence—Worldwide; more extensively reported in North America and Europe because of better reporting systems. Salmonellosis is classified as a foodborne disease because contaminated food, mainly of animal origin, is the predominant mode of transmission. Only a proportion of cases are recognized clinically; in industrialized countries, as few as 1% of clinical cases are reported. The incidence rate of infection is highest in infants and young children. Epidemiologically, *Salmonella* gastroenteritis may occur in small outbreaks in the general population. About 60%–80% of all cases occur sporadically; however, large outbreaks in hospitals, institutions for children, restaurants and nursing homes are not uncommon, usually arising from food contaminated at its source, or less often through handling by an ill person or a carrier; person-to-person spread can also occur. An epidemic in the USA that involved 25 000 cases resulted from a non-chlorinated municipal water supply; the largest known single epidemic due to improperly pasteurized milk affected 285 000 persons.

4. Reservoir—Domestic and wild animals, including poultry, swine, cattle, rodents and pets such as iguanas, tortoises, turtles, terrapins, chicks and other baby poultry, dogs, cats, hamsters, and hedgehogs; also humans, i.e. patients, convalescent carriers and—especially—mild and unrecognized cases. Chronic carriers are rare in humans but prevalent in animals, including birds.

Occurrence in animal products is significant in most—if not all—countries. In 2005, investigators in the USA examining 40 000 random samples of meat including chicken, pork and beef, found 5.7% of all samples and 33% of poultry positive for *Salmonella*. Highest positive prevalence is often found in poultry products—some European countries have found up to 40–50% of poultry samples to be positive.

5. Mode of transmission—Ingestion of the organisms in food derived from infected animals, contaminated by feces of an infected animal or person. Food sources include contaminated raw and undercooked eggs/egg products, raw milk/milk products, contaminated water, meat/meat products, poultry/poultry products, and contaminated produce. Contact with infected animals and/or their environments may lead to infection with *Salmonella*. Pets and unsterilized pharmaceuticals of animal origin are potential sources of infection. Several outbreaks of salmonellosis have been traced to consumption of raw fruits and vegetables that were contaminated in the kitchen or in their growing environment. Infection is transmitted to farm animals by feeds and fertilizers prepared from contaminated meat scraps, tankage, fish meal and bones; the infection spreads by bacterial multiplication during rearing and slaughter. In addition, person-to-person fecal-oral transmission is possible, especially when diarrhea is present; infants and stool-incontinent adults pose a greater risk of transmission than do asymptomatic carriers. With several serotypes, a few organisms ingested in vehicles that buffer gastric acid can suffice to cause infection, but over 100 to 1000 organisms are usually required. Newer risk assessment modeling has enabled the preparation of dose-response curves, reflecting the fact that the infection process should be viewed as a probability of infection related to the dose ingested. These models suggest a 10–20% probability for infection with a dose of 100 organisms, and a 60–80% probability for infection at 1 000 000 organisms.

Epidemics are usually traced to foods such as: processed meat products; inadequately cooked poultry/poultry products; uncooked or lightly cooked foods containing eggs/egg products; raw milk and dairy products, including dried milk; and foods contaminated by an infected food handler. Epidemics may also be traced to foods such as meat and poultry products processed or prepared with contaminated utensils or on work surfaces contaminated in previous use. *S. Enteritidis* infection of chickens and eggs has caused outbreaks and single cases, and is responsible for the majority of cases of this serotype in North America. The organisms can multiply in a variety of foods, especially milk, to attain very high infective doses; temperature abuse of food during preparation and cross-contamination during food handling are the most important risk factors. Hospital epidemics tend to be protracted, with organisms persisting in the environment; they often start with contaminated food and continue through person-to-person transmission via the hands of personnel or contaminated instruments. Maternity units with infected (at times asymptomatic) infants can be sources of further spread. Fecal contamination of non-chlorinated public water supplies has caused extensive outbreaks. Geographically widespread outbreaks have been identified due to ingestion of tomatoes or melons from single suppliers, and from commercially processed foods including frozen pot pies, peanut butter, and a dry puffed vegetable snack. Dry dog food and pet treats, such as pig ears, have been sources of recent human outbreaks of *Salmonella* infections, suggesting that contaminated pet products may be an under-recognized source of human infections. Outbreaks are often linked to the use of manure for fertilizer or contamination of irrigation water with manure.

6. Incubation period—From 6 to 72 hours, usually about 12–36 hours. Longer incubation periods of up to 16 days have been documented, and may not be uncommon following low-dose ingestion.

7. Period of communicability—Throughout the course of infection; extremely variable, usually several days to several weeks. A temporary carrier state may continue for months, especially in infants. Depending on the serotypes, approximately 1% of infected adults and 5% of children under 5 may excrete the organism for 1 year.

8. Susceptibility—Susceptibility is general and usually increased by achlorhydria, antacid treatment, gastrointestinal surgery, prior or current broad-spectrum antibiotherapy, neoplastic disease, immunosuppressive treatment and other debilitating conditions including malnutrition. Severity of the disease is related to serotype, number of organisms ingested, and host factors. While gastroenteritis caused by non-typhoidal *Salmonella* is usually self-limiting, immunosuppressed patients, including HIV-infected persons, are at risk for recurrent non-typhoidal *Salmonella* septicemia. In such cases antimicrobial treatment is advised. Septicemia in people with sickle-cell disease increases the risk of focal systemic infection, e.g. osteomyelitis.

9. Methods of control—

    A. Preventive measures:

        1) Investigate potential to limit prevalence in flocks or herds affected. In some countries a radical policy of eradication of chicken flocks found positive for *Salmonella* has resulted in significantly lower salmonellosis incidence in the human population.

2) Decrease contamination with animal feces of foods consumed with no or minimal cooking, including through limited use of animal waste for fertilizer.

3) Investigate the potential for animal (e.g. chicken) vaccination with mutant *Salmonella* or attenuated *Salmonella* vaccine strains, to reduce colonization or increase immune response in chicken.

4) Educate all food handlers about the importance of a) handwashing before, during and after food preparation; b) refrigerating prepared foods in small containers; c) thoroughly cooking all foodstuffs derived from animal sources, particularly poultry, pork, egg products and meat dishes; d) avoiding recontamination within the kitchen after cooking is completed; and e) maintaining a sanitary kitchen and protecting prepared foods against rodent and insect contamination.

5) Educate the public against consuming raw or incompletely cooked eggs (e.g. eggs "over easy" or "sunny side up," eggnogs, and homemade ice cream), and using dirty or cracked eggs.

6) Use pasteurized or irradiated egg products to prepare dishes in which eggs would otherwise be pooled before cooking, or when the dish containing eggs is not subsequently cooked.

7) Establish the facilities for, and encourage the use of, food irradiation for meats and eggs.

8) Exclude individuals with diarrhea from food handling and from care of hospitalized patients, the elderly and children.

9) Educate known carriers on the need for careful handwashing after defecation (and before handling food), and discourage them from handling food for others as long as they shed organisms.

10) Recognize the risk of *Salmonella* infections in pets and other animals, particularly those which may be handled closely by small children. Thorough handwashing is recommended after handling animals and pet foods and after cleaning animal enclosures.

11) Inspect for sanitation and adequately supervise abattoirs, food-processing plants, feed-blending mills, egg grading stations and butcher shops.

12) Establish *Salmonella* control programs (feed control, cleaning and disinfection, vector control and other sanitary and hygienic measures).

13) Adequately cook or heat-treat (including by pasteurization or irradiation) animal-derived foods prepared for animal consumption (e.g. meat or bone or fish meal and pet foods) to eliminate pathogens; follow by measures to avoid recontamination.

B. *Control of patient, contacts and the immediate environment:*

1) Report to local health authority: Obligatory case report, Class 2 (see *Reporting*).

2) Isolation: Proper handwashing should be stressed. For hospitalized patients, enteric precautions in handling feces and contaminated clothing and bed linen. Exclude symptomatic individuals from food handling and from direct care of infants and young children, the elderly, and immunocompromised and institutionalized patients. Exclusion of asymptomatic infected individuals is indicated for those with questionable hygienic habits, and may be required by local or state regulations. When exclusion is mandated, release to return to work handling food or in patient care generally requires 2 consecutive negative stool cultures for *Salmonella* collected not less than 24 hours apart; if antibiotics have been given, the initial culture should be taken at least 48 hours after the last dose.

3) Concurrent disinfection: Of feces and articles soiled therewith. In communities with adequate sewage disposal systems, feces can be discharged directly into sewers without preliminary disinfection. Terminal cleaning.

4) Quarantine: Not applicable.

5) Immunization of contacts: Not applicable.

6) Investigation of contacts and source of infection: Culture stools of household contacts who are involved in food handling, direct patient care, or care of young children or elderly people in institutional settings.

7) Specific treatment: For uncomplicated enterocolitis, none generally indicated except rehydration and electrolyte replacement with oral rehydration solution (see *Cholera*, 9B7). Antibiotics may not eliminate the carrier state and may lead to resistant strains or more severe infections. However, infants aged up to 2 months, the elderly, the debilitated, those with sickle-cell disease, persons infected with HIV and/or patients with continued/high fever or manifestations of extra-intestinal infection should receive antibiotherapy. Antimicrobial resistance of non-typhoidal salmonellae is variable; in adults, ciprofloxacin is highly effective, but its use is not approved for children; ampicillin or amoxicillin may also be used. Trimethoprim-sulfamethoxazole and chloramphenicol are alternatives when antimicrobial-resistant strains are involved. Patients infected with HIV may require lifelong treatment to prevent *Salmonella* septicemia.

An important recent development is the emergence of multi-resistant *S. Typhimurium* DT (Definitive phage-Type) 104. These strains are usually resistant to ampicillin, chloramphenicol, streptomycin, sulfonamide and tetracycline, and genes associated with these resistance properties are chromosomally encoded. The emergence of *S. Typhimurium* DT104 may have been linked to the use of antimicrobial agents in agriculture, especially in intensive calf rearing or aquaculture. An important antibiotic resistance gene cluster has been shown to transfer horizontally to other *Salmonella* serovars, including *S. Agona*, *S. Albany*, and *S. Newport*.

C. Epidemic measures: See *Foodborne diseases*, *Staphylococcal food intoxication*, *Typhoid fever* 9C. Search for a history of food handling errors, such as use of unsafe raw ingredients, inadequate cooking, time-temperature abuses and cross-contamination. In *S. Enteritidis* outbreaks in which dishes containing eggs are implicated, trace back to the egg source; reporting to the ministry of agriculture is advised.

D. Disaster implications: A danger in a situation with mass feeding and poor sanitation.

E. International measures: WHO Collaborating Centres provide support as required. More information can be found at:

<http://www.who.int/collaboratingcentres/database/en/>

Also see the *WHO Golden Rules for Safe Food Preparation* and the *WHO Five Keys to Safer Food Manual (2007)*; further information can be found at:

<http://www.who.int/foodsafety/publications/consumer/manual_keys.pdf>

- and the WHO Global Salm-Surv Network

<http://www.who.int/salmsurv>

SCABIES   ICD-9 033.0; ICD-10 B86
(Sarcoptic itch, Sarcoptic acariasis)
[CCDM19: M. Eberhard, F. Ndowa, J. Watson]
[CCDM18: F. Ndowa]

1. Identification—A parasitic infestation of the skin caused by a mite whose penetration is visible as papules, vesicles or tiny linear burrows containing the mites and their eggs. Lesions are prominent around finger webs, anterior surfaces of wrists and elbows, anterior axillary folds, belt line, thighs and external genitalia in men; nipples, abdomen and the lower portion of the buttocks are frequently affected in women. In infants, the head, neck, palms and soles may be involved; these areas are usually spared in older individuals. Itching is intense, especially at night, but complications are limited to lesions secondarily infected by scratching. In immunodeficient individuals and in senile patients, infestation often appears as a generalized dermatitis more widely distributed than the burrows, with extensive scaling and sometimes vesiculation and crusting ("Norwegian" or "crusted" scabies); the usual severe itching may be reduced or absent. When scabies is complicated by beta-hemolytic streptococcal infection, there is a risk of acute glomerulonephritis.

Diagnosis may be established by recovery from a burrow and microscopic identification of the mite, eggs, or mite feces (scybala). Care should be taken to choose lesions for scraping or biopsy that have not been excoriated by repeated scratching. Prior application of mineral oil facilitates collecting the scrapings and examining them under a cover slip. Applying ink to the skin and then washing it off will disclose the burrows.

2. **Etiologic agent**—*Sarcoptes scabiei* var *hominis*, a mite.

3. **Occurrence**—Widespread. Causes of epidemics are not clear but past epidemics were attributed to poverty, poor sanitation and crowding due to war, mass movement of people and economic crises. Recent epidemics have affected people of all socioeconomic levels and standards of personal hygiene. Endemic in many developing countries.

4. **Reservoir**—Humans; Other *Sarcoptes* species and other animal mites, including other forms of *S. scabiei*, can live but not reproduce on humans; such infestations are self-limiting.

5. **Mode of transmission**—Transfer of parasites commonly occurs through prolonged direct contact with infested skin and also during sexual contact. Transfer from undergarments and bedclothes occurs only if these have been contaminated by infested persons immediately beforehand. Mites can burrow beneath the skin surface in about 1 hour. Persons with the crusted ("Norwegian") scabies syndrome are highly contagious because of the large number of mites present in the exfoliating scales.

6. **Incubation period**—In persons without previous exposure, 2–6 weeks before onset of itching. Persons who have been previously infested develop symptoms 1–4 days after re-exposure.

7. **Period of communicability**—Until mites and eggs are destroyed by treatment, ordinarily after 1 or occasionally 2 courses of treatment a week apart. Crusted scabies is highly contagious, and can require multiple treatment with one or more agents to eliminate an infestation.

8. Susceptibility—Some resistance is suggested; fewer mites succeed in establishing themselves on persons previously infested than on those with no prior exposure. Immunologically compromised persons, including those with HIV, are susceptible to hyperinfestation.

9. Methods of control—

A. *Preventive measures:* Educate the public and medical community on mode of transmission, early diagnosis and treatment of infested patients and contacts.

B. *Control of patient, contacts and the immediate environment:*

1) Report to local health authority: Official report not ordinarily justifiable, Class 5 (see *Reporting*).

2) Isolation: Exclude infested individuals from school or work until the day after treatment. For hospitalized patients, contact isolation for 24 hours after start of effective treatment. Twenty-four hours may be insufficient in crusted scabies because viable mites can remain on the patient after a single treatment; in this case an alternative isolation approach is suggested in institutional outbreaks: 10-day quarantine of index patient.

3) Concurrent disinfestation: Laundering underwear, clothing and bedsheets worn or used by the patient in the 48 to 72 hours prior to treatment, using hot cycles of both washer and dryer, will kill mites and eggs, but may not be needed for most infestations. Laundering bedding and clothing is important for patients with crusted scabies because potential for fomite transmission is high.

4) Quarantine: Not applicable.

5) Immunization of contacts: Not applicable.

6) Investigation of contacts and source of infestation: Search for unreported or unrecognized cases among companions and household members; single infestations in a family are uncommon. Treat prophylactically those who have had skin-to-skin contact with infested persons (including family members and sexual contacts).

7) Specific treatment: The treatment of choice, particularly for children and pregnant or nursing women, is topical 5% permethrin. Other topical therapies are 10% Crotamiton or 1% lindane (gamma benzene hexachloride). Because of concerns about neurologic toxicity, lindane should be used only in patients who cannot tolerate or have failed treatment with safer medication, is contraindicated in premature neonates, and must be used with caution in infants, children, the elderly, persons with other skin conditions, persons weigh-

ing less than 50 kg (110 lbs), and pregnant women. More recently comparable cure rates to topical agents have been demonstrated with a single dose or two doses repeated at a 2-week interval of oral ivermectin 200 mg/kg body weight, although ivermectin is not licensed for this indication. Both tetraethylthiuram monosulfide (carbamyl) in 5% solution and emulsion of benzyl benzoate have been used as scabicides. A combination of benzyl benzoate and oral ivermectin may prove useful in HIV-infected persons with severe scabies. Resistance has been reported for all scabicides. Treatment details vary with the drug.

Topical agents are applied to the whole body except the head, left on for the prescribed time, and then washed off as directed. On the following day, a cleansing bath is taken and a change made to fresh clothing and bedclothes. All affected members of a household or close community should be treated at the same time to avoid re-infestation. Itching may persist for 1–2 weeks; this should not be regarded as a sign of drug failure or re-infestation. Over-treatment is common and should be avoided because of toxicity of some of these agents, especially gamma benzene hexachloride.

In about 5% of cases, a repeat course of treatment with oral ivermectin may be necessary after 7–10 days if eggs survived the initial treatment. Multiple courses of treatment with one or more scabicides may be necessary for patients with crusted scabies. Close supervision of all treatment, including bathing, is necessary.

C. Epidemic measures:

1) Provide treatment and educate infested individuals and others at risk. Cooperation of non-health authorities is often needed.
2) Coordinated mass treatment.
3) Case-finding efforts are extended to screen whole families, military units or institutions, with segregation of infested individuals if possible.
4) Soap and facilities for mass bathing and laundering are essential. Tetmosol® soap, where available, may help prevent infestation.

D. Disaster implications: A potential nuisance in situations of overcrowding.

E. International measures: None.

SCHISTOSOMIASIS   ICD-9 120; ICD-10 B65
(Bilharziasis, Snail fever)
[CCDM19: M. Eberhard]
[CCDM18: D. Engels]

1. Identification—A blood fluke (trematode) infection with adult male and female worms living within mesenteric or vesical veins of the host over a life span of many years. Eggs produce minute granulomata and scars in organs where they lodge or are deposited. Symptoms are related to the number and location of the eggs in the human host: *Schistosoma mansoni* and *S. japonicum* give rise primarily to hepatic and intestinal pathology, and early signs and symptoms include diarrhea, abdominal pain and hepatosplenomegaly. *S. japonicum* can also cause CNS disease, with Jacksonian seizures. *S. haematobium* gives rise to urinary manifestations, and early signs and symptoms include dysuria, urinary frequency and hematuria at the end of urination; CNS disease has, rarely, been reported.

The WHO-recommended case definitions in endemic areas are a) For urinary schistosomiasis: visible hematuria or positive reagent strip for hematuria, or with eggs of *S. haematobium* in urine (confirmed case); b) For intestinal schistosomiasis: non-specific abdominal symptoms, blood in stool, hepato(spleno)megaly (suspected case), or presence of eggs in stools (confirmed case).

The most important effects of schistosomiasis are the late complications that arise from chronic infection: liver fibrosis, portal hypertension and its sequelae, and possibly colorectal malignancy in the intestinal forms; and obstructive uropathy, superimposed bacterial infection, infertility and bladder cancer in the urinary form. Eggs can be deposited at ectopic sites, including the brain, spinal cord, skin, pelvis and vulvovaginal areas.

The larvae of certain schistosomes of birds and mammals may penetrate the human skin and cause a dermatitis, sometimes known as "swimmer's itch"; these schistosomes do not mature in humans. Such infections may be prevalent among bathers in lakes in many parts of the world. However, the clinical entity of "seabather's eruption", a pruritic dermatitis that appears principally where the bathing suit has been worn, has been shown to be caused by the larval stage of some jellyfish species, and not by a schistosome.

Definitive diagnosis of schistosomiasis depends on demonstration of eggs in biopsy specimens, in the stool by direct smear or on a Kato thick smear, or in urine by the examination of a urine sediment or Nuclepore® filtration. Urine filtration is especially useful for *S. haematobium* infections. Useful immunological tests include immunoblot analysis, the circumoval precipitin test, IFA and ELISA with egg or adult worm antigen, and RIA with purified egg or adult antigens; positive results on serological antibody detection tests could be indicative of prior infection and are not proof of current infection. More recently, various assays developed to detect schistosome antigens directly in serum or urine have proved useful in detecting current infection, and in assessing cure after treatment.

2. Infectious agents—*Schistosoma mansoni*, *S. haematobium* and *S. japonicum* are the major species causing human disease. *S. mekongi*, *S. malayensis*, *S. intercalatum* and *S. mattheei* are of importance only in limited areas.

3. Occurrence—*S. mansoni* is found in Africa (including Madagascar); the Arabian Peninsula; Brazil, Suriname and Venezuela in South America; and in some Caribbean islands. *S. haematobium* is found in Africa (including Madagascar) and the Middle East. *S. japonicum* is found in China, the Philippines and Sulawesi (Celebes) in Indonesia; no new cases have been found in Japan since 1978 after an intensive control program. *S. mekongi* is found in the Mekong River area of Cambodia and the Lao People's Democratic Republic. *S. intercalatum* occurs in parts of western Africa, including Cameroon, Chad, the Democratic Republic of Congo, Gabon, and Sao Tome. *S. malayensis* is known only from peninsular Malaysia. Human infection with the bovine parasite *S. mattheei* has been reported from southern Africa.

4. Reservoir—Humans are the principal reservoir of *S. haematobium*, *S. intercalatum* and *S. mansoni*, although the latter has been reported to occur in rodents. Humans, dogs, cats, pigs, cattle, water buffalo and wild rodents are potential hosts of *S. japonicum*; their relative epidemiological importance varies in different regions. *S. malayensis* appears to be a rodent parasite that occasionally infects humans. Epidemiological persistence of the parasite depends on the presence of an appropriate snail as intermediate host—i.e. species of the genera *Biomphalaria* for *S. mansoni*; *Bulinus* for *S. haematobium*, *S. intercalatum* and *S. mattheei*; *Oncomelania* for *S. japonicum*; *Neotricula* for *S. mekongi*; and *Robertsiella* for *S. malayensis*.

5. Mode of transmission—Infection is acquired from freshwater containing free-swimming larval forms (cercariae) that have developed in snails. The eggs of *S. haematobium* leave the mammalian body mainly in the urine, those of the other species in the feces. The eggs hatch in water and the liberated larvae (miracidia) penetrate into suitable freshwater snail intermediate hosts. After several weeks, the cercariae emerge from the snail and penetrate human skin, usually while the person is in contact with infected water—e.g. working, swimming or wading. Cercariae then enter the bloodstream, are carried to blood vessels of the lungs, migrate to the liver, develop to maturity, then migrate to veins of the abdominal or pelvic cavity.

Adult forms of *S. mansoni*, *S. japonicum*, *S. mekongi*, *S. mattheei* and *S. intercalatum* usually remain in mesenteric veins; those of *S. haematobium* usually migrate through anastomoses into the vesical plexus of the urinary bladder. Eggs are deposited in venules and escape into the lumen of the bowel or urinary bladder, or end up lodging in other organs, including the liver and the lungs.

6. Incubation period—Acute systemic manifestations (Katayama fever) may occur in primary infections 2–6 weeks after exposure, immediately preceding and during initial egg deposition. Acute systemic manifestations are uncommon, but can occur with *S. haematobium* infections.

7. Period of communicability—Not communicable from person to person; persons with schistosomiasis may spread the infection by discharging eggs in urine and/or feces into bodies of water for as long as they excrete eggs. It is common for human infections with *S. mansoni* and *S. haematobium* to last in excess of 10 years. Infected snails will release cercariae for as long as they live, a period that may last from several weeks to about 3 months.

8. Susceptibility—Susceptibility is universal; any immunity developing as a result of infection is variable and not yet fully investigated.

9. Methods of control—

A. Preventive measures:

1) Treat patients in endemic areas with praziquantel to relieve suffering and prevent disease progression. Regularly treat high-risk groups—such as school-age children, women of childbearing age, or special occupational groups in endemic areas—with presumptive curative doses. A height-measuring pole (<http://whqlibdoc.who.int/trs/WHO_TRS_912.pdf>) has been tested in Africa and facilitates praziquantel dosage.

2) Educate the public in endemic areas to seek treatment early and regularly, and to protect themselves.

3) Dispose of feces and urine so that viable eggs will not reach bodies of freshwater containing intermediate snail hosts. Though difficult, control of animals infected with *S. japonicum* is desirable.

4) Improve irrigation and agriculture practices; reduce snail habitats by removing vegetation, by draining and filling, or by lining canals with concrete.

5) Treat snail-breeding sites with molluskicides. Cost may limit the use of these agents.

6) Individual protection: prevent exposure to contaminated water (e.g. by wearing rubber boots). To minimize cercarial penetration after brief or accidental water exposure, vigorously and completely towel dry skin surfaces that are wet with suspected water. Apply 70% alcohol immediately to the skin to kill surface cercariae.

7) Provide water for drinking, bathing and washing clothes from sources free of cercariae or treated to kill them. Effective measures for inactivating cercariae include water treatment with iodine or chlorine. Allowing water to stand 48–72 hours before use is also effective.

8) Travelers visiting endemic areas should be advised of the risks and informed about preventive measures.

B. Control of patient, contacts and the immediate environment:

1) Report to local health authority: in selected endemic areas; in many countries, not a reportable disease, Class 3 (see *Reporting*).
2) Isolation: Not applicable.
3) Concurrent disinfection: Sanitary disposal of feces and urine.
4) Quarantine: Not applicable.
5) Immunization of contacts: Not applicable.
6) Investigation of contacts and source of infection: Examine contacts for infection from a common source.
7) Specific treatment: Praziquantel is the drug of choice against all species. Alternative drugs are oxamniquine for *S. mansoni*, and metrifonate for *S. haematobium*.

C. Epidemic measures: Examine for schistosomiasis and treat all who are infected, but especially those with disease and/or moderate to heavy intensity of infection; pay particular attention to children. Provide clean water, warn people against contact with water potentially containing cercariae, and prohibit contamination of water. Treat areas that have high snail densities with molluskicides.

D. Disaster implications: None.

E. International measures: WHO Collaborating Centres provide support as required. More information can be found at:

http://www.who.int/collaboratingcentres/database/en/

Further information may be found at:

http://www.who.int/tdr/diseases/schisto/default.htm

SEVERE ACUTE RESPIRATORY SYNDROME ICD-10 U04.9 (provisional)
(SARS)
[CCDM19: A. Merianos]
[CCDM18: D. Heymann]

1. Identification—A severe respiratory infection thought to have originated in the Guangdong Province of China, with emergence into human populations sometime in November 2002. The 2003 epidemic was characterized by "super spreading events" that seeded outbreaks in Canada; China (originating in Guangdong Province and spreading to major cities in other areas, including Beijing, Taipei and the Special Administrative Region of Hong Kong); Singapore; and Viet Nam. The disease spread internationally along major airline routes, and resulted in 8 098 SARS cases in 26 countries, with 774 deaths. Transmission occurred primarily in hospitals and among families and contacts of hospital workers. The last reported case of SARS occurred in China in April 2004, associated with a cluster of cases linked to a laboratory worker, and since then there has been no evidence of SARS coronavirus (SARS-CoV) circulating in human populations.

It remains very difficult to predict when or whether SARS will re-emerge in epidemic form. China has implemented strict market and food safety and other measures to prevent the transmission of SARS-like coronaviruses from animal hosts to humans. However, clustering of SARS-like illness in persons exposed to potential animal hosts, among health care workers, or among others exposed to a health care facility remain important sentinel events that may indicate the re-emergence of SARS (WHO SARS alert).

The diagnosis of SARS requires both a compatible clinical illness and definitive laboratory tests for SARS-CoV infection independently verified at a WHO International SARS Reference and Verification Network laboratory, as the risk of false-positive test results is very high. WHO recommends that testing for SARS-CoV is only undertaken when there is compelling clinical and/or epidemiological evidence that SARS may be the cause of an individual case or cluster of acute respiratory illness.

Symptoms and signs of SARS are non-specific, with a spectrum of disease ranging from severe respiratory illness to milder or atypical presentations. SARS should be considered in the differential diagnosis in an individual presenting with fever $\geq 38°C$ (100.4°F), symptoms of lower respiratory tract illness (cough, dyspnea or shortness of breath), with radiological evidence of lung infiltrates consistent with pneumonia or adult respiratory distress syndrome (ARDS), or autopsy findings consistent with pneumonia or ARDS without an identifiable cause and in whom no alternative diagnosis can fully explain the illness. Severe cases develop rapidly progressing respiratory distress and oxygen desaturation, coinciding with peak viremia at 10 days after onset of illness, with about 20% requiring intensive care. Mild and atypical presentations are likely to be missed unless there is supportive epidemiological and laboratory evidence suggesting a SARS-CoV infection.

The clinical spectrum and course of SARS vary, appearing to depend on immunological factors. Based on an analysis of data from Canada, China, the Special Administrative Region of Hong Kong, Singapore, Viet Nam and the USA during the 2003 epidemic, the case-fatality ratio of SARS is estimated to range from 0% to more than 50% depending on the age group affected and reporting center, with a crude global CFR of approximately

9.6%. Various studies have associated higher mortality with male gender and the presence of co-morbidities.

The WHO has published guidance on the laboratory diagnosis of SARS:

a) *Summary of the discussion and recommendations of the SARS Laboratory Workshop* (October 2003), which can be found at:
http://www.who.int/csr/sars/guidelines/en/SARSLab meeting.pdf

b) *WHO SARS International Reference and Verification Laboratory Network: Policy and Procedures in the Inter-Epidemic Period* (January 2004), which can be found at:
http://www.who.int/csr/resources/publications/en/ SARSReferenceLab.pdf

A variety of diagnostics tests are available. The reliability of diagnostic tests for SARS-CoV infection depends on the type of clinical specimens collected, and the timing and mode of collection. Respiratory samples—ideally nasopharyngeal aspirates—and stool samples should be routinely collected for nucleic acid detection by RT-PCR or virus isolation during the first and second weeks of illness, as these specimens are most likely to yield virus. During the SARS epidemic, the overall sensitivity of the RT-PCR was around 70% within the first days after disease onset. A confirmed positive PCR for SARS requires at least 2 different clinical specimens (e.g. nasopharyngeal and stool); or the same type clinical specimen collected on 2 or more days during illness (e.g. 2 or more nasopharyngeal aspirates); or 2 different assays; or repeat PCR using a new extract from the original clinical sample on each occasion of testing. Acute and convalescent phase sera should also be collected at least 8 days apart for serology (e.g. IF, ELISA, Western blots and neutralization tests).

Laboratories performing SARS tests must adopt strict quality control procedures, use standardized test protocols and reagents, and independently verify their results for initial cases/clusters in non-epidemic periods. All sporadic cases testing positive at a national laboratory, and at least one case in any new (independent) chain of human transmission, should be independently verified by a WHO International SARS Reference and Verification Network laboratory.

2. Infectious agent—SARS is caused by a coronavirus similar, on electron microscopy, to animal coronaviruses. It is stable in feces and urine at room temperature for at least 1–2 days, and for up to 4 days in stools from patients who manifest diarrhea. The SARS virus loses infectivity after exposure to different commonly used disinfectants and fixatives.

Heating at 56°C (132.8°F) kills SARS-CoV at approximately 10 000 units per 15 minutes.

3. Occurrence—Major outbreaks of SARS occurred during the period between November 2002 and July 2003 in Canada, China (including Hong Kong Special Administrative Region and Taiwan), Singapore and Viet Nam. The virus is known to have been transported by infected humans to over 20 additional sites in Africa, the Americas, Asia, Australia, Europe, the Middle East and the Pacific. On July 5, 2003, WHO reported that person-to-person transmission of the SARS virus had been interrupted at all outbreak sites. Intensified surveillance detected four subsequent additional outbreaks, all but one associated with breaches in laboratory biosafety. Single cases were reported in laboratory workers in Singapore and Taipei (Taiwan, China) in 2003. In December 2003, the first of what was thought to be four sporadic community-acquired SARS cases were reported from Guangdong Province, China, three of which were attributed to exposure to animal or environmental sources. No further community-acquired infections were reported, but in April 2004 a cluster of nine cases, seven of which were associated with one chain of transmission linked to a laboratory worker and with hospital spread, were reported in Anhui Province and Beijing, China. Two additional cases were detected as part of a serosurvey of contacts at the facility.

4. Reservoir—Cave-dwelling bats in the genus *Rhinolophus* (Chinese horseshoe bats) are a reservoir of SARS-like coronaviruses closely related to those responsible for the SARS epidemic. These SARS-like coronaviruses display greater genetic variation than SARS-CoV isolated from humans or from the Himalayan masked palm civet (Paguma larvata), which is considered the main source of animal-to-human transmission. Initial studies in Guangdong Province, China, showed similar coronaviruses in civets and a small number of other wildlife species sold in wet markets.

For cases of SARS to reappear, the virus has to re-emerge from one of three sources: an animal source, a laboratory accident, or undetected transmission cycles in human populations. The laboratory-associated outbreaks of SARS highlight the importance of strict adherence to biosafety procedures and practices for laboratory work with SARS-CoV. WHO strongly recommends Biosafety Level 3 (BSL3) as the appropriate containment level for working with live SARS-CoV material.

5. Mode of transmission—In 2002, SARS-CoV-like viruses are thought to have been introduced into the human population from wildlife hosts. SARS is usually transmitted from person to person by direct contact, by fomites, and by respiratory droplets. Caring for or living with an infected person, or having direct contact with respiratory secretions, body fluids and excretions of a case of SARS, are high-risk exposures in the absence of appropriate levels of infection control. In one recorded instance, the virus is thought to have been transmitted by some environmental vehicle, possibly aerosolized sewerage or transport of sewerage by mechanical vectors.

6. Incubation period—From 2 to 10 days (mean of 5 days), with isolated reports of longer incubation periods.

7. Period of communicability—Not yet completely understood. Epidemiological and virological studies and clinical follow-up during the 2003 epidemic indicated that transmission does not occur before onset of clinical signs and symptoms, and that maximum period of communicability is less than 21 days. Health workers are at greatest risk of transmission, especially before the diagnosis of SARS is made and when involved in aerosol-generating procedures such as intubation or nebulization. Health care settings have been sites of SARS amplification, serving as a major entry points of the disease into the community.

8. Susceptibility—Unknown, but assumed to be universal. Race and gender appear not to alter susceptibility. Because of the small numbers of cases reported among children during the SARS epidemic, and differences in the intensity of exposure between adults and children, it has not been possible to assess the influence of age on susceptibility.

9. Methods of control—

    A. Preventive measures:

        Preventive measures include preparedness planning for the detection, investigation, containment and control of unexplained clusters of acute respiratory disease. Curative health services should develop clinical algorithms to assist clinicians in assessing patients with acute febrile respiratory infection for their risk of SARS, based on the national and global risk assessment of SARS re-emergence. The *WHO guidelines for the global surveillance of SARS, October 2004* and the *WHO SARS Risk Assessment and Preparedness Framework* provide detailed guidance on SARS alert and triage of acute respiratory illness in the current epidemiological situation. It is unlikely that sporadic cases of SARS will be detected unless a patient with an atypical pneumonia gives a history of one or more of the following:

        i) Exposure to an animal host.

        ii) SARS-CoV related laboratory work.

        iii) Travel to southern China or another area with increased likelihood of animal-to-human transmission of SARS-CoV-like viruses from wildlife or other animal reservoirs.

        In the post-epidemic period, SARS is a diagnosis by exclusion of more usual causes of severe respiratory disease (see WHO SARS alert cases).

        1) Identify all suspect and probable cases using the WHO case definitions for SARS.

Persons who arrive at health care facilities and require SARS assessment must be rapidly diverted by triage nurses to a separate area to minimize transmission to other health care workers (HCWs), patients and visitors, and—if tolerated—must be given a face mask to wear, preferably one that provides filtration of expired air.

HCWs involved in the triage process should wear a face mask (N/R/P 95/99/100 or FFP 2/3 or equivalent national manufacturing standard) with eye protection, and wash hands before and after contact with any patient, after activities likely to cause contamination, and after removing gloves. Triage and waiting areas need to be adequately ventilated, with at least 12 air exchanges per hour (ACH).

Soiled gloves, stethoscopes and other equipment must be treated with care, as they have the potential to spread infection. Broad-spectrum disinfectants of proven antiviral activity, such as fresh bleach solutions, must be widely available at appropriate concentrations, and must be used according to manufacturers' instructions.

2) Isolation of persons under investigation for SARS and health care infection control:

Persons under investigation for SARS cases should be isolated and accommodated as follows, in descending order of preference:

- Negative pressure rooms with door closed
- Single room with its own bathroom facilities
- Cohort placement in an area with an independent air supply
- Exhaust system and bathroom facilities
- Cohort patients with the same diagnosis.

If this is not possible, keep patient beds at least 1 meter apart. Airborne precaution rooms can be naturally or mechanically ventilated, with adequate air change rate of at least 12 ACH and controlled direction of airflow. If an independent air supply is not feasible, air conditioning should be turned off and windows opened (if away from public places) for good ventilation.

Strict standard and airborne precautions for infection control must be applied to avoid direct contact with body fluids and respiratory droplets, and for aerosols; all staff, including ancillary staff, must be fully trained in infection control and must use appropriate personal protective equipment (PPE) as follows:

- A particulate respirator at least as protective as a NIOSH-certified N95, EU FFP2 or equivalent (NRP 95/99/100 or

FFP 2/3 or equivalent manufacturing standard or standard applicable to the country of manufacture) as the minimum level of respiratory protection required for HCWs performing aerosol-generating procedures, and:

- Single pair of gloves
- Eye protection (face shield, goggles)
- Disposable gown
- Fluid-resistant apron
- Footwear that can be decontaminated.

Disposable equipment should be used wherever possible in the treatment and care of patients with SARS, and disposed of appropriately. If medical devices are to be reused, they must be sterilized according to manufacturers' instructions. Surfaces should be cleaned with broad-spectrum disinfectants of proven antiviral activity.

Movement of patients outside the isolation unit should be avoided. If moved, patients should wear a face mask, if tolerated. Visits should be kept to a minimum and personal protective equipment used under supervision.

Handwashing with access to clean water is crucial before and after contact with any patient, after activities likely to cause contamination, and after removing gloves. Alcohol-based skin disinfectants can be used if there is no obvious contamination with organic material.

Particular attention should be paid to interventions such as use of nebulizers, chest physiotherapy, bronchoscopy or gastroscopy, and other interventions that may disrupt the respiratory tract or place the health care worker in close proximity to the patient and to potentially infected secretions.

All sharp and cutting instruments must be handled promptly and safely; patients' linen must be prepared on site for the laundry staff and placed into biohazard bags.

3) Contact tracing:

A contact is a person who cared for, lived with, or had direct contact with the respiratory secretions, body fluids and/or excretion (e.g. feces) of, any confirmed case of SARS or person under investigation (WHO SARS alert case). Contact tracing must be systematic for contacts during an agreed period prior to the onset of symptoms in the index case.

B. Control of patients, contacts and the immediate environment:

1) Report to WHO: SARS is a notifiable disease under the International Health Regulations (2005), Class 1 (see *Reporting*).
2) Patient management:

Hospitalize under isolation or with cohort patients with the same diagnosis, keeping patient beds at least 1 meter apart.

Obtain samples (nasopharyngeal aspirate, blood, serum, stool and urine) to exclude standard causes of pneumonia, including atypical causes. Consider the possibility of co-infection with SARS-CoV and carry out appropriate chest radiography. Obtain other samples to aid clinical diagnosis of SARS, including: white blood cell count; platelet count; creatinine phosphokinase; liver function tests; urea; electrolytes; and C-reactive protein.

At the time of admission, prescription of antibiotics for the treatment of community-acquired pneumonia is recommended until diagnoses of treatable causes of ARDS have been excluded. Numerous antibiotherapies have been tried for treatment of SARS, with no clear effect. Inflammatory cytokine responses ("cytokine storms") might be involved in the immunopathological damage in SARS patients. Ribavirin with or without use of steroids and other combination therapies were used in patients during the SARS epidemic, but their effectiveness has not been proven. Severe adverse reactions to ribavirin use and long-term sequelae, such as avascular necrosis of the hip associated with prolonged high-dose steroid use, were observed.

3) Contact management:

Give information on the signs, symptoms, and means of transmission of SARS to each contact.

Place under active surveillance for 10 days, and train contacts in self-monitoring for fever and recording temperature daily. Stress to the contact that the most consistent first symptom to appear in SARS is fever.

Ensure the contact is visited or telephoned daily by a member of the public health care team to determine whether fever or other signs and symptoms of SARS are developing.

If the contact develops fever or other SARS signs and symptoms, follow-up examination should be conducted at a suitable health care facility, under appropriate levels of infection control.

If the suspect or probable SARS case has been removed from surveillance because an alternative diagnosis can fully explain the illness, contacts can also be removed from surveillance and discharged from follow-up.

Voluntary home quarantine of asymptomatic contacts was used routinely as a control measure in some of the affected cities during the 2003 epidemic before the period of communicability and characteristics of viral excretion were well described; however, its efficacy in reducing transmission was not formally evaluated. In light of strong epidemiological and virological evidence that SARS-CoV transmission occurs after the onset of symptoms, contact health monitoring without quarantine is a preferable intervention.

C. Epidemic Measures:

Establish a multi-sectoral national SARS advisory group to oversee control measures.

Traditional public health measures, including active case finding, case isolation, strict adherence to infection control in health care settings, contact tracing, fever monitoring and enhanced surveillance, were successful in controlling the spread of SARS.

Ensure adequate triage facilities and clearly indicate to the general public where they are located and how they can be accessed.

During the SARS outbreaks of 2003, the perception of risk of infection by the general population was far greater than the actual risk of infection. Outbreak risk communication and community education should be an integral part of epidemic control measures.

Establish telephone hotlines or other means of dealing with enquiries from the general public, health professionals and the media, and ensure that the means of access to this resource are clearly provided to all stakeholders.

D. Disaster Implications:

During the SARS epidemic, transmission was amplified in health care settings, placing severe strain on curative and public health systems. As with other emerging infections, severe adverse economic impact and socioeconomic consequences on society have been shown to occur.

E. International Measures:

SARS is a notifiable disease under the International Health Regulations (2005). Should SARS re-emerge, WHO will provide regular information updates and evidence-based travel recommendations, effective in limiting the international spread of infection, in accordance with the IHR. A global response facilitating exchange of information among scientists, clinicians and public health experts has been shown to be effective in providing information and effective evidence-based policies and strategies.

SHIGELLOSIS ICD-9 004; ICD-10 A03
(Bacillary dysentery)
[CCDM19: E. Mintz]
[CCDM18: C. Chaignat]

1. Identification—An acute bacterial disease involving the distal small intestine and colon, characterized by loose stools of small volume accompanied by fever, nausea and sometimes toxemia, vomiting, cramps and tenesmus. In typical cases, the stools contain blood and mucus (dysentery) resulting from mucosal ulcerations and confluent colonic crypt microabscesses caused by the invasive organisms; many cases present with watery diarrhea. Convulsions may be an important complication in young children. Bacteremia is uncommon. Severity and case-fatality rate vary with the host (age and pre-existing nutritional state) and the serotype. *Shigella dysenteriae* type 1 (Shiga bacillus) spreads in epidemics and is often associated with serious disease and complications including toxic megacolon, intestinal perforation and the hemolytic uremic syndrome; case-fatality rates have been as high as 20% among hospitalized cases even in recent years. Mild and asymptomatic infections occur; illness is usually self-limited, lasting on average 4–7 days. Many infections with *S. sonnei* result in a short clinical course and an almost negligible case-fatality rate except in immunocompromised hosts. Certain strains of *S. flexneri* can cause a reactive post-infectious arthropathy (formerly known as Reiter syndrome), especially in persons who are genetically predisposed by having HLA-B27 antigen.

Isolation of *Shigella* from feces or rectal swabs provides bacteriological diagnosis. Prompt laboratory processing of specimens and use of appropriate media (differential, low selectivity—MacConkey agar—together with high selectivity XLD or S/S agar) increase the likelihood of *Shigella* isolation. Isolation of *S. dysenteriae* type 1 requires special efforts, since this organism is inhibited by some selective media, including S/S agar. Outside the human body, *Shigella* remains viable only for a short period, which is why stool specimens must be processed rapidly after collection. Infection is usually associated with large numbers of fecal leukocytes detected through microscopic examination of stool mucus stained with methylene blue or Gram.

2. Infectious agents—The genus *Shigella* comprises 4 species or serogroups:

Group A: *S. dysenteriae*
Group B: *S. flexneri*
Group C: *S. boydii*
Group D: *S. sonnei*.

Groups A, B and C are further divided into 15, 15, and 19 serotypes and subtypes, respectively, designated by Arabic numbers and lower case letters (e.g. *S. flexneri* 2a). *S. sonnei* (Group D) consists of a single serotype. A specific virulence plasmid is necessary for the epithelial cell invasiveness manifested by *Shigellae*.

3. Occurrence—Worldwide; shigellosis causes an estimated 600 000 deaths per year. Two-thirds of the cases, and most of the deaths, are in children under 10. Illness in infants under 6 months is unusual. Secondary attack rates in households can be as high as 40%. Outbreaks occur in crowded conditions and where personal hygiene is poor, such as in prisons, institutions for children, day care centers, mental hospitals and crowded refugee camps, as well as among men who have sex with men. Shigellosis is endemic in both tropical and temperate climates; reported cases represent only a small proportion of cases, even in developed areas. The geographical distribution of the 4 *Shigella* serogroups is different, as is their pathogenicity.

More than one serotype is commonly present in a community; mixed infections with other intestinal pathogens also occur. In general, *S. flexneri*, *S. boydii* and *S. dysenteriae* account for most isolates from developing countries. *S. dysenteriae* type 1 is of particular concern in developing countries and complex emergency situations where huge outbreaks can occur. *S. sonnei* is most common in industrialized countries, where the disease is generally less severe. Multidrug-resistant *Shigellae* (including *S. dysenteriae* 1) with considerable geographical variations have appeared worldwide, in relation with the widespread use of antimicrobial agents.

4. Reservoir—The only significant reservoir is humans, although prolonged outbreaks have occurred in primate colonies.

5. Mode of transmission—Mainly by direct or indirect fecal-oral transmission from a symptomatic patient or a short-term asymptomatic carrier. Infection may occur after the ingestion of contaminated food or water, as well as from person to person. The infective dose can be as low as 10-100 organisms. Individuals primarily responsible for transmission include those who fail to clean hands and under fingernails thoroughly after defecation. They may spread infection to others directly by physical contact, or indirectly by contaminating food. Transmission via drinking or recreational water may occur as the result of direct fecal contamination; flies can transfer organisms from latrines to uncovered food items.

6. Incubation period—Usually 1-3 days, but may range from 12 to 96 hours; up to 1 week for *S. dysenteriae* 1.

7. Period of communicability—During acute infection and until the infectious agent is no longer present in feces, usually for 4 weeks after illness. Asymptomatic carriers may transmit infection; very rarely, the carrier state may persist for months or longer. Appropriate antimicrobial treatment usually reduces duration of carriage to a few days.

8. Susceptibility—Susceptibility is general, infection following ingestion of a small number of organisms; in endemic areas the disease is more severe in young children than in adults, among whom many infections may be asymptomatic. The elderly, the debilitated and the malnourished of all ages are particularly susceptible to severe disease and death. Breast-feeding is protective for infants and young children. Studies with experimental serotype-specific live oral vaccines and parenteral polysaccharide conjugate vaccines show protection of short duration (1 year) against infection with the homologous serotype.

9. **Methods of control**—General measures to improve hygiene are important, but often difficult to implement because of cost. An organized effort to promote careful handwashing with soap and water is the single most important control measure to decrease transmission rates in most settings.

The potentially high case-fatality rate in infections with *S. dysenteriae* 1, coupled with antibiotic resistance, calls for measures comparable to those for typhoid fever, including the need to identify the source(s) of all infections. In contrast, an isolated infection with *S. sonnei* in a private home would not deserve such an approach. Common-source foodborne or waterborne outbreaks require prompt investigation and intervention whatever the infecting species. Institutional outbreaks may require special measures, including separate housing for cases and new admissions, a vigorous program of supervised handwashing, and repeated cultures of patients and attendants. The most difficult outbreaks to control are those that involve groups of young children (not yet toilet-trained) or the mentally disabled, and those where there is an inadequate supply of water. Closure of affected day care centers may lead to placement of infected children in other centers with subsequent transmission in the latter, and is not by itself an effective control measure.

A. *Preventive measures:* Same as those listed under *Typhoid fever*, 9A1–9A10, except that no commercial vaccine is available.

B. *Control of patient, contacts and the immediate environment:*

1) Report to local health authority: Case report obligatory in many countries, Class 2 (see *Reporting*). Recognition and report of outbreaks in childcare centers and institutions are especially important.

2) Isolation: During acute illness, enteric precautions. Because of the small infective dose, patients with known *Shigella* infections should not be employed to handle food or to provide child or patient care until 2 successive fecal samples or rectal swabs (collected 24 or more hours apart, but not sooner than 48 hours after discontinuance of antimicrobials) are found to be *Shigella*-free. Patients must be told of the importance and effectiveness of handwashing with soap and water after defecation as a means of curtailing transmission of *Shigella*.

3) Concurrent disinfection: Of feces and contaminated articles. In communities with an adequate sewage disposal system, feces can be discharged directly into sewers without preliminary disinfection. Terminal cleaning.

4) Quarantine: Not applicable.

5) Management of contacts: Whenever feasible, ill contacts should be excluded from food handling and the care of children or patients until diarrhea ceases and 2 successive negative stool cultures are obtained at least 24 hours apart and at least 48 hours after discontinuation of antibiotics. Thorough handwashing after defecation and before handling food or caring for children or patients is essential if such contacts are unavoidable.

6) Investigation of contacts and source of infection: The search for unrecognized mild cases and convalescent carriers among contacts may be unproductive, and seldom contributes to the control of an outbreak. Cultures of contacts should generally be confined to food handlers, attendants and children in hospitals, and other situations where the spread of infection is particularly likely.

7) Specific treatment: Fluid and electrolyte replacement is important when diarrhea is watery or there are signs of dehydration (see *Cholera*, 9B7). Antibiotics, selected according to the prevailing antimicrobial sensitivity pattern of where cases occur, shorten the duration and severity of illness and the duration of pathogen excretion. They should be used in individual cases if warranted by the severity of illness or to protect contacts (e.g. in day care centers or institutions) when epidemiologically indicated. During the past 50 years *Shigellae* have shown a propensity to acquire resistance against newly introduced antimicrobials that were initially highly effective. Multidrug resistance to most of the low-cost antibiotics (ampicillin, trimethoprim-sulfamethoxazole) is common, and the choice of specific agents will depend on the antibiogram of the isolated strain or on local antimicrobial susceptibility patterns. In many areas, high prevalence of *Shigella* resistance to trimethoprim-sulfamethoxazole, ampicillin and tetracycline (NB tetracycline cannot be used in children less than eight years of age) has resulted in a reliance on fluoroquinolones such as ciprofloxacin as first line treatment, but resistance to these has also occurred. Azithromycin may also be considered as an alternative antimicrobial for the treatment of shigellosis, especially in pediatric infections. The use of anti-motility agents such as loperamide is contraindicated in children and generally discouraged in adults, since these drugs may prolong illness. If administered in an attempt to alleviate the severe

cramps that often accompany shigellosis, anti-motility agents should be limited to 1 or at most 2 doses, and should never be given without concomitant antimicrobial therapy.

C. Epidemic measures:

1) Report at once to the local health authority any group of cases of acute diarrheal disorder, even in the absence of specific identification of the causal agent.
2) Investigate water, food, and milk supplies, and use general sanitation measures.
3) Prophylactic administration of antibiotics is not recommended.
4) Publicize the importance of handwashing after defecation; provide soap and individual paper towels if otherwise not available.

D. Disaster implications:

A potential problem where personal hygiene and environmental sanitation are deficient (see *Typhoid fever*); *S. dysenteriae* type 1 is of particular concern.

E. International measures:

WHO Collaborating Centres provide support as required. More information can be found at <http://www.who.int/collaboratingcentres/database/en/>.

SMALLPOX   ICD-9 050; ICD-10 B03
[CCDM19: I. Damon, M. Lim, C. Roth]
[CCDM18: D. Heymann]

The last naturally acquired case of smallpox in the world occurred in October 1977 in Somalia; global eradication was certified 2 years later (1979) by WHO, and sanctioned by the World Health Assembly (WHA) in May 1980. Except for a laboratory-associated smallpox infection that caused a limited outbreak after a laboratory accident at the University of Birmingham, England, in 1978, no further cases have been identified. All known variola virus stocks are held under security in two places: at CDC, Atlanta, GA, USA; and at the State Research Centre of Virology and Biotechnology, Koltsovo, Novosibirsk Region, Russia. In response to concerns that live variola virus may be needed for research in the event that smallpox should re-emerge as result of accidental or intentional release, in May 1999 the WHA authorized the retention of virus at the laboratories in Russia and the USA for the purposes of essential research. The WHA reaffirmed that destruction of all the remaining virus stocks is still the Organization's ultimate goal, and has appointed a group of experts to determine and oversee the research that must be carried out before the virus can be destroyed. WHO has also set up a biosafety inspection program for the two laboratories where official stocks are kept, to make sure they are secure and research can be carried out safely.

Because of increasing concerns about the potential for deliberate use of clandestine supplies of variola virus, it is important that health care workers become familiar with the clinical and epidemiological features of smallpox and how it can be distinguished from chickenpox. Laboratory confirmation of variola virus from suspect smallpox patients is performed at the two WHO Collaborating Centre laboratories where the virus stocks are held, using appropriate biosafety containment practices. For more information on the deliberate use of infectious agents to cause harm, see the section on *Deliberate use*.

1. Identification—Smallpox was a systemic viral disease generally presenting with a characteristic skin eruption. Preceding the appearance of the rash was a prodrome of sudden onset, with high fever (40°C/104°F), malaise, headache, prostration, severe backache and occasional abdominal pain and vomiting—a clinical picture that resembled influenza. After 2–4 days, the fever began to fall, and a deep-seated rash developed in which individual lesions containing infectious virus progressed through successive stages of macules, papules, vesicles, pustules, then crusted scabs that fell off 3–4 weeks after the appearance of the rash. The lesions first appeared on the face and extremities, including the palms and soles, and subsequently on the trunk—the so-called centrifugal rash distribution. They were well-circumscribed, and at the same stage of development in a given area.

Two types of smallpox were recognized during the 20th century: *variola minor* (including a genetically and biologically distinct subgroup described as alastrim), which had a case fatality rate of less than 1%; and *variola major*, which had a fatality rate among unvaccinated populations of 20–50% or more (30% on average). Fatalities normally occurred between the fifth and seventh day, occasionally as late as the second week. Fewer than 3% of variola major cases experienced a fulminant hemorrhagic course, characterized by a severe prodrome, prostration, and bleeding into the skin and mucous membranes; such hemorrhagic cases were rapidly fatal. In hemorrhagic smallpox the usual vesicular rash did not appear, and the disease might have been confused with severe leukemia, meningococcemia, or idiopathic thrombocytopenic purpura. The rash of smallpox could also be significantly modified in previously vaccinated persons, to the extent that only a few highly atypical lesions might be seen. In such cases, prodromal illness was not modified, but the maturation of lesions was accelerated, with crusting by the tenth day.

Smallpox was most frequently confused with chickenpox, in which skin lesions commonly occur in successive crops with several stages of maturity visible at the same time. The chickenpox rash is more abundant on covered than on exposed parts of the body, and is centripetal rather than centrifugal. Smallpox was indicated by a clear-cut prodromal illness; the more or less simultaneous appearance of all lesions when the fever broke; the similarity of appearance of all lesions in a given area rather than successive crops; and the more deep-seated lesions, often involving sebaceous glands and scarring of the pitted lesions (whereas chickenpox lesions are superficial, not well circumscribed and manifested with irregular borders, and chickenpox rash is usually pruritic). Smallpox lesions were virtually never seen at the apex of the axilla; and chickenpox lesions were rarely, if ever, seen on the palms and soles of the feet—a distribution characteristic of smallpox in many cases.

Outbreaks of variola minor were recognized by low case-fatality rates in the late 19th century. Although the rash was like that in ordinary smallpox, patients generally experienced less severe systemic reactions, and hemorrhagic cases were virtually unknown.

Prior to eradication, laboratory confirmation of smallpox used isolation of the virus on chorioallantoic membranes or tissue culture from the scrapings of lesions, from vesicular or pustular fluid, from crusts, and sometimes from blood during the febrile prodrome. Electron microscopy or immunodiffusion technique often permitted a rapid provisional diagnosis—though eradication was made possible on the basis of clinical, not laboratory, diagnosis. Molecular methods, such as PCR, are now available for rapid diagnosis of smallpox and other orthopoxvirus infections. Should smallpox infection be suspected, immediate communication by national authorities to WHO is imperative, for advice on appropriate laboratories for diagnosis.

2. Infectious agent—Variola virus, a species of *Orthopoxvirus*.

3. Occurrence—Formerly a worldwide disease; no known human cases since 1978.

4. Reservoir—As epidemiologically described in the 19th and 20th centuries, smallpox was exclusively a human disease, with no known animal or environmental reservoir. Currently, the virus is maintained only in two WHO-designated laboratories.

5. Mode of transmission—Infection usually occurred via the respiratory tract (droplet spread) or skin inoculation. The conjunctivae or the placenta were occasional portals of entry.

6. Incubation period—From 7–19 days; commonly 10–14 days to onset of illness and 2–4 days more to onset of rash.

7. Period of communicability—From the time of development of the earliest rash lesions to disappearance of all scabs; about 3 weeks. Risk of transmission appears to have been highest in the first week after appearance of the earliest lesions, through droplet spread from the oropharyngeal enanthem and subsequent oropharyngeal excretion of virus.

8. Susceptibility—Susceptibility among the unvaccinated is universal.

9. Methods of control—Control of smallpox was based on identification and isolation of cases, vaccination (vaccinia virus) of contacts and those living in the immediate vicinity (ring vaccination), surveillance of contacts (including daily monitoring of temperature), and isolation of those contacts in whom fever develops.

Because of the relatively long period of incubation for smallpox, vaccination within a 4-day period after exposure prevented or attenuated clinical illness.

Should a non-varicella, smallpox-like case be suspected, **IMMEDIATE TELEPHONE COMMUNICATION WITH LOCAL NATIONAL HEALTH AUTHORITIES IS OBLIGATORY. NATIONAL HEALTH AUTHORITIES SHOULD INFORM WHO IMMEDIATELY.**

Further information can be found at:

http://www.who.int/csr/disease/smallpox

VACCINIA   ICD-9 051.0; ICD-10 B08.0

Vaccinia virus is the live, fully-replicative, orthopoxvirus immunizing agent used to eradicate smallpox. Discovery of vaccinia-variants causing human infection in the Indian subcontinent and in South America (Brazil) has led to the consideration that vaccine may have "escaped" into animal populations; alternatively, these occurrences may be indicative of the origins of vaccinia virus. Vaccinia virus has been genetically engineered and biologically derived into candidate vaccines (some are in clinical trials), with low potential for spread to non-immune contacts.

Vaccination with licensed (fully-replicative) smallpox vaccine is recommended for all laboratory workers at high risk of contracting infection, such as those who directly handle cultures or animals contaminated or infected with vaccinia or other orthopoxviruses that infect humans. It may also be considered for other health care personnel who are at lower risk of infection, such as doctors and nurses whose contact with these viruses is limited to contaminated dressings. WHO does not recommend vaccination in the general public, because the risk of death (1 per 1 000 000 doses) or serious side-effects is greater than the known risk of infection with smallpox.

Vaccination is contraindicated in persons with deficient immune systems, persons with eczema or certain other dermatitis disorders, and pregnant women. Vaccine immune globulin can be obtained for laboratory workers in the USA through the CDC Drug Service (1-404-639-3670), and in other industrialized countries from public health agencies. Vaccination should be repeated unless a major reaction (one that is indurated and erythematous 7 days after vaccination) or "take" has developed.

Booster vaccinations are recommended within 10 years in categories for which vaccine is recommended. WHO maintains a supply of the vaccine seed lot (vaccinia virus strain Lister Elstree) at the WHO Collaborating Centre for Smallpox Vaccine at the National Institute of Public Health and Environmental Protection in Bilthoven, The Netherlands. WHO also maintains a stockpile of vaccine should an outbreak occur.

MONKEYPOX   ICD-9 051.9; ICD-10 B04

Human monkeypox is a sporadic zoonotic infection first identified in 1970 from remote rural villages in central and western African rainforest countries, as smallpox disappeared. Clinically, the disease closely resembles ordinary or modified smallpox, but lymphadenopathy is a more prominent feature in many cases, and occurs in the early stage of the disease. Pleomorphism and "cropping" similar to that seen in chickenpox are observed in 20% of patients. The natural history of the disease is unclear; humans, primates and squirrels appear to be involved in the enzootic cycle. The disease affects all age groups; children under 16 have historically constituted the greatest proportion of cases. The case-fatality rate among children not vaccinated against smallpox ranges from 1% to 14%. Smallpox vaccination protects against infection in some instances, and in some others mitigates clinical manifestations; recent studies suggest the protection provided by childhood smallpox vaccination is waning in the general populations at risk since the cessation of smallpox vaccination in the 1980s. Between 1970 and 1994, over 400 cases of monkeypox were reported from western and central Africa; the Democratic Republic of the Congo (DRC; formerly Zaire) accounted for about 95% of reported cases during a 5-year surveillance period from 1981 to 1986. Poor public health infrastructure and other factors complicate accurate case reporting. In the late 1990s, a prolonged outbreak of human monkeypox was recognized in DRC: it has been postulated that lack of vaccination and an epizootic allowed multiple virus transmission events to humans across the species barrier. In 2003, a prolonged and efficient, chain of human-to-human transmission was described, also in DRC.

In the 1980s about 75% of reported cases of human monkeypox were attributable to contact with affected animals; in recent outbreaks it appears that a larger number of cases were attributable to person-to-person contact. The longest chain of person-to-person transmission was 7 reported serial cases, but serial transmission usually does not extend beyond secondary. Epidemiological data suggest a secondary attack rate of about 8%. Most cases have occurred either singly or in clusters in small remote villages, usually in tropical rainforest where the population has multiple contacts with several types of wild animals. Ecological studies in the 1980s point to squirrels (*Funisciurus* and *Heliosciurus*), abundant among the oil palms surrounding the villages, as a significant local reservoir host. Maintenance of an animal reservoir and animal contact is required to sustain the disease among humans. Thus, human infection may be controllable by education to limit contact with infected cases and potentially infected animals. A recent (2003) introduction of monkeypox in the USA, related to importation and sale of exotic animals from western Africa as pets, resulted in infection of north American prairie dogs and at least 50 probable and confirmed human cases, mainly among prairie dog owners and animal handlers. Evaluation of the species associated with the shipment of imported animals demonstrated monkeypox virus in terrestrial giant pouched Gambian rats (*Cricetomys* sp.), squirrels (*Funisciurus* but not *Heliosciurus* spp.) and dormice (*Graphiurus* spp.). A thorough investigation of this outbreak led to the understanding that at least two genetically distinct clades of monkeypox exist, with different human clinical and epidemiologic manifestations. To date, West African clade monkeypox manifests without apparent human-to-human transmission, and without human mortality; whereas the Congo Basin clade is associated with human-to-human transmission and case fatalities historically reported at an average of approximately 10% in unvaccinated persons.

Monkeypox virus is a species of the genus *Orthopoxvirus*, with biological properties and a genome distinct from variola virus. The 2003 outbreak in the USA clearly demonstrates potential for monkeypox to be a public health threat outside enzootic areas; and there is evidence that disease has also emerged in nature outside of historic "known" enzootic areas. Full evaluation of the ecology, epidemiology, and virology associated with monkeypox outbreaks in endemic areas will enable understanding of prevention and control measures. Currently, due to adverse event profiles and anticipated clinical and epidemiologic risk-benefit ratios, cross-protective prophylactic vaccination with "smallpox vaccine" (fully replicative vaccinia) is not routinely recommended by WHO. Smallpox (vaccinia) vaccination was, however, used as an outbreak response intervention in the USA in 2003. A WHO Technical Advisory Committee on monkeypox has recently recommended continued studies of human monkeypox—in particular, intensified prospective surveillance and ecological studies.

SPOROTRICHOSIS
[CCDM19: M. Brandt]
[CCDM18: A. M. Kimball]

ICD-9 117.1; ICD-10 B42

1. Identification—A fungal disease, usually of the skin, often of an extremity, which begins as a nodule. As the nodule grows, lymphatics draining the area become firm and cord-like and form a series of nodules, which in turn may soften and ulcerate. Osteoarticular, pulmonary and multifocal infections are rare, except as regards multifocal infections for patients with HIV infection. Fatalities are uncommon.

Culture of a biopsy, pus or exudate confirms the diagnosis. Organisms are rarely visualized by direct smear. Biopsied tissue should be examined with fungal stains.

2. Infectious agent—*Sporothrix schenckii*, a dimorphic fungus.

3. Occurrence—Reported worldwide; an occupational disease of farmers, gardeners and horticulturists. The disease is characteristically sporadic and relatively uncommon. An epidemic among gold miners in South Africa involved some 3 000 people; fungus was growing on mine timbers. Contact with infected cats was an exposure risk in a Brazilian outbreak in 2003.

4. Reservoir—Soil, decaying vegetation, wood, moss and hay.

5. Mode of transmission—Introduction of fungus through the skin pricks from thorns or barbs, handling of sphagnum moss or slivers from wood or lumber. Outbreaks have occurred among children playing in baled hay, and adults working with it. Pulmonary sporotrichosis presumably arises through inhalation of conidia. Persons handling sick cats are an occupational risk group.

6. Incubation period—The lymphatic form develops 1 week to 3 months after injury.

7. Period of communicability—Person-to-person transmission has only rarely been documented.

8. Susceptibility—Unknown.

9. Methods of control—

A. *Preventive measures:* Treat lumber with fungicides in industries where disease occurs. Wear gloves and long sleeves when working with sphagnum moss and when gardening, and use personal protection when handling sick cats.

B. *Control of patient, contacts and the immediate environment:*

1) Report to local health authority: Official report not ordinarily justifiable, Class 5 (see *Reporting*).
2) Isolation: Not applicable.
3) Concurrent disinfection: Discharges and dressings. Terminal cleaning.
4) Quarantine: Not applicable.
5) Immunization of contacts: Not applicable.
6) Investigation of contacts and source of infection: Seek undiagnosed and untreated cases.
7) Specific treatment: Orally administered saturated solution of potassium iodide (increased drop by drop from 1-2 ml to 4-6 ml),

given 3 times daily or itraconazole are effective in lymphocutaneous infection. In extracutaneous forms, amphotericin B is the drug of choice, but itraconazole is also useful.

C. Epidemic measures: Determine source to limit future exposures. In the South African epidemic, mine timbers were sprayed with a mixture of zinc sulfate and triolith in order to control the epidemic.

D. Disaster implications: None.

E. International measures: None.

STAPHYLOCOCCAL DISEASES
[CCDM19: Editorial Board]
[CCDM18: F. Waldvogel]

Staphylococci produce a variety of syndromes, with clinical manifestations ranging from a single pustule to sepsis and death. A pus-containing lesion (or lesions) is the primary clinical finding, and abscess formation is the typical pathological manifestation; production of toxins may also lead to staphylococcal diseases, as in toxic shock syndrome. Virulence of bacterial strains varies greatly. The most important human pathogen is *Staphylococcus aureus*. Most strains ferment mannitol and are coagulase-positive. However, coagulase-negative strains are increasingly important, especially in bloodstream infections among patients with intravascular catheters or prosthetic materials, in female urinary tract infections, and in nosocomial infections.

Staphylococcal disease has different clinical and epidemiological patterns in the general community, in newborns, in menstruating women and among hospitalized patients; each will be presented separately. Staphylococcal food poisoning, an intoxication and not an infection, is also discussed separately (see *Foodborne intoxications*, section I, *Staphylococcal*).

I. STAPHYLOCOCCAL DISEASE
IN THE COMMUNITY
BOILS, CARBUNCLES,
FURUNCLES, ABSCESSES   ICD-9 680, 041.1;
ICD-10 L02; B95.6-B95.8

IMPETIGO	ICD-9 684, 041.1; ICD-10 L01
CELLULITIS	ICD-9 682.9; ICD-10 L03
STAPHYLOCOCCAL SEPSIS	ICD-9 038.1; ICD-10 A41.0-A41.2
STAPHYLOCOCCAL PNEUMONIA	ICD-9 482.4; ICD-10 J15.2
ARTHRITIS	ICD-9 711.0, 041.1; ICD-10 M00.0
OSTEOMYELITIS	ICD-9 730, 041.1; ICD-10 M86
ENDOCARDITIS	ICD-9 421.0, 041.1; ICD-10 133.0

1. **Identification**—The common bacterial skin lesions are impetigo, folliculitis, furuncles, carbuncles, abscesses and infected lacerations. The basic lesion of impetigo is described in section II, 1; a distinctive "scalded skin" syndrome is associated with certain strains of *Staphylococcus aureus*, which elaborate an epidermolytic toxin. Other skin lesions are localized and discrete. Constitutional symptoms are unusual; if lesions extend or are widespread, fever, malaise, headache and anorexia may develop. Usually, lesions are uncomplicated, but seeding of the bloodstream may lead to pneumonia, lung abscess, osteomyelitis, sepsis, endocarditis, arthritis or meningitis. In addition to primary skin lesions, staphylococcal conjunctivitis occurs in newborns and the elderly. Staphylococcal pneumonia is a well-recognized complication of influenza. Staphylococcal endocarditis and other complications of staphylococcal bacteremia may result from parenteral use of illicit drugs, or nosocomially from intravenous catheters and other devices. Embolic skin lesions are frequent complications of endocarditis and/or bacteremia.

Coagulase-negative staphylococci may cause sepsis, meningitis, endocarditis or urinary tract infections, and are increasing in frequency, usually in connection with prosthetic devices or indwelling catheters.

Diagnosis is confirmed by isolation of the organism.

2. **Infectious agent**—Various coagulase-positive strains of *Staphylococcus aureus*. Most strains of staphylococci may be characterized through molecular methods such as pulsed-field gel electrophoresis, phage type, or antibiotic resistance profile; epidemics are caused by relatively few specific strains. The majority of clinical isolates of *Staphylococcus aureus*, whether community- or hospital-acquired, are resistant to penicillin G, and multiresistant (including methicillin-resistant) strains have become widespread. Evidence suggests that slime-producing strains of coagulase-negative staphylococci may be more pathogenic, but the data are inconclusive. *S. saprophyticus* is a common cause of urinary tract infection in young women.

3. **Occurrence**—Worldwide. Highest incidence is in areas where hygiene conditions (especially the use of soap and water) are sub-optimal and people are crowded; common among children, especially in warm

weather. The disease occurs sporadically and as small epidemics in families and summer camps, with various members developing recurrent illness due to the same staphylococcal strain (hidden carriers).

4. Reservoir—Humans; rarely animals.

5. Mode of transmission—The major site of colonization is the anterior nares; 20%–30% of the general population are nasal carriers of coagulase-positive staphylococci. Autoinfection is responsible for at least one-third of infections. Persons with a draining lesion or purulent discharge are the most common sources of epidemic spread. Transmission is through contact with a person who has a purulent lesion or is an asymptomatic (usually nasal) carrier of a pathogenic strain. Some carriers are more effective disseminators of infection than others. The role of contaminated objects has been overstressed; hands are the most important instrument for transmitting infection. Airborne spread is rare, but has been demonstrated in patients with associated viral respiratory disease.

6. Incubation period—Variable and indefinite.

7. Period of communicability—As long as purulent lesions continue to drain or the carrier state persists. Autoinfection may continue for the period of nasal colonization or duration of active lesions.

8. Susceptibility—Immune mechanisms depend mainly on an intact opsonization/phagocytosis axis involving neutrophils. Susceptibility is greatest among the newborn and the chronically ill. Elderly and debilitated people, drug abusers, and those with diabetes mellitus, cystic fibrosis, chronic renal failure, agammaglobulinemia, disorders of neutrophil function (e.g. agranulocytosis, chronic granulomatous disease), neoplastic disease and burns are particularly susceptible. Use of steroids and antimetabolites also increases susceptibility.

9. Methods of control—

   A. *Preventive measures:*

   1) Educate the public and health personnel in personal hygiene, especially handwashing and the importance of not sharing toilet articles.
   2) Treat initial cases in children and families promptly.

   B. *Control of patient, contacts and the immediate environment:*

   1) Report to local health authority: Obligatory report of outbreaks in schools, summer camps and other population groups; also any recognized concentration of cases in the community for many industrialized countries. No individual case report, Class 4 (see *Reporting*).

2) Isolation: Not practical in most communities; infected people should avoid contact with infants and debilitated people.
3) Concurrent disinfection: Place dressings from open lesions and discharges in disposable bags; dispose of these in a practical and safe manner.
4) Quarantine: Not applicable.
5) Immunization of contacts: Not applicable.
6) Investigation of contacts and source of infection: Search for draining lesions; occasionally, determination of nasal carrier status of the pathogenic strain among family members or health care workers (as appropriate) is useful.
7) Specific treatment: In localized skin infections, systemic antimicrobials are not indicated unless infection spreads significantly or complications ensue; local skin cleaning followed by application of an appropriate topical antimicrobial (such as mupirocin, 4 times a day) is adequate. Avoid wet compresses, which may spread infection; hot dry compresses may help localized infections. Incise abscesses to permit drainage of pus and possible removal of foreign bodies. For severe staphylococcal infections, use penicillinase-resistant penicillin; if there is hypersensitivity to penicillin, use a cephalosporin active against staphylococci (unless there is a history of immediate hypersensitivity to penicillin) or a macrolide. In severe systemic infections, choice of antibiotics should be governed by results of susceptibility tests on isolates. Vancomycin is the treatment of choice for severe infections caused by coagulase-negative staphylococci and methicillin-resistant *S. aureus*; prompt parenteral treatment is important.

Strains of *Staphylococcus aureus* with high-level resistance to vancomycin and other glycopeptide antibiotics are reported from many countries worldwide. These are usually recovered from patients treated with vancomycin for extended periods (months), and escalate in some healthcare settings.

C. *Epidemic measures:*

1) Search for and treat those with clinical illness, especially those with draining lesions; strict personal hygiene with emphasis on handwashing. Culture for nasal carriers of the epidemic strain and treat locally with mupirocin—and, if unsuccessful, orally administered antimicrobials.
2) Investigate unusual or abrupt prevalence increases in community staphylococcal infections for a possible common source, e.g. an unrecognized hospital epidemic.

D. *Disaster implications:* None.

E. *International measures:* WHO Collaborating Centres can provide technical support as required. More information can be found at:

<http://www.who.int/collaboratingcentres/database/en/>

II. STAPHYLOCOCCAL DISEASE IN HOSPITAL NURSERIES

IMPETIGO NEONATORUM	ICD-9 684, 041.1; ICD-10 L00
STAPHYLOCOCCAL SCALDED SKIN SYNDROME (SSS, Ritter disease)	ICD9-695.8
ABSCESS OF THE BREAST	ICD-9 771.5, 041.1; ICD-10 P39.0

1. Identification—Impetigo or pustulosis of the newborn and other purulent skin manifestations are the staphylococcal diseases most frequently acquired in nurseries. Characteristic skin lesions develop secondary to colonization of the nose, umbilicus, circumcision site, rectum or conjunctivae. Colonization of these sites with staphylococcal strains is a normal occurrence and does not imply disease.

Lesions most commonly occur in diaper and intertriginous areas, but also elsewhere on the body. They are initially vesicular, rapidly turning seropurulent, surrounded by an erythematous base; bullae may form (bullous impetigo). Rupture of pustules favors their spread. Complications are unusual, although lymphadenitis, furunculosis, breast abscess, pneumonia, sepsis, arthritis, osteomyelitis and others have been reported.

Though uncommon, staphylococcal scalded skin syndrome (SSSS or Ritter disease, pemphigus neonatorum) may occur; clinical manifestations range from diffuse scarlatiniform erythema to generalized bullous desquamation. Like bullous impetigo, it is caused by strains of *S. aureus*, usually phage type II, which produce an epidermolytic toxin.

2. Infectious agent—See *Staphylococcal disease in the community* (Section I, 2).

3. Occurrence—Worldwide. Problems occur mainly in hospitals, are promoted by lax aseptic techniques, and are exaggerated by development of antibiotic-resistant strains (hospital strains).

4. Reservoir—See *Staphylococcal disease in the community* (Section I, 4).

5. Mode of transmission—Primary spread by hands of hospital personnel; rarely airborne.

6. Incubation period—Commonly 4–10 days; disease may not occur until several months after colonization.

7. Period of communicability—See *Staphylococcal disease in the community* (Section I, 7).

8. Susceptibility—Susceptibility of newborns appears to be general. For the duration of colonization with pathogenic strains, infants remain at risk of disease.

9. Methods of control—

    A. Preventive measures:

        1) Use aseptic techniques when necessary, and wash hands before contact with each infant in nurseries.

        2) Personnel with minor lesions (pustules, boils, abscesses, paronychia, conjunctivitis, severe acne, otitis external or infected lacerations) must not be permitted to work in nurseries.

        3) Surveillance and supervision through an active hospital infection control committee, including a regular system for investigating, reporting and reviewing hospital-acquired infections. Illness developing after discharge from hospital must also be investigated and recorded, preferably through active surveillance of all discharged newborns after about 1 month.

        4) Some advocate routine application of antibacterial substances such as gentian violet, acriflavine, chlorhexidine or bacitracin ointment to the umbilical cord stump while in the hospital.

    B. Control of patient, contacts and the immediate environment:

        1) Report to local health authority: Obligatory report of epidemics; no individual case report, Class 4 (see *Reporting*).

        2) Isolation: Without delay, place all known or suspected cases in the nursery on contact isolation precautions.

        3) Concurrent disinfection: See *Staphylococcal disease in the community* (Section I, 9B3).

        4) Quarantine: Not applicable.

        5) Immunization of contacts: Not applicable.

        6) Investigation of contacts and source of infection: See epidemic measures in 9C.

        7) Specific treatment: Localized impetigo: cleanse skin and apply a topical antibiotic such as mupirocin ointment (4 times a day); widespread lesions may be treated orally with an anti-staphylococcal antimicrobial such as cephalexin or cloxacillin. Serious infections require parenteral treatment

(Section I, 9B7). Nasal decontamination with mupirocin is indicated to prevent recurrence.

C. Epidemic measures:

1) The occurrence of 2 or more concurrent cases of staphylococcal disease related to a nursery or a maternity ward is presumptive evidence of an outbreak and warrants investigation. Culture all lesions to determine antibiotic resistance pattern and type of epidemic strain. Laboratories should keep clinically important isolates for 6 months before discarding them, so as to support possible epidemiological investigation using antibiotic sensitivity patterns or pulsed-field gel electrophoresis.

2) In nursery outbreaks, institute isolation precautions for cases and contacts until all have been discharged. Use a rotational system ("cohorting") where one unit (A) is filled and subsequent babies are admitted to another nursery (B) while the initial unit (A) discharges infants and is cleaned before new admissions. If facilities are present for baby in-rooming, this may reduce risk. Colonized or infected infants should be grouped in another cohort. Assignments of nursing and other ward personnel should be restricted to specific cohorts.

   Before admitting new patients, wash cribs, beds and other furniture with an approved disinfectant. Autoclave instruments that enter sterile body sites, wipe mattresses, and thoroughly launder bedding and diapers (or use disposable diapers).

3) Examine *all* patient care personnel for draining lesions anywhere on the body. Perform an epidemiological investigation, and if one or more personnel are associated with the disease, culture nasal specimens from them and all others in contact with infants. It may become necessary to exclude and treat all carriers of the epidemic strain until cultures are negative. Treatment of asymptomatic carriers is directed at suppressing the nasal carrier state, usually through local application of appropriate antibiotic ointments to the nasal vestibule, sometimes with concurrent systemic rifampicin for 3–9 days.

4) Investigate adequacy of nursing procedures, especially availability of handwashing facilities. Emphasize strict handwashing; if facilities are inaccessible or inadequate, consider use of a hand antiseptic agent (e.g. alcohol-based) at the bedside. Personnel assigned to infected or colonized infants should not work with non-colonized newborns.

D. Disaster implications: None.

      E. *International measures:* WHO Collaborating Centres provide support as required. More information can be found at:
         <http://www.who.int/collaboratingcentres/database/en/>

III. STAPHYLOCOCCAL DISEASE ON HOSPITAL MEDICAL AND SURGICAL WARDS   ICD-9 998.5; ICD-10 T81.4

    1. Identification—Lesions vary from simple furuncles or stitch abscesses to extensively infected bedsores or surgical wounds, septic phlebitis, acute or chronic osteomyelitis, pneumonia, meningitis, endocarditis or sepsis. Post-operative staphylococcal disease is a constant threat to the convalescence of the hospitalized surgical patient. The increasing complexity of surgical operations, greater organ exposure and more prolonged anesthesia promote entry of staphylococci. Increased use of prosthetic devices and indwelling catheters accounts for increased incidence of nosocomial staphylococcal infections. A toxic state can complicate infection (toxic shock syndrome) if the strain produces toxins (this is an ever-present risk). Frequent and sometimes injudicious use of antimicrobials has increased the prevalence of antibiotic-resistant staphylococci. Verification depends on isolation of *Staphylococcus aureus*, associated with a clinical illness compatible with the bacteriological findings.

    2. Infectious agent—*Staphylococcus aureus*; see section I, 2. Resistance to penicillin occurs in 95% of strains and increasing proportions are resistant to semi-synthetic penicillins (e.g. methicillin), aminoglycosides (e.g. gentamicin), and quinolones.

    3. Occurrence—Worldwide. Staphylococcal infection is a major form of acquired sepsis in the general wards of hospitals. Attack rates may assume epidemic proportions, and community spread may occur when hospital-infected patients are discharged.

    4., 5., 6., and **7. Reservoir, Mode of transmission, Incubation period** and **Period of communicability**—See *Staphylococcal disease in the community* (Section I, 4, 5, 6, and 7).

    8. Susceptibility—See section I. Widespread use of continuous intravenous treatment with indwelling catheters and parenteral injections has opened new portals of entry for infectious agents.

    9. Methods of control—

        A. *Preventive measures:*

           1) Educate hospital medical staff to use common, narrow-spectrum antimicrobials for simple staphylococcal infections for short periods, and to reserve certain antibiotics for

specific situations (e.g. reserve cephalosporins for penicillin-resistant staphylococcal infections, and vancomycin for beta-lactam resistant staphylococcal infections).

2) A hospital infection control committee must enforce strict aseptic technique and provide programs to monitor nosocomial infections.

3) Change sites of IV needle infusions every 48 hours; establish a monitoring system for the examination of central venous lines.

B. Control of patient, contacts and the immediate environment:

1) Report to local health authority: Obligatory report of epidemics; no individual case report, Class 4 (see *Reporting*).

2) Isolation: Whenever staphylococci are known or suspected to be abundant in draining pus or the sputum of a patient with pneumonia, the patient should be placed in a private room. This is not required when wound drainage is scanty, provided an occlusive dressing is used and care is taken in changing dressings to prevent environmental contamination. Health care workers must practice appropriate handwashing, gloving and gowning techniques.

3) Concurrent disinfection: See *Staphylococcal disease in the community* (Section I, 9B3).

4) Quarantine: Not applicable.

5) Immunization of contacts: Not applicable.

6) Investigation of contacts and source of infection: Not practical for sporadic cases (see 9C).

7) Specific treatment: Appropriate antimicrobials as determined through antibiotic sensitivity tests. Life-threatening infections should be treated with vancomycin pending test results.

C. Epidemic measures:

1) The occurrence of 2 or more cases with epidemiological association is sufficient to suspect epidemic spread, and to initiate investigation.

2) See section II, 9C3.

3) Review and enforce rigid aseptic techniques.

D. Disaster implications: None.

E. International measures: WHO Collaborating Centres can provide technical support as required. More information can be found at:
<http://www.who.int/collaboratingcentres/database/en/>

IV. TOXIC SHOCK SYNDROME
ICD-9 785.5;
ICD-10 A48.3

Toxic shock syndrome (TSS) is a severe illness characterized by sudden onset of high fever, vomiting, profuse watery diarrhea and myalgia, followed by hypotension and—in severe cases—shock. An erythematous "sunburn-like" rash is present during the acute phase, about 1–2 weeks after onset, with desquamation of the skin, especially of palms and soles. Fever is usually high (39°C/102°F), with hypotension, and 3 or more of the following organ systems are involved:

- GI,
- Muscular (severe myalgia and/or creatine phosphokinase level more than twice the normal upper limit),
- Mucous membranes (vaginal, pharyngeal and/or conjunctival hyperemia),
- Renal (blood urea nitrogen or creatinine more than twice normal and/or sterile pyuria),
- Hepatic (AST or ALT more than twice normal),
- Hematological (platelets 100 000/mm^3; SI units 100×109/L), or
- CNS (disorientation or alterations in consciousness without focal neurological signs).

Blood, throat and CSF cultures are negative for pathogens; the recovery of *S. aureus* from any of these sites does not invalidate a case. Serological tests for Rocky Mountain spotted fever, leptospirosis and measles are negative.

Most cases of TSS have been associated with strains of *S. aureus*-producing toxic shock syndrome toxin 1. These strains, rarely present in vaginal cultures from healthy women, are regularly recovered from women with menstrually-associated TSS or in those with TSS after gynecological surgery.

Although almost all early cases of TSS occurred in women during menstruation, and most with vaginal tampon use, only 55% of cases now reported are associated with menses. Other risk factors include use of contraceptive diaphragms and vaginal contraceptive sponges, and infection following childbirth or abortion. Instructions for sponge use, advising that these should not be left in place for more than 30 hours, must be heeded. A growing number of cases in men and women have shown *S. aureus* isolated from focal lesions of skin, bone, the respiratory tract and surgical sites. No source of infection could be found in one-third of cases, where rash is often scant or undetectable.

Menstrual TSS can be prevented by avoiding use of highly absorbent vaginal tampons; risk may be reduced by using tampons intermittently (that is, not all day and all night throughout the period), and using less absorbent tampons. Women who develop a high fever and vomiting or diarrhea during menstruation must discontinue tampon use immediately and consult a physician. It is not known when those who have had an episode of menstrual TSS can safely resume tampon use.

A TSS virtually identical to that occurring with *S. aureus* infection occurs with infection caused by group A beta-hemolytic streptococci.

Treatment of TSS is largely supportive. Efforts should be made to eradicate potential foci of *S. aureus* infection through drainage of wounds, removal of vaginal or other foreign bodies (e.g. wound packing), and use of beta-lactam resistant anti-staphylococcal drugs. Clindamycin may help reduce toxin production.

STREPTOCOCCAL DISEASES CAUSED BY GROUP A (BETA HEMOLYTIC) STREPTOCOCCI ICD-9 034, 035, 670; ICD-10 A49.1, J02.0, A38, L01.0, A46, 085

(Streptococcal sore throat, Streptococcal infection, Scarlet fever, Impetigo, Erysipelas, Puerperal fever, Rheumatic fever)
[CCDM19: C. Van Beneden]
[CCDM18: E. Kaplan]

1. Identification—Group A streptococci cause a variety of diseases. The most frequently encountered conditions are streptococcal pharyngitis/tonsillitis, or sore throat (ICD-9 034.0; ICD-10 J02.0) and streptococcal superficial skin infections such as impetigo (ICD-9 684) or pyoderma (ICD-9 686.0). Other acute infections include scarlet fever (ICD-9 034.1/ICD-10 A38), puerperal fever (ICD-9 670/ICD-10 O85), septicemia, erysipelas (ICD 9 035), cellulitis, mastoiditis, otitis media, pneumonia, peritonsillitis, wound infections, and, rarely, necrotizing fasciitis and a toxic shock-like syndrome. One or other form of clinical disease often predominates during outbreaks.

Symptoms may be minimal or absent; patients with streptococcal sore throat typically exhibit sudden onset of fever, exudative tonsillitis or pharyngitis (sore throat), and tender, enlarged anterior cervical lymph nodes. The pharynx, the tonsillar pillars and soft palate may be injected and edematous; petechiae may be present against a background of diffuse redness. Coincident or subsequent otitis media or peritonsillar abscess may occur. Possible non-suppurative complications include acute rheumatic fever (an average of 19 days following pharyngitis) and acute glomerulonephritis (1–5 weeks or an average of 10 days following pharyngitis or skin infection). Rheumatic heart (valvular) disease occurs days to weeks after acute streptococcal infection, and Sydenham chorea several months following infection.

Streptococcal skin infection (pyoderma, impetigo) is usually superficial and may proceed through vesicular, pustular and encrusted stages. Scarlatiniform rash is unusual, and rheumatic fever is not a sequel;

however, glomerulonephritis may occur later, usually 3 weeks after the skin infection.

Scarlet fever is a form of streptococcal disease characterized by a skin rash, occurring when the infecting strain produces a pyrogenic exotoxin (erythrogenic toxin) and the patient is sensitized, but not immune, to the toxin. Clinical characteristics may include all symptoms associated with a streptococcal sore throat (or with a streptococcal wound, skin or puerperal infection) as well as enanthem, strawberry tongue and exanthem. The rash is usually a fine erythema, commonly punctate, blanching on pressure, often felt (like sandpaper) better than seen, and appearing most often on the neck, chest, folds of the axilla, elbow, groin and inner surfaces of the thighs.

Typically, the scarlet fever rash does not involve the face, but there is flushing of the cheeks and circumoral pallor. High fever, nausea and vomiting often accompany severe infections. During convalescence, desquamation of the skin occurs at the tips of fingers and toes, and less often over wide areas of trunk and limbs, including palms and soles; it is more pronounced where the exanthem was severe. The case-fatality rate in some parts of the world has occasionally been as high as 3%. Scarlet fever may be followed by the same sequelae as streptococcal sore throat.

Erysipelas is an acute skin infection characterized by fever, constitutional symptoms, leukocytosis and a red, tender, edematous spreading lesion of the skin, typically with a definite raised border. The central point of origin tends to clear as the periphery extends. Face and legs are common sites. Recurrences are frequent and disease is more common among persons with underlying skin conditions. The disease has a good prognosis with early diagnosis and treatment, but may be especially severe in patients suffering from debilitating disease. Erysipelas due to group A streptococci is to be distinguished from erysipeloid caused by *Erysipelothrix rhusiopathiae*, a localized cutaneous infection (typically without fever or systemic symptoms) seen primarily as an occupational disease of people handling freshwater fish or shellfish, infected swine or turkeys or their tissues or—rarely—sheep, cattle, chickens or pheasants.

Perianal cellulitis due to group A streptococci has been recognized more frequently in the past decade and, though it occurs among all ages, is primarily a disease of early childhood. It can also result in disease outbreaks.

Streptococcal puerperal fever is an acute disease, usually febrile, with local and general symptoms/signs of bacterial invasion of the genital tract and sometimes the bloodstream in the postpartum or post-abortion patient. Case-fatality rate is low when streptococcal puerperal fever is adequately treated. Puerperal infections may be caused by organisms other than hemolytic streptococci; they are clinically similar but differ bacteriologically and epidemiologically (See *Staphylococcal disease*).

Recognition of streptococcal toxic shock syndrome (STSS) in people with invasive group A streptococcal infection increased in the late 1980s and early 1990s, and probably increased over that period of time (in the years between 1998 and 2007, however, active surveillance in the USA indicates that rates of STSS and necrotizing fasciitis (see below) have been fairly stable). Predominant clinical features include hypotension and any of the following: renal impairment; thrombocytopenia; disseminated intra-vascular coagulation (DIC); SGOT or bilirubin elevation; adult respiratory distress syndrome; a generalized erythematous macular rash; or soft-tissue necrosis (necrotizing fasciitis). STSS may occur with either systemic or focal (throat, skin, lung sites) group A streptococcal infections. Mortality rate of STSS is high (35-40%); rapid diagnosis, aggressive management and early use of appropriate antibiotics are critical.

Streptococci of other groups can produce infections in humans. Beta-hemolytic organisms of group B found in the human vagina may cause neonatal sepsis and suppurative meningitis (see group B streptococcal disease of the newborn), as well as urinary tract infections, postpartum endometritis, and other systemic disease in adults, especially those with diabetes mellitus. Group D organisms (including enterococci), hemolytic or nonhemolytic, are involved in bacterial endocarditis and urinary tract infections. Groups C and G have produced outbreaks of streptococcal tonsillitis, usually food-borne; their role in sporadic cases is less well-defined, but they can both cause invasive diseases similar to group A infections. Glomerulonephritis has followed group C infections, but has very rarely been reported after group G infection; neither group is known to cause rheumatic fever. Group C and G pharyngeal infections are more common in adolescents and young adults. Alpha-hemolytic streptococci are also a common cause of bacterial endocarditis.

Provisional laboratory findings for group A streptococcal disease are based on the isolation of the organisms from affected tissues on blood agar or other appropriate media, or on identification of group A streptococcal antigen in pharyngeal secretions (the rapid antigen detection test). Colony morphology and the production of clear beta-hemolysis on blood agar made with sheep's blood identify streptococci on cultures; inhibition by special antibiotic discs containing bacitracin (0.02–0.04 units) constitutes tentative identification. Specific serogrouping procedures provide defini-tive identification. Antigen detection tests also allow rapid identification, demonstrating a rise in serum antibody titer (antistreptolysin O, antihy-aluronidase (not commercially available), anti-DNA-ase B) between acute and convalescent stages of illness; high titers may persist for several months.

In the USA, current recommended practice is to first do a rapid antigen detection test (high specificity but low sensitivity) or a throat culture and, if this is positive, assume the patient has a group A streptococcal infection. If the result of a rapid test used in a child or adolescent is negative or equivocal, a throat culture should be done to guide management and prevent superfluous use of antibiotics.

2. Infectious agent—*Streptococcus pyogenes*, group A streptococci, of over 130 serologically distinct types that vary by geographic and time distributions. Distinct group A streptococcal serotypes are increasingly being identified through *emm* typing—a system that determines the *emm* gene which encodes the M serospecificity of the organism. Group A streptococci producing skin infections usually differ serologically from those associated with throat infections. In scarlet fever, three immunologically different types of erythrogenic toxin (pyrogenic exotoxins A, B and C) have been demonstrated. In STSS, 80% of isolates produce pyrogenic exotoxin A. While beta-hemolysis is characteristic of group A streptococci, strains of groups B, C and G are often also beta-hemolytic. Phenotypically mucoid strains have been involved in recent outbreaks of rheumatic fever.

3. Occurrence—Streptococcal pharyngitis/tonsillitis and scarlet fever are common in temperate zones, well recognized in semitropical areas, and less frequently recognized in tropical climates. Unapparent infections are at least as common in tropical as in temperate zones. In North America and Europe, streptococcal diseases may be endemic, epidemic or sporadic. Streptococcal pharyngitis is unusual before the age of 2-3 years; this peaks in age group 6–12, and declines thereafter. Cases of GAS pharyngitis occur year round but peak in colder seasons; GAS infections peak in later winter and spring. Group A streptococcal infections caused by specific types of M protein (M-types) have frequently been associated with the development of acute glomerulonephritis after pharyngeal infection.

Acute rheumatic fever (ARF) may occur as a non-suppurative complication following streptococcal pharyngitis/tonsillitis. In developing countries ARF tends to occur sporadically. Rheumatic fever remains a great health problem in the developing world and is a major cause of cardiovascular disease. It is estimated that 15.6 million people worldwide have rheumatic heart disease, and that 470 000 new cases of rheumatic fever occur each year.

Acute rheumatic fever has virtually disappeared from industrialized countries. However, in North America, a resurgence of ARF in scattered communities occurred in the mid-1980s. People aged between three and 15 years and military and school populations have been most often affected. Many reported cases have followed infections by specific group A serotypes, such as M-types 1, 3, 5, 6 and 18, particularly among highly mucoid strains of M18. The highest incidence, during late winter and spring, corresponds to that of pharyngitis.

In the USA, of the estimated 9 000–12 000 annual cases of severe (invasive) group A streptococcal infection, 1 000–1 850 patients die. Approximately 6% and 7% of those with invasive infection develop STSS and necrotizing fasciitis respectively. The burden of invasive group A strep infections in the developing world is not well described.

The highest incidence of streptococcal impetigo occurs in young children in the latter part of the hot season in hot climates. Nephritis following skin infections is associated with a limited number of streptococcal M-types (among which are types 2, 49, 55, 57, 58, 59, 60) that generally differ from those associated with nephritis following infections of the upper respiratory tract.

Geographical and seasonal distribution of erysipelas are similar to those for scarlet fever and streptococcal sore throat; erysipelas is most common in infants and those over 20. Occurrence is sporadic, even during epidemics of streptococcal infection.

Reliable morbidity data do not exist for puerperal fever. In industrialized countries, morbidity and mortality have declined, although epidemics may still occur in institutions where aseptic technique is faulty.

4. Reservoir—Humans.

5. Mode of transmission—Large respiratory droplets or direct contact with patients or carriers; extremely rarely through indirect contact through objects. Individuals with acute upper respiratory tract (especially nasal) infections are particularly likely to transmit infection. Casual contact rarely leads to infection. In populations where impetigo is prevalent, group A streptococci may be recovered from normal skin for 1-2 weeks before skin lesions develop; the same strain may appear in the throat (without clinical evidence of throat infection), usually late in the course of the skin infection.

Anal, vaginal, skin and pharyngeal carriers have been responsible for nosocomial outbreaks of serious streptococcal infection, particularly following surgical procedures. Many such outbreaks have been traced to operating room personnel or other health care workers. Identification of the carrier often involves intensive epidemiological and microbiological investigation; eradication of the carrier state is often difficult, typically requires a different antibiotic regimen than that used for treatment of disease, and may require multiple courses of specific antibiotic regimens (see 9, B7). Dried streptococci reaching the air via contaminated items (floor dust, lint from bedclothes, handkerchiefs) may be viable, but apparently do not infect mucous membranes and intact skin.

Explosive outbreaks of streptococcal sore throat may follow ingestion of contaminated food. Milk and milk products have been associated most frequently with food-borne outbreaks; egg salad and similar preparations have recently been implicated. Contamination of milk or egg products by humans appears to be the important source of food-borne episodes; infected food preparers are often implicated as the original source of infection. Group B organisms that cause human and bovine disease differ biochemically, but group A streptococci may be transmitted to cattle from human carriers, then spread through raw milk from these cattle. Milk-borne group C outbreaks have been traced to infected cows. Food-borne outbreaks of group G streptococcal pharyngitis have also been reported.

6. Incubation period—Short, usually 1-3 days, rarely longer.

7. Period of communicability—In untreated, uncomplicated cases, 10-21 days; in untreated conditions with purulent discharges, weeks or months. With adequate penicillin treatment, transmissibility of group A streptococcal pharyngitis generally ends within 24 hours. Patients with untreated streptococcal pharyngitis may carry the organism for weeks or months, usually in decreasing numbers; contagiousness for these patients decreases sharply in 2–3 weeks after onset of infection.

8. Susceptibility—Susceptibility to streptococcal pharyngitis/tonsillitis and scarlet fever is general, although many people develop either antitoxin- or type-specific antibacterial immunity, or both, through unapparent infection. Antibacterial immunity develops against the specific M-type of group A *Streptococcus* that induced infection, and may last for years. Antibiotic therapy may interfere with the development of type-specific immunity. No differences in susceptibility have been defined for men and women; reported racial differences probably relate to environmental factors.

Repeated attacks of pharyngitis/tonsillitis or other disease due to different types of streptococci are not uncommon. However, when a child or adolescent experiences multiple episodes of culture- or rapid test-positive acute pharyngitis within a period of months to years, it is most likely that this person is a pharyngeal carrier of group A *Streptococcus* who is actually experiencing viral pharyngitis. Immunity against erythrogenic toxin, and hence against rash, develops within a week after onset of scarlet fever and is usually permanent; second attacks of scarlet fever are rare, but may occur because of the three immunological forms of toxin. Some degree of passive immunity to group A streptococcal disease occurs in newborns with trans-placental maternal type specific antibodies. Patients who had one attack of rheumatic fever have a significant risk of recurrence of rheumatic fever, often with further cardiac damage following group A streptococcal infections. Individuals who had erysipelas appear predisposed to subsequent attacks. Recurrence of glomerulonephritis is unusual, perhaps because very few M-types are "nephritogenic."

9. Methods of control—

 A. Preventive measures:

   1) Educate the public, parents and health workers about modes of transmission and the importance of hand hygiene; about the relationship of streptococcal infection to acute rheumatic fever, Sydenham chorea, rheumatic heart disease and glomerulonephritis; and about the need for prompt diagnosis and completion of the full course of antibiotics prescribed for streptococcal infections.
   2) Provide easily accessible laboratory facilities for recognition of group A hemolytic streptococci.
   3) Pasteurize milk, and exclude infected people from handling milk likely to become contaminated.

4) Prepare other potentially dangerous foods just prior to serving, or adequately refrigerate in small quantities at 4°C (39°F) or less.

5) Exclude people with skin lesions from food handling.

6) Secondary prevention of complications: To prevent streptococcal re-infection and possible recurrence of rheumatic fever or chorea among patients with acute rheumatic fever, monthly injections of long-acting benzathine penicillin G (or daily penicillin orally in compliant patients) should be given for at least 5 years (for those with mild mitral regurgitation, at least 10 years; for those with severe valve disease or after valve surgery, life-long prophylaxis is recommended). Those who do not tolerate penicillin may be given sulfadiazine orally, or erythromycin if necessary. Prophylactic IM or oral penicillin may be used in some patients with recurrent erysipelas.

B. Control of patient, contacts and the immediate environment:

1) Report to local health authority: Obligatory report of epidemics, Class 4. Acute rheumatic fever and/or STSS reportable in some localities, Class 3 (see *Reporting*).

2) Isolation: Drainage and secretion precautions may be terminated after 24 hours' effective antibiotic therapy; antibiotics should be continued for 10 days to avoid development of rheumatic heart disease.

3) Concurrent disinfection: Of purulent discharges and all articles soiled therewith. Terminal cleaning.

4) Infection control: Critical assessment of adherence to infection control practices should be undertaken in group A streptococcal outbreaks in facilities housing highly vulnerable populations (e.g., nursing homes and acute and long-term rehabilitation facilities). Outbreaks in such facilities are often due to, or perpetuated by, poor routine infection control practices.

5) Quarantine: Not applicable.

6) Immunization of contacts: Not applicable; efforts are currently underway to develop a vaccine against group A *Streptococcus,* but at time of writing in early 2008 it is not likely that one will be available in the near future.

7) Investigation of contacts and source of infection: Culture from symptomatic contacts. Search for and treat carriers in situations where contacts may be at high risk for developing sequelae of group A streptococcal infections (e.g. evidence of streptococcal infection in families with multiple cases of rheumatic fever or streptococcal TSS; occurrence of cases of rheumatic fever or acute nephritis in a population group

such as a school; outbreaks of post-operative wound or postpartum infections). Identification and treatment of carriers may also be undertaken in well-documented epidemics of severe streptococcal infection, such as outbreaks of invasive group A streptococcal infections among nursing home residents, in order to halt ongoing transmission among a highly vulnerable population.

8) Specific treatment for disease: Penicillin; several forms: benzathine penicillin G, IM (treatment of choice), or oral penicillin G or penicillin V (which is more absorbable). To date there has never been a documented penicillin-resistant strain of group A beta-hemolytic streptococci. Treatment must provide adequate penicillin levels for 10 days. While antibiotics may shorten clinical illness somewhat, it is also recognized that patients with streptococcal pharyngitis improve in 3–4 days without antibiotics. Appropriate antibiotic use reduces the frequency of suppurative complications and prevents the development of most cases of acute rheumatic fever. It may also reduce the risk of acute glomerulonephritis after pharyngeal infection (not confirmed for acute nephritis after skin infections) and prevent further spread of the organism in the community. Erythromycin is the preferred treatment for penicillin sensitive patients, but strains resistant to this antibiotic have been reported (up to 38%), most notably in Asia and Europe. Clindamycin or a cephalosporin can be used when penicillin and erythromycin are contraindicated (e.g. because of allergy or resistance). Sulfonamides do not eliminate streptococci from the throat, nor do they prevent non-suppurative complications. Many group A streptococcal strains are resistant to the tetracyclines, and these should not be used against streptococcal pharyngitis.

C. Epidemic measures:

1) Determine source and manner of spread (person-to-person or single-source outbreaks due to contaminated milk or food). Single-source food-borne or nosocomial outbreaks can often be traced to an individual with an acute or persistent streptococcal infection, or who is carrying streptococci (nose, throat, skin, vagina or perianal area), through identification of the M-type or *emm* type of the streptococcus.

2) Investigate promptly any unusual grouping of cases to identify possible common sources, such as contaminated milk or foods.

3) For extensive or protracted outbreaks in special close contact groups (e.g. military recruits, day care centers, nursing

homes), it may be necessary to administer penicillin to the entire group to terminate spread. In these settings, the benefits of such widespread use of antibiotics should be carefully weighed against the potential side effects.

D. Disaster implications: Patients with thermal burns or wounds are highly susceptible to streptococcal infections of the affected area.

E. International measures: WHO Collaborating Centres provide support as required. More information can be found at: <http://www.who.int/collaboratingcentres/database/en/>

GROUP B STREPTOCOCCAL SEPSIS OF THE NEWBORN

ICD-9 771.8; ICD-10 P36.0

[CCDM18: O. Lincetto]
[CCDM19: D. Heymann]

1. Identification— Human subtypes of group B streptococci (*S. agalactiae*) produce invasive disease in the newborn of 2 distinct forms. Early onset disease (from 1–7 days), with sepsis, pneumonia and less frequently meningitis, osteomyelitis or septic arthritis, is acquired in utero or during delivery. Late onset disease (7 days to several months) is acquired in about half the cases through person-to-person contact, and presents mostly as meningitis or sepsis. Premature babies are more susceptible to Group B streptococci infection than full-term babies, but most babies who get disease from these streptococci (75%) are full term. Advances in neonatal care have led to a fall in the case fatality rate from 50% to 4%. Survivors may have speech, hearing or visual problems, psychomotor retardation, or seizure disorders if there has been meningeal involvement.

2. Infectious agents— *Streptococcus agalactiae*, Group B is the cause of sepsis in the newborn. About 10%–30% of pregnant women harbor group B streptococci in the genital tract, and about 1% of their offspring may develop symptomatic infection. Group B streptococci found in bovine mastitis are not a cause of this disease.

3. Occurrence—Thought to occur worldwide, but most study at time of writing in early 2008 is occurring in North America and Europe.

4. Reservoir—Humans; commonly found in the gastrointestinal, reproductive and urinary tracts.

5. Mode of transmission—Transmitted to infants during the intrapartum period, especially to infants delivered at <37 weeks, and/or when rupture of membranes occurs 18 hours prior to delivery.

6. Incubation period—From one to six days after birth.

7. Period of communicability—Intrapartum period, during delivery; especially high risk with premature birth and/or rupture of membranes >18 hours prior to delivery, or when mother has fever during labor.

8. Susceptibility—High risk in premature infants.

9. Methods of control—

A. *Preventive measures:* Two preventive approaches have been used successfully.

1) Risk-based method: identify candidates for intrapartum chemoprophylaxis according to the presence of any of the following intrapartum risk factors for early-onset disease:

- Delivery at <37 weeks
- Intrapartum temperature >38.0°C (>100.4°F)
- Rupture of membranes for 18 hours or more.

2) Screening-based method: screen all pregnant women for vaginal and rectal GBS colonization between 35 and 37 weeks' gestation, and offering women with colonization intrapartum antibiotics during labor. In both cases, women with GBS bacteriuria during the current pregnancy, or who previously gave birth to an infant with early-onset GBS disease, are candidates for intrapartum antibiotic prophylaxis.

Compelling evidence for a strong protective effect of the screening-based method relative to the risk-based strategy has led to the current recommendation in many countries of prenatal screening by vaginal-rectal culture for group B streptococcus colonization at 35–37 weeks' gestation, and chemoprophylaxis for all pregnant women identified as GBS carriers at the time of labor or rupture of membranes. Women whose culture results are unknown at the time of delivery should be managed according to the risk-based method.

B. *Control of patient, contacts and the immediate environment:*

1) Report to local health authority: Official report not ordinarily justified, Class 5 (see *Reporting*).
2) Isolation: In hospitals and institutions patients should be isolated, especially in maternity wards and nurseries.
3) Concurrent disinfection: Infection control measures (for more information, see the chapter on *Infection control*).

4) Quarantine: Not applicable.

5) Immunization of contacts: A vaccine for pregnant women to stimulate antibody production against invasive disease in newborns is under development.

6) Investigation of contacts and source of infection: Treat mothers who carry infection.

7) Specific treatment: The administration to women colonized with group B streptococci of intravenous penicillin or ampicillin at the onset of and throughout labor interrupts transmission to newborn infants, decreasing infection and mortality. Penicillin is the preferred agent in women without penicillin allergy. No GBS isolates with confirmed resistance to penicillin or ampicillin have been observed to date. Alternative regimens for allergic women include clindamycin, erythromycin and cefazolin. Routine use of antimicrobial prophylaxis for newborns whose mothers received intrapartum chemoprophylaxis for GBS infection is not recommended, although therapeutic use of these agents is appropriate for infants with clinically suspected sepsis.

C. Epidemic measures: None.

D. Disaster implications: None.

E. International measures: None.

DENTAL CARIES OF EARLY CHILDHOOD, STREPTOCOCCAL   ICD-9 521.0; ICD-10 K02
(Nursing bottle caries, Baby bottle tooth decay)
[CCDM18: P. Petersen]

While the cause of dental caries in young children is multifactorial, the subject is included in this section because of the involvement of a streptococcal species.

In early childhood a characteristic pattern of dental caries occurs, in which maxillary primary incisors are routinely affected with carious lesions, but mandibular primary incisors are rarely involved; involvement of other primary teeth varies. Because of the association of this pattern with a specific feeding habit, the process was called nursing bottle caries or baby bottle tooth decay, but it also occurs in children using feeding cups.

Streptococcus mutans is present in these carious lesions. These Gram-positive facultative anerobes produce caries in young experimental animals in the presence of dietary sugar. They are members of the *viridans* group of streptococci; hemolysis of blood agar is usually alpha or gamma.

They require a non-shedding oral surface for colonization, and are common residents of dental plaque.

Early childhood caries occur worldwide, with highest prevalence in developing countries. Disadvantaged children, regardless of ethnicity or culture, and those with low birthweight, are most frequently involved; enamel hypoplasia, which may occur because of compromised nutritional status during formative stages of primary dentition, is often associated. The main reservoir from which infants acquire *mutans* streptococci is the mother; strains isolated from mothers and their babies show similar or identical bacteriocin profiles and identical plasmid or chromosomal DNA patterns.

Mother-to-child transmission occurs through transfer of infected saliva by kissing the baby on the mouth or, more likely, by moistening the nipple or pacifier, or by tasting food on the baby's spoon before serving it. Colonization by maternal organisms largely depends on inoculum size; mothers with extensive dental caries usually have high levels of *mutans* streptococci in their saliva.

To prevent dental caries of early childhood, promote good oral hygiene in mothers and encourage early weaning from the bottle. Counsel parents and caretakers about the dangers of dental caries from milk and beverages containing sugar, and of transferring saliva to a baby's mouth when mothers and other caretakers have untreated carious teeth.

STRONGYLOIDIASIS   ICD-9 127.2; ICD-10 B78
[CCDM19: M. Eberhard, A. Gabrielli, L. Savioli]
[CCDM18: L. Savioli]

1. Identification—An often-asymptomatic helminthic infection of the duodenum and upper jejunum. Clinical manifestations include transient dermatitis when larvae of the parasite penetrate the skin on initial infection; cough, rales and sometimes demonstrable pneumonitis when larvae pass through the lungs; or abdominal symptoms caused by the adult female worm in the intestinal mucosa. Symptoms of chronic infection may be mild or severe, depending on the intensity of infection.

Classic symptoms include abdominal pain (usually epigastric, often suggesting peptic ulcer), diarrhea and urticaria; sometimes also nausea, weight loss, vomiting, weakness and constipation. Intensely pruritic dermatitis (larva currents) radiating from the anus may occur, as can stationary wheals lasting 1–2 days, as well as a migrating serpiginous rash moving several centimeters per hour across the trunk. Rarely, intestinal autoinfection with increasing worm burden may lead to disseminated strongyloidiasis with wasting, pulmonary involvement and death, particularly but not exclusively in the immunocompromised host. In these cases, secondary Gram-negative sepsis is common. Eosinophilia is usually moderate (10%–25%) in the chronic stage and in those with intercurrent infections, especially persons infected with human T-cell lymphotrophic virus (HTLV-1) or HIV, and those receiving chemotherapy for malignancies, but may be normal or low with dissemination.

Diagnosis entails identifying larvae in concentrated stool specimens (motile in freshly passed feces), in the agar plate method, in duodenal aspirates or, occasionally, in sputum. Ruling out the diagnosis may require repeat examinations. Held at room temperature for 24 hours or more, feces may show developing stages of the parasite, including rhabditiform (non-infective) and filariform (infective) larvae (these must be distinguished from larvae of hookworm species) and free-living adults. Serological tests based on larval stage antigens are positive in 80%–85% of infected patients.

2. Infectious agents—*Strongyloides stercoralis* and *S. fulleborni*, nematodes.

3. Occurrence—Throughout tropical and temperate areas; more common in warm, wet regions. Prevalence in endemic areas is not accurately known. May be prevalent in residents of institutions where personal hygiene is poor. Human infection with *S. fulleborni* has been reported only in Africa and in Papua New Guinea.

4. Reservoir—Humans are the principal reservoir of *S. stercoralis*, with occasional transmission of dog and cat strains to humans. Nonhuman primates are the reservoir of *S. fulleborni* in Africa. Person-to-person transmission may also occur.

5. Mode of transmission—Infective (filariform) larvae develop in feces or moist soil contaminated with feces; penetrate the skin; enter the venous circulation; and are carried to the lungs. They penetrate capillary walls, enter the alveoli, ascend the trachea to the epiglottis and descend into the digestive tract to reach the upper part of the small intestine, where development of the adult female is completed.

The adult worm, a parthenogenetic female, lives embedded in the mucosal epithelium of the intestine, especially the duodenum, where eggs are deposited. These hatch and liberate rhabditiform (non-infective) larvae that migrate into the intestinal lumen, exit in feces and develop after reaching the soil into either infective filariform larvae (which may infect the same or a new host) or free-living male and female adults. The free-living fertilized females produce eggs that hatch and liberate rhabditiform larvae, which may become filariform larvae within 24–36 hours. In some individuals, rhabditiform larvae may develop to the infective stage before leaving the body and penetrate through the intestinal mucosa or perianal skin; resulting autoinfection can cause persistent infection for many years.

6. **Incubation period**—2-4 weeks from penetration of the skin by filariform larvae until rhabditiform larvae appear in the feces; the period until symptoms appear is indefinite and variable.

7. **Period of communicability**—As long as living worms remain in the intestine; up to 35 years in cases of autoinfection.

8. **Susceptibility**—Susceptibility is universal. Acquired immunity has been demonstrated in laboratory animals but not in humans. Patients with malignant disease or on immunosuppressive medication, and HIV-infected patients with AIDS, are at risk of dissemination.

9. **Methods of control**—

   A. *Preventive measures:*

      1) Dispose of human feces in a safe manner.
      2) Pay strict attention to hygienic habits, including use of footwear in endemic areas.
      3) Rule out suspected strongyloidiasis before initiating immunosuppressive treatment.
      4) Examine and treat infected dogs, cats and monkeys in contact with humans.

   B. *Control of patient, contacts and the immediate environment:*

      1) Report to local health authority: Official report not ordinarily justifiable, Class 5 (see *Reporting*).
      2) Isolation: Not applicable.
      3) Concurrent disinfection: Safe disposal of feces.
      4) Quarantine: Not applicable.
      5) Immunization of contacts: Not applicable.
      6) Investigation of contacts and source of infection: Members of the same household or institution should be examined for evidence of infection.
      7) Specific treatment: Because of the potential for autoinfection and dissemination, all infections, regardless of worm burden, should be treated. Ivermectin 200 micrograms/kg or 200 micrograms/kg/day for 2 days is the regimen of choice; thiabendazole 25 mg/kg twice a day for 3-7 days or albendazole 400 mg once or twice daily for 3 days are less efficient alternatives. Repeated courses of treatment may be required.

   C. *Epidemic measures:* Not applicable; a sporadic disease.

   D. *Disaster implications:* None.

   E. *International measures:* None.

SYPHILIS

I. VENEREAL SYPHILIS

ICD-9 090-096;
ICD-10 A50-A52

(Lues)
[CCDM19: F. Ndowa, T. Peterman]
[CCDM18: G. M. Antal]

1. **Identification**—An acute and chronic treponemal disease characterized clinically by a primary lesion, a secondary eruption involving skin and mucous membranes, long periods of latency, and late lesions of skin, bone, viscera, the central nervous system (CNS) and the cardiovascular system. The primary lesion (chancre) usually appears about 3 weeks after exposure as an indurated, painless ulcer with a serous exudate at the site of initial invasion. Invasion of the bloodstream precedes the initial lesion; a firm, non-fluctuant, painless satellite lymph node (bubo) commonly follows.

Infection may occur without a clinically evident external chancre; e.g. in the rectum or on the cervix. After 4–6 weeks, even without specific treatment, the chancre begins to involute and, in most cases, a generalized secondary eruption appears, often accompanied by mild constitutional symptoms. A symmetrical maculopapular rash involving the palms and soles, with associated lymphadenopathy, is classic. Secondary manifestations resolve spontaneously within weeks to 12 months; all untreated cases will go on to latent infection for weeks to years, and one-third will exhibit tertiary syphilis signs and symptoms. In the early years of latency, there may be recurrence of infectious lesions of the skin and mucous membranes.

CNS disease, manifested as acute syphilitic meningitis, may occur at any time in secondary or early latent syphilis, later as meningovascular syphilis, and finally as paresis or tabes dorsalis. Latency sometimes continues throughout life. In other, unpredictable instances, 5–20 years after initial infection, other symptoms occur, including disabling lesions in the aorta (cardiovascular syphilis) or gummas in the skin, viscera, bone and/or mucosal surfaces. Death or serious disability rarely occurs during early stages; late manifestations shorten life, impair health and limit occupational efficiency. The widespread use of antimicrobials has decreased the frequency of late manifestations. Concurrent HIV infection may increase the risk of CNS syphilis; neurosyphilis must be considered in the differential diagnosis of HIV-infected individuals with CNS symptoms.

Fetal infection results in congenital syphilis and occurs with high frequency in pregnant women with untreated early syphilis infections. It frequently causes abortion or stillbirth and may cause infant death through preterm delivery of low birthweight infants, or from generalized systemic disease. Congenital infection may result in late manifestations that include involvement of the CNS with occasional stigmata such as Hutchinson teeth (small, wide-spaced, grayish incisors), saddlenose, saber shins (periostitis), interstitial keratitis and deafness. Congenital syphilis can be asymptomatic, especially in the first weeks of life.

The laboratory diagnosis of syphilis is usually made through serological testing of blood (and CSF when indicated). To aid in excluding biological false-positive reactions, reactive tests with non-treponemal antigens (e.g. rapid plasma regain, or RPR; or Venereal Disease Research Laboratory [VDRL]) should be confirmed by tests using treponemal antigens (i.e. FTA-Abs [fluorescent treponemal antibody absorbed] or TPHA [*T. pallidum* hemagglutinating antibody]), when available. For screening newborns, serum is preferred over cord blood, which produces more false-positive reactions. Primary and secondary syphilis can be confirmed through darkfield or phase-contrast examination, or direct fluorescence (FA) antibody staining of exudates from lesions or aspirates from lymph nodes (if no antibiotic has been administered). Serological tests are often non-reactive during the early primary stage; a darkfield examination of all genital ulcerative lesions can be useful, particularly in suspected early seronegative primary syphilis. *T. pallidum* polymerase chain reaction (PCR) tests have become an adjunct to darkfield microscopy in the diagnosis of syphilitic chancre.

2. Infectious agent—*Treponema pallidum*, subsp. *pallidum*, a spirochete.

3. Occurrence—Widespread; in industrialized countries sexually active young people are primarily involved, but with some epidemiological variation: for example, median age in the USA is 35, and in the UK, 41% of cases are in persons over 34. Racial differences in incidence reflect social rather than biological factors. Syphilis is usually more prevalent in urban than rural areas, and in some cultures, in males more than in females. After some decline in the late 1970s and early 1980s, then again in the late 1990s, incidence has increased again in recent years, notably in western Europe and the USA among men who have sex with men. This may be an indicator of increased sexual behavior in the era of antiretroviral treatments for HIV infection.

4. Reservoir—Humans.

5. Mode of transmission—Direct contact with infectious exudates from obvious or concealed moist, early lesions of skin, and with mucous membranes of infected people during sexual contact; exposure nearly always occurs during oral, anal or vaginal intercourse. Transmission by kissing or fondling children with early congenital disease occurs rarely. Transplacental infection of the fetus occurs during pregnancy in an infected woman.

Transmission can occur through blood transfusion if the donor is in the early stages of disease. Infection through contact with contaminated articles may be theoretically possible, but is extraordinarily rare. Health professionals have developed primary lesions on the hands following unprotected clinical examination of infectious lesions.

6. **Incubation period**—10 days to 3 months, usually 3 weeks.

7. **Period of communicability**—Communicability exists when moist mucocutaneous lesions of primary and secondary syphilis are present. The distinction between the infectious primary and secondary stages and the noninfectious early latent stage of syphilis is somewhat arbitrary with regard to communicability, since primary and secondary stage lesions may not be apparent to the infected individual. Lesions of secondary syphilis may recur with decreasing frequency up to 4 years after infection, but transmission of infection is rare after the first year. In many countries, infectious early syphilis is usually defined as ending after the first year of infection.

Transmission of syphilis from mother to fetus is most probable during early maternal syphilis, but can occur throughout the latent period. Infected infants may have moist mucocutaneous lesions that are more widespread than in adult syphilis and are a potential source of infection.

8. **Susceptibility**—Susceptibility is universal, though only approximately 30% of exposures result in infection. Infection leads to gradual development of immunity against *T. pallidum* and, to some extent, against heterologous treponemes; immunity often fails to develop because of early treatment in the primary and secondary stages. Concurrent HIV infection may reduce the normal host response to *T. pallidum*.

9. **Methods of control**—

   A. **Preventive measures:** (applicable to all STIs). Emphasis on early detection and effective treatment of patients with transmissible syphilis and their contacts should not preclude search for persons with latent syphilis to prevent relapse and disability due to late manifestations.

   1) Educate the community in general health promotion measures; provide health and sex instruction that teaches the means of preventing sexually transmitted infections, including the use of condoms, reducing the number of sexual partners, and establishing mutually monogamous relationships. Syphilis serology must be included in the workup of all cases of STD and should be a routine part of prenatal examination. Congenital syphilis is prevented through serological examination in early pregnancy, and again in late pregnancy, and at delivery in high prevalence populations; treat those who are reactive.
   2) Protect the community by preventing and controlling STDs in sex workers and their clients, and by discouraging unprotected sex, especially if there are multiple sexual partners

and anonymous or casual sexual activity. Teach methods of personal prevention applicable before and during exposure, especially the correct and consistent use of condoms.
3) Provide health care facilities for early diagnosis and treatment of STIs; encourage their use through education of the public about symptoms of STIs and modes of spread; make these services culturally appropriate and readily accessible and acceptable, regardless of economic status. Establish intensive case-finding programs that include interviewing patients and partner notification; for syphilis, repeated serological screening within special populations with known high incidence of STIs. Test patients who have syphilis for other STIs including HIV.

B. Control of patient, contacts and the immediate environment:

1) Report to local health authority: Case report of early infectious syphilis and congenital syphilis is required in most countries, Class 2 (see *Reporting*); laboratories must report reactive serology and positive darkfield examinations in many areas. Confidentiality of the individual must be safeguarded.
2) Isolation: For hospitalized patients, universal precautions for blood and body secretions. Patients should refrain from sexual intercourse until treatment is completed and lesions disappear; to avoid re-infection, they should refrain from sexual activity with previous partners until the partners have been examined and treated.
3) Concurrent disinfection: Not applicable in adequately treated cases; avoid contact with discharges from open lesions and articles soiled therewith.
4) Quarantine: Not applicable.
5) Immunization of contacts: Not applicable.
6) Investigation of contacts and source of infection: A fundamental feature of programs for syphilis control is the interviewing of patients to identify sexual contacts from whom infection was acquired in addition to those whom the patient may have infected. Trained interviewers obtain best results. The stage of disease determines which partners should be notified and tested: a) for primary syphilis, all sexual contacts during the 3 months preceding onset of symptoms; b) for secondary syphilis, contacts during the 6 months preceding onset of symptoms; c) for early latent syphilis, those of the preceding year, if time of primary and secondary lesions cannot be established; d) for late and late latent syphilis, marital partners, and children of infected mothers; and e) for congenital syphilis, all members of the immediate family. All

identified sexual contacts of confirmed cases of early syphilis exposed within 90 days of examination should receive treatment. Patients and their partners must be encouraged to obtain HIV counseling and testing.

If adequate and appropriate treatment of the mother prior to the last month of pregnancy cannot be established, all infants born to seroreactive mothers should be treated with penicillin.

7) Specific treatment: Long-acting penicillin G (benzathine penicillin), 2.4 million units in a single IM dose on the day that primary, secondary or early latent syphilis is diagnosed; this assures effective treatment even if the patient fails to return. Alternative treatment for non-pregnant patients allergic to penicillin: either doxycycline PO, 100 mg twice/day for 14 days, or tetracycline PO, 500 mg 4 times/day for 14 days—though tetracycline and doxycycline cannot be used in children less than eight years of age. Serological testing is important to ensure adequate treatment; tests are repeated at 3 and 6 months after treatment and later as needed. In HIV-infected patients, tests are repeated at 3, 6, 9, 12, and 24 months, and at 3-month intervals thereafter. A 4-fold titer rise indicates a need for re-treatment. In a small percentage of patients treated for primary or secondary syphilis, non-treponemal tests may remain positive despite repeated treatment. Failure of non-treponemal tests to decline 4-fold by 3 months after treatment for primary or secondary syphilis identifies those at risk of treatment failure. Careful evaluation of prior treatment and additional evaluation may be required. CSF analysis should be considered (increased risk of neurosyphilis) in case of treatment failure and infection with HIV, or in the presence of neurological findings.

Increased dosages and longer periods of treatment (benzathine penicillin G 7.2 million units total, as 3 doses of 2.4 million units IM at 1-week intervals) are indicated for late stages of syphilis. For neurosyphilis, aqueous crystalline penicillin G 18–24 million units a day administered as 3–4 million units IV every four hours for 10–14 days. An alternative treatment is procaine penicillin 2–4 million units IM daily, plus probenecid PO, 500 mg, 4 times/day, both for 10–14 days. Success in treatment must be verified by following serological titers and appropriate CSF examinations every 6 months until CSF cell count is normal.

Penicillin-sensitive pregnant women should have their allergy confirmed with skin tests (major and minor penicillin determinants) if test antigens are available. Patients with confirmed penicillin allergy can be desensitized and given the appropriate dose of penicillin. For others unable to take penicillin, ceftriaxone 1 gram intravenously or intramuscularly every day for 10 days provides identical cure rates.

For early congenital syphilis, aqueous crystalline penicillin G 50 000 units/kg/dose, given IV or IM every 12 hours during the first 7 days of life, then every 8 hours thereafter for another 10–14 days. An alternative is procaine penicillin G 50 000 units/kg/dose IM once per day for 10 days. For late congenital syphilis, if the CSF is normal without neurological involvement, children can be treated as for latent syphilis. If the CSF is abnormal, treatment for neurosyphilis is required: 200 000–300 000 units/kg/day of aqueous crystalline penicillin G at 50 000 units/kg/dose every 4–6 hours for 10–14 days.

C. Epidemic measures: Intensification of measures outlined under 9A and 9B. In protracted epidemics in selected populations (e.g. commercial sex workers) that remain refractory to standard interventions, mass treatment of the at-risk population may be considered.

D. Disaster implications: None.

E. International measures:

1) Examine groups of adolescents and young adults who move from areas of high prevalence for treponemal infections.
2) Adhere to agreements among nations as to records, provision of diagnostic and treatment facilities and contact interviews at seaports for foreign merchant seamen (e.g. Brussels Agreement).
3) Provide for rapid international exchange of information on contacts.
4) WHO Collaborating Centres provide support as required. More information can be found at:
   http://www.who.int/collaboratingcentres/database/en/

II. NONVENEREAL ENDEMIC SYPHILIS   ICD-9 104.0; ICD-10 A65
(Bejel, Njovera)

1. Identification—An acute disease of limited geographic distribution, characterized clinically by an eruption on skin and mucous membranes, usually without an evident primary sore. Mucous patches of the mouth are often the first lesions, soon followed by moist papules in skinfolds and by drier lesions of the trunk and extremities. Other early skin lesions are macular or papular, often hypertrophic, and frequently circinate; lesions resemble those of venereal syphilis. Plantar and palmar hyperkeratoses occur frequently, often with painful fissuring; alopecia and patchy depigmentation/hyperpigmentation of the skin are common. Inflammatory or destructive lesions of skin, long bones and nasopharynx are late manifestations. Unlike venereal syphilis, bejel rarely shows neurological or cardiovascular involvement. The case-fatality rate is low. Darkfield examination can demonstrate organisms in lesions during early disease. Serological tests for syphilis are reactive in the early stages and remain so for many years, then gradually tend toward reversal; response to treatment is as in venereal syphilis.

2. Infectious agent—*Treponema pallidum*, subsp. *endemicum*, a spirochete indistinguishable from that of syphilis except through molecular testing.

3. Occurrence—A common disease of childhood in localized areas with poor socioeconomic conditions and primitive sanitary and dwelling arrangements. Low level transmission in a few foci in the eastern Mediterranean including the Middle East; major foci exist in the Sahel region of Africa.

4. Reservoir—Humans.

5. Mode of transmission—Direct or indirect contact with infectious early lesions of skin and mucous membranes; the shared use of eating and drinking utensils and generally unsatisfactory hygienic conditions favor the latter. Congenital transmission does not occur.

6. Incubation period—From 2 weeks to 3 months.

7. Period of communicability—Until moist eruptions of skin and mucous patches disappear; sometimes several weeks or months.

8. Susceptibility—Body contact, predominantly at an early age (3 to 15 years). Reports of congenital infections are anecdotal.

9. Methods of control—

   A. Preventive measures: See *Yaws*, 9A.

   B. Control of patient, contacts and the immediate environment:

      1) Report to local health authority: In selected endemic areas; in most countries not a reportable disease, Class 3 (see *Reporting*).
         2), 3), 4), 5), 6) and 7) Isolation, Concurrent disinfection, Quarantine, Immunization of contacts, Investigation of contacts and source of infection, and Specific treatment: See *Yaws*, 9B, applicable to all non-venereal treponematoses.

   C. Epidemic measures: Intensification of preventive and control activities.

D. Disaster implications: None.

E. International measures: See *Yaws*, 9E. WHO Collaborating Centres provide support as required. More information can be found at:
http://www.who.int/collaboratingcentres/database/en/

TAENIASIS   ICD-9 123; ICD-10 B68

TAENIA SOLIUM
  TAENIASIS
    INTESTINAL FORM   ICD-9 123.0; ICD-10 B68.0
(Pork tapeworm)
TAENIA SAGINATA

TAENIASIS   ICD-9 123.2; ICD-10 B68.1
(Beef tapeworm)
CYSTICERCOSIS   ICD-9 123.l; ICD-10 B69
(Cysticerciasis, *Taenia solium* cysticercosis)
[CCDM19: M. Eberhard, J. Schlundt]
[CCDM18: D. Engels, J. Schlundt]

1. Identification—Taeniasis is an intestinal infection with the adult stage of large tapeworms; cysticercosis is a tissue infection with the larval stage of one species, *Taenia solium*. Clinical manifestations of infection with the adult worm, if present, are variable, and may include nervousness, insomnia, anorexia, weight loss, abdominal pain and digestive disturbances. Except for the annoyance of having segments of worms emerging from the anus, many infections are asymptomatic. Taeniasis is usually a nonfatal infection, but the larval stage of *T. solium* may cause fatal cysticercosis.

Cysticercosis is the larval infection of humans with the pork tapeworm. It may produce serious somatic disease, usually involving the CNS. When eggs or proglottids of the pork tapeworm are swallowed by humans, the eggs hatch in the small intestine and the larvae migrate to the subcutaneous tissues, striated muscles, and other tissues and vital organs of the body, where they form cysticerci. Consequences may be grave when larvae localize in the eye, CNS or heart. In the presence of somatic cysticercosis, epileptiform seizures, headache, signs of intracranial hypertension or psychiatric disturbances strongly suggest cerebral involvement. CNS cysticercosis, or neurocysticercosis, may cause serious disability, but with a relatively low case-fatality rate.

Infection with an adult tapeworm is diagnosed by identification of proglottids (segments), eggs or antigens of the worm in the feces or on anal swabs. Eggs of *T. solium* and *T. saginata* cannot be differentiated morphologically. Specific diagnosis is based on the morphology of the scolex (head) and/or gravid proglottids.

Specific serological tests should support the clinical diagnosis of cysticercosis. Subcutaneous cysticerci may be visible or palpable; microscopic examination of an excised cysticercus confirms the diagnosis. Cysticercosis in intracerebral and other tissues may be recognized by CAT scan or MRI, or by X-ray when the cysticerci are calcified.

2. Infectious agents—*Taenia solium*, the pork tapeworm, causes both intestinal infection with the adult worm and extraintestinal infection with the larvae (cysticerci). *T. saginata*, the beef tapeworm, only causes intestinal infection with the adult worm in humans.

3. Occurrence—Worldwide; particularly frequent wherever beef or pork is eaten raw or insufficiently cooked, and where sanitary conditions allow pigs and cattle to have access to human feces. Prevalence is highest in parts of Latin America, Africa, south and southeastern Asia and eastern Europe, and infection is common in immigrants from these areas. In Latin America, seroprevalence levels in endemic villages have been reported to be 10-25%. In some of the *T. solium* endemic regions this tapeworm is considered responsible for over 10% of acute case admission to neurological wards. Transmission of *T. solium* is rare in Canada, the USA, western Europe and most parts of Asia and the Pacific. Although fecal-oral transmission related to imported *T. solium* infections has been reported with increasing frequency in the USA, infection is unlikely to spread significantly in countries with good sanitation.

4. Reservoir—Humans are the definitive host of both species of taenia; cattle are the intermediate hosts for *T. saginata* and pigs for *T. solium*. East African countries report among the highest prevalence of swine cysticercosis; in parts of Tanzania, prevalence is reported to reach 37%.

5. Mode of transmission—Eggs of *T. saginata* passed in the stool of an infected person are infectious only to cattle, in the flesh of which the parasites develop into *Cysticercus bovis*, the larval stage of *T. saginata*. In humans, infection follows ingestion of raw or undercooked beef containing cysticerci; in the intestine, the adult worm develops attached to the jejunal mucosa.

Intestinal infection due to *T. solium* in humans follows ingestion of raw or undercooked infected pork ("measly pork"), with subsequent development of the adult worm in the intestine. Human cysticercosis occurs either by direct transfer of *T. solium* eggs from the feces of people harboring an adult worm to their own mouth (autoinfection) or to the mouth of another individual, or indirectly by ingestion of food or water contaminated with eggs. When humans or pigs ingest eggs of *T. solium*, the embryos escape from the shells and penetrate the intestinal wall into lymphatics or blood vessels, and thence to the various tissues, where they develop to produce cysticercosis.

6. Incubation period—Symptoms of cysticercosis may appear from weeks to 10 years or more after infection. Eggs appear in the stool 8–12 weeks after infection with the adult *T. solium* tapeworm, and 10–14 weeks after infection with *T. saginata*.

7. Period of communicability—*T. saginata* is not directly transmitted from person to person, but *T. solium* may be. Eggs of both species are disseminated into the environment as long as the worm remains in the intestine, sometimes more than 30 years; eggs may remain viable in the environment for months.

8. Susceptibility—Susceptibility is general. No apparent resistance follows infection; the presence of more than one tapeworm in a person has rarely been reported.

9. Methods of control—

A. Preventive measures:

1) Cysticercosis can be well controlled using current technology; the most cost-effective approach to eradication is by public education and sanitary measures.
2) Educate the public to prevent fecal contamination of soil, water, and human and animal food; to avoid use of sewage effluents for pasture irrigation; and to cook beef and pork thoroughly.
3) Identification and immediate treatment or institution of enteric precautions for people harboring adult *T. solium* is essential to prevent human cysticercosis. *T. solium* eggs are infective immediately on leaving the host, and may produce severe human illness. Appropriate measures are necessary to protect patients from infecting themselves and their contacts.
4) Freezing pork or beef at a temperature below −5°C (23°F) for more than 4 days kills the cysticerci effectively. Irradiation is very effective at 1 kGy.
5) Inspection of carcasses of cattle and swine will detect only a proportion of those that are infected; these should be condemned, irradiated or processed into cooked products.
6) Prevent swine access to latrines and human feces. Consider use of a new swine vaccine to control *T. solium* in the animals.

B. Control of patient, contacts and the immediate environment:

1) Report to local health authority: Selectively reportable, Class 3 (see *Reporting*).
2) Isolation: Not applicable. Stools of patients with untreated taeniasis due to *T. solium* may be infective (see 9A2).
3) Concurrent disinfection: Dispose of feces in a sanitary manner; emphasize strict sanitation, with handwashing after defecating and before eating, especially for *T. solium*.
4) Quarantine: Not applicable.
5) Immunization of contacts: Not applicable.
6) Investigation of contacts and source of infection: Evaluate symptomatic contacts.
7) Specific treatment: Praziquantel is effective in the treatment of *T. saginata* and *T. solium* intestinal infections. Niclosamide, no longer widely available, is an alternative. Patients with active CNS cysticercosis may benefit from treatment with praziquantel or albendazole under hospitalization; a short course of corticosteroids is usually given to control cerebral edema due to dying cysticerci. Although a recent Cochrane review suggests that treatment of CNS cysticercosis with praziquantel or albendazole is not justified by the evidence, debate continues, and in fact some patients with active CNS cysticercosis may benefit. Where cysticidal treatment is not indicated, symptomatic treatment, such as with anti-epileptic drugs, may bring relief. In some cases surgical intervention may be needed to relieve symptoms.

C. Epidemic measures: Not applicable.

D. Disaster implications: None.

E. International measures: WHO Collaborating Centres provide support as required. More information can be found at: <http://www.who.int/collaboratingcentres/database/en/>

ASIAN TAENIASIS

Human infections with a *T. saginata*-like tapeworm, acquired by eating uncooked liver and other viscera of pigs, have been reported in Taiwan (China), Indonesia, the Republic of Korea, the Philippines and Thailand. In experimental studies this organism produced cysticerci only in the viscera of pigs, cattle, goats and monkeys. It is unknown if human cysticercosis occurs with this species. This organism is now classified as a species *T. asiatica*.

TETANUS
ICD-9 037; ICD-10 A35

(Lockjaw)
(Obstetrical tetanus: ICD-10 A34)
[CCDM19: M.P. Joyce]
[CCDM18: J. Vandelaer]

1. Identification—An acute disease induced by an exotoxin of the tetanus bacillus, which grows anerobically at the site of an injury. The disease is characterized by painful muscular contractions, primarily of the masseter and neck muscles, secondarily of trunk muscles. A common first sign suggestive of tetanus in older children and adults is abdominal rigidity, though rigidity is sometimes confined to the region of injury. Generalized spasms occur, frequently induced by sensory stimuli; typical features of the tetanic spasm are the position of opisthotonos and the facial expression known as "risus sardonicus." History of an injury or apparent portal of entry may be lacking. Case-fatality rate ranges from 10% to over 80% depending on age and quality of care available, is highest in infants and the elderly, and varies inversely with the length of the incubation period and the availability of experienced intensive care unit personnel and resources.

Attempts at laboratory confirmation are of little help. The organism is rarely recovered from the site of infection, and usually there is no detectable antibody response.

2. Infectious agent—*Clostridium tetani*, the tetanus bacillus.

3. Occurrence—Worldwide. The disease is more common in agricultural regions and in areas where contact with animal excreta is more likely and immunization is inadequate. Parenteral use of drugs by addicts, particularly intramuscular or subcutaneous use, can result in individual cases and occasional circumscribed outbreaks. In 2006, an estimated 290 000 people worldwide died of tetanus, most of them in Asia, Africa and South America. Over 250 000 of these deaths were due to tetanus neonatorum, dealt with in a separate section below. In rural and tropical areas people are especially at risk, and tetanus neonatorum (see below) is common. There is some inconclusive evidence that at high altitude the risk for tetanus could be lower. The disease is sporadic and relatively uncommon in most industrialized countries.

4. Reservoir—Intestines of horses and other animals, including humans, in which the organism is a harmless normal inhabitant. Soil or fomites contaminated with animal and human feces. Tetanus spores, ubiquitous in the environment, can contaminate wounds of all types.

5. Mode of transmission—Tetanus spores are usually introduced into the body through a puncture wound contaminated with soil, street dust or animal or human feces; through lacerations, burns and trivial or unnoticed wounds; or by injected contaminated drugs (e.g. street drugs).

Tetanus occasionally follows surgical procedures, which include circumcision and abortions performed under unhygienic conditions. The presence of necrotic tissue and/or foreign bodies favors growth of the anerobic pathogen. Cases have followed injuries considered too trivial for medical consultation.

6. Incubation period—Usually 3-21 days, although it may range from 1 day to several months, depending on the character, extent and location of the wound; average 10 days. Most cases occur within 14 days. In general, shorter incubation periods are associated with more heavily contaminated wounds, more severe disease, and a worse prognosis.

7. Period of communicability—No direct person-to-person transmission.

8. Susceptibility and resistance—Susceptibility is general. Active immunity is induced by tetanus toxoid and persists for at least 10 years after full immunization; transient passive immunity follows injection of tetanus immune globulin (TIG) or tetanus antitoxin (equine origin). Infants of actively immunized mothers acquire passive immunity that protects them from neonatal tetanus. Recovery from tetanus may not result in immunity; second attacks can occur and primary immunization is indicated after recovery.

9. Methods of control—

   A. Preventive measures:

     1) Educate the public on the necessity for complete immunization with tetanus toxoid, the hazards of puncture wounds and closed injuries that are particularly liable to be complicated by tetanus, and the potential need after injury for active and/or passive prophylaxis.

     2) Universal active immunization with adsorbed tetanus toxoid (TT), which gives durable protection for at least 10 years; after the initial basic series has been completed, single booster doses elicit high levels of immunity. In children under 7, the toxoid is generally administered together with diphtheria toxoid and pertussis vaccine as a triple (DTP or DTaP) antigen, or as double (DT) antigen when contraindications to pertussis vaccine exist. Preparations that include other antigens including *Haemophilus influenzae* type b conjugate vaccines (DTP-Hib), Hepatitis B vaccine (DTP-HB), and/or inactivated polio vaccine are also available in some countries.

       Tetanus and diphtheria (Td) vaccine is used for children

older than seven years. For adolescents and adults up to age 64, and where available, combined tetanus, diphtheria and acellular pertussis (Tdap) vaccine can be safely used as a single dose and for boosting as part of wound prophylaxis. In countries with incomplete immunization programs for children, all pregnant women should receive 2 doses of tetanus toxoid in the first pregnancy, with an interval of at least 1 month, and with the second dose at least 2 weeks prior to childbirth, in order to prevent maternal and neonatal tetanus. Booster doses may be necessary to ensure ongoing protection (see below).

Non-absorbed ("plain") tetanus toxoid vaccines, as opposed to alum adjuvant tetanus toxoid preparations, are less immunogenic for primary immunization or booster shots. Minor local reactions following tetanus toxoid injections are relatively frequent; severe local and systemic reactions are infrequent but do occur, particularly after excessive numbers of prior doses have been given.

a) The schedule recommended for tetanus immunization in childhood is the same as for diphtheri. The schedule recommended in developing countries is at least 3 primary doses IM at 6, 10 and 14 weeks of age; and a DTP booster at 18 months to 4 years.

The following schedules are recommended for use in industrialized countries (some countries may recommend different ages or dosages):

i) Recommended immunization schedule for persons aged 0–18 Years.

The first 3 doses are given at 4- to 8-week intervals beginning when the infant is 6 to 8 weeks of age; a fourth dose is given 6–12 months after the third dose. This schedule should not entail restarting immunizations because of delays in administering scheduled doses. A fifth dose is given at 4–6 years, prior to school entry; this dose is not necessary if the fourth dose was given after the fourth birthday. If the pertussis component of DTP is contraindicated, diphtheria and tetanus toxoids for children (DT) should be substituted. A booster dose with an adult formulation, Tdap (or Td if Tdap is unavailable), is recommended at 11–18 years of age.

ii) Previously unvaccinated persons aged 7 years.

Because adverse reactions may increase with age, a preparation with a reduced concentration of diphtheria toxoid (adult Td) is usually given after the seventh birthday for booster doses.

For a previously unimmunized person, a primary 3-dose series of adsorbed tetanus and diphtheria toxoids (Td) is advised. Two doses are given at 4- to 8-week intervals, and the third dose is given 6 months to 1 year after the second dose. If the person is aged 10 years or older, a dose of Tdap may be substituted for a single Td dose in the series. Limited data from Sweden suggest that the 3-dose Td regimen may not induce protective diphtheria antibody levels in most adults, and additional doses may be needed.

iii) Active protection should be maintained by administering a dose of Td every 10 years thereafter. A one-time dose of Tdap may be substituted for the next Td dose in persons ages 19–64 years, for added protection against pertussis.

b) While tetanus toxoid is recommended for universal use regardless of age, it is especially important for workers in contact with soil, sewage and domestic animals; members of the military forces; policemen and others with greater than usual risk of traumatic injury; adults with diabetes mellitus; older adults who are currently at highest risk for tetanus and tetanus-related mortality; and women of reproductive age and newborns. Vaccine-induced maternal immunity is important in preventing maternal and neonatal tetanus.

c) Active protection should be maintained by administering booster doses of Td every 10 years. A dose of Tdap may be substituted for Td.

d) For children and adults who are severely immunocompromised or infected with HIV, tetanus toxoid is indicated in the same schedule and dose as for immunocompetent persons, even though the immune response may be suboptimal.

3) Prophylaxis in wound management: Tetanus prophylaxis in patients with wounds is based on careful assessment of whether the wound is clean or contaminated, the immunization status of the patient, proper use of tetanus toxoid and/or TIG (see table below), wound cleaning, and—where required—surgical debridement and the proper use of antibiotics.

a) Those who have been completely immunized and who sustain minor and uncontaminated wounds require a booster dose of toxoid only if more than 10 years have elapsed since the last dose was given. For major and/or contaminated wounds, a single booster injection of tetanus toxoid (preferably as Td or Tdap) should be administered promptly on the day of injury if the patient has not received tetanus toxoid within the preceding 5 years.

b) Persons who have not completed a full primary series of tetanus toxoid require a dose of toxoid as soon as possible following the wound, and may require passive immunization with human TIG if the wound is a major one and/or if it is contaminated with soil containing animal excreta. DTP/DTaP, DT or Td, as determined by the age of the patient and previous immunization history, should be used at the time of the wound, and ultimately to complete the primary series.

Passive immunization with at least 250 IU of human-derived TIG IM (or 1 500 to 5 000 IU of antitoxin of animal origin if globulin is not available), regardless of the patient's age, is indicated for patients with other than clean, minor wounds and a history of no, unknown or fewer than 3 previous tetanus toxoid doses. When tetanus toxoid and TIG or antitoxin are given concurrently, separate syringes and separate sites must be used.

When antitoxin of animal origin is given, it is essential to avoid anaphylaxis by first injecting 0.02 ml of a 1:100 dilution in physiologic saline intradermally, with a syringe containing adrenaline on hand. Pretest with a 1:1000 dilution if there has been prior animal serum exposure, together with a similar injection of physiologic saline as a negative control. If after 15–20 minutes there is a wheal with surrounding erythema at least 3 mm larger than the negative control, it is necessary to desensitize the individual.

Antibiotics may theoretically prevent the multiplication of *C. tetani* in the wound and thus reduce production of toxin, but this does not obviate the need for prompt treatment of the wound together with appropriate immunization.

Summary Guide to Tetanus Prophylaxis in Routine Wound Management[1]

History of tetanus immunization (doses)	Clean, minor wounds		All other wounds	
	Td[2]	TIG	Td[2]	TIG
Uncertain or <3	Yes	No	Yes	Yes
3 or more	No[3]	No	No[4]	No

[1]Important details are to be found in the text.

[2]For children under seven years, DTaP or DTP (DT, if pertussis vaccine contraindicated) are preferred to tetanus toxoid alone. For children aged seven years or older, Td is preferred to tetanus toxoid alone. For adolescents and adults aged up to 64, tetanus toxoid as Tdap is preferred where available, if the patient has not previously been vaccinated with Tdap.

[3]Yes, if ≥ 10 years since most recent dose.

[4]Yes, if ≥ 5 years since most recent dose. More frequent boosters are not needed and can accentuate side-effects.

B. Control of patient, contacts and the immediate environment:

1) Report to local health authority: Case report required in most countries, Class 2 (see *Reporting*).
2) Isolation: Not applicable.
3) Concurrent disinfection: Not applicable.
4) Quarantine: Not applicable.
5) Immunization of contacts: Not applicable.
6) Investigation of contacts and source of infection: Case investigation to determine circumstances of injury.
7) Specific treatment: TIG IM in doses of 3 000-6 000 IU. If immunoglobulin is not available, tetanus antitoxin (equine origin) in a single large dose should be given IV following appropriate testing for hypersensitivity. Metronidazole, the most appropriate antibiotic in terms of recovery time and case-fatality, should be given for 7-14 days in large doses; this also allows for a reduction in the amount of muscle relaxants and sedatives required. The wound should be debrided widely if possible. Wide debridement of the umbilical stump in neonates is not indicated. Maintain an adequate airway and employ sedation as indicated; muscle relaxant drugs, together with tracheotomy or nasotracheal intubation and mechanically assisted respiration, may be lifesaving. Active immunization should be initiated concurrently with treatment.

C. Epidemic measures:
In the rare outbreak, search for contaminated street drugs or other common-use injections.

D. Disaster implications: Social upheaval (military conflicts, riots) and natural disasters (floods, hurricanes, earthquakes) that cause many traumatic injuries in non-immunized populations will result in an increased need for TIG or tetanus antitoxin and toxoid for injured patients.

E. International measures: Up-to-date immunization against tetanus is advised for international travelers.

TETANUS NEONATORUM   ICD-9 771.3; ICD-10 A33

Tetanus neonatorum is a serious health problem in many developing countries where maternity care services are limited and immunization against tetanus is inadequate. In the past 10 years the incidence of tetanus neonatorum has declined considerably in many developing countries, thanks to improved training of birth attendants and immunization with tetanus toxoid for women of childbearing age. Despite this decline, WHO estimated in 2006 that tetanus neonatorum still caused about 257 000 deaths, mainly in the developing world. Most newborn infants with tetanus are born to non-immunized mothers delivered by an untrained birth attendant outside a hospital.

The disease usually occurs through introduction of tetanus spores via the umbilical cord, during delivery through the use of an unclean instrument to cut the cord, or after delivery by "dressing" the umbilical stump with substances heavily contaminated with tetanus spores, frequently as part of natal rituals.

In neonates, inability to nurse is the most common presenting sign. Tetanus neonatorum is typified by a newborn infant who sucks and cries well for the first few days after birth but subsequently develops progressive difficulty and then inability to feed because of trismus, generalized stiffness with spasms or convulsions and opisthotonos. The average incubation period is about 6 days, with a range from 3 to 28 days. Overall, case-fatality rates for neonatal tetanus are very high, exceeding 80% among cases with short incubation periods. Neurological sequelae including mild retardation occur in 5% to over 20% of those children who survive.

Prevention of tetanus neonatorum can be achieved through a combination of 2 approaches:

1) Improving maternity care, with emphasis on increasing the tetanus toxoid immunization coverage of women of childbearing age (especially pregnant women) and clean deliveries
2) Increasing the proportion of deliveries attended by trained attendants. Important control measures include licensing of midwives, providing professional supervision and education as to methods, equipment and techniques of asepsis in childbirth, and educating mothers, relatives and attendants in the practice of strict asepsis of the umbilical stump of newborn infants. The latter is especially important in many areas where strips of bamboo are used to sever the umbilical cord,

or where ashes, cow dung poultices or other contaminated substances are traditionally applied to the umbilicus. In those areas, any woman of childbearing age visiting a health facility should be screened and offered immunization, no matter what the reason for the visit.

Non-immunized pregnant women should receive at least 2 doses of tetanus toxoid, preferably as Td, according to the following schedule: the first dose at initial contact or as early as possible during pregnancy; the second dose 4 weeks after the first and preferably at least 2 weeks before delivery. A third dose could be given 6–12 months after the second, or during the next pregnancy. An additional 2 doses should be given at annual intervals, or during subsequent pregnancies. One of the five doses of tetanus toxoid should be given as Tdap where available, ideally while the mother is immediately postpartum or between pregnancies.

A total of 5 doses of tetanus toxoid protects the previously unimmunized woman throughout the entire childbearing period. Women whose infants have a risk of neonatal tetanus, but who themselves have received 3 or 4 doses of DTP/DTaP as children, need only receive 2 doses of tetanus toxoid during each of their first 2 pregnancies.

TOXOCARIASIS   ICD-9 128.0; ICD-10 B83.0
(Visceral larva migrans [VLM], Larva migrans visceralis, Ocular larva migrans, *Toxocara [canis] [cati]* infection)
[CCDM19: M. Eberhard, A. Gabrielli, L. Savioli]
[CCDM18: A. Montresor]

1. Identification—A chronic infection and usually mild disease, predominantly of young children but increasingly recognized in adults, caused by migration of larval forms of *Toxocara* species in the organs and tissues. A rarer but more serious visceral larva migrans (VLM) syndrome is caused by larval forms of *Baylisascaris*. It is characterized by eosinophilia of variable duration, hepatomegaly, hyperglobulinemia, pulmonary symptoms, and fever. With an acute and heavy infection, the WBC count may reach 100 000/mm³ or more (SI units more than 100×10^9/L), with 50%–90% eosinophils. Symptoms may persist for a year or longer; symptomatology is related to total parasite load. Pneumonitis, chronic abdominal pain, a generalized rash and focal neurological disturbances may occur, as may endophthalmitis (caused by larvae entering the eye), usually in older children; this can result in loss of vision in the affected eye (ocular larva migrans). Retinal lesions must be differentiated from retinoblastoma and other retinal masses. The disease is rarely fatal.

Differential diagnosis includes larval ascariasis (which has a shorter duration) and strongyloidiasis (longer duration). Ocular larva migrans should be distinguished from retinoblastoma and toxoplasmosis.

Exposure to dog feces, a history of pica, and suggestive laboratory findings orient the diagnosis, which is confirmed by serology. ELISA is the test of choice: testing with larval-stage antigens is highly sensitive and specific in visceral larva migrans and in ocular infections. Western blotting procedures can be used to increase specificity of the ELISA screening test. Other tests are also available.

2. Infectious agents—*Toxocara canis* and *T. cati*, predominantly the former; *Baylisascaris*, predominately *B. procyonis*.

3. Occurrence—Worldwide. Severe disease occurs sporadically and affects mainly children aged 14–40 months, but also in older age groups. Siblings often have eosinophilia or other evidence of light or residual infection. Serological studies in asymptomatic children have shown a wide range in different populations. Internationally, seroprevalence ranges from lows of 0%–4% in Germany and urban Spain (Madrid) to 83% in some Caribbean subpopulations. Adults are less often acutely infected. *Baylisascaris* has been reported in humans in North America, and occurs in raccoons in Europe, Japan, and elsewhere.

4. Reservoir—Dogs and cats, for *T. canis* and *T. cati*, respectively, and raccoons for *B. procyonis*. Puppies are infected by transplacental and transmammary migration of larvae, and pass eggs in their stools by the time they are 3 weeks old. Infection among bitches may end or become dormant with sexual maturity; with pregnancy, however, *T. canis* larvae become active and infect the fetuses, and also newborn pups through milk. Similar though less marked differences apply for cats; older animals are less susceptible than young ones.

5. Mode of transmission—For most infections in children, by direct or indirect transmission of infective *Toxocara* eggs from contaminated soil to the mouth, directly by contact with infected soil, or indirectly by eating unwashed raw vegetables. Some infections may occur through ingestion of larvae in raw liver from infected chickens, cattle and sheep.

Eggs are shed in feces of infected dogs and cats; up to 30% of soil samples from certain parks in the UK and the USA contained eggs; in certain parks in Japan, up to 75% of sandboxes contained eggs. Eggs require 1–3 weeks' incubation to become infective, but remain viable and infective in soil for many months to more than a year; they are adversely affected by desiccation.

After ingestion, embryonated eggs hatch in the intestine; larvae penetrate the wall and migrate to the liver and other tissues via the lymphatic and circulatory systems. From the liver, larvae spread to other tissues, particularly the lungs and abdominal organs (visceral larva migrans) or the eyes (ocular larva migrans), and induce granulomatous lesions. The parasites cannot replicate in the human or other end-stage hosts; viable larvae may remain in tissues for years, usually in the absence of symptomatic disease. When the tissues of end-stage hosts are eaten, the larvae may be infective for the new host. *Baylisascaris* is similar to *Toxocara*, except that larvae of *Baylisascaris* can grow in the human host, to more than 1 mm in length.

6. **Incubation period**—In children, weeks or months, depending on intensity of infection, re-infection, and sensitivity of the patient. Ocular manifestations may occur as late as 4-10 years after initial infection. In infections through ingestion of raw liver, very short incubation periods (hours or days) have been reported.

7. **Period of communicability**—No direct person-to-person transmission.

8. **Susceptibility**—Lower incidence in older children and adults relating mainly to lesser exposure. Re-infection can occur.

9. **Methods of control**—

   A. *Preventive measures:*

   1) Educate the public, especially pet owners, concerning sources and origin of the infection; the need for removal of pet feces from public areas such as parks and proper collection and disposal of pet feces in the immediate vicinity of the house; the particular danger of pica; the danger of exposure to areas contaminated with feces of untreated puppies; and the danger of ingestion of raw or undercooked liver from animals exposed to dogs or cats. Parents of toddlers should be made aware of the risk associated with pets in the household and how to minimize them.
   2) Prevent contamination of soil by dog and cat feces in areas immediately adjacent to houses and children's play areas, especially in urban areas and multiple housing projects. Encourage cat and dog owners to practice responsible pet ownership, including prompt removal of pets' feces from areas of public access, particularly play areas. Children's sandboxes/sandpits offer an attractive site for defecating cats; cover when not in use. Control stray dogs and cats; ensure that raccoons do not live in close proximity to human dwellings.
   3) De-worm dogs and cats, beginning at 3 weeks of age, repeated 3 times at 2-week intervals, and every 6 months thereafter. Also treat lactating bitches. Dispose of feces passed as a result of treatment, as well as other stools, in a sanitary manner.
   5) Always wash hands after handling soil and before eating.
   6) Teach children not to put dirty objects into their mouths.

   B. *Control of patient, contacts and the immediate environment:*

   1) Report to local health authority: Official report not ordinarily justifiable, Class 5 (see *Reporting*).

2) Isolation: Not applicable.

3) Concurrent disinfection: Not applicable.

4) Quarantine: Not applicable.

5) Immunization of contacts: Not applicable.

6) Investigation of contacts and source of infection: Search for site of infection of index case; identify others exposed. Intensify preventive measures (see 9A). Treatment of asymptomatic, ELISA positive individuals is not indicated; treatment may be considered for those with hypereosinophilia.

7) Specific treatment: diethylcarbamazine is the drug of choice. To reduce the intensity of allergic reactions induced by dying larvae, dosage is commonly commenced at 1 mg/kg twice daily and raised progressively to 3 mg/kg twice daily for 10–21 days. Alternative drugs are: albendazole (400 mg daily for 10–21 days or 10–15 mg/kg/day for 10–21 days); mebendazole (100 mg daily for 10-21 days); and thiabendazole (50 mg/kg daily in three divided doses for 7–28 days). Mebendazole or albendazole are the anthelminthics of choice because of relative safety; effectiveness of anthelminthics is questionable at best. For *Baylisascaris*, no drug has been demonstrated effective, although albendazole, started as soon as possible, may prevent clinical disease and is recommended for children with known exposure. Mebendazole, levamisole or ivermectin could be tried if albendazole is not available. Steroid therapy may be helpful, especially in ocular or CNS infection.

C. Epidemic measures: Not applicable.

D. Disaster implications: None.

E. International measures: None.

GNATHOSTOMIASIS   ICD-9 128.1; ICD-10 B83.1

Another visceral larva migrans, common in Thailand and elsewhere in southeastern Asia, is caused by *Gnathostoma spinigerum*, a nematode parasite of dogs, cats, and large carnivores, such as tigers and leopards. Following ingestion of undercooked fish, frogs, poultry or snakes containing third stage larvae, the parasites migrate through the tissue of humans or animals, forming transient inflammatory lesions or abscesses in various parts of the body, including the subcutaneous tissue, where they cause a typical painless, migrating, intermittent edema. Larvae may also invade the brain, producing focal cerebral lesions associated with eosinophilic pleocytosis. Diagnosis is suggested by a history of eating raw poultry and fish (such as "sashimi" in Japan, "somfak" in Thailand or "ceviche" in Central and South America) and by clinical and laboratory findings (eosinophilia); diagnosis is confirmed by ELISA test. Although no clear recommendation is available, albendazole 400 mg twice daily for 21 days has produced good cure rates. Mebendazole 300 mg daily for 5 days has also been shown to have some effect. Infection can be prevented by thoroughly cooking poultry and fish.

CUTANEOUS LARVA MIGRANS
ICD-9 126; ICD-10 B76.9

DUE TO *ANCYLOSTOMA BRAZILIENSE*
ICD-9 126.2; ICD-10 B76.0

DUE TO *ANCYLOSTOMA CANINUM*
ICD-9 126.8; ICD-10 B76.0
(Creeping eruption)

Infective larvae of dog and cat hookworms, *Ancylostoma caninum* and *A. braziliense* and *A. caninum*, cause a dermatitis called "creeping eruption", that affects utility workers, gardeners, children, sea-bathers and others who come in contact with damp sandy soil contaminated with dog and cat feces; in the USA, most prevalent in the southeastern areas. The larvae enter the skin and migrate intracutaneously for long periods; eventually they may penetrate to deeper tissues. Each larva causes a serpiginous track, advancing several millimeters to a few centimeters a day, with intense itching especially at night. The cutaneous disease is self-limited, with spontaneous cure after weeks or months. Freezing the area with ethyl chloride spray can kill individual larvae. Thiabendazole is effective as a topical ointment; a single dose of albendazole 400 mg or a single dose of ivermectin 12 mg is effective systemically. A 7-day course of albendazole 400 mg daily prevents recurrence. *A. caninum* larvae may migrate to the small intestine where they cause eosinophilic enteritis; these zoonotic infections respond to treatment with pyrantel pamoate, mebendazole or albendazole.

TOXOPLASMOSIS
ICD-9 130; ICD-10 B58

CONGENITAL TOXOPLASMOSIS
ICD-9 771.2; ICD-10 P37.1

[CCDM19: M. Eberhard, J. Jones, F. Meslin, H. V. Nielsen]
[CCDM18: F. van Knapen]

1. Identification—A systemic coccidian protozoan disease. Infections are frequently asymptomatic, or present as acute disease with lymphadenopathy only, or resemble infectious mononucleosis, with fever, lymphadenopathy and lymphocytosis persisting for days or weeks. Development of an immune response decreases parasitemia, but *Toxoplasma* cysts remaining in the tissues contain viable organisms. These cysts may reactivate if the immune system becomes compromised. Among immuno-deficient individuals, including HIV-infected patients, primary or reactivated infection may cause a maculopapular rash, generalized skeletal muscle involvement, cerebritis, chorioretinitis, pneumonia, myocarditis, and/or death. Cerebral toxoplasmosis is a frequent component of AIDS.

Infections with genetically distinct subtypes have been described, predominantly in South America, with fatal outcome in otherwise immunocompetent patients. An increased occurrence of chronic chorioretinitis in acquired toxoplasmosis has also been described in this region.

A primary infection during early pregnancy may lead to fetal infection with death of the fetus or manifestations such as chorioretinitis, brain damage with intracerebral calcification, hydrocephaly, microcephaly, fever, jaundice, rash, hepatosplenomegaly, xanthochromic CSF and convulsions evident at birth or shortly thereafter. Later in pregnancy, maternal infection results in milder or subclinical fetal disease with delayed manifestations, such as recurrent or chronic chorioretinitis. In immunosuppressed pregnant women who are *Toxoplasma*-seropositive, a reactivation of latent infection may result in congenital toxoplasmosis, though this is thought to be a rare event.

Diagnosis is based on clinical signs and supportive serological results, demonstration of the agent in body tissues or fluids by biopsy or necropsy, or isolation in animals or cell culture. Rising antibody titers are corroborative of active infection; the presence of specific IgM and/or rising IgG titers in sequential sera of newborns is conclusive evidence of congenital infection. The presence of IgA is also helpful in determining infection in newborns. High IgG antibody levels may persist for years with no relation to active disease.

2. Infectious agent—*Toxoplasma gondii*, an intracellular coccidian protozoan that completes its sexual life cycle phase in cats, and which belongs to the family Sarcocystidae, in the class Sporozoa.

3. Occurrence—Worldwide in mammals and birds. Infection in humans is common.

4. Reservoir—The definitive hosts of *T. gondii* are cats and other felines, which acquire infection mainly from eating infected mammals (especially rodents) or birds, and probably also from oocysts in soil contaminated with cat feces, acquired during licking/grooming. Felines alone harbor parasites in the intestinal tract, where the sexual stage of the protozoan life cycle occurs, resulting in excretion of oocysts in feces for 10–20 days, and rarely longer.

The intermediate hosts of *T. gondii* include sheep, goats, rodents, swine, cattle, chickens and other birds; all may carry an infective stage of *T. gondii* encysted in tissue, especially muscle and brain. Tissue cysts remain viable for long periods, perhaps lifelong. Cattle seem to be only minimally affected by natural *Toxoplasma* infection.

5. Mode of transmission—Transplacental infection occurs in humans when a pregnant woman has rapidly dividing cells (tachyzoites) circulating in the bloodstream, usually during primary infection. Children may become infected by ingesting infective oocysts from dirt in sandboxes, playgrounds and yards in which cats have defecated. Infections arise from eating raw or undercooked infected meat containing tissue cysts (pork, mutton or wild game, very rarely beef); ingesting infective oocysts in food like raw vegetables; or ingesting water contaminated with feline feces. Presumed inhalation of sporulated oocysts was associated with one outbreak; another was associated epidemiologically with consumption of raw goat milk. Infection may occur through blood transfusion or organ transplantation from an infected donor.

6. Incubation period—From 10 to 23 days from ingestion of undercooked meat in one common source outbreak; 5–20 days in another outbreak associated with cats.

7. Period of communicability—No direct person-to-person transmission except *in utero*. Oocysts shed by cats sporulate and become infective 1–5 days later, and may remain infective in water or moist soil for over a year. Cysts in the flesh of infected animals remain infective throughout the period during which the meat is edible and uncooked.

8. Susceptibility—Susceptibility to infection is general, but immunity is readily acquired and most infections are asymptomatic. Duration and degree of immunity are unknown but they are assumed to be long-lasting or permanent; antibodies persist for years, probably for life. Patients undergoing cytotoxic or immunosuppressive treatment and HIV-infected patients are at high risk of developing illness from reactivated infection.

9. Methods of control—

A. Preventive measures:

1) Educate pregnant women about preventive measures:

   a) Use irradiated meats or cook them to 66°C (150°F) before eating. Freezing meat down to −20°C (−4°F) for 24 hours is a good alternative. Carefully wash/clean raw vegetables before eating.
   b) Unless they are known to have antibodies to *T. gondii*, pregnant women must avoid cleaning litter pans and must avoid contact with cats of unknown feeding history.

They must wear gloves during gardening, and wash hands thoroughly after work and before eating.

c) Raw fruits and vegetables should be peeled or thoroughly washed before eating.

2) Wash hands thoroughly before eating and after handling raw meat, or after contact with soil possibly contaminated with cat feces. Cutting boards, dishes, counters, and utensils should be washed after contact with raw meat.

3) Cats should be fed dry, canned or boiled food and discouraged from hunting (i.e. kept as indoor pets only).

4) Dispose of cat feces and litter daily (before sporocysts become infective). Feces can be flushed down the toilet, burned, or deeply buried. Disinfect litter pans daily by scalding; wear gloves or wash hands thoroughly after handling potentially infective material. Dispose of dried litter without shaking, to avoid aerial dispersal of oocysts.

5) Control stray cats and prevent their access to sandboxes and sand piles used by children for play. Keep sandboxes covered when not in use.

6) Avoid drinking untreated water.

7) *Toxoplasma*-seropositive patients who have a CD4+ T-lymphocyte count <100/uL should be administered prophylaxis against toxoplasmic encephalitis. A double-strength tablet daily dose of trimethoprim-sulfamethoxazole is the preferred regimen.

8) Patients with AIDS who experience symptomatic toxoplasmosis must receive prophylactic treatment throughout life with pyrimethamine, sulfadiazine and folinic acid.

B. Control of patient, contacts and the immediate environment:

1) Report to local health authority: Not ordinarily required, but reportable in some countries to facilitate further epidemiological understanding of the disease, Class 3 (see *Reporting*).

2) Isolation: Not applicable.

3) Concurrent disinfection: Not applicable.

4) Quarantine: Not applicable.

5) Immunization of contacts: Not applicable.

6) Investigation of contacts and source of infection: In congenital cases, determine antibody titers in mother and child; in acquired cases, determine antibody titers in members of the household, and common exposure to cat feces, soil, untreated water, raw meat or unwashed vegetables.

7) Specific treatment: Treatment not routinely indicated for a healthy immunocompetent host, except for confirmed initial infection during pregnancy or presence of active chorioretinitis, myocarditis or other organ involvement. Pyrimethamine com-

bined with sulfadiazine and folinic acid (to avoid bone marrow depression) for 4 weeks is the preferred treatment for those with severe symptomatic disease. Clindamycin has been used in addition to these agents to treat ocular toxoplasmosis. In ocular disease, systemic corticosteroids are indicated when irreversible loss of vision can occur from lesions of the macula, papillomacular bundle, or optic nerve.

Treatment of pregnant women is problematic. Spiramycin is commonly used to prevent placental infection; pyrimethamine and sulfadiazine should be considered if ultrasound, PCR of amniotic fluid, or other investigations indicate that fetal infection has occurred. Because of concerns about possible teratogenicity, pyrimethamine should not be given during the first 16 weeks of pregnancy; sulfadiazine may be administered alone in this case. Infants whose mothers had primary infections or were HIV positive during pregnancy should be treated with pyrimethamine-sulfadiazine-folinic acid during their 1st year of life or until congenital infection is ruled out, in an attempt to prevent chorioretinitis and other sequelae. At time of writing in early 2008, there is as yet no international consensus on the correct management of infants born to HIV infected mothers who are seropositive for *Toxoplasma*.

C. Epidemic measures: None.

D. Disaster implications: None.

E. International measures: The EU zoonosis directive (92/117 EEG) mentions toxoplasmosis under category B (collection of data in Member States when available). WHO Collaborating Centres provide support as required. More information can be found at:

   http://www.who.int/collaboratingcentres/database/en/

TRACHOMA

ICD-9 076; ICD-10 A71

[CCDM19: Editorial Board]
[CCDM18: S. Resnikoff]

1. **Identification**—A chlamydial conjunctivitis of insidious or abrupt onset; the infection may persist for a few years if untreated, but the characteristic lifetime duration of active disease in hyperendemic areas is the result of frequent reinfection. The disease is characterized by the presence of lymphoid follicles and diffuse conjunctival inflammation

(papillary hypertrophy), particularly on the tarsal conjunctiva lining the upper eyelid. The inflammation produces superficial vascularization of the cornea (pannus) and scarring of the conjunctiva, which increases with the severity and duration of inflammatory disease.

The marked conjunctival scarring causes in-turning of eyelashes and lid deformities (trichiasis and entropion), which in turn cause chronic abrasion of the cornea and scarring with visual impairment and blindness later in adult life. Secondary bacterial infections frequently occur in populations with endemic trachoma and contribute to the communicability and severity of the disease.

Early trachoma in some developing countries is an endemic childhood disease. Early stages of trachoma may be indistinguishable from conjunctivitis caused by other bacteria (including genital strains of *Chlamydia trachomatis*). Differential diagnosis includes molluscum contagiosum nodules of the eyelids, toxic reactions to chronically administered eye drops, and chronic staphylococcal lid-margin infection. An allergic reaction to contact lenses (giant papillary conjunctivitis) may produce a trachoma-like syndrome with tarsal nodules (giant papillae), conjunctival scarring, and corneal pannus.

Laboratory diagnosis is made through Giemsa-stained smears for the detection of intracellular chlamydial elementary bodies in epithelial cells of conjunctival scrapings; IF examination after methanol fixation of the smear; detection of chlamydial antigen by EIA or DNA by probe; or isolation of the agent in special cell culture.

2. Infectious agent—*Chlamydia trachomatis* serovars A, B, Ba and C. Some strains are indistinguishable from those of chlamydial conjunctivitis; serovars B, Ba and C have been isolated from genital chlamydial infections.

3. Occurrence—Worldwide, as an endemic disease, most often of poor rural communities in developing countries. In endemic areas, trachoma presents in childhood, then subsides in adolescence, leaving varying degrees of potentially disabling scarring. Blinding trachoma is still widespread in the Middle East, northern and sub-Saharan Africa, parts of the Indian subcontinent, southeastern Asia and China. Pockets of blinding trachoma also occur in Latin America, Australia (among Aboriginals), and the Pacific islands.

The disease occurs among population groups with poor hygiene, poverty and crowded living conditions, particularly in dry, dusty regions. The late complications of trachoma (in-turned lids and corneal scarring) occur in older people who had infectious trachoma in childhood; these people are rarely infectious.

4. Reservoir—Humans.

5. Mode of transmission—Through direct contact with infectious ocular or nasopharyngeal discharges on fingers, or indirect contact with contaminated fomites such as towels, clothes and nasopharyngeal discharges from infected people and materials soiled therewith. Flies, especially *Musca sorbens* in Africa and the Middle East, contribute to the spread of the disease. In children with active trachoma, *Chlamydia* can be recovered from the nasopharynx and rectum, but the trachoma serovars do not appear to have a genital reservoir in endemic communities.

6. **Incubation period**—From 5 to 12 days (based on volunteer studies).

7. **Period of communicability**—As long as active lesions are present in the conjunctivae and adnexal mucous membranes; this may last a few years. Concentration of the agent in the tissues is greatly reduced with cicatrization, but increases again with reactivation and recurrence of infective discharges. Infectivity ceases within 2–3 days of the start of antibiotherapy, long before clinical improvement.

8. **Susceptibility**—Susceptibility is general; while there is no absolute immunity conferred by infection, the severity of active disease due to reinfection gradually decreases over the childhood years, and active infection is no longer seen in older children or young adults. In endemic areas, children have active disease more frequently than adults. The severity of disease is often related to living conditions, particularly poor hygiene; exposure to dry winds, dust and fine sand may also contribute. Although studies have shown that vaccines could prevent infection and reduce severity of infection, considerations of cost and time-limited effectiveness preclude their use.

9. **Methods of control**—

   A. *Preventive measures:*

   1) Educate the public on the need for personal hygiene, especially the risk of common-use towels.
   2) Improve basic sanitation, including availability and use of soap and water; encourage washing the face; avoid common-use towels.
   3) Provide adequate case-finding and treatment facilities, with emphasis on preschool children.
   4) Conduct epidemiological investigations to determine important factors in the occurrence of the disease for specific situations.

   B. *Control of patient, contacts and the immediate environment:*

   1) Report to local health authority: Case report required in some countries of low endemicity, Class 2 (see *Reporting*).
   2) Isolation: Not practical in most areas where the disease occurs. For hospitalized patients, drainage and secretion precautions.

3) Concurrent disinfection: Of eye and nasal discharges and contaminated articles.
4) Quarantine: Not applicable.
5) Immunization of contacts: Not applicable.
6) Investigation of contacts and source of infection: Members of family, playmates and schoolmates.
7) Specific treatment: In areas where the disease is severe and highly prevalent, mass treatment of the whole population, especially children, with oral azithromycin (20 mg/kg up to 1 gram, once or twice a year) or topical tetracycline ointment (twice daily for 6 weeks).

C. Epidemic measures: In regions of hyperendemic prevalence, mass treatment campaigns have been successful in reducing severity and frequency when associated with education in personal hygiene, especially cleanliness of the face, and improvement of the sanitary environment, particularly a good water supply.

D. Disaster implications: None.

E. International measures: WHO Collaborating Centres provide support as required. More information can be found at:

<http://www.who.int/collaboratingcentres/database/en/>

For further information, please contact the WHO/Alliance for the Global Elimination of blinding Trachoma.

TRENCH FEVER   ICD-9 083.1; ICD-10 A79.0
(Quintana fever)
[CCDM18: D. Raoult]

1. Identification—A typically non-fatal, febrile bacterial septicemic disease varying in manifestations and severity, characterized by headache, malaise, pain, and tenderness, especially on the shins. Onset is either sudden or slow, with a fever that may be relapsing (usually with a 5-day periodicity), typhoid-like, or limited to a single febrile episode lasting several days. Splenomegaly is common; a transient macular rash may occur. Symptoms may continue to recur many years after the primary infection, which may be sub-clinical with organisms circulating in the blood for months, with or without recurrence of symptoms. Bacteremia, osteomyelitis and bacillary angiomatosis can occur in immunocompromised patients, especially those with HIV infection. Endocarditis has been associated with trench fever infections, especially among homeless or alcoholic individuals.

Laboratory diagnosis is made by culture of patient blood on blood or chocolate agar under 5% CO_2. Microcolonies are visible after 8–21 days incubation at 37°C (98.6°F). Infection evokes genus-specific antibodies detectable by serological tests. ELISA tests are highly sensitive and an IFA test is commercially available.

2. Infectious agent—*Bartonella quintana* (formerly *Rochalimaea quintana*).

3. Occurrence—Epidemics occurred in Europe during World Wars I and II, among those living in crowded, unhygienic conditions; the disease is encountered especially among the homeless and persons infested with lice. Endemic foci have been detected in Burundi, Ethiopia, France, Mexico, Peru, Poland, Russia, USA and North Africa. Two forms of infection were documented during the 1990s in France and USA: an opportunistic febrile infection in patients with HIV infection (sometimes presenting as bacillary angiomatosis; see *Bartonella infections* and *Cat scratch disease*); and a louse-borne febrile disease in homeless or alcoholic individuals, the so-called "urban trench fever" which may be associated with endocarditis.

4. Reservoir—Humans. The intermediate host and vector is the body louse, *Pediculus humanus corporis*. The organism multiplies extracellularly in the gut lumen for the duration of the insect's life, which is approximately 5 weeks after hatching. No trans-ovarial transmission occurs. Cat fleas and ticks may also be infected.

5. Mode of transmission—Not directly transmitted from person to person. People are infected by inoculation of the organism in louse feces through a break in the skin. Infected lice begin to excrete infectious feces 5–12 days after ingesting infective blood; this continues for the remainder of their lifespan. The disease spreads when lice leave abnormally hot (febrile) or cold (dead) bodies in search of a normothermic host.

6. Incubation period—Generally 7–30 days.

7. Period of communicability—Organisms may circulate in the blood (thus infecting lice) for weeks, months or years, and may recur with or without symptoms. A history of trench fever is a permanent contraindication to blood donation.

8. Susceptibility—Susceptibility is general. The degree of post-infection immunity to either re-infection or disease is unknown.

9. Methods of control—

    A. Preventive measures: Delousing procedures: Dust clothing and body with an effective insecticide.

B. Control of patient, contacts and the immediate environment:

1) Report to local health authority so that an evaluation of louse infestation in the population may be made and appropriate measures taken; Class 3 (see *Reporting*).
2) Isolation: None after delousing.
3) Concurrent disinfection: Treat louse-infested clothing to kill the lice.
4) Quarantine: Not applicable.
5) Immunization of contacts: Not applicable.
6) Investigation of contacts and source of infection: Search bodies and clothing of people at risk for the presence of lice; delouse if indicated.
7) Specific treatment: tetracyclines for 2–4 weeks (note that tetracyclines cannot be used in children less than eight years of age). Patients should first be evaluated carefully for endocarditis, as this will change the duration and follow-up of antibiotherapy. Relapse may occur, despite antibiotherapy, in both immunocompromised and immunocompetent patients.

C. Epidemic measures: Systematic application of residual insecticide to clothing of all people in affected population (see 9A).

D. Disaster implications: Risk is increased when louse-infested people are forced to live in crowded, unhygienic shelters (see 9B1).

E. International measures: WHO Collaborating Centres provide support as required. More information can be found at:

<http://www.who.int/collaboratingcentres/database/en/>

TRICHINELLOSIS   ICD-9 124; ICD-10 B75
(Trichiniasis, Trichinosis)
[CCDM19: M. Eberhard]
[CCDM18: D. Engels]

1. Identification—A disease caused by an intestinal roundworm whose larvae (trichinae) migrate to and become encapsulated in the muscles. Clinical illness in humans is highly variable and can range from inapparent infection to a fulminating, fatal disease, depending on the number of larvae ingested. Sudden appearance of muscle soreness and pain together with edema of the upper eyelids and fever are early characteristic signs. These are sometimes followed by sub-conjunctival, sub-ungual and retinal hemorrhages, pain and photophobia. Thirst, profuse sweating, chills, weakness, prostration and rapidly increasing eosinophilia may follow shortly after the ocular signs.

Gastrointestinal symptoms, such as diarrhea due to the intra-intestinal activity of the adult worms, may precede the ocular manifestations. Remittent fever is usual, sometimes as high as 40°C (104°F); fever terminates after 1–6 weeks, depending on intensity of infection. Cardiac and neurological complications may appear in the third to sixth week; in the most severe cases, death due to myocardial failure may occur in either the first to second week, or between the fourth and eighth weeks.

Serological tests and marked eosinophilia may aid in diagnosis. Biopsy of skeletal muscle, taken more than 10 days after infection (most often positive after the fourth or fifth week of infection), frequently provides conclusive evidence of infection, by demonstrating the uncalcified parasite cyst.

2. Infectious agent—*Trichinella spiralis*, an intestinal nematode. Separate taxonomic designations have been accepted for isolates found in the Arctic (*T. nativa*) and Palaearctic (*T. britovi*), in carnivore mammals and sometimes wild boar and domestic pigs in Europe and Asia), in Africa (*T. nelsoni*) and in several regions of the world (*T. pseudospiralis*).

3. Occurrence—Worldwide, but variable in incidence, depending in part on practices of eating and preparing pork or wild animal meat, and the extent to which the disease is recognized and reported. Cases are usually sporadic and outbreaks localized, often resulting from eating sausage and other meat products containing pork, or from sharing meat from Arctic mammals. Several outbreaks have been reported in France and Italy through infected horse meat.

4. Reservoir—Swine, dogs, cats, horses, rats and many wild animals, including foxes, wolves, bears, moose, mountain lions, polar bears, wild boar and marine mammals in the Arctic, and hyena, jackal, lion and leopard in the tropics. A new species (*T. zimbabwensis*) has been found in farmed crocodiles; health risks for humans consuming crocodile meat are unknown.

5. Mode of transmission—Consumption of raw or insufficiently cooked flesh of animals containing viable encysted larvae, chiefly pork and pork products and beef products, such as hamburger, adulterated intentionally or inadvertently with raw pork. In the epithelium of the small intestine, larvae develop into adults. Gravid female worms then produce larvae, which penetrate the lymphatics or venules and are disseminated via the bloodstream throughout the body. The larvae become encapsulated in skeletal muscle.

6. Incubation period—Systemic symptoms usually appear about 8–15 days after ingestion of infected meat; this varies from 5 to 45 days depending on the number of parasites involved. GI symptoms may appear within a few days.

7. Period of communicability—Not transmitted directly from person to person. Animal hosts remain infective for months, and their meat stays infective for appreciable periods unless cooked, frozen or irradiated to kill the larvae (see 9A).

8. Susceptibility—Susceptibility is universal. Infection results in partial immunity.

9. Methods of control—

    A. Preventive measures:

1) Educate the public on the need to cook all fresh pork and pork products and meat from wild animals at a temperature and for a time sufficient to allow all parts to reach at least 71°C (160°F), or until meat changes from pink to grey, which allows a sufficient margin of safety. This should be done unless it has been established that these meat products have been processed either by heating, curing, freezing or irradiation adequate to kill trichinae.

2) Grind pork in a separate grinder, or clean the grinder thoroughly before and after processing other meats.

3) Adopt regulations to encourage commercial irradiation processing of pork products. Testing carcasses for infection with a digestion technique is useful, as is immunodiagnosis of pigs with an approved ELISA test.

4) Adopt and enforce regulations that allow only certified trichinae-free pork to be used in raw pork products that have a cooked appearance, or in products that are traditionally not heated sufficiently in final preparation to kill trichinae.

5) Adopt laws and regulations to require and enforce the cooking of garbage and offal before feeding to swine.

6) Educate hunters to cook the meat of walrus, seal, wild boar, bear and other wild animals thoroughly.

7) Freezing temperatures maintained throughout the mass of the infected meat are effective in inactivating trichinae; holding pieces of pork up to 15 cm thick at a temperature of −15°C (5°F) for 30 days or −25°C (−13°F) or lower for 10 days will effectively destroy all common types of trichinae cysts. Hold thicker pieces at the lower temperature for at least 20 days. These temperatures will not inactivate the cold-resistant Arctic strains (*T. nativa* and possibly *T. britovi*) found in walrus and bear meat and—rarely—in swine. For *T. nativa*, meat must be heated at more than 60°C (140°F) for a duration related to the thickness of the meat.

8) Exposure of pork cuts or carcasses to low-level gamma irradiation effectively sterilizes and, at higher doses, kills encysted trichinae.

B. Control of patient, contacts and the immediate environment:

1) Report to local health authority: Case report required in most countries, Class 2 (see *Reporting*).
2) Isolation: Not applicable.
3) Concurrent disinfection: Not applicable.
4) Quarantine: Not applicable.
5) Immunization of contacts: Not applicable.
6) Investigation of contacts and source of infection: Check family members and persons who have eaten meat suspected as the source of infection. Dispose of any remaining suspected food.
7) Specific treatment: Albendazole or mebendazole are effective in the intestinal stage and in the muscular stage. Corticosteroids are indicated only in severe cases to alleviate symptoms of inflammatory reaction when the CNS or heart is involved; however, they delay elimination of adult worms from the intestine. In rare situations where infected meat is known to have been consumed, prompt administration of anthelminthic treatment may prevent development of symptoms.

C. Epidemic measures: Epidemiological study to determine the common food involved. Confiscate remainder of suspected food and correct faulty practices. Eliminate infected herds of swine.

D. Disaster implications: None.

E. International measures: WHO Collaborating Centres provide support as required. More information can be found at:

<http://www.who.int/collaboratingcentres/database/en/>

TRICHOMONIASIS   ICD-9 131; ICD-10 A59
[CCDM19: M. Eberhard, F Ndowa]
[CCDM18: L. Savioli]

1. Identification—A common and persistent protozoan infection of the genitourinary tract, characterized in women by vaginitis, with small petechial or sometimes punctate hemorrhages on the cervix ("strawberry cervix"), and a profuse, thin, foamy, greenish-yellow discharge with foul odor. The disease may cause urethritis or cystitis but is frequently asymptomatic; it may also cause obstetric complications and may facilitate

HIV infection. In men, the infectious agent invades the prostate, urethra or seminal vesicles; it often causes only mild symptoms, but may cause as much as 5%-10% of nongonococcal urethritis in some areas.

Trichomoniasis often coexists with gonorrhea. In some studies, up to 40% of persons with gonorrhea have concurrent trichomoniasis. The majority of women with trichomoniasis also have bacterial vaginosis. A full assessment for STI pathogens ("STI check") must be carried out when trichomoniasis is diagnosed.

Diagnosis is through identification of the motile parasite, either by microscopic examination of discharges or by culture, which is more sensitive. The organisms can be seen on a Papanicolaou smear. PCR testing is available but is insufficiently reliable for routine use, particularly in women; it is, however, probably superior to culture in men.

2. Infectious agent—*Trichomonas vaginalis*, a flagellate protozoan.

3. Occurrence—Widespread; a frequent disease, primarily of adults, with the highest incidence among females 16-35 years. Overall, about 20% of females may become infected during their reproductive years.

4. Reservoir—Humans.

5. Mode of transmission—Through contact with vaginal and urethral discharges of infected people during sexual intercourse.

6. Incubation period—4-20 days, average 7 days; many people are symptom-free carriers for years.

7. Period of communicability—For the duration of the persistent infection, which may last years.

8. Susceptibility—Susceptibility to infection is general, but clinical disease is seen mainly in females.

9. Methods of control—

    A. *Preventive measures:* Educate the public to seek medical advice whenever there is an abnormal discharge from the genitalia, and to refrain from sexual intercourse until investigation and treatment of self and partner(s) are completed. Promotion of "safer sex" behavior, including condom use, is recommended for all sexual contacts where mutual monogamy is not the case.

    B. *Control of patient, contacts and the immediate environment:*

        1) Report to local health authority: Official report not ordinarily justifiable, Class 5 (see *Reporting*).

2) Isolation: Avoid sexual relations during period of infection and treatment.
3) Concurrent disinfection: Not applicable; the organism does not withstand drying.
4) Quarantine: Not applicable.
5) Immunization of contacts: Not applicable.
6) Investigation of contacts and source of infection: Evaluate sexual partners for other STIs and treat concurrently.
7) Specific treatment: oral metronidazole, tinidazole or ornidazole is effective in both male and female patients; contraindicated during the first trimester of pregnancy. Clotrimazole produces symptomatic relief and may cure up to 50% of patients. Concurrently treat sexual partner(s) to prevent reinfection. Cases of metronidazole resistance have been reported, and should be treated with higher doses of metronidazole or tinidazole. Appropriate protocols must be followed when determining further treatment for refractory trichomoniasis. Although intravaginal paromomycin has been successfully used, severe side effects including mucosal ulceration and pain have been reported, and its use requires caution.

C. Epidemic measures: None.

D. Disaster implications: None.

E. International measures: None.

TRICHURIASIS
ICD-9 127.3; ICD-10 B79
(Trichocephaliasis, Whipworm disease)
[CCDM19: M. Eberhard, A. Gabrielli, L. Savioli]
[CCDM18: L. Savioli]

1. **Identification**—A nematode infection of the large intestine, usually asymptomatic. Heavy infections may cause bloody, mucoid stools and diarrhea. Rectal prolapse, clubbing of fingers, hypoproteinemia, anemia and growth retardation may occur in heavily infected children.

Diagnosis is made through demonstration of eggs in feces, or sigmoidoscopic observation of worms attached to the wall of the lower colon in heavy infections. Eggs must be differentiated from those of *Capillaria* species.

2. **Infectious agent**—*Trichuris trichiura* (*Trichocephalus trichiurus*) or human whipworm, a nematode.

3. **Occurrence**—Worldwide, especially in warm, moist regions.

4. **Reservoir**—Humans. Animal whipworms do not infect humans.

5. **Mode of transmission**—Indirect, particularly through pica (eating of non-food items, in this context especially soil) or ingestion of contaminated vegetables; no immediate person-to-person transmission. Eggs passed in feces require a minimum of 10–14 days in warm moist soil to become infective. Hatching of larvae follows ingestion of infective eggs from contaminated soil, attachment to the mucosa of the cecum and proximal colon, and development into mature worms. Eggs appear in the feces 70–90 days after ingestion of embryonated eggs; symptoms may appear much earlier.

6. **Incubation period**—Indefinite.

7. **Period of communicability**—Several years in untreated carriers.

8. **Susceptibility**—Susceptibility is universal.

9. **Methods of control**—

   A. *Preventive measures:*

   1) Educate all members of the family, particularly children, in the use of toilet facilities.
   2) Provide adequate facilities for feces disposal.
   3) Encourage satisfactory hygienic habits, especially handwashing before food handling; avoid ingestion of soil by thorough washing of vegetables and other foods contaminated with soil.
   4) WHO recommends a "preventive chemotherapy" strategy focused on treatment of high-risk groups at regular intervals, for the control of morbidity due to soil-transmitted helminth (STH) infections, including ascariasis, trichuriasis and hookworm disease. Recommended drugs and dosages are single-dose mebendazole (500 mg) or albendazole (400 mg, half dose for children 12-24 months). Action to be taken is differentiated according to prevalence of any STH infection (infection with at least one STH) among school-age children (children aged 6-15 years):

Recommended treatment strategy for STH in preventive chemotherapy[a]

Category	Prevalence of infection among school-age children	Action to be taken	
High-risk community	≥50%	Treat all school-age children (enrolled and not enrolled) twice each year[b]	Also treat with the same frequency: • Preschool children (aged 1–5) • Women of childbearing age including women in the 2nd and 3rd trimesters and lactating women • Adults at high risk in certain occupations (e.g. tea pickers and miners)
Low-risk community	≥20% and <50%	Treat all school-age children (enrolled and not enrolled) once a year	Also treat with the same frequency: • Preschool children (aged 1–5) • Women of childbearing age including women in the 2nd and 3rd trimester and lactating women • Adults at high risk in certain occupations (e.g. tea pickers and miners)

[a]When prevalence of any STH infection is less than 20%, large-scale preventive chemotherapy interventions are not recommended. Affected individuals should be dealt with on a case-by-case basis.

[b]If resources are available, a third drug distribution intervention might be added. In this case the appropriate frequency of treatment would be every 4 months.

Extensive monitoring has shown no significant ill effects of administration to pregnant women, however women in the 1st trimester should not be treated as a precautionary measure. Administration of anthelminthics to very young children (1–2 years old) is safe, provided some key recommendations are followed: a) children should never be forced to swallow tablets; b) tablets should be crushed and mixed with water that is safe for drinking; and c) treatment should be supervised by trained personnel.

B. Control of patient, contacts and the immediate environment:

1) Report to local health authority: Official report not ordinarily justifiable, Class 5 (see *Reporting*). Advise school health authorities of unusual frequency in school populations.
2) Isolation: Not applicable.
3) Concurrent disinfection: Sanitary disposal of feces.
4) Quarantine: Not applicable.
5) Immunization of contacts: Not applicable.
6) Investigation of contacts and source of infection: Examine feces of all symptomatic members of the family group, especially children and playmates.
7) Specific treatment: Single-dose oral mebendazole (500 mg) or albendazole (400 mg, half dose for children 12–24 months). Single-dose ivermectin 200 micrograms/kg is an alternative. For all drugs, longer treatment courses (up to 3 days) are required in heavy infections. On theoretical grounds, pregnant women should not be treated in the first trimester unless there are specific medical or public health indications.

C. Epidemic measures: Not applicable.

D. Disaster implications: None.

E. International measures: None.

TRYPANOSOMIASIS   ICD-9 086; ICD-10 B56-B57

I. AFRICAN
TRYPANOSOMIASIS ICD-9 086.3-086.5; ICD-10 B56
(Sleeping sickness)
[CCDM19: P. Simarro]
[CCDM18: J. Jannin]

1. Identification—A systemic protozoal disease, always fatal without treatment. There are two forms of the disease. The gambiense or chronic form, which may run a course of several years, is due to *Trypanosoma brucei gambiense*, and is found in Western and Central Africa (ICD-9 086.3; ICD-10 B56.0); the rhodesiense or acute form, which used to be lethal within weeks or months, is due to *Trypanosoma. Brucei rhodesiense*, and is located in Eastern and Southern Africa (ICD-9 086.4; ICD-10 B56.1).

In the early stage, a painful chancre, originating as a papule and evolving into a nodule, may be found at the primary tsetse fly bite site (more frequent in *rhodesiense* disease); there may also be fever, intense head-ache, insomnia, painless enlarged lymph nodes, local edema, rash, and unspecific cardiac symptoms. In the late stage, after the parasite crosses the blood-brain barrier, neurological signs are added, such as disturbances of circadian rhythm, sensory disturbances, endocrine dysfunction, disorders of tonus and mobility, abnormal movements, mental changes or psychiatric disorders. Neurological symptoms are correlated to the damaged areas of the CNS.

Diagnosis, which cannot be based on clinical symptoms only, relies on finding trypanosomes in blood, lymph or eventually CSF. Parasite-concentration techniques are always required in gambiense, and less often in rhodesiense disease: in blood, capillary tube centrifugation or minianion exchange centrifugation; in CSF, single modified centrifugation or double centrifugation. Inoculation on laboratory rats or mice is sometimes useful in rhodesiense disease. Standard bioclinical parameters such as anemia may provide indirect evidence of trypanosomiasis. IgM concentrations in *T. b. gambiense* patients can be increased up to 16 times as a result of polyclonal, non-specific B-cell activation. The accompanying poly-specific immune response leads to production of non-trypanosome specific antibodies and auto-antibodies, e.g. against fibrin, fibrinogen, DNA, red blood cells, thymocyte antigens and CNS components such as myelin, galacto-cerebrosides and neurofilament. *T. b. gambiense*-specific IgG and IgM antibodies are present in high concentrations and are mainly directed against the variable surface glycoprotein of the parasite. They are detectable by ELISA or immunofluorescence, using purified trypanosomal glycoproteins or whole trypanosomes of selected antigen types. Molecular diagnostic tests are available using different targets.

The screening test of choice for *T. b. gambiense* is the card agglutination test for trypanosomiasis (CATT), a simple 5-minute test based on the agglutination of whole, fixed and stained trypanosomes in the presence of specific antibodies. The control programs in areas where *T. b. gambiense* is endemic use it for seroscreening of at-risk populations. There is no seroscreening test available for *T. b. rhodesiense*.

Diagnosis should be followed by CSF exams (WBC and parasites) to determine the involvement (late stage) or not (early stage) of the CNS.

2. Infectious agents—Extracellular hemoflagellates subspecies of *T. brucei*: *Trypanosoma brucei gambiense* and *Trypanosoma brucei rhodesiense*. There are no morphological criteria for subspecies differentiation. Clinically, acute cases contracted in eastern and southern Africa have been considered due to *T. b. rhodesiense,* whereas chronic cases infected in western and central Africa are have been considered due to *T. b. gambiense*. It is now possible to differentiate both subspecies by molecular biology.

3. Occurrence—The disease is confined to tropical Africa between 15°N and 20°S latitude, corresponding to the distribution of the tsetse fly.

The annual incidence of cases reported to WHO is 12 000–15 000. WHO estimates some 50 000 to 70 000 people are currently infected per year, with up to 60 million people in 36 countries at risk of contracting the disease. The gambiense form of the disease represents 95% of the total cases reported. Sleeping sickness, which occurs at over 250 foci in the poorest rural areas of some of the least industrialized countries, ranks high in terms of disability-adjusted life years (DALY).

Outbreaks can occur when human-fly contact is intensified, when reservoir hosts introduce trypanosome human-infective strains into a tsetse-infested area, or when populations are displaced into endemic areas.

4. Reservoir—In *T. b. gambiense* infection, humans are the major reservoir; however, the role of domestic and wild animals is not clear. Wild animals, especially bushbucks and antelopes, and cattle and other domestic animals are the chief reservoirs for *T. b. rhodesiense*.

5. Mode of transmission—Through the bite of infective *Glossina*, the tsetse fly. Six species are the main vectors in nature. The riverine species are vectors for *T. b. gambiense*: *G. palpalis*, *G. fuscipes* and *G. tachinoides*. The wooden savannah species are vectors of *T. b. rhodesiense*: *G. morsitans*, *G. pallidipes* and *G. swynnertoni*. The fly is infected by ingesting blood of a human or animal that carries trypanosomes. The parasite multiplies in the fly for 12–30 days, depending on temperature and other factors, until infective forms develop in the salivary glands. Once infected, a tsetse fly remains infective for life (average 3 months, but as long as 10 months); infection is not passed from generation to generation in flies. Congenital transmission can occur in humans. Transmission by blood transfusion is possible. Direct mechanical transmission by blood on the proboscis of *Glossina* and other biting insects, such as horseflies, or in laboratory accidents, is possible.

6. Incubation period—Symptoms usually appear within 3 days to a few weeks after infection with *T. b. rhodesiense*, but they may not be apparent for several months with *T. b. gambiense* infection, which has a longer incubation period of up to several months or even years.

7. Period of communicability—Communicable to the tsetse fly as long as the parasite is present in the blood of the infected person or animal. Parasitemia in humans occurs in waves of varying intensity in untreated cases, and occurs at all stages of the disease.

8. Susceptibility—Susceptibility is general. Occasional inapparent or asymptomatic infections have been documented with both *T. b. gambiense* and *T. b. rhodesiense*. Spontaneous recovery in cases with the gambiense form without CNS involvement has been claimed, but has not been confirmed.

9. **Methods of control—**

A. *Preventive measures:* Selection of appropriate prevention methods must be based on knowledge of the local ecology of vectors and infectious agents. In a given geographic area, priority must be given to one or more of the following:

   1) Educate the public on personal protective measures against tsetse fly bites—this has limited impact because tsetse flies bite during the day at the workplace. Bednets are not useful.
   2) Reduce the parasite population by screening and diagnosing exposed populations and treating those infected. This is mainly effective for *T. b. gambiense*, where humans are the main reservoir.
   3) Reduce the parasite population by diagnosing and treating cattle. This is mainly effective for *T. b. rhodesiense*, where cattle is the main reservoir
   4) Destroy vector tsetse fly habitats if useful; indiscriminate destruction of vegetation is not recommended.
   5) Reduce the tsetse fly population by appropriate use of traps and screens, impregnated with insecticide or otherwise; by local use of residual insecticide; or by sequential aerial spraying of insecticide by helicopter or fixed-wing aircraft. Sterile insect technique has been successfully used to eradicate tsetse from Unguja island in Zanzibar.
   6) Check for the disease in case of blood donation from those that have visited or lived in endemic areas in Africa.

B. *Control of patient, contacts and the immediate environment:*

   1) Systematic screening of exposed populations in each *T. b. gambiense* focus, aimed at identifying asymptomatic infections at an early stage. Early diagnosis reduces both the risk of sequelae and the late-stage drug-related risks, and helps stop transmission.

      Regular surveillance in local health centers and villages for both rhodesiense and gambiense areas.

      Report to local health authority: In selected endemic areas, establish records of prevalence and encourage control measures; not a reportable disease in most countries, Class 3 (see *Reporting*).
   2) Isolation: Not recommended. Prevent tsetse flies from feeding on patients with trypanosomes in their blood.
   3) Concurrent disinfection: Not applicable.
   4) Quarantine: Not applicable.
   5) Immunization of contacts: Not applicable.

6) Investigation of contacts and source of infection: If the case is a member of a tour group or a family, others in the group or family should be alerted and investigated.

7) Specific treatment:

Treatment differs according to form and phase of the disease. If diagnosis occurs early in the initial phase, chances of cure are high. Treatment of the neurological phase requires drugs that can cross the blood-brain barrier. If started too late, treatment cannot prevent irreversible neurological damage. Early diagnosis allows low-risk early stage treatment on an outpatient basis; but the disease is notoriously difficult to treat in the neurological stage. Available medicines for this stage are difficult to manufacture and complicated to administer. While some people tolerate drugs well, in others fatal complications are common. Problems of drug resistance have increasingly been reported in several countries.

Four drugs—suramin, pentamidine, melarsoprol, and elforine—are registered for treatment of African trypanosomiasis. Development work on nifurtimox, a drug registered for Chagas disease, is underway to support "label extension" for African trypanosomiasis for use in combination regimens. All 5 drugs are available through WHO, the only provider, and are fee of charge through donation programs.

Pentamidine (IM. 4mg/kg/d for 7 days) is used for early stages of *T. b. gambiense*, and Suramin (IV. 20mg/Kg/week for 5 weeks) for early stages of *T. b. rhodesiense* infections. Late-stage disease, with CNS involvement, requires inpatient treatment with a drug that can cross the blood-brain barrier. Available medicines suffer from a range of difficulties, including substantial toxicity and lengthy or complicated parenteral administrations. Increasing rates of treatment failure have been observed in some foci of *T. b. gambiense*

Melarsoprol is an arsenical derivate drug used to treat both forms at the neurological stage (IV, 2.2 mg/Kg/d for 10 days for the gambiense disease, and three series of daily injections for three days with intervening rest periods of seven days for the rhodesiense form). Reactive encephalopathy occurs in 5–10% of treatments; this is the main adverse effect of melarsoprol and is often fatal. This drug must be administered on an inpatient basis, in the intensive care unit if possible.

Eflornithine (slow IV perfusion 100 mg/kg/6 hours for 14 days) is used for late-stage *T. b. gambiense* infection. This drug is difficult to administer under field conditions. Although it can have fatal complications, it is safer than melarsoprol. Pafuramidine, an oral treatment for early stage infection, is also in clinical development.

Patients must be followed up for at least one and preferably 2 years after treatment to assess drug efficacy.

C. *Epidemic measures:* Mainly for *T. b. rhodesiense*: mass surveys, urgent treatment for identified infections, and tsetse fly control. If epidemics recur despite initial control measures, the measures recommended in 9A must be pursued more vigorously.

D. *Disaster implications:* None.

E. *International measures:* The Pan-African Tsetse and Trypanosomosis Eradication Campaign is an Africa Union program to promote and coordinate anti-trypanosomiasis efforts of governments in countries where the vector and the disease are present. WHO is leading a human African trypanosomiasis surveillance and control program providing capacity building as well as technical and logistical support (diagnosis reagents and equipment, drugs, training) to countries where the disease is endemic, and carrying out surveillance and control activities and improving reporting of the disease. WHO Collaborating Centres provide support as required. More information can be found at:
  http://www.who.int/collaboratingcentres/database/en/

Further information on trypanosomiasis can be found at:
  http://www.who.int/trypanosomiasis_african/en/
  http://www.who.int/mediacentre/factsheets/fs259/en/
  http://www.who.int/tdr/diseases/tryp/default.htm

II. AMERICAN TRYPANOSOMIASIS   ICD-9 086.2; ICD-10 B57
(Chagas disease)
[CCDM19: M. Eberhard, A. Moore]
[CCDM18: R. Salvatella Agrelo]

1. Identification—The acute disease, with variable fever, lymphadenopathy, malaise, and hepatosplenomegaly, generally occurs in children—although the majority of infections are asymptomatic or paucisymptomatic. In 20%–30% of infections, irreversible chronic manifestations generally appear later in life. An inflammatory response at the site of infection (chagoma) may last up to 8 weeks. Unilateral bipalpebral-edema (Romana's sign) occurs in a small percentage of acute cases. Life-threatening or fatal manifestations include myocarditis and meningoencephalitis.

Chronic irreversible sequelae include myocardial damage with cardiac dilatation, arrhythmias and major conduction abnormalities, and intestinal tract involvement with megaesophagus and megacolon. Megavisceral manifestations occur mainly in central Brazil. The prevalence of megaviscera and cardiac involvement varies according to regions; the latter is not as common north of Ecuador as in southern areas. In AIDS patients, acute myocarditis and severe multifocal or diffuse meningoencephalitis with necrosis and hemorrhage occur as relapses of chronic infection. Reactivation of chronic Chagas disease may also occur with non-AIDS immunosuppression, and is characterized by skin lesions, blood parasitemia, and often, acute myocarditis. CNS involvement is not usually seen.

Infection with *Trypanosoma rangeli* occurs in foci of endemic Chagas disease extending from Central America to Colombia and Venezuela; prolonged parasitemia occurs, sometimes co-existing with *T. cruzi* flagellates (with which *T. rangeli* shares reservoir hosts)—no clinical manifestations attributable to *T. rangeli* have been noted.

Diagnosis of Chagas disease in the acute phase is established through demonstration of the organism in blood (rarely, in a lymph node or skeletal muscle) by direct examination or after hemoconcentration, culture or xenodiagnosis (feeding noninfected triatomid bugs on the patient and finding the parasite in the bugs' feces several weeks later).

Parasitemia is most intense during febrile episodes early in the course of infection. In the chronic phase, xenodiagnosis and blood culture on diphasic media may be positive, but other methods rarely reveal parasites. Parasites are differentiated from those of *T. rangeli* by their shorter length (20 micrometers *vs.* 36 micrometers) and larger kinetoplast. Serologic tests are valuable for individual diagnosis as well as for screening purposes.

2. Infectious agent—*Trypanosoma cruzi* (*Schizotrypanum cruzi*), a protozoan that occurs in humans as a hemoflagellate (trypomastigote) and as an intracellular parasite (amastigote) without an external flagellum.

3. Occurrence—The disease is confined to the Western Hemisphere, with wide geographic distribution in rural Mexico and Central and South America. However, progress in reduction of vector- and blood-borne transmission in endemic countries, together with migration of chronically infected people to nonendemic countries, is changing the epidemiology of the disease. Based on limited data from seroprevalence studies among blood donors and other populations, it is estimated that at least 100 000 people in north America are infected with *T. cruzi*, mainly immigrants from endemic countries.

4. Reservoir—Humans and over 150 domestic and wild mammals species, including dogs, cats, rats, mice, marsupials, edentates, rodents, chiroptera, carnivores, primates and others.

5. Mode of transmission—Infected vectors—i.e. blood-sucking species of Reduviidae (cone-nosed bugs or kissing bugs), especially various species from the genera *Triatoma*, *Rhodnius* and *Panstrongylus*— have the trypanosomes in their feces. Defecation occurs during feeding; infection of humans and other mammals occurs when the freshly excreted bug feces contaminate conjunctivae, mucous membranes, abrasions or skin wounds (including the bite wound). The bugs become infected when they feed on a parasitemic animal; the parasites multiply in the bugs' gut. Transmission may also occur by blood transfusion: there are increasing numbers of infected donors in cities because of migration from rural areas. Organisms may also cross the placenta to cause congenital infection (in 2% to 8% of pregnancies for those infected); transmission through breastfeeding seems highly unlikely, so there is currently no reason to restrict breastfeeding by chagasic mothers. Transmission through ingestion of food or drink contaminated with triatomine feces has also been reported. Accidental laboratory infections occur occasionally; transplantation of organs from chagasic donors presents a growing risk of *T. cruzi* transmission.

6. Incubation period—Symptoms usually become apparent within 1 to 3 weeks after vector bite and exposure but may be delayed if infected through blood transfusion. About 5–14 days after bite of insect vector; 30–40 days if infected through blood transfusion.

7. Period of communicability—Organisms are regularly present in the blood during the acute period and may persist in very small numbers throughout life in symptomatic and asymptomatic people. The vector becomes infective 10–30 days after biting an infected host; gut infection in the bug persists for life (as long as 2 years).

8. Susceptibility—All ages are susceptible, but the acute disease is usually more severe in younger people. Immunosuppressed people, especially those with AIDS, are at risk of serious infections and complications.

9. Methods of control—

   A. Preventive measures:

   1) Educate the public on mode of spread and methods of prevention.
   2) Systematically attack vectors infesting poorly constructed houses and houses with thatched roofs, using effective insecticides with residual action (spraying or use of insecticidal paints or fumigant canisters).
   3) Construct or repair living areas to eliminate lodging places for insect vectors and shelter for domestic and wild reservoir animals. In certain areas, palm trees close to houses often harbor infested bugs and can be considered a risk factor.
   4) Use bednets (preferably insecticide-impregnated) in houses infested by the vector.
   5) Screen blood and organ donors living in or coming from endemic areas, using appropriate serological tests, to prevent infection by transfusion or transplants, as required by law in most countries in the Americas.

B. Control of patient, contacts and the immediate environment:

1) Report to local health authority: In selected endemic areas; not a reportable disease in most countries, Class 3 (see *Reporting*).
2) Isolation: Not generally practical. Blood and body fluid precautions for hospitalized patients.
3) Concurrent disinfection: Not applicable.
4) Quarantine: Not applicable.
5) Immunization of contacts: Not applicable.
6) Investigation of contacts and source of infection: Search thatched roofs, bedding and rooms for vectors. All family members of a case should be examined. Infants born to mothers with known seropositive status should be evaluated for congenital infection. Serological tests and blood examinations on all blood and organ donors implicated as possible sources of transfusion- or transplant-acquired infection.
7) Specific treatment: Benznidazole, a 2-nitroimidazole derivative, and nifurtimox, a nitrofurfurylidene derivative, have proven effective in acute cases. These drugs are available from major hospitals in endemic areas. Randomized controlled trials show that benznidazole substantially and significantly modifies parasite-related outcomes compared to placebo among young persons with chronic, asymptomatic infection. Treatment is recommended for acute and congenital cases, for children with chronic asymptomatic infection, and for reactivated infection in immunocompromised patients. Many experts also offer treatment to asymptomatic adults; the same applies for chronic asymptomatic *T. cruzi* infection. The potential of trypanocidal treatment in Chagas disease among asymptomatic, chronically infected persons is under evaluation.

C. Epidemic measures: In areas of high incidence, field survey to determine distribution and density of vectors and animal hosts and implementation of measures described under 9A.

D. Disaster implications: None.

E. International measures: Although triatomine vectors are still responsible for most human infections, successful programs based on application of residual insecticides have substantially reduced transmission by this route in the "Southern Cone" of South America. Uruguay, Chile, and parts of Brazil have been certified free of vector-borne transmission. Further research and implementation efforts are necessary in the Amazon, Andean and Central American regions, where transmission occurs through both domiciliated and non-domiciliated vectors. Many Latin

American countries have made considerable progress in improving blood safety. In 10 of the 17 endemic countries, more than 99% of the blood supply is screened by at least one assay for *T. cruzi* antibodies.

Further information can be found at:

http://www.who.int/tdr/diseases/chagas/default.htm

TUBERCULOSIS   ICD-9 010-018; ICD-10 A15-A19
(TB, TB disease)
[CCDM19: A. Buff, M. Raviglione]
[CCDM18: M. Raviglione]

1. Identification—A mycobacterial disease with over nine million new infections and 1.7 million deaths (including 230 000 among HIV-associated tuberculosis cases) every year, tuberculosis (TB) is a major global cause of disability and death, especially in developing countries. The disease begins, in virtually all cases, with exposure to an infectious human source, and subsequent infection that usually goes un-noticed. This can be detected through tuberculin skin testing (TST) sensitivity and/or one of the newer interferon-gamma release assays (IGRA). These tests become positive after 2–6 weeks.

Initial infection generally causes no outward clinical manifestations. This latent infection state is characterized by small microscopic lesions in the lungs that commonly heal, leaving no residual changes other than occasional small pulmonary or tracheo-bronchial lymph node calcifications. Less than 10% of those otherwise healthy persons infected will eventually develop active disease during their lifetime. Among persons who develop active disease, half will develop disease within the first 2 years following infection; over 90% of infected individuals will never develop active TB. Appropriate treatment of latent TB infection can reduce the lifetime risk of TB disease.

In some individuals, initial TB infection may progress rapidly to active tuberculosis; this is called primary TB disease. Rapid clinical progression is more common among infants, in whom the disease is often disseminated (e.g. miliary) or meningeal, and in the immunosuppressed, such as HIV-infected persons. Treatment of latent TB infection in these individuals and other susceptible populations is highly effective in preventing development of TB disease.

Active pulmonary TB may arise from endogenous reactivation of a latent focus originating from the initial sub-clinical infection or from exogenous re-infection. Demonstration of acid-fast bacilli (AFB) in stained smears from sputum or other body fluids in a clinical and epidemiological situation suggestive of TB allows a presumptive diagnosis of active TB disease, and justifies initiation of anti-tuberculosis treatment. Fluorescent microscopy enhances sensitivity compared to standard microscopy by about 10%. Isolation of organisms of *Mycobacterium tuberculosis* complex on culture confirms diagnosis and also permits determination of drug susceptibility of the infecting organism. Traditional egg- or agar-based media for culturing mycobacteria include Löwenstein-Jensen and Middle-brook 7H10. In modern laboratories, liquid culture media for isolation and nucleic acid probes for speciation accelerate timing of diagnosis confirmation to 2–3 weeks. In the absence of bacteriological confirmation, active disease can be presumed if clinical, histological or radiological evidence is suggestive of TB and other likely diseases can be ruled out. Diagnosis of TB among persons living with HIV/AIDS is further complicated by frequent atypical presentations and a tendency to smear-negative disease.

Extrapulmonary TB occurs less commonly than pulmonary TB, but in up to one third of all cases. Children and persons with immunodeficiencies, such as those with HIV infection and AIDS, have a higher risk of extrapulmonary TB, but pulmonary disease remains the most common type worldwide, even in these more susceptible groups, and often occurs simultaneously with extrapulmonary diseases. TB may affect any organ or tissue; in order of frequency, TB tends to affect lymph nodes, pleura, the genito-urinary tract, bones and joints, meninges, the gastro-intestinal tract and peritoneum, and the pericardium.

Cough, fatigue, fever, night sweats, weight loss, and pleuritic pain are common signs and symptoms associated with pulmonary TB disease. Localizing symptoms, including hemoptysis, and hoarseness (which can be associated with laryngeal TB), can become prominent in advanced stages. Globally, the classification of pulmonary TB for treatment purposes is based primarily on the presence or absence of acid-fast bacilli (AFB) in the sputum. A smear positive for AFB is indicative of high infectiousness. Non-specific signs and symptoms, such as fever, night sweats, weight loss and fatigue, may occur early. In most cases, cough appears, initially non-productive and later accompanied by purulent sputum. In some cases, hemoptysis ensues as a result of the rupture of small vessels inside a growing cavity. Chest radiography most commonly reveals pulmonary infiltrates and cavitations in the upper segments of the lung lobes. In prolonged disease, fibrotic changes with volume loss can be seen. Approximately 65% of patients with untreated sputum smear-positive pulmonary TB will die within 5 years of diagnosis.

Immunocompetent persons who have been infected with *Mycobacterium tuberculosis* complex usually have a delayed-type (cellular) hypersensitivity reaction to 5 IUs of purified protein derivative (PPD) tuberculin. Among persons with active TB disease, up to 25% may have no reaction to PPD tuberculin. Therefore, a negative tuberculin skin test (TST) result does not exclude TB disease in a person with signs and symptoms consistent with TB. Persons suspected to have TB disease should have a full diagnostic evaluation, including a chest radiograph and three sputum specimens collected for AFB smear and culture. Sputum specimens should be collected at least 8 hours apart, and at least one should be an early morning specimen.

Interpretation of the TST induration size is important because it determines the need to start treatment for latent TB infection (also referred to as chemoprophylaxis or preventive therapy). In the USA, a positive TST result is defined as an induration with a transverse diameter of 5, 10, or 15 mm based on the person's risk of exposure to TB disease and risk of progression from latent TB infection to disease. An induration of ≥5 mm is considered positive among persons who are HIV-infected; are recent contacts of a person with TB disease; have fibrotic changes on chest radiograph consistent with old TB disease; or are immunosuppressed. An induration of ≥10 mm is considered positive among persons who are recent arrivals (<5 years) from high-prevalence countries; injecting drug users; residents and employees of high-risk congregate settings (e.g., prisons, institutions, homeless shelters); and persons with high-risk clinical conditions (e.g., silicosis, diabetes mellitus, chronic renal failure or hemodialysis, gastrectomy, or carcinoma of the head or neck). Any reaction of 15 mm or more should be considered positive among low-risk persons. Generally, testing is not recommended for persons at low risk.

Skin tests for anergy (i.e., control antigens) are no longer recommended, even for high-risk patients. In many industrialized low-incidence TB countries, including the USA, routine skin testing of all children for TB is no longer recommended; children to be tested include those suspected of having active TB disease and those exposed to an infectious case. If treatment for latent TB infection will be initiated, targeted tuberculin skin testing can be provided to immigrants, including children, from high-incidence countries, as well as other high-risk groups such as incarcerated, homeless, or HIV-infected persons.

In some persons with latent TB infection, delayed-type hypersensitivity to PPD tuberculin may wane with time. When persons are tested many years after initial TB infection, they may show a negative reaction (i.e. negative TST result); however, the skin test can "boost" their ability to react subsequently to tuberculin PPD, causing a positive reaction to subsequent tests. This boosting phenomenon can persist for up to several years and might be incorrectly interpreted as recent infection. Boosting has also been reported in persons who have received the Bacille Calmette-Guérin (BCG) vaccine. To prevent misinterpretation, a two-step skin testing procedure can distinguish between reactions due to new boosting and those due to recent TB infection. If the reaction to the first TST is classified as negative, a positive reaction to a second test 1–3 weeks later probably represents a boosted reaction. On the basis of this second result, the person should be classified as previously infected and treated for latent TB infection as indicated. If the second test is also negative, the person should be classified as uninfected with TB. Two-step skin testing should be used for initial skin testing of adults who will be retested periodically (e.g. health care workers), who are not known to have a prior positive TST result, and who have not had a documented TST result in the previous year or so. Treatment for latent TB infection generally does not change future TST results; therefore, persons with positive TST results should not have repeat skin testing. Persons with prior positive TST results and subsequent exposure to a person with infectious TB disease should have a clinical evaluation to exclude active TB disease.

In the last few years, two in vitro interferon-gamma release assays (IGRAs) have become available: QuantiFERON-TB Gold ® (Cellestis ltd, Carnegie, Australia), done on whole blood, and T-SPOT.TB ® (Offord Immunotec, Oxford, UK) done on purified blood cells. These tests measure the release of interferon-gamma by T lymphocytes in response to stimulation with TB-specific antigens. They are highly specific, with reduced cross-reactivity with BCG and other mycobacteria, and at least as sensitive as TST in detecting active disease and latent infection.

In addition, IGRAs do not trigger a boosting effect because the tests do not expose persons to antigens. In direct comparisons, the 80% sensitivity of IGRAs has been statistically similar to that of the TST for detecting infection in persons with untreated culture-confirmed TB as a surrogate for latent TB infection. However, their true sensitivity for latent TB infection, particularly in certain populations (e.g. children and immunocompromised persons) has not been determined. IGRAs, as with the TST, cannot differentiate TB infection from TB disease. A diagnosis of latent TB infection requires that active TB disease be excluded.

Similar to the TST, impaired immune function can decrease the sensitivity of IGRAs. Consequently, the performance of IGRAs might be decreased and the rate of indeterminate results increased for persons with HIV infection, undernourishment, immunosuppression, hematologic disorders (e.g., leukemia, lymphoma), specific malignances, diabetes, silicosis, and chronic renal failure. As with a negative TST result, a negative or indeterminate IGRA result alone might not be sufficient to exclude *M. tuberculosis* infection in these persons.

IGRAs are being integrated into routine clinical and public health practice in many regions of the world. In the USA, IGRAs have been recommended for use in all circumstances in which the TST is currently used, including contact investigations, evaluation of recent immigrants, and sequential testing surveillance programs for infection control (e.g., healthcare workers). IGRAs can be used in place of the TST, but are not recommended for use in addition to the TST (simultaneously or sequentially).

When the epidemiological and clinical evidence suggests TB disease, demonstration of AFB in smears from sputum or other body fluids is a presumptive diagnosis of TB disease and justifies initiation of anti-TB treatment. Isolation and identification of *M. tuberculosis* by culture confirms the diagnosis and permits determination of drug-susceptibility patterns. In the absence of bacteriological culture confirmation, TB disease can be diagnosed if clinical, histological, or radiological evidence is suggestive of TB disease and other likely disease processes have been excluded.

2. Infectious agents—*Mycobacterium tuberculosis* complex. This includes *M. tuberculosis, M. bovis* (the "bovine tubercle bacillus", historically an important cause of TB transmitted from infected cows through unpasteurized milk), *M. africanum*, and *M. canettii* (the latter two responsible for a small number of cases in Africa). Occasionally, *M. microti, M. caprae* and *M. pinnipedii* have also caused human disease. Other mycobacteria occasionally produce disease clinically indistinguishable from tuberculosis; the causal agents can be identified only through culture and speciation. *M. tuberculosis* is a thin aerobic organism, usually neutral on Gram's stain, but acid-fast (it cannot be decolorized by acid alcohol once stained). Its genome has been fully sequenced, and contains over 4 000 genes.

3. Occurrence—Worldwide, all countries are affected; 9.15 million new infections occurred in 2006, of which some 61% were officially reported. Over 95% of infections are in developing countries, where TB remains a dominant cause of morbidity and mortality. The highest rates per capita are in Africa, especially the eastern and southern sub-regions (up to 1 000 per 100 000 population), but the highest numbers are reported in Asia (nearly 60% of all cases). In high incidence settings, morbidity is highest among adult males. In most industrialized countries, downward trends of mortality and morbidity in place for nearly a century reversed in the mid-1980s, when incidence of TB stagnated or began to increase. This phenomenon, still observed today in some northern European countries, is due to a number of factors, including immigration from high incidence areas, HIV infection, and deteriorated socio-economic conditions among the poorest segments of the population, besides dismantling of TB control services. In regions with declining TB incidence, TB mortality and morbidity rates increase with age. Morbidity and mortality rates are also higher among impoverished, disadvantaged, and minority populations, and are usually higher in urban areas.

The global estimated incidence of TB peaked around 2004–2005, and estimated incidence is now stable or decreasing in six of nine WHO epidemiological regions. The 22 highest-burden TB countries account for approximately 80% of the estimated number of new TB cases arising each year; for these 22 countries, the estimated case rate was 174 cases per 100 000 persons in 2005.

The prevalence of latent TB infection, detected by TST, increases with age. It is estimated that one third of the human population is infected today. The incidence of infection, expressed as annual risk of infection, in industrialized countries has declined rapidly in recent decades; in the USA, the annual risk of new infection is estimated to average about 10/100 000 people at most, although segments of the population in the USA and other industrialized countries may have a relatively high annual risk of new infection. In areas where human infections with non-tuberculous myco-bacteria are prevalent, cross-reactions can complicate interpretation of the TST reaction.

In the low incidence areas of USA and many other industrialized countries, most TB disease in adults results from reactivation of latent foci remaining from an initial infection. However, in some large urban areas, about one-third of TB disease cases may result from recent infection. Micro-epidemics have been reported in closed spaces, such as nursing homes, shelters for the homeless, hospitals, schools, prisons, and during long-haul-flights.

From 1989 to the early 1990s, outbreaks of multidrug-resistant TB (MDR-TB), defined as resistance to at least isoniazid and rifampicin, have been recognized in settings where HIV-infected persons are congregated (hospitals, prisons, drug treatment clinics and HIV residences). These outbreaks were associated with high fatality rates and transmission of *M. tuberculosis* to other patients and health care workers. Strict enforce-ment of infection control guidelines, proactive case finding, intensive contact investigations, and ensuring completion of appropriate treatment regimens have been effective in stopping and preventing MDR TB outbreaks. In a 2008 report, WHO estimated that 4.8% of all TB cases worldwide were due to MDR strains; in some countries, particularly those in Eastern Europe and Central Asia, up to 20% of new cases and 60% of previously treated cases were MDR TB. Three countries—China, India, and Russia—accounted for 57% of the overall estimated incidence of MDR TB.

Recently, extensively resistant forms of TB (XDR-TB) have emerged, especially in settings where the use of second-line drugs has been widespread and poorly managed, and where the capacity to diagnose drug resistance exists. XDR-TB is defined as MDR-TB plus resistance to any fluoroquinolone and any of the three injectable drugs, amikacin, kanamy-cin and capreomycin. In a 2005–2006 outbreak of XDR TB in KwaZulu Natal, South Africa, 52 of 53 (98%) patients died, and median survival was 16 days from date of diagnosis. In a laboratory study published in 2007, over 6% of all MDR TB isolates worldwide met the definition for XDR TB.

HIV-associated TB (TB/HIV) is frequent in Africa and a few other settings. Worldwide, more than 700 000 TB cases a year were estimated to be due to HIV in 2006, with over 230 000 deaths a year. For HIV-infected persons, the annual risk of TB disease has been estimated at 2%–13%, based on CD4 cell count, and the cumulative risk is well over 50%.

Human infection with *M. bovis*, the bovine tubercle bacillus, continues to be a problem in areas where the disease in cattle is poorly controlled, and unpasteurized milk or dairy products are consumed raw. In some industrialized countries, TB disease caused by *M. bovis* accounts for approximately 1% of all reported TB cases.

4. **Reservoir**—Primarily humans, rarely other primates; except for *M. bovis,* which is found in cattle and a variety of other mammals.

5. Mode of transmission—Exposure to tubercle bacilli in airborne, aerosolized droplet nuclei, that measure 1–5 microns in diameter, and are produced by persons with pulmonary or high respiratory tract tuberculosis (e.g. laryngeal) during forceful expiratory efforts (e.g. coughing, singing or sneezing). The droplet nuclei are inhaled by a vulnerable contact into the pulmonary alveoli. Here, the aerosolized particles containing *M. tuberculosis* are ingested by alveolar macrophages, initiating a new infection.

The balance between number and virulence of the microorganisms and the bactericidal activity of the macrophages determines the capacity to contain the infection. The risk of exposure and subsequent infection is linked with the intimacy and duration of the contact, the ventilation in the shared environment, and the degree of contagiousness of the index case. Health care workers are at high risk of exposure during aerosolizing procedures such as bronchoscopy, intubation, and autopsy. Laryngeal TB disease is highly contagious, but rare. Direct invasion through mucous membranes or breaks in the skin can occur but are extremely rare. Bovine tuberculosis, also a rare event, results from exposure to tuberculous cattle; exposure to *M. bovis* usually occurs through ingestion of unpasteurized contaminated milk or dairy products, and sometimes through airborne spread from cattle to farmers and animal handlers. Except for rare situations where there is a draining sinus, extrapulmonary tuberculosis (other than laryngeal) is generally not communicable.

6. Incubation period—Two to 10 weeks from infection to demonstrable primary lesion or significant TST reaction and positivity of IGRA. IGRAs are expected to be positive by 10 weeks from infection, but the actual time from infection to IGRA conversion has not been adequately studied. Less than 10% of infected persons will develop TB disease in their lifetimes; half of those will develop TB disease within 2 years after initial infection. Latent TB infection can persist for a lifetime. HIV infection and other immunosuppressive conditions increase the subsequent risk of progressive pulmonary or extrapulmonary TB and shorten the interval for the development of TB disease following infection.

7. Period of communicability—Theoretically, as long as viable tubercle bacilli are discharged in the sputum. Effective antimicrobial chemotherapy usually eliminates communicability within 2–4 weeks, although *M. tuberculosis* can still be cultured from sputum. Some untreated or inadequately treated patients (e.g. "chronic cases") with TB disease can be intermittently AFB sputum-positive, and therefore contagious, for years. Studies from the United States and Canada suggest that persons with smear-negative, culture-positive pulmonary TB can be contagious and can transmit infection to other persons. Children with primary TB generally are not contagious.

The degree of communicability depends on intimacy and duration of the exposure, the number of bacilli discharged, infectivity of the bacilli, adequacy of ventilation, exposure of bacilli to sun or ultraviolet light, and opportunities for aerosolization through coughing, sneezing, talking or singing— or, for health care workers, during aerosolizing procedures.

8. Susceptibility—The risk of infection with the tubercle bacillus is directly related to the degree of exposure and less to genetic or other host factors. However, HIV-infected persons may have a higher risk of infection following exposure. The first 12–24 months after infection constitute the period of greatest risk for the development of clinical TB disease. The risk of developing disease is highest in children under 3, lowest in school-aged children, and high again among adolescents and young adults, the very old and the immunocompromised. Population groups not previously exposed to TB appear to have greater susceptibility to new infection and disease. Reactivation of long-latent infection accounts for a large proportion of TB disease cases in older people. Among infected persons, susceptibility to reactivation and TB disease is markedly increased by HIV infection and other forms of immunosuppression, and among the underweight or undernourished, people with a debilitating disorder (e.g. diabetes, chronic renal failure, some forms of cancer, silicosis, or gastrectomy), and substance users. Tobacco smokers and alcoholics are also at increased risk of TB morbidity and mortality.

For adults co-infected with HIV and latent TB, the lifetime risk of developing active TB disease rises from an estimated 10% to up to 50%. This phenomenon has resulted in a parallel pandemic of HIV/AIDS and TB disease where HIV prevalence is high: in some sub-Saharan African areas, where 10%–15% of the adult population are co-infected with both HIV and TB, annual TB disease rates have increased 5- to 10-fold between the start of the HIV/AIDS pandemic in the 1980s and today. In some countries in eastern and southern Africa, the HIV seroprevalence among TB cases may be as high as 70–80%.

9. Methods of control—

   A. Preventive measures:

   1) The best prevention of TB is prompt diagnosis and treatment, especially of infectious sputum smear-positive cases, as patients are rendered non-infectious within 2–4 weeks after starting an effective regimen. Establishment of active case-finding through contact investigations, and provision of adequate treatment facilities for infectious cases, are key to reducing transmission. This normally requires a well-functioning and coordinated TB program operating at the lowest health administrative authority level (e.g., district level), under the guidance of national program norms and standards, providing training and supervision, and monitoring performance.

2) Ensure clinical, laboratory, and radiology facilities for prompt identification of suspects and examination of patients and contacts. Ensure provision of the four essential anti-TB drugs (see below) and medical facilities for early and complete treatment of cases and people at high risk of infection, including beds for those needing hospitalization due to severe, advanced disease.

Among persons presenting with signs and symptoms consistent with TB disease in high-incidence countries, direct microscopy sputum examination for AFB can detect as much as 50%–65% of infectious pulmonary TB. In most situations, direct microscopy is the most cost-effective method of case finding, and this is the first priority in developing countries. However, culture, especially using liquid media to accelerate detection, is today recommended to identify TB among HIV-infected people and MDR-TB. In fact, due to the emergence of MDR-TB in most countries, ideally all initial isolates should be submitted to drug susceptibility testing. In countries currently with limited resources and laboratory capacity, drug susceptibility testing should be performed at least among cases needing re-treatment, such as treatment failures and defaulters of previous treatment. In countries with adequate resources, all cases should have culture confirmation and drug susceptibility testing. To face the management challenge of MDR-TB more effectively, WHO has recently recommended the use of molecular, PCR-based methods for rapid detection of isoniazid and rifampicin resistance. These methods, called "line-probe assays" (LPSa), can be used directly on the sputum produced by sputum-smear positive cases and reveal the presence of MDR-TB within a few hours, thus shortening time to diagnosis and start of proper treatment.

3) Educate the public regarding mode of spread, methods of control, and importance of early diagnosis and continued adherence to treatment.

4) Reduce or eliminate social conditions that increase the risk of infection and progression to disease.

5) Establish and maintain effective TB infection control programs in institutional settings where healthcare is provided and where immunocompromised patients (e.g., HIV-infected persons) congregate (including hospitals, drug treatment programs, prisons, nursing homes, and homeless shelters).

6) Treating latent TB infections (TLTBI, also called preventive chemotherapy or chemoprophylaxis) with isoniazid (INH) for 6–9 months has been effective in preventing the progression of latent TB infection to TB disease in up to 90% of adherent individuals. Studies in adults with HIV infection

have shown the effectiveness of alternative regimens including 4 months of daily rifampicin and 3 months of isoniazid and rifampicin. A shorter course (2 months) of rifampicin and pyrazinamide has been associated with severe and even fatal hepatotoxicity, and is not currently recommended for general use. It is essential to rule out active TB disease before starting treatment for latent TB infection, especially in immunocompromised persons such as HIV-infected individuals, in order to avoid inadvertently treating active disease with a 1- or 2-drug regimen that would encourage the development of drug resistance. Because of the risk of isoniazid-associated hepatitis, isoniazid is not routinely advised for persons with active liver disease.

In the USA, 9 months of daily INH (twice weekly if directly observed therapy is available) is the recommended treatment for all persons with latent TB infection without contraindications; 4 months of daily rifampin (RIF) is an acceptable alternative. RIF is contraindicated in HIV-infected persons being treated with certain combinations of antiretroviral drugs (protease inhibitors or non-nucleoside reverse transcriptase inhibitors [NNRTI]). WHO and UNAIDS recommend a preventive treatment with 6 months of daily isoniazid for all HIV-infected individuals after careful exclusion of active disease.

Persons started on TLTBI must be informed of possible adverse effects (e.g. hepatitis, drug fever or severe rash), reminded of these possibilities, and checked for symptoms monthly, prior to prescription refills; they should be advised to discontinue treatment and seek medical advice if suggestive symptoms develop. Baseline liver function tests are important in patients with signs, symptoms or history of liver disease, and in those who abuse alcohol. Avoiding or discontinuing isoniazid generally is advised for persons with serum aspartate aminotransferase levels more than 5 times the upper limit of normal values (3 times if symptoms suggest hepatic dysfunction). Supervised treatment should be used when possible (e.g. prisons, drug treatment programs, schools). Not more than 1 month's supply of medication should be given at any one time, and patients should be queried at least monthly about adverse effects. Among persons taking INH, 10%–20% can have asymptomatic elevation of serum liver enzymes and 0.1%–0.15% can develop clinical hepatitis. Factors that can increase the rate or severity include alcohol consumption, underlying liver disease, or concurrent use of liver-metabolized medications. Peripheral neuropathy occurs in less than 0.2% of persons and is more likely in the presence of other conditions associated with neuropathy (e.g., diabetes, HIV infection, renal failure, and alcohol abuse). Pyridoxine (vitamin B6) supplementation is recommended to prevent peripheral neuropathy in persons at increased risk for this complication.

Among persons taking RIF, 0.6% can have hepatotoxicity, as evidenced by transient asymptomatic hyperbilirubinemia, and 6% can have cutaneous reactions, such as pruritis with or without a rash. Orange discoloration of body fluids is expected and harmless; soft contact lenses can be permanently stained. RIF interacts with a number of drugs and accelerates hepatic metabolism; as a result, RIF reduces the concentrations of methadone, warfarin, oral contraceptives, and phenytoin.

Baseline hepatic transaminases are important in persons with a known or suspected history of liver disease, alcohol abuse, HIV infection, or pregnancy. Routine periodic laboratory tests are recommended for persons who had abnormal initial results or who are at high risk for hepatic disease. Laboratory testing is recommended for any persons on treatment who have symptoms suggestive of hepatitis (e.g., fatigue, weakness, malaise, anorexia, nausea, vomiting, abdominal pain, pale stools, dark urine, chills) or who have signs of jaundice. At the start of treatment and at each monthly visit for medication refills, persons should be advised not to wait until a clinic visit to stop treatment, and to seek medical attention immediately if symptoms of hepatitis develop.

During pregnancy, it may be wise to postpone treatment for latent TB infection until after delivery, except in high-risk individuals, where it should be administered with caution. If INH treatment is prescribed for pregnant women or in the immediate post-partum period, monthly routine hepatic transaminases should be monitored. INH daily or twice weekly (using directly observed therapy) is the preferred regimen supplementation with 50 mg of pyridoxine (vitamin B6) is recommended. Breastfeeding is not contraindicated.

Mass TLTBI is unsuitable in most communities unless there is a well-organized program to supervise and encourage adherence to treatment and unless a high rate of cure can be achieved among patients with active TB disease. However, vulnerable groups, such as the HIV-infected, may be targeted for selective, large-scale treatment. Infants and children under 5 years of age with latent TB infection have been recently infected and are therefore at high risk for progression to disease. Risk of INH-related hepatitis in infants, children, and adolescents is minimal and routine monitoring of liver enzymes is not necessary. If resources allow, directly observed therapy should be considered.

Treating latent TB infection in contacts (especially in pediatric and HIV-infected contacts) is the highest public health priority after finding and curing active TB cases. Mass treatment for latent TB infection is unrealistic and unsuitable in most communities unless (a) high detection and cure rates are first being achieved among persons with TB disease; (b) contact investigations are thorough, with recently infected persons routinely completing treatment; and (c) there is a well-organized program to supervise and ensure adherence to treatment.

7) Persons infected with HIV should be screened for TB at the time their HIV infection is identified; they should start TLTBI if they have been tested positive with TST or IGRA and if active TB disease has been carefully ruled out through proper medical history and examination, including chest radiography. Conversely, all people with evidence of TB disease should be counseled and tested for HIV infection, and offered the option of antiretroviral treatment and all other support measures for HIV-infected persons.

8) In industrialized countries where BCG immunization is not routinely carried out, selective TST and TLTBI may be considered for groups at high risk of TB infection and/or HIV infection, including health care workers and groups such as prison inmates and injecting drug users; this may also be considered for foreign-born persons from areas of high tuberculosis prevalence, and possibly for travelers to and from high-prevalence areas. Prior BCG immunization may complicate interpretation of a positive skin test in a child or recently immunized adult. Since skin test reactions from BCG wane over time, strongly positive reactions or significant increases in reactivity should be considered indicative of TB infection. Targeted testing, standard interpretation of TST, and TLTBI are recommended regardless of prior history of BCG vaccination.

9) For contacts with TB infection from infectious cases with known drug-resistant strains, treatment regimens have been based on in vitro data, extrapolation from treatment of active TB disease, and expert opinion rather than controlled clinical trials. None of the potential regimens has been fully evaluated for efficacy. For persons who are likely to be infected with drug-resistant strains and are at high risk of developing TB disease, treatment regimens that include at least 2 drugs to which the mycobacteria from the source patient are known to be susceptible should be considered for 6–12 months duration. Clinical evaluations and chest radiographs

every 3-6 months for the first 2 years is an alternative strategy to treatment with unproven drug regimens.

10) Provide public health nursing and outreach services to patients; ensure each patient receives directly observed therapy for TB disease; ensure contact investigations are conducted to identify and treat latent TB infection among contacts.

11) Persons with HIV infection should have tuberculin skin testing or an IGRA at their first clinical evaluation; HIV-infected persons with a positive TST result (≥5 mm induration) or IGRA should start treatment for latent TB infection as soon as active TB disease has been excluded. In the USA, 9 months of INH is the recommended treatment for HIV-infected persons with latent TB infection; RIF is generally contraindicated in persons who are taking protease inhibitors and NNRTIs. Conversely, all persons with TB infection or disease should receive HIV counseling and testing where available.

12) Case-control and contact studies consistently show that BCG is protective against TB meningitis and disseminated disease in children under 5. Some controlled trials indicate that protection may persist for as long as 20 years in high-incidence situations; others have shown no protection at all. Meta-analyses on BCG effectiveness provide conflicting results. Ongoing efforts to develop a vaccine more effective than BCG have identified candidate vaccines that are currently undergoing testing in humans for safety and immunogenicity. Because the risk of infection is low in many industrialized countries, BCG is not used routinely in these settings; BCG may be considered for children with a negative PPD skin test who cannot be placed on preventive therapy but have continuous exposure to people with untreated or ineffectively treated active disease, or are continuously and irremovably exposed to patients infected by organisms resistant to isoniazid and rifampicin. In countries with high TB prevalence, WHO recommends BCG vaccination for newborns as part of the routine immunization program. A live-attenuated vaccine, BCG is contraindicated in persons with immunodeficiency disorders, including infants and children with symptomatic HIV infection, because of the risk of disseminated BCG disease. In settings where HIV services for mothers and infants are limited, BCG vaccine should continue to be given at birth to all infants regardless of HIV exposure. WHO recommends close follow-up of infants known to be born to HIV-infected mothers and who receive BCG at birth, in order to identify and treat BCG-related complications. In settings with adequate HIV services that

could allow for early identification and administration of antiretroviral therapy to HIV-infected infants, consideration should be given to delaying BCG vaccination in infants born to mothers known to be HIV-infected until the infants are confirmed to be HIV negative. Re-vaccination at older ages is regarded as an intervention for which evidence of efficacy is controversial, and WHO does not recommend it.

BCG immunization of uninfected (TST-negative) people induces tuberculin reactivity in approximately half of those vaccinated. Tuberculin reactivity and protection vary. Protection varies markedly in different field trials, and is probably related to immunological characteristics of population, quality of vaccine, BCG strain, and prevalence of environmental mycobacteria.

13) Eliminate bovine tuberculosis among dairy cattle, through tuberculin testing and slaughtering of positive reactors; pasteurize or boil milk and dairy products for human consumption.

14) A number of social and economic conditions and their consequences have been associated with a high risk of developing TB among those infected; these include malnutrition, silicosis among those working in industrial plants and mines, indoor air pollution, smoking and alcohol abuse. Interventions aiming at reducing the prevalence of such conditions will also benefit TB control.

B. Control of patient, contacts and the immediate environment:

1) Report to local public health authorities when diagnosis is suspected: obligatory case report in most countries, Class 2 (see *Reporting*). Case reports must state whether the case is bacteriologically confirmed (AFB smear positive or culture positive) or if diagnosis was based on clinical and/or radiographic findings, and whether the case was previously treated. Public health authorities must maintain a register of cases requiring treatment, and must be actively involved with planning and monitoring the course of treatment.

2) Isolation: For pulmonary tuberculosis, control of infectivity is most efficiently achieved through prompt specific drug treatment, usually leading to disappearance of vital organisms in the sputum in 2–4 weeks and full sputum clearance within 4–8 weeks. Hospitalization is necessary only for patients with severe illness requiring hospital-level care, and for those whose medical or social circumstances make treatment at home impossible. Where available, adult patients with sputum smear-positive pulmonary TB who reside in congregate settings should be placed in an airborne

infection isolation room with negative pressure ventilation, with at least six air exchanges per hour. Patients should be taught to cover both mouth and nose when coughing or sneezing. Face masks, such as the cloth or paper surgical masks, prevent spread of bacilli from the wearer to others by capturing the large wet particles expelled, but do not protect the wearer from inhaling infectious droplets nuclei in the air. Persons entering rooms where TB patients reside should wear personal respiratory protective devices capable of filtering particles of less than a micron in diameter, such as N95 face respirators. Patients whose sputum is bacteriologically negative, who do not cough, and who are known to be on adequate chemotherapy (known or probable drug susceptibility and clear clinical response to treatment) do not require isolation, nor do children with active TB disease with negative sputum smears and no cough, as they are not contagious. For patients with MDR TB, sputum culture conversion to negative is generally recommended for discontinuing isolation precautions.

Adolescents should be managed as adults. The need to adhere to the prescribed chemotherapeutic regimen must be emphasized repeatedly to all patients. Proper patient education, counseling and support must be provided to ensure that drug regimens are taken as prescribed. Supervision of drug administration through a health care worker or a recognized community worker to ensure that daily doses are taken as prescribed, including directly observed therapy, is essential for all patients. In resource-limited settings, directly observed therapy should be prioritized for persons with suspected drug resistance, a previous history of poor adherence to treatment, or who live in conditions where relapse would result in exposure of many other susceptible persons.

3) Concurrent disinfection: Hand-washing and good housekeeping practices must be maintained according to policy. Because TB has an airborne mode of transmission, no special precautions are necessary for handling fomites. Decontamination of air is achieved by ventilation; this may be supplemented by filtration and ultraviolet light.

4) Quarantine: Recently, the emergence of highly drug-resistant forms of TB (MDR-TB, XDR-TB) has raised the issue of application of quarantine measures to enforce isolation. WHO strongly recommends that governments ensure, as their top priority, that every patient has access to high quality TB diagnosis and treatment for TB and drug-resistant forms of TB. It also fully supports the rights and responsibilities of TB patients as recommended in the Patients' Charter for TB Care. In this regard, if a patient willfully refuses treatment

and is a danger to the public as a result, the serious threat posed by XDR-TB (and MDR-TB) means that limiting that individual's human rights may be necessary to protect the wider public. Therefore, interference with freedom of movement when instituting quarantine or isolation for a communicable disease such as MDR-TB and XDR-TB may be necessary for the public good, and could be considered legitimate under international human rights law. This must be viewed as a last resort, and justified only after all voluntary measures to isolate such a patient have failed.

A key factor in determining if the necessary protections exist when rights are restricted is that each one of the five criteria of the Siracusa Principles must be met (but these should be of a limited duration, and subject to review and appeal). The Siracusa principles are as follows:

- The restriction is provided for and carried out in accordance with the law.
- The restriction is in the interest of a legitimate objective of general interest.
- The restriction is strictly necessary in a democratic society to achieve the objective.
- There are no less intrusive and restrictive means available to reach the same objective.
- The restriction is based on scientific evidence and not drafted or imposed arbitrarily, i.e. in an unreasonable or otherwise discriminatory manner.

5) Management and investigation of contacts and source of infection: Investigation of potentially exposed contacts is recommended at the time of diagnosis. TST or IGRA tests for all household members and other close contacts are recommended. If the initial TST or IGRA result is negative, a repeat TST or IGRA should be performed at least 8–10 weeks after exposure to the person with TB disease has ended or they are no longer considered contagious. Clinical evaluation and a chest radiograph should be obtained for contacts with a positive TST ($\geq$5 mm induration) or IGRA result to exclude TB disease. Treatment of latent TB infection is indicated (see 9.A.6.) for contacts with positive TST or IGRA results. In addition, close contacts at high risk of developing TB disease (i.e., children younger than 5 years and persons with HIV infection) should be started on presumptive treatment (i.e., "window prophylaxis") until the post-exposure TST or IGRA result is available. In many developing countries, investigation of household contacts is limited to sputum microscopy

of those contacts who have symptoms suggestive of TB disease.

6) Specific treatment: principles of case management are included in the WHO's Stop TB Strategy. Its first component, "Pursue DOTS expansion" (where "DOTS" is the WHO-recommended 5-element package for TB control), explicitly describes adequate approaches to diagnosis, treatment, and patient monitoring. Such approaches should be implemented by all care providers, regardless of whether they work in governmental facilities or in the non-state sector (e.g. non-governmental organizations, faith-based organizations, academic institutions, private practice, etc.). They are also described in the International Standards of TB Care. Community participation is also integral part of this strategy, as it supports adherence to treatment and, possibly, early detection of suspects, cases and contacts.

Adequate patient support to ensure that all drugs are taken as prescribed, including directly observed therapy, is highly effective in achieving cure and is recommended for treatment of TB disease worldwide. Patients with TB disease must be promptly treated with an appropriate combination of antimicrobial drugs. In pulmonary TB cases, sputum smears and cultures must be monitored at regular intervals.

For all TB cases, WHO and the International Standards of TB Care recommend a treatment regimen of 2 months of daily doses of INH, RIF, pyrazinamide (PZA), and ethambutol (EMB), followed by 4 months of daily or intermittent (three times a week) INH and RIF. All treatment should be supervised or directly observed to ensure medication ingestion by the patient; this regimen is known as short-course chemotherapy. If treatment cannot be directly observed in the continuation phase, 6 months of INH and EMB can be substituted in place of 4 months of INH and RIF. However, this regimen is a weaker alternative as it increases chances of relapse and failure.

Some recommend that treatment could be extended to 9 months for patients with cavitary lung disease or who remain sputum smear or culture positive after 3 months on appropriate therapy. After drug susceptibility results become available, a specific drug regimen can be selected if the patient has a drug-resistant strain.

In HIV-infected patients, concomitant treatment for TB and antiretroviral therapy has several challenges, including adherence to multiple medications, overlapping medication side effects, immune reconstitution inflammatory syndrome (IRIS), and drug-drug interactions. The key interactions are those between the rifamycin antibiotics and four classes of antiretroviral drugs: protease inhibitors, NNRTIs, CCR5-receptor antagonists, and integrase inhibitors. Two of the antiretroviral drug classes, the nucleoside analogues (excluding zidovudine) and enfuvirtide (a parenteral entry inhibitor) do not have significant interactions with the rifamycins. Because of the complexity of treating TB and HIV concomitantly, these patients should be treated by or in close consultation with a clinician with expertise in management of both TB and HIV.

If sputum culture fails to become negative after 3 months of standard treatment or reverts to positive after a series of negative results, or if clinical response is poor, examination of the patient's drug adherence and repeat drug-susceptibility testing is indicated. Treatment failure can be due to irregular or interrupted drug regimens, drug malabsorption, the presence of a drug-resistant strain, or a combination of these factors. A change in supervision practices is required if the problem is irregular or interrupted drug regimens. If drug-susceptibility testing is available, at least 2 new drugs to which the organisms are susceptible should be added to the original drug regimen; a single new drug should never be added to a failing regimen. Adding a single new drug to a failing regimen increases the risk of developing resistance to the new drug and can further complicate clinical management. If the organisms are resistant to INH or RIF, treatment should continue for at least 18 months after cultures have become negative to ensure a cure has been obtained. Expert consultation is advised for the proper management of patients with MDR TB and XDR TB.

WHO recommends children receive the same regimens as adults with minor modifications; susceptibility of the causal organism can often be inferred from the drug-susceptibility pattern of the adult source patient's isolate. Children with pulmonary or extrapulmonary TB can be treated with INH, RIF, PZA, and EMB for 2 months, followed by INH and RIF for 4 months. If treatment cannot be directly observed in the continuation phase, 6 months of INH and EMB can be substituted in place of 4 months of INH and RIF. Children with TB meningitis or HIV co-infection should be treated for a minimum of 9 months. In some countries, EMB generally is not used until the child is old enough for color vision to be checked (usually when aged 5 years or more), although it can be added to the regimen of children with more severe disease. A recent review indicates, however, that EMB can be safely added to the regimen of children at a dose of 20 mg/kg daily. Children with meningitis, miliary disease, bone/joint disease or HIV infection should be treated for 9 to 12 months.

For further details of case management in children, see *Guidance for national tuberculosis programmes on the management of tuberculosis in children*, which can be found at:

   <http://whqlibdoc.who.int/hq/2006/WHO_HTM_TB_ 2006.371_eng.pdf>.

All drugs can cause adverse reactions. Thoracic surgery is rarely indicated, but has been used successfully in certain MDR and XDR TB cases with focal pulmonary disease and adequate pulmonary function. Patients in whom surgery is considered should have several months of adequate treatment before resection, and should continue treatment for 12–24 months following surgery. For WHO guidance on details of case management (including MDR- and HIV-associated TB), see *Treatment of tuberculosis: Guidelines for national programmes* (WHO/CDS/TB/2003.313), which can be found at:

   <http://whqlibdoc.who.int/hq/2003/WHO_CDS_TB_2003. 313.pdf>

For US-specific case management advice, see *Treatment of tuberculosis: American Thoracic Society, CDC, and Infectious Diseases Society of America*, which can be found at:

   <http://www.cdc.gov/MMWR/PDF/rr/rr5211.pdf>

Monitoring of treatment response necessitates symptom evaluation and in pulmonary cases, sputum-smear microscopy and culture monthly, or at least after 1, 2, 5, and 6 months. In developing countries where smear microscopy is still the only readily available tool, the latter plan is most common. Radiological abnormalities may persist for months after a bacteriological response, often with permanent scarring, and monitoring by serial chest radiographs is thus neither useful nor recommended for evaluation of response. An end-of-treatment chest X-ray in patients with pulmonary or pleural TB may help show new baseline anatomy and will document findings for future comparison.

WHO strongly recommends that cohort analysis of treatment outcomes include all patients registered for treatment. The 6 mutually exclusive categories of treatment results are: bacteriologically proven cure; treatment completion (without bacteriological evidence of cure); failure (smear positive at month 5 after treatment start); default; death; and transfer to other administrative units. Cohort analysis allows proper evaluation of treatment program performance and prompts corrective measures when unacceptable levels of treatment failures, deaths, and defaulting occur.

C. **Epidemic measures:** Prompt diagnosis and treatment of each person with contagious TB disease; active case finding for secondary cases of TB disease among contacts; identification and treatment of TB infections among contacts; in pediatric TB patients, an intensive search for and treatment of the source patient; airborne infection precautions.

D. **Disaster implications:** TB care and control are not a priority in the acute phase of an emergency when mortality rates are high. A TB control program should be considered when there is a high prevalence of TB disease, basic needs are provided for, essential clinical services and supplies are available, and death rates have been reduced to less than 1 per 10 000 persons per day. TB control programs in these settings should be integrated with the national or host country TB control program to ensure acceptable standards and outcomes are met. For WHO guidance, see *Tuberculosis care and control in refugee and displaced populations: An interagency field manual*, which can be found at:

<http://whqlibdoc.who.int/publications/2007/9789241595421_eng.pdf>.

E. **International measures:** In industrialized countries, a high proportion of new disease cases arise among foreign-born persons, especially those from high prevalence areas. The annual proportion of new cases born abroad has been growing steadily, and today is around 60% in some industrialized countries. Surveillance allows the identification of those at excess risk. Among the at-risk population, screening allows individuals to benefit from curative and preventive interventions. These include:

i) Adequate notification systems (physician and laboratory reports) to identify populations at risk
ii) Smears, culture and other diagnostic procedures, followed by curative/preventive interventions for symptomatic persons with latent TB infection or TB disease
iii) Provision of culturally and socially sensitive curative and preventive services for persons with TB disease; ensured follow-up of interventions
iv) Ongoing evaluation of the efficiency and efficacy of interventions.
   Further information can be found at:

<http://www.who.int/topics/tuberculosis/en/>
<http://www.cdc.gov/tb/>
<http://www.who.int/gtb/>
<http://www.stoptb.org>.

DISEASES DUE TO OTHER
MYCOBACTERIA   ICD-9 031; ICD-10 A31
(Mycobacterioses, Non-tuberculous mycobacterial disease)

Mycobacteria other than the *M. tuberculosis* complex organisms and *M. leprae* are ubiquitous and can produce disease in humans. These acid-fast bacilli have in the past been variously termed environmental, atypical, unclassified mycobacteria, non-tuberculous mycobacteria (NTM), or mycobacteria other than tuberculosis (MOTT). Of more than 90 identified species, only about 15 are recognized as pathogenic to humans. The NTMs are often classified based on their growth characteristics in solid media. Some grow rapidly and within 7 days (*M. abscessus, M. chelonae, M. fortuitum*). Others grow more slowly, usually in 2–3 weeks (*M. avium, M. kansasii, M. ulcerans, M. marinum*).

Clinical syndromes associated with the pathogenic species of mycobacteria can be classified broadly as follows:

1) Disseminated disease—often in the presence of severe immunodeficiency—*M. avium, M. kansasii, M. haemophilum, M. genavense*. Presenting symptoms include fever, weight loss, fatigue. Diagnosis can be obtained through isolation in blood, liver or bone marrow culture.

2) Pulmonary disease resembling tuberculosis—*M. kansasii, M. avium* complex (*M. intracellulare, M. abscessus, M. xenopi, M. simian, M. malmoense*.

3) Lymphadenitis (primarily cervical)—*M. avium* complex, *M. scrofulaceum, M. kansasii*.

4) Skin ulcers and surgical would infections—*M. ulcerans* (see *Buruli ulcer*), *M. fortuitum, M. chelonae, M. abscessus, M. marinum*. These infections may appear as nodular or ulcerating; at times, they spread along the lymphatics.

5) Post-traumatic wound infections—*M. fortuitum, M. chelonae, M. abscessus, M. marinum, M. avium* complex.

5) Crohn's disease—*M. paratuberculosis* has been suggested as the causative agent in some cases of regional enteritis; incorrect diagnosis of inflammatory bowel disease may delay diagnosis and treatment of TB disease of the bowel, and worsening of disease if immunosuppressive drugs are used inadvertently.

6) Nosocomial disease: surgical wound infections and catheter-related infections (bacteremia, peritonitis, post-injection abscesses)—*M. fortuitum, M. chelonae, M. abscessus*.

The epidemiology of the diseases attributable to these organisms has not been well delineated, but the organisms have been found in soil, milk, and water; other factors, such as host tissue damage and immunodeficiency, may predispose to infection. With the exception of organisms causing skin lesions, there is no evidence of person-to-person transmission. A single isolation from sputum or gastric washings can occur in the absence of signs or symptoms of clinical disease. Multiple isolations of NTM from respiratory specimens, in the absence of illness or other specific pathology, may be evidence of commensal colonization (e.g. with *M. gordonae*), with no clinical significance. A single positive culture from a wound or tissue is generally considered diagnostic.

In general, the diagnosis of disease requiring treatment is based on repeated isolations of many colonies from symptomatic patients with progressive illness. Where human infections with NTM are prevalent, cross-reactions may interfere with the interpretation of TST for *M. tuberculosis* infection, but less so if IGRAs are used. Chemotherapy is relatively effective against *M. kansasii* and *M. marinum* disease, but traditional anti-tuberculosis drugs (especially PZA) may not be effective for other NTM. Some cases of failure of TB treatment, in settings with limited facilities for culture and drug susceptibility testing, may in fact be cases of disease with NTM, which are commonly resistant to standard TB drugs. Drug susceptibility tests on the isolated organism will help select an effective drug combination. In general, pulmonary disease due to *M. avium* can be treated with ethambutol, rifabutin plus a macrolide, while that due to *M. kansasii* responds to rifampicin, isoniazid and ethambutol. Surgery should be given more consideration than in TB, especially when the disease is localized. Cutaneous diseases caused by rapidly growing NTM can be treated with clarithromycin and/or amikacin, depending on the extent of skin disease. Skin infection caused by *M. marinum* is treated with a combination of clarithromycin and ethambutol, usually for 3–4 months.

Disseminated *Mycobacterium avium* infection is a major problem in HIV-infected persons; in the past it was considered poorly amenable to treatment. Drug regimens containing clarithromycin and ethambutol, with possible addition of rifabutin lasting for at least 12–18 months, have shown therapeutic potential. Weekly azythromycin is recommended for prophylaxis against disseminated *M. avium* infection among severely immunocompromised AIDS patients. AIDS patients are also susceptible to disseminated infection caused by *M. kansasii*. Treatment consists of daily rifampicin, isoniazid and ethambutol.

Further information can be found at:

<http://www.thoracic.org/sections/publications/statements/pages/mtpi/nontuberculous-mycobacterial-diseases.html>

TULAREMIA   ICD-9 021; ICD-10 A21
(Rabbit fever, Deer-fly fever, Ohara disease, Francis disease)
[CCDM19: M. Chu, P. Mead, A. Sjöstedt]
[CCDM18: A. Sjöstedt]

1. Identification—A zoonotic bacterial disease with diverse clinical manifestations related to route of introduction and virulence of the disease agent. The onset of disease is typically sudden and influenza-like, with high fever, chills, fatigue, general body aches, headache, and nausea. Most often it presents as an indolent skin ulcer at the site of introduction of the organism, together with swelling of the regional lymph nodes (ulceroglandular type). There may be one or more enlarged and painful lymph nodes that may suppurate without visible primary ulcer (glandular type). Ingestion of contaminated food or water may produce a painful pharyngitis (with or without ulceration), abdominal pain, diarrhea and vomiting (oropharyngeal type). Inhalation of infectious material may be followed by respiratory involvement (often described as typhoidal type) or evidenced by a primary septicemia; bloodborne organisms may localize in the lung and pleural spaces. The conjunctival sac is a rare route of introduction that results in a clinical disease of painful purulent conjunctivitis with regional lymphadenitis (oculoglandular type). Pneumonia may complicate all clinical types and requires prompt identification and specific treatment to prevent development of serious symptoms.

The infectious agent is found in habitats limited to the Northern hemisphere. Three subspecies with differing virulence cause human disease. The most virulent form, *Francisella tularensis* subsp. *tularensis* (Jellison type A), is found in North America, with a case-fatality rate, before the introduction of efficacious antibiotic regimens, of up to 30%. With appropriate antibiotic therapy, the case fatality rate is low. The more prevalent and less virulent form found in North America and elsewhere is caused by *F. tularensis* subsp. *holarctica* (Jellison type B); patients recover, even without treatment, with few fatalities. The third and rarest form is associated with the mildest presentation, caused by infection with *F. tularensis* subsp. *novicida*, which is typically associated with waterborne acquired infection. Clinically, because of buboes and/or severe pneumonia, tularemia may be confused with plague, as well as other infectious diseases including staphylococcal and streptococcal infections, cat-scratch fever, and tuberculosis.

Diagnosis is most commonly clinical and confirmed by a titer rise in specific serum antibodies that usually appear during the second week of the disease. Using tube-agglutination, cross-reactions occur with *Brucella* species, whereas ELISA-based serological testing for reactivity to *F. tularensis* is highly specific. Examination of ulcer exudate, lymph node and other clinical specimens by FA test or identification of bacterial DNA by polymerase chain reaction may provide rapid diagnosis. Diagnostic biopsy of acutely infected lymph nodes should be done only under the cover of specific therapy, since it will often induce bacteremia. The causative

662 / TULAREMIA

bacteria can be cultured on special media such as cysteine-glucose blood agar, agar supplemented with thiol-iron, or through inoculation of laboratory animals with material from lesions, blood or sputum as appropriate with presentation. The subspecies are differentiated by their chemical reactions: type A organisms ferment glycerol and convert citrulline to ornithine. Extreme care must be exercised to avoid laboratory transmission of highly infectious aerosolized organisms; culture identification is performed only in reference laboratories and most cases are diagnosed serologically. *F. tularensis* subsp. *novicida* grows more robustly, and does not require cysteine for growth.

2. Infectious agent—*Francisella tularensis* is, a small, faintly-staining, Gram-negative non-motile coccobacillus. All isolates are serologically homogeneous, but are differentiated epidemiologically and biochemically into *F. tularensis* subsp. *tularensis* (Jellison type A), with an LD_{50} in rabbits of fewer than 10 bacteria, or *F. tularensis* subsp. *holarctica* (Jellison type B) with an LD_{50} in rabbits of greater than 10^6 bacteria. *F. tularensis* subsp. *novicida* typically does not kill rabbits.

3. Occurrence—Tularemia occurs throughout North America and in many parts of continental Europe, Russia, China and Japan. In North America, most cases occur from May through August, but cases are reported throughout the year. *F. tularensis* subsp. *tularensis* organisms, restricted to North America, are common in rabbits and are frequently transmitted by tick bite. *F. tularensis* subsp. *holarctica* strains commonly occur in mammals other than rabbits in North America; strains are found in voles, muskrats, rabbits, hares, water rats in Eurasia, and rabbits in Japan. Clinicians should also be aware of tularemia associated with handling of sick pets (dogs, cats, hamsters) and exotic animals (prairie dogs, monkeys).

4. Reservoir—Wild animals, especially rabbits, hares, voles, muskrats, beavers and some domestic animals; also various hard ticks. A rodent-mosquito cycle has been described for *F. tularensis* subsp. *holarctica* in the Scandinavian countries and Russia.

5. Mode of transmission—Arthropod bites including those of the wood tick *Dermacentor andersoni*, the dog tick *D. variabilis*, the lone star tick *Amblyomma americanum*, less commonly the deer fly *Chrysops discalis* and, in Russia and Sweden, various mosquito species; through inoculation of skin, conjunctival sac or oropharyngeal mucosa with contaminated water, blood or tissue while handling infected carcasses (e.g. skinning, dressing or performing necropsies); by handling or ingesting insufficiently cooked meat of infected animals; by drinking contaminated water; by inhalation of dust from contaminated soil, grain or hay, or from contaminated animal pelts and paws; and by handling sick pet animals. Laboratory infections frequently present as respiratory tularemia.

6. Incubation period—Related to size of inoculum; usually 3–5 days (range 1–14 days).

7. Period of communicability—No direct person-to-person transmission. The infectious agent may be found in the blood of untreated patients during the first 2 weeks of disease, and in lesions for a month or more. Flies can be infective for 14 days, and ticks throughout their lifetime (about 2 years). Rabbit meat frozen at −15°C (5°F) has remained infective for over 3 years.

8. Susceptibility—All ages are susceptible, and long-term immunity follows recovery; reinfection is extremely rare and has been reported only in laboratory staff.

9. Methods of control—

A. *Preventive measures:*

1) Educate the public to avoid bites of ticks, flies and mosquitoes, for example by using long sleeves and repellents, and to avoid contact with untreated water where infection prevails among wild animals.
2) Use impervious gloves when skinning or handling animals, especially rabbits. Cook the meat of wild rabbits and rodents thoroughly. Avoid handling such meat together with vegetables.
3) Use universal precautions in direct handling of small animals (especially pets) that are exhibiting signs and symptoms of illness.
4) Live attenuated vaccines applied intradermally by scarification are used extensively in Russia, and to a limited extent for occupational risk groups in some other countries, such as Sweden and United States.
5) Take appropriate precautions (using facemasks, gowns and impervious gloves, and carrying out work under Class II biosafety cabinets) when handling cultures of *F. tularensis*.

B. *Control of patient, contacts and the immediate environment:*

1) Report to local health authority: In selected endemic areas; in many countries not a reportable disease, Class 3 (see *Reporting*).
2) Isolation: Secretion precautions for open lesions and universal precautions during patient care.
3) Concurrent disinfection: Of discharges from ulcers, lymph nodes or conjunctival sacs.
4) Quarantine: Not applicable.
5) Immunization of contacts: Not indicated.

6) Investigation of contacts and source of infection: Important in each case, with search for the origin of infection.

7) Specific treatment: Aminoglycosides (gentamicin or strepto-mycin) are the drugs of choice in serious infections. Tetra-cyclines, also widely used effectively as prophylaxis and treatment, are associated with higher relapse rates (and cannot be used in children less than eight years of age). Recent experience of treatment with ciprofloxacin has shown excellent efficacy and is a preferred treatment if oral treatment is used. Many antibiotics, including all beta-lactam antibiotics and modern cephalosporins, are ineffective for treatment, and many isolates show resistance to macrolides. Treatment with aminoglycosides or ciprofloxacin should last 10–14 days, and tetracyclines for 21 days.

C. Epidemic measures: Search for sources of infection related to arthropods, animal hosts, water, and environments soiled by small mammals, including hay. Control measures as indicated in 9A.

D. Disaster implications: None.

E. International measures: None.

F. Measures in the case of deliberate use: Tularemia is consid-ered to be a potential agent for deliberate use, particularly if used as an aerosol threat. As is true of plague, cases acquired by inhalation present as primary pneumonia. Such cases require prompt identification and specific treatment to prevent a fatal outcome. All diagnosed cases, and especially clusters of pneu-monia due to *F. tularensis*, must be reported immediately to the health department for appropriate investigation.

For more information on the deliberate use of infectious agents to cause harm, see the section on *Deliberate use*.

TYPHOID FEVER   ICD-9 002.0; ICD-10 A01.0
(Enteric fever, Typhus abdominalis)
PARATYPHOID FEVER
ICD-9 002.1-002.9; ICD-10 A01.1-A01.4
[CCDM19: E. Mintz, S. Sodha]
[CCDM18: C. Chaignat]

1. Identification—A systemic bacterial disease with insidious onset of sustained fever, marked headache, malaise, anorexia, relative bradycardia, splenomegaly, nonproductive cough in the early stage of the illness, rose spots on the trunk in 25% of white-skinned patients and constipation more often than diarrhea in adults. The clinical picture varies from mild illness with low-grade fever to severe clinical disease with abdominal discomfort and multiple complications. Severity is influenced by factors such as strain virulence, quantity of inoculum ingested, duration of illness before adequate treatment, age and previous exposure to vaccination.

Unapparent or mild illnesses occur, especially in endemic areas; 60%–90% of patients with typhoid fever do not receive medical attention or are treated as outpatients. Mild cases show no systemic involvement; the clinical picture is that of a gastroenteritis (see *Salmonellosis*). Non-sweating fevers, mental dullness, slight deafness and parotitis may occur. Peyer patches in the ileum can ulcerate, with intestinal hemorrhage or perforation (about 1% of cases), especially late in untreated cases. Severe forms with altered mental status have been associated with high case-fatality rates. The case-fatality rate of 10%–20% observed in the pre-antibiotic era can fall below 1% with prompt antimicrobial therapy. Depending on the antimicrobials used, 15%–20% of patients may experience relapses (generally milder than the initial clinical illness).

Paratyphoid fever, caused by *Salmonella enterica* subsp. *enterica* serovars Paratyphi. A, B, and C (commonly *S*. Paratyphi A, B and C), presents a similar clinical picture. Serovar Paratyphi B refers to the invasive biotype that is associated with paratyphoid fever. A tartrate fermenting variant, referred to as serovar Paratyphi B var L(+) tartrate+, or var. Java, is associated with routine gastrointestinal disease. Since the distinction between these two biovars is currently based on a single phenotypic trait, they can be easily confused. The ratio of disease caused by *Salmonella enterica* subsp. *enterica* serovar Typhi (commonly *S. Typhi*, the latter not italicized) to that caused by *S. Paratyphi* A and B is estimated to be about 4:1. Relapses occur in approximately 3%–4% of cases. *S. Paratyphi* C infections are rare.

The causal organisms can be isolated from blood early in the disease, and from urine and feces after the first week. Blood culture is the diagnostic mainstay for typhoid fever, but bone marrow culture provides the most sensitive method for bacteriological confirmation even in patients who have already received antimicrobials. Because of limited sensitivity and specificity, serological tests based on agglutinating antibodies (Widal) are generally of little diagnostic value. New rapid sero-diagnostic tests based upon the detection of specific antibodies appear very promising, but their current sensitivity and specificity limit usefulness in routine practice.

2. Infectious agents—In the recently proposed nomenclature for *Salmonella* the agent formerly known as *S. typhi* is called *S. enterica* subsp. *enterica* serovar Typhi (commonly *S. Typhi*). Paratyphoid fever is caused mainly by *S. Paratyphi* A and Paratyphi B, but also by Paratyphi C in rare cases. Note that each of the Paratyphi serotypes belongs to a different O-group of Salmonella referred to in its name; S. Typhi belongs to O-group D.

3. Occurrence—Worldwide, the annual estimated incidence of typhoid fever is about 22 million cases with approximately 200 000 deaths. Most of the burden of the disease occurs in the developing world. The burden is sporadic in industrialized countries; currently most cases in the industrialized world are acquired during travel in endemic areas. Paratyphoid fever occurs sporadically or in limited outbreaks, probably more frequently than reports suggest. Of the 3 serotypes, Paratyphi A is most common, Paratyphi B is less frequent, and Paratyphi C is extremely rare. In parts of China and Pakistan, more cases have been reported as caused by *S. Paratyphi* than by *S. Typhi*.

4. Reservoir—Humans for both typhoid and paratyphoid; questionably, domestic animals for paratyphoid. Family contacts may be transient or permanent carriers. A carrier state may follow acute illness or mild or even sub-clinical infections. In most parts of the world, short-term fecal carriers are more common than urinary carriers. The chronic carrier state is most common (2%–5%) among persons infected during middle age, especially women; carriers frequently have biliary tract abnormalities including gallstones, with *S. Typhi* located in the gallbladder. The chronic urinary carrier state may occur with schistosome infections or kidney stones.

5. Mode of transmission—Ingestion of food and water contaminated by feces and urine of patients and carriers. Important vehicles in some countries include shellfish (particularly oysters) from sewage-contaminated beds, raw fruit, vegetables fertilized by night soil and eaten raw, and contaminated milk/milk products (usually contaminated through hands of carriers). Flies may infect foods in which the organism then multiplies to infective doses (those are reportedly lower for typhoid than for paratyphoid bacteria). Epidemiological data suggest that, while waterborne transmission of *S. Typhi* usually involves small inocula, food-borne transmission is associated with large inocula and high attack rates over short periods. Sexual transmission of typhoid fever from an asymptomatic carrier has been documented.

6. Incubation period—Depends on inoculum size and on host factors; from 3 days to over 60 days— usual range 8–14 days; the incubation period for paratyphoid fever is 1–10 days.

7. Period of communicability—As long as bacilli appear in excreta, usually from the first week throughout convalescence; variable thereafter (commonly 1–2 weeks for paratyphoid). About 10% of untreated typhoid fever patients discharge bacilli for 3 months after onset of symptoms; 2%–5% become permanent carriers. Fewer persons infected with paratyphoid organisms may become permanent gallbladder carriers.

8. Susceptibility—Susceptibility is general and is increased in individuals with gastric achlorhydria. One study has suggested that susceptibility may be increased in persons who are HIV-positive. Relative specific immunity follows recovery from clinical disease, unapparent infection and active immunization. In endemic areas, typhoid fever is most common in preschool children and children 5–19.

9. **Methods of control—**

   A. *Preventive measures:* Prevention is based on access to safe water and proper sanitation, as well as adherence to safe food-handling practices.

   1) Educate the public regarding the importance of hand-washing. Provide suitable hand-washing facilities, particularly for food handlers and attendants involved in the care of patients and children.
   2) Dispose of human feces safely, and maintain fly-proof latrines. Where culturally appropriate, encourage use of sufficient toilet paper to minimize finger contamination. Under field conditions, dispose of feces by burial at a site distant and downstream from the source of drinking water.
   3) Protect, purify and chlorinate public water supplies, provide safe private supplies, and avoid possible backflow connections between water and sewer systems. For individual and small group protection, and during travel or in the field, treat water chemically or by boiling.
   4) Control flies by screening and use of insecticidal baits and traps or, where appropriate, spraying with insecticides. Control fly-breeding through frequent garbage collection and disposal, and through fly control measures in latrine construction and maintenance.
   5) Use scrupulous cleanliness in food preparation and handling; refrigerate as appropriate. Pay particular attention to the storage of salads and other foods served cold. These provisions apply to home and public eating-places. If uncertain about sanitary practices, select foods that are cooked and served hot, and fruit that is peeled by the consumer.
   6) Pasteurize or boil all milk and dairy products. Supervise the sanitary aspects of commercial milk production, storage and delivery.
   7) Enforce suitable quality-control procedures in industries that prepare food and drink for human consumption. Use chlorinated water for cooling during canned food processing.
   8) Limit the collection and marketing of shellfish to supplies from approved sources. Boil or steam (for at least 10 minutes) before serving.
   9) Instruct the community, patients, convalescents and carriers in personal hygiene. Emphasize hand-washing as a routine practice after defecation and before preparing, serving or eating food.

10) Encourage breast-feeding throughout infancy; boil all milk and water used for infant feeding.

11) Typhoid carriers should be excluded from handling food and from providing patient care. Identify and supervise typhoid carriers; culture of sewage may help in locating them. Chronic carriers should not be released from supervision and restriction of occupation until local or state regulations are met, often not until 3 consecutive negative cultures are obtained from authenticated fecal specimens (and urine in areas endemic for schistosomiasis), at least 1 month apart and at least 48 hours after antimicrobial therapy has stopped. Fresh stool specimens are preferred to rectal swabs. It has been suggested that at least 1 of the 3 consecutive negative stool specimens should be obtained by purging.

Administration of 750 mg of ciprofloxacin or 400 mg of norfloxacin twice daily for 28 days provides successful treatment of carriers in 80–90% of cases. Limited studies have suggested 14–21 days of treatment to be equally efficacious. Follow-up cultures are necessary to confirm cure.

12) Immunization for typhoid fever is not routinely recommended in non-endemic areas except for those subject to unusual occupational exposure to enteric infections (e.g. clinical microbiology technicians) and household members of known carriers. WHO recommends vaccination for people who travel to endemic high-risk areas and school-age children living in endemic areas where typhoid fever control is a priority. Vaccination of high-risk populations is considered the most promising strategy for the control of typhoid fever. No vaccines for paratyphoid fever are currently available.

An oral, live vaccine using *S. Typhi* strain Ty21a (requiring 3 or 4 doses, 2 days apart) and a parenteral vaccine containing the single dose polysaccharide Vi antigen are available; these are as protective as the whole cell bacteria vaccine (which has been removed from the market) and much less reactogenic. However, Ty21a should not be used in patients receiving antibiotics until 24 hours or more after the last antibiotic dose. Booster doses every 2 to 5 years, according to vaccine type, are desirable for those at continuing risk of infection. In field trials, oral Ty21a conferred partial protection against paratyphoid B, but not as well as it protected against typhoid. Neither vaccine is licensed for children less than 2 years old; Ty21a is only licensed for children 6 years old and older in the US, but is licensed for younger children in other countries.

A new Vi vaccine conjugated to a nontoxic recombinant *Pseudomonas aeruginosa* exotoxin A (rEPA) was shown in Vietnam to have more than 90% efficacy, and to be potentially immunogenic in younger children. This promising new vaccine has not yet been licensed.

B. Control of patient, contacts and the immediate environment:

1) Report to local health authority: Obligatory case report in most countries, Class 2 (see *Reporting*).

2) Isolation: Enteric precautions while ill; hospital care is desirable during acute illness. Release from supervision by local health authority based on not fewer than 3 consecutive negative cultures of feces (and urine in patients with schistosomiasis) at least 24 hours apart, at least 48 hours after any antimicrobials, and not earlier than 1 month after onset. If any of these is positive, repeat cultures at monthly intervals during the 12 months following onset until at least 3 consecutive negative cultures are obtained.

3) Concurrent disinfection: Of feces, urine and articles soiled therewith. In communities with adequate sewage disposal systems, feces and urine can be disposed of directly into sewers without preliminary disinfection. Terminal cleaning.

4) Quarantine: Not applicable.

5) Immunization of contacts: Routine administration of typhoid vaccine is of limited value for family, household and nursing contacts who have been or may be exposed to active cases; it should be considered for those who may be exposed to carriers on a prolonged basis. There is no effective immunization for paratyphoid fever.

6) Investigation of contacts and source of infection: Determine actual or probable source of infection of every case through search for unreported cases, carriers or contaminated food, water, milk or shellfish. All members of travel groups in which a case has been identified should be followed.

   The presence of elevated antibody titers to purified Vi polysaccharide is highly suggestive of the typhoid carrier state, especially in the setting of an epidemiologically consistent history. Identification of the same phage type or molecular subtype in the carrier and in organisms isolated from patients suggests a possible chain of transmission.

   Consideration should be given to obtaining 2 negative feces and urine cultures, taken at least 24 hours apart, from household and close contacts before allowing them to be employed in sensitive occupations (e.g. as food handlers).

7) Specific treatment: Evidence suggests that fluoroquinolones are the drug of choice in adults. However, recent emergence of decreased susceptibility, and frank resistance to fluoroquinolones in both *S. Typhi* and *S. Paratyphi* A, restricts widespread and indiscriminate use in primary care facilities and mandates

antimicrobial testing of all isolates. If local strains are known to be sensitive to traditional first-line antibiotics, oral chloramphenicol, amoxicillin or trimethoprim-sufoxazole (particularly in children) should be used in accordance with local antimicrobial sensitivity patterns. Ceftriaxone, a parenteral once-daily antibiotic, is useful in patients with dulled perceptions or those with complications such that oral antibiotics cannot be used. Short-term, high-dose corticosteroid treatment, combined with specific antibiotics and supportive care, reduces mortality in critically ill patients (see 9A11 for treatment of carrier state). Patients with concurrent schistosomiasis must also be treated with praziquantel to eliminate possible schistosome carriage of *S. Typhi*. Patients with confirmed intestinal perforation need intensive care as well as surgical intervention. Early intervention is crucial, as morbidity rates increase with delayed surgery after perforation.

Strains resistant to chloramphenicol and other recommended antimicrobials have become prevalent in several areas of the world. Most isolates from southern and southeastern Asia, the Middle East and northeastern Africa in the 1990s carry an R factor plasmid encoding resistance to those antimicrobial agents that were previously the mainstay of oral treatment, including chloramphenicol, ampicillin and trimethoprim/sufamethoxazole. Resistance to fluoroquinolones continues to emerge rapidly, especially in Asia. For treatment of Salmonella infections resistant to Nalidixic Acid, Erythromycin seems to be effective.

C. *Epidemic measures:*

1) Search intensively for the case/carrier who is the source of infection, and for the vehicle (water or food) through which infection was transmitted.
2) Selectively eliminate suspected contaminated food. Pasteurize or boil milk, or exclude milk supplies and other foods suspected on epidemiological evidence, until safety is ensured.
3) Chlorinate suspected water supplies adequately under competent supervision, or avoid use. All drinking water must be chlorinated, treated with iodine, or boiled before use.
4) Use of vaccine should be considered before or during an outbreak; a protective efficacy of over 70% was recently obtained among immunized school-age children during an outbreak in China.

D. *Disaster implications:* With disruption of usual water supply and sewage disposal, and of controls on food and water, transmission and large-scale outbreaks of typhoid fever may occur if there are active cases or carriers in a displaced population. Efforts are advised to restore safe drinking-water supplies and excreta disposal facilities. Selective immunization of stabilized groups such as school children, prisoners and utility, municipal or hospital personnel may be helpful.

E. International measures:

1) For typhoid fever: Immunization is advised for international travelers to endemic areas, especially if travel is likely to involve exposure to unsafe food and water, or close contact in rural areas to indigenous populations. Immunization is not a legal requirement for entry into any country.
2) WHO Collaborating Centres provide support as required. More information can be found at:

   <http://www.who.int/collaboratingcentres/database/en/>

TYPHUS FEVER ICD-10 A75
[CCDM19: Editorial Board]
[CCDM18: D. Raoult]

I. EPIDEMIC LOUSE-BORNE
   TYPHUS FEVER   ICD-9 080; ICD-10 A75
(Louse-borne typhus, Typhus exanthematicus, Classic typhus fever)

1. Identification—A rickettsial disease with variable onset; often sudden and marked by headache, chills, prostration, fever and general pains. A macular eruption appears on the fifth to sixth day, initially on the upper trunk, followed by spread to the entire body, but usually not to the face, palms or soles. The eruption is often difficult to observe on black skin. Toxemia is usually pronounced, and the disease terminates by rapid defervescence after about 2 weeks of fever. The case-fatality rate increases with age and varies from 10% to 40% in the absence of specific treatment. Mild infections may occur without eruption, especially in children and people partially protected by prior immunization. The disease may recrudesce years after the primary attack (Brill-Zinsser disease, ICD-9 081.1; ICD-10 A75.1); this form of disease is milder, has fewer complications, and has a lower case-fatality rate.

The IF test is most commonly used for laboratory confirmation, but it does not discriminate between louse-borne and murine typhus (ICD-9 081.0;

ICD-10 A75.2) unless the sera are differentially absorbed with the respective rickettsial antigen prior to testing. Blood can be collected on filter paper that are forwarded to a reference laboratory. Other diagnostic methods are EIA, PCR, immunohistochemical staining of tissues, CF with group specific or washed type-specific rickettsial antigens, and the toxin neutralization test. Sending lice to a reference laboratory for PCR testing may help detect an outbreak. Antibody tests usually become positive in the second week.

2. **Infectious agent**—*Rickettsia prowazekii*.

3. **Occurrence**—In colder areas where people may live under unhygienic conditions and are infested with lice. Explosive epidemics may occur during war and famine. Endemic foci exist in the mountainous regions of Mexico, in Central and South America, in central and eastern Africa and numerous countries in Asia. Recent outbreaks have been observed in Burundi and Rwanda. This rickettsia exists as a zoonosis of flying squirrels (*Glaucomys volans*) in the USA, and there is serological evidence that humans have been infected from this source, possibly via the squirrel flea.

4. **Reservoir**—Humans are the reservoir and are responsible for maintaining the infection during inter-epidemic periods. Although not a major source of human disease, sporadic cases may be associated with flying squirrels.

5. **Mode of transmission**—The body louse, *Pediculus humanus corporis*, is infected by feeding on the blood of a patient with acute typhus fever. Patients with Brill-Zinsser disease (see Identification, above) can infect lice, and may serve as foci for new outbreaks in louse-infested communities. Infected lice excrete rickettsiae in their feces, and usually defecate at the time of feeding. People are infected by rubbing feces or crushed lice into the bite or into superficial abrasions. Inhalation of infective louse feces in dust may account for some infections. Transmission from the flying squirrel is presumed to be through the bite of the squirrel flea, but this has not been documented.

6. **Incubation period**—From 1 to 2 weeks, commonly 12 days.

7. **Period of communicability**—The disease is not directly transmitted from person to person. Patients are infective for lice during the febrile illness, and possibly for 2–3 days after the temperature returns to normal. Infected lice pass rickettsiae in their feces within 2–6 days after the blood-meal; they are infective earlier if crushed. The louse invariably dies within 2 weeks after infection; rickettsiae may remain viable in the dead louse for weeks.

8. **Susceptibility**—Susceptibility is general. One attack usually confers long-lasting immunity.

9. **Methods of control—**

A. *Preventive measures:*

1) Apply an effective residual insecticide powder at appropriate intervals by hand or power blower to clothes and persons of populations living under conditions favoring louse infestation. The insecticide used should be effective on local lice.
2) Improve living conditions with provisions for bathing and washing clothes.
3) Treat prophylactically those who are subject to risk, by application of residual insecticide to clothing (dusting or impregnation).

B. *Control of patient, contacts and the immediate environment:*

1) Report to local health authority: Report of louse-borne typhus fever required as a Disease under Surveillance by WHO, Class 1 (see *Reporting*).
2) Isolation: Not required after proper delousing of patient, clothing, living quarters and household contacts.
3) Concurrent disinfection: Appropriate insecticide powder applied to clothing and bedding of patient and contacts; launder clothing and bedclothes. Lice tend to leave abnormally hot or cold bodies in search of a normothermic clothed body. If death from louse-borne typhus occurs before delousing, delouse the body and clothing by thorough application of an insecticide.
4) Quarantine: Susceptible persons infested with lice and exposed to typhus fever should ordinarily be quarantined for 15 days, if possible, after application of an insecticide with residual effect.
5) Management of contacts: All immediate contacts should be kept under surveillance for 2 weeks.
6) Investigation of contacts and source of infection: Every effort should be made to trace the infection to the immediate source.
7) Specific treatment: A single dose of doxycycline 200 mg will normally cure patients (though doxycycline cannot be used in children less than eight years of age). When faced with a seriously ill patient with possible typhus, suitable treatment should be started without waiting for laboratory confirmation.

C. *Epidemic measures:* The best measure for rapid control of typhus is application of an insecticide with residual effect to all contacts. Where louse infestation is known to be widespread, systematic application of residual insecticide to all people in the community is indicated. Treatment of cases in an epidemic may also decrease the spread of disease. In epidemics, individuals may protect themselves by wearing silk or plastic clothing tightly fastened around wrists, ankles and neck, and impregnating clothes with repellents or permethrin.

D. Disaster implications: Typhus can be expected to be a significant problem in louse-infested populations in endemic areas if social upheavals and crowding occur.

E. International measures:

1) Notification by governments to WHO and to adjacent countries of the occurrence of a case or an outbreak of louse-borne typhus fever in an area previously free of the disease.
2) International travelers: No country currently requires immunization against typhus for entry.
3) Louse-borne typhus is a Disease under Surveillance by WHO. WHO Collaborating Centres provide support as required. More information can be found at:

    <http://www.who.int/collaboratingcentres/database/en/>

F. Measures in case of deliberate use: R. prowazekii has been produced as a possible bioweapon and was used before World War II. It is infectious by aerosol, with a high case-fatality rate. The initial reference treatment of any suspected case is a single dose of 200 mg of doxycycline.

  For more information on the deliberate use of infectious agents to cause harm, see the section on *Deliberate use*.

II. ENDEMIC FLEA-BORNE
TYPHUS FEVER   ICD-9 081.0; ICD-10 A75.2
(Murine typhus, Shop typhus)

  1. Identification—A rickettsial disease the course of which resembles that of louse-borne typhus, but is milder. The case-fatality rate for all ages is less than 1%, but increases with age. Absence of louse infestation, geographic and seasonal distribution, and sporadic occurrence of the disease help differentiate it from louse-borne typhus. For laboratory diagnosis, see section I, 1.

  2. Infectious agents—*Rickettsia typhi* (*Rickettsia mooseri*); *R. felis*.

  3. Occurrence—Worldwide. Found in areas where people and rats occupy the same buildings. Multiple cases may occur in the same household.

  4. Reservoir—Rats, mice and possibly other small mammals. Infection is maintained in nature by a rat-flea-rat cycle where rats are the reservoir (commonly *Rattus rattus* and *R. norvegicus*) but infection is inapparent. A closely-related organism, *Rickettsia felis*, has been found to pass from cat to cat flea to opossum or other animals in North America, Europe and Africa. Both *rickettsiae* are transmitted transovarially.

5. Mode of transmission—Infective rat fleas (usually *Xenopsylla cheopis*) defecate rickettsiae while sucking blood; this contaminates the bite site and other fresh skin wounds. Occasionally, a case may follow inhalation of dried infective flea feces.

6. Incubation period—From 1 to 2 weeks, commonly 12 days.

7. Period of communicability—Not directly transmitted from person to person. Once infected, fleas remain so for life (up to 1 year), and transfer infection to their progeny.

8. Susceptibility—Susceptibility is general. One attack confers immunity.

9. Methods of control—

    A. Preventive measures:

        1) To avoid increased exposure of humans, wait until flea populations have first been reduced by insecticides, before instituting rodent control measures (see *Plague*, 9A2-9A3, 9B6).
        2) Apply insecticide powders with residual action to rat runs, burrows and harborages.

    B. Control of patient, contacts and the immediate environment:

        1) Report to local health authority: Case report obligatory in most countries, Class 2 (see *Reporting*).
        2) Isolation: Not applicable.
        3) Concurrent disinfection: Not applicable.
        4) Quarantine: Not applicable.
        5) Immunization of contacts: Not applicable.
        6) Investigation of contacts and source of infection: Search for rodents or opossums (North America) around premises or home of patient.
        7) Specific treatment: See *Rocky Mountain Spotted Fever*.

    C. Epidemic measures: In endemic areas with numerous cases, use of a residual insecticide effective against rat or cat fleas will reduce the flea index and the incidence of infection in humans.

    D. Disaster implications: Cases can be expected when people, rats and fleas are forced to co-exist in close proximity, but murine typhus has not been a major contributor to disease rates in such situations.

E. International measures: WHO Collaborating Centres provide support as required. More information can be found at:

<http://www.who.int/collaboratingcentres/database/en/>

III. SCRUB TYPHUS   ICD-9 081.2; ICD-10 A75.3
(Tsutsugamushi disease, Mite-borne typhus fever)

1. Identification—A rickettsial disease often characterized by a primary "punched out" skin ulcer (eschar) corresponding to the site of attachment of an infected mite. An acute febrile onset follows within several days, along with headache, profuse sweating, conjunctival injection and lymphadenopathy. Late in the first week of fever, a dull red maculopapular eruption appears on the trunk, extends to the extremities, and disappears in a few days. Cough and X-ray evidence of pneumonitis are common. Without antibiotherapy, fever lasts for about 14 days. The case-fatality rate in untreated cases varies from 1% to 60%, according to area, strain of infectious agent, and previous exposure to disease; it is consistently higher among older people.

Definitive diagnosis is made by isolation of the infectious agent by inoculating the patient's blood into mice. Serological diagnosis is complicated by antigenic differences of various strains of the causal rickettsia; the IF test is the preferred technique, but EIAs are also available. Many cases develop a positive Weil-Felix reaction with the Proteus OXK strain.

2. Infectious agent—*Orientia tsutsugamushi* with multiple, serologically distinct strains.

3. Occurrence—Central, eastern and southeastern Asia; from southeastern Siberia and northern Japan to northern Australia and Vanuatu, as far west as Pakistan, to as high as 3 000 meters (10 000 feet) above sea level in the Himalaya Mountains, and particularly prevalent in northern Thailand. Acquired by humans in one of innumerable small, sharply-delimited typhus islands (some covering an area of only a few square feet), where infectious agent, vectors and suitable rodents exist simultaneously. Occupational infection is restricted mainly to adult workers (males more than females) who frequent overgrown terrain or other mite-infested areas, such as forest clearings, reforested areas, new settlements, or even newly irrigated desert regions. Epidemics occur when susceptibles are brought into endemic areas, especially in military operations in which 20%–50% of troops have been infected within weeks or months.

4. Reservoir—Infected larval stages of trombiculid mites; *Leptotrombidium akamushi*, *L. deliensis* and related species (varying with area) are the most common vectors for humans. Infection is maintained by transovarian passage in mites.

5. Mode of transmission—Through the bite of infected larval mites; nymphs and adults do not feed on vertebrate hosts.

6. Incubation period—From 6 to 21 days, usually 10–12 days.

7. Period of communicability—No direct person-to-person transmission.

8. Susceptibility—Susceptibility is general. An attack confers prolonged immunity against the homologous strain of *O. tsutsugamushi* but only transient immunity against heterologous strains. Heterologous infection results in mild disease within a few months, but produces typical illness after a year or so. Second and even third attacks of naturally-acquired scrub typhus (usually benign or inapparent) occur among people who spend their lives in endemic areas, or who have not been completely treated (see below). No experimental vaccine has been effective.

9. Methods of control—

A. Preventive measures:

1) Prevent contact with infected mites through personal prophylaxis against the mite vector, achieved by impregnating clothes and blankets with miticidal chemicals (permethrin and benzyl benzoate) and application of mite repellents (diethyltoluamide) to exposed skin surfaces.
2) Eliminate mites from the specific sites through application of chlorinated hydrocarbons, such as lindane, dieldrin or chlordane, to ground and vegetation in environs of camps, mine buildings and other populated zones in endemic areas.
3) In a small group of volunteers in Malaysia, the administration of 7 weekly doses of doxycycline (200 mg/week in a single dose) was an effective prophylactic regimen, but doxycyline cannot be used in children less than eight years of age.

B. Control of patient, contacts and the immediate environment:

1) Report to local health authority: In selected endemic areas (clearly differentiated from murine and louse-borne typhus). In many countries, not a reportable disease, Class 3 (see *Reporting*).
2) Isolation: Not applicable.
3) Concurrent disinfection: Not applicable.
4) Quarantine: Not applicable.
5) Immunization of contacts: Not applicable.
6) Investigation of contacts and source of infection: None (see 9C).

7) Specific treatment: One of the tetracyclines orally in a loading dose, followed by divided doses daily until patient is afebrile (average 30 hours). Chloramphenicol is equally effective and should be given if tetracyclines are contraindicated (see section I, 9B7). NB tetracycline and doxycyline cannot be used in children less than eight years of age. If treatment is started within the first 3 days of illness, recrudescence is likely unless another course of antibiotic is given after an interval of 6 days. In Malaysia single doses of doxycycline (5 mg/kg) were effective when given on the seventh day, and in the Pescadores Islands (China, province of Taiwan) when given on the fifth day; earlier administration was associated with some relapses. Azithromycin and rifampicin have also been used successfully in pregnant patients.

C. *Epidemic measures:* Rigorously employ procedures described in this section, 9A1–9A2 above, in the affected area; daily observation of all people at risk for fever and appearance of primary lesions; institute treatment on first indication of illness.

D. *Disaster implications:* Only if refugee centers are sited in or near a "typhus island."

E. *International measures:* WHO Collaborating Centres provide support as required. More information can be found at:

<http://www.who.int/collaboratingcentres/database/en/>

WARTS, VIRAL ICD-9 078.1; ICD-10 B07
(Verruca vulgaris, Common wart, Condyloma acuminatum, Papilloma venereum)

1. **Identification**—A viral disease manifested by diverse skin and mucous membrane lesions. These include:

- The common wart, a circumscribed, hyperkeratotic, rough-textured, painless papule, varying in size from a pinhead to large masses.
- Filiform warts, elongated, pointed, delicate lesions that may reach 1 cm in length.
- Laryngeal papillomas on vocal cords and the epiglottis in children and adults.
- Flat warts, smooth, slightly elevated, usually multiple lesions varying in size from 1 mm to 1 cm.
- Venereal warts (condyloma acuminatum), cauliflower-like fleshy growths, most often seen in moist areas in and around the genitalia,

around the anus and within the anal canal, which must be differentiated from condyloma lata of secondary syphilis.

- Flat papillomas of the cervix.
- Plantar warts, flat, hyperkeratotic and often painful lenous of lesions of the plantar surface of the feet.

Both laryngeal papillomas and genital warts have occasionally become malignant. The warts in epidermodysplasia verruciformis occur usually on the torso and upper extremities, usually appearing in the first decade of life; they often undergo malignant transformation to squamous cell carcinomas in young adulthood.

The diagnosis is usually based on the typical lesion. If there is doubt, the lesion should be excised and examined histologically.

2. Infectious agent—Human papillomavirus (HPV) of the papovavirus group of DNA viruses (the human wart viruses). At least 70 HPV types have been associated with specific manifestations, and more than 20 types of HPV can infect the genital tract. Most genital HPV infections are asymptomatic, subclinical, or unrecognized. Visible genital warts are usually caused by HPV types 6 or 11: they can also cause warts on the uterine cervix and in the vagina, urethra, and anus, and are sometimes symptomatic. Other HPV types in the anogenital region, types 16, 18, 31, 33, and 35, have been strongly associated with cervical dysplasia; they have been associated also with vulvar, penile, and anal squamous intraepithelial neoplasia (i.e. squamous cell carcinoma in situ, bowenoid papulosis, erythroplasia of Queyrat, or Bowen disease of the genitalia). Type 7 is associated with warts in meat handlers and veterinarians. Types 5 and 8 are associated with epidermodysplasia verruciformis.

3. Occurrence—Worldwide.

4. Reservoir—Humans.

5. Mode of transmission—Usually through direct contact. Warts may be auto-inoculated, such as by razors in shaving; contaminated floors are frequently incriminated as the source of infection. Condyloma acuminatum is usually sexually transmitted; laryngeal papillomata in children are probably transmitted during passage of the infant through the birth canal. The viral types in the genital and respiratory tracts are the same.

6. Incubation period—About 2–3 months; range is 1–20 months.

7. Period of communicability—Unknown, probably at least as long as visible lesions persist.

8. Susceptibility—Common and flat warts are most frequently seen in young children, genital warts in sexually active young adults, and plantar warts in school-age children and teenagers. The incidence of warts is increased in immunosuppressed patients.

9. **Methods of control—**

   A. *Preventive measures:* Avoid direct contact with lesions on another person.

   B. *Control of patient, contacts and the immediate environment:*

      1) Report to local health authority: None, Class 5 (see *Reporting*).
      2) Isolation: Not applicable.
      3) Concurrent disinfection: Not applicable.
      4) Quarantine: Not applicable.
      5) Immunization of contacts: Not applicable.
      6) Investigation of contacts and source of infection: Sexual contacts of patients with venereal warts should be examined and treated if indicated.
      7) Specific treatment: Warts usually regress spontaneously within months to years. Treatment of the affected individual will decrease the amount of wart virus available for transmission. If treatment is indicated, use freezing with liquid nitrogen for lesions on most of the body surface; salicylic acid plasters and curettage for plantar warts; and 10%–25% podophyllin in tincture of benzoin, trichloroacetic acid or liquid nitrogen for readily accessible genital warts—except in pregnant females. For widespread genital lesions, 5-fluorouracil has been helpful. Intralesional recombinant interferon alpha-2b has been effective in treatment of condyloma acuminatum, and is approved for this use. Surgical removal or laser treatment is required for laryngeal papillomata. Cesarean section may be considered if genital papillomatosis is very extensive.
      8) Microscopic examination of cells (Papanicolaou smears) is an effective method for detecting cellular abnormalities associated with malignancy in women. Surgical intervention for cervical cancer is curative if the intervention is done early in the disease. See also the section on Vaccination in the *Cervical Cancer* section of the *Malignant neoplasms associated with infectious agents* chapter.

   C. *Epidemic measures:* Usually a sporadic disease.

   D. *Disaster implications:* None.

   E. *International measures:* None.

YAWS
(Framboesia tropica)

ICD-9 102; ICD-10 A66

[CCDM19: Editorial Board]
[CCDM18: G. Antal]

1. Identification—A chronic relapsing nonvenereal treponematosis, characterized by highly contagious, primary and secondary cutaneous lesions and non-contagious, tertiary/late destructive lesions. The typical initial lesion (mother yaw) is a papilloma on the face or extremities (usually the leg), persisting for weeks or months, and painless unless secondarily infected. This proliferates slowly and may form a framboesial (raspberry) lesion, or undergo ulceration (ulceropapilloma). Secondary disseminated or satellite papillomata and/or papules and squamous macules appear before or shortly after healing of the initial lesion in successive crops, often accompanied by periostitis of the long bones (saber shin) and fingers (polydactylitis), with mild constitutional symptoms. In the dry season, papillomatous crops are usually restricted to the moist skinfolds and papules/macular lesions predominate. Painful and usually disabling papillomata and hyperkeratosis on palms and soles may appear in early and in late stages. Lesions heal spontaneously; relapses may occur after periods of latency.

The late stage, with destructive lesions of skin and bone, occurs in about 10%–20% of untreated patients, usually 5 or more years after infection. Unlike what happens in syphilis, the brain, eyes, heart, aorta and abdominal organs are not involved. Congenital transmission does not occur; the infection is rarely if ever fatal, but can be very disfiguring and disabling. Diagnosis is confirmed through darkfield or direct FA microscopic examination of exudates from primary or secondary lesions. Nontreponemal serological tests for syphilis— e.g. VDRL (Venereal Disease Research Laboratory) and RPR (rapid plasma reagin)— become reactive during the initial stage, remain so during the early infection, and tend to become non-reactive after many years of latency, even in the absence of specific treatment; in some patients, they remain reactive at low titer for life. Treponemal serological tests—e.g. FTA-ABS (fluorescent treponemal antibody absorbed) and MHA-TP (microhemagglutination assay for antibody to Treponema pallidum)—usually remain reactive for life despite adequate treatment.

2. Infectious agent—*Treponema pallidum*, subsp. *pertenue*, a spirochete.

3. Occurrence—Predominantly a disease of children living in rural humid tropical areas; more frequent in males. Mass penicillin treatment campaigns in the 1950s and 1960s dramatically decreased worldwide prevalence but yaws has re-emerged in parts of equatorial and western Africa, with scattered foci of infection persisting in Latin America, the Caribbean islands, southeastern Asia and some South Pacific islands. In

September 2006, India declared yaws elimination, with zero cases reported since 2004. Yaws should be considered in the evaluation of a reactive syphilis serology in any person who has emigrated from an endemic area.

4. Reservoir—Humans and possibly higher primates.

5. Mode of transmission—Principally through direct contact with exudates of early skin lesions of infected people. Indirect transmission through contamination from scratching, skin-piercing articles and flies on open wounds is probable, but of unknown importance. Climate influences the morphology, distribution and infectiousness of the early lesions, both being greater in warm and humid regions.

6. Incubation period—From 2 weeks to 3 months.

7. Period of communicability—Variable; may extend intermittently over several years when moist lesions are present. The infectious agent is not usually found in late destructive lesions.

8. Susceptibility—No evidence of natural or racial resistance. Infection results in immunity to reinfection and may offer some protection against infection by other pathogenic treponemes.

9. Methods of control—

  A. Preventive measures: The following apply to yaws and other nonvenereal treponematoses. Although present techniques cannot differentiate the infectious agents, differences observed among clinical syndromes are unlikely to result from epidemiological or environmental factors alone.

  1) General health promotion measures; health education of the public about the value of better sanitation, including liberal use of soap and water and the importance of improving social and economic conditions over a period of years to reduce incidence. Improve access to health services.
  2) Organize intensive control activities on a community level suitable to the local problem; examine entire populations, and treat patients with active or latent disease. Treatment of asymptomatic contacts is beneficial, and WHO recommends treating the entire population when the prevalence rate for active disease is above 10%; if prevalence is 5%–10%, treat patients, contacts and all children below 15; if 5%, treat active cases plus household and other contacts. Periodic clinical resurveys and continuous surveillance are essential for success.

3) Serological surveys for latent cases, particularly in children, to prevent relapses and development of infective lesions that maintain the disease in the community.
4) Provide facilities for early diagnosis and treatment as part of a plan in which mass control campaigns (See 9A2) are eventually consolidated into permanent local health services.
5) Treat disfiguring and incapacitating late manifestations.

B. Control of patient, contacts and the immediate environment:

1) Report to local health authority: In selected endemic areas; in many countries not a reportable disease, Class 3 (see *Reporting*). Differentiation of venereal and nonvenereal treponematoses, with proper reporting of each, has particular importance in the evaluation and consolidation of mass campaigns.
2) Isolation: Avoid intimate contact and contamination of the environment until lesions are healed.
3) Concurrent disinfection: Care in disposal of discharges and articles contaminated therewith.
4) Quarantine: Not applicable.
5) Immunization of contacts: Not applicable.
6) Investigation of contacts and source of infection: Treat all family contacts; those with no active disease should be regarded as latent cases. In low-prevalence areas, treat all active cases, all children and close contacts of infectious cases.
7) Specific treatment: Penicillin. For patients 10 years or older with active disease and contacts, a single injection of benzathine penicillin G, 1.2 million units IM; 0.6 million units for patients under 10 years.

C. Epidemic measures: Active mass treatment programs in areas of high prevalence. Essential features are:

1) Examining a high percentage of the population through field surveys.
2) Extending treatment of active cases to family and community contacts based on the demonstrated prevalence of active yaws.
3) Surveys at yearly intervals for 1–3 years, as part of the established rural public health activities of the country.

D. Disaster implications: None observed, but potentially a risk in refugee or displaced populations in endemic areas without hygienic facilities.

E. International measures: To protect countries against risk of reinfection where active mass treatment programs are in progress, adjacent countries in the endemic area should institute suitable measures against yaws. Movement of infected people across frontiers may require supervision (see *Syphilis*, section I, 9E). WHO Collaborating Centres provide support as required. More information can be found at:

<http://www.who.int/collaboratingcentres/database/en/>

YELLOW FEVER   ICD-9 060; ICD-10 A95
[CCDM19: E. Staples]
[CCDM18: C. Roth, R. Shope]

1. Identification—Acute infectious viral disease of short duration and varying severity. The mildest cases may be clinically indeterminate; typical attacks are characterized by sudden onset of fever, chills, headache, backache, generalized muscle pain, prostration, nausea and vomiting. The pulse may be slow and weak out of proportion to the elevated temperature (Faget sign). Leukopenia appears early and is most pronounced about the fifth day. Most infections resolve at this stage. Approximately 15% of cases progress after a brief remission of hours to a day into the ominous stage of intoxication, manifested by jaundice and hemorrhagic symptoms including epistaxis, gingival bleeding, hematemesis (coffee-ground or black), and melaena. Elevated liver enzymes, abnormalities in clotting factors, albuminuria, and anuria may occur as a result of liver and renal failure. The overall case-fatality rate is 20%–50%.

Laboratory diagnosis is through isolation of virus from blood by inoculation (suckling mice, mosquitoes or cell cultures); through demonstration of viral antigen in the blood by ELISA or in tissues, especially liver, by use of labeled specific antibodies; and through demonstration of viral RNA in blood and tissue by PCR or hybridization probes. PCR or hybridization probes can also be used to distinguish acute infections with yellow fever virus from recent vaccination. Serological diagnosis includes demonstrating specific IgM in early sera or a rise in titer of specific antibodies in paired acute and convalescent sera. Demonstration of a rise in IgM level in the 2nd serum is also preferable. Serological cross-reactions occur with other flaviviruses.

2. Infectious agent—The virus of yellow fever, of the genus *Flavivirus* and family Flaviviridae.

3. Occurrence—Yellow fever has three transmission cycles: a sylvatic or jungle cycle that involves *Aedes* or *Haemagogus* mosquitoes and nonhuman primates; an intermediate cycle involving humans and various *Aedes spp* in savannah regions of Africa; and an urban cycle involving humans and mainly *Aedes aegypti* mosquitoes. Sylvatic transmission is restricted to tropical regions of Africa and Latin America, where a few hundred cases occur annually, most often among occupationally exposed young adult males in forested or transitional areas. The intermediate transmission cycle involves humans in humid or semi-humid areas of Africa, where infected mosquitoes feed on both monkeys and humans, resulting in small-scale epidemics. Historically, urban yellow fever occurred in main cities of the Americas, causing large epidemics. At time of writing in early 2008, a large urban outbreak of yellow fever has not been seen in over 50 years in the Americas—though a small urban outbreak was believed to occur in Bolivia during 1999. In Africa, urban outbreaks still occur. Re-infestation with *Ae. aegypti* may put many cities at risk of renewed urban yellow fever transmission.

In Africa, the endemic zone is located between 15°N and 10°S latitude, and encompasses 33 countries with a combined population of over 500 million. Nine countries in the tropical region of South America and the Caribbean islands also have endemic disease. While no recent cases have been identified, yellow fever disease and transmission has been documented previously in Europe and North and Central America. There is no evidence that yellow fever has ever been present in Asia.

4. **Reservoir**—In urban areas, humans and *Aedes* mosquitoes; in forest areas, vertebrates other than humans, mainly nonhuman primates and possibly marsupials, and forest mosquitoes. Trans-ovarial transmission of the infection in mosquitoes has been documented, but its contribution to maintenance of infection is unknown. Humans have no essential role in transmission of jungle yellow fever, but are the primary amplifying host in the urban cycle.

5. **Mode of transmission**—In urban and certain rural areas, the bite of infective *Aedes spp.* mosquitoes. In South American forests, the bite of several species of forest mosquitoes, *Haemagogus spp.* and *Sabethes spp.* In Africa, *Ae. africanus* is the principal vector in the monkey population, while semi-domestic *Aedes spp.*, such as *Ae. furcifer, Ae. luteocephalus,* and *Ae. simpsoni complex,* transmit the virus from monkeys to humans. *Ae. simpsoni* was also believed to be responsible as the person-to-person vector during large epidemics in Ethiopia. While *Ae. albopictus* is a relatively inefficient vector for yellow fever transmission, its recent territorial expansion raises concern about this species as a potential bridging vector for sylvatic and urban cycles of yellow fever.

6. **Incubation period**—From 3 to 6 days.

7. **Period of communicability**—Blood of patients is infective for mosquitoes shortly before onset of fever and for the first 3–5 days of illness; however the virus has been found in the blood up to 17 days after illness onset. The disease is highly communicable where many susceptible people and abundant vector mosquitoes coexist; it is not communicable through contact or common vehicles. The extrinsic incubation period in *Ae. aegypti* is 9–12 days at the usual tropical temperatures. Once infected, mosquitoes remain so for life.

8. Susceptibility—Recovery from yellow fever is followed by lasting immunity; second attacks are unknown. Mild unapparent infections are common in endemic areas. Transient passive immunity in infants born to immune mothers may persist for up to 6 months. In natural infections, antibodies appear in the blood within the first week.

9. Methods of control—

A. Preventive measures:

1) Institute a program for active immunization of all people 9 months or older who are at risk of becoming infected due to residence, occupation or travel. A single subcutaneous injection of a vaccine containing viable attenuated yellow fever 17D strain virus, cultivated in chick embryo, is effective in >95% of recipients. Antibodies appear 7–10 days after immunization and may persist for at least 30–35 years, though immunization or re-immunization within 10 years is required by the *International Health Regulations* for travel from endemic areas.

Of the 44 countries identified as having endemic yellow fever, 33 are using yellow fever vaccine in national immunization schedules, with 43% coverage. Since 1989, WHO has recommended that at-risk countries in the endemic-epidemic belt of Africa incorporate yellow fever vaccine into their routine childhood immunization programs (EPI). Of the 33 at-risk African countries, 22 have introduced YF in EPI; overall yellow fever EPI immunization coverage was 66% (range of 30% to 95%) in 2006, up from 22% in 2002. The vaccine can be given any time after 6 months of age, and can be administered with other antigens such as measles vaccine. The vaccine is contraindicated in the first 4 months of life, and should be considered for those aged 4–9 months only if the risk of exposure is judged to exceed the risk of vaccine-associated encephalitis, the main complication in this age group. The vaccine is not recommended during pregnancy or breastfeeding unless the risk of disease is believed to be higher than the theoretical risk to the fetus or infant. There is no evidence of major malformations occurring in the fetus secondary to the vaccine. However, one study observed lower rates of maternal seroconversion; checking antibody titers or re-immunizing women after delivery or termination may therefore be warranted. There is insufficient evidence to permit a definitive statement on whether the vaccine would pose a risk for humans infected with HIV. Limited data suggest the vaccine may be tolerated in individuals with asymptomatic disease, but the vaccine is not currently recommended for individuals with symptomatic HIV, and a waiver clause therefore applies.

Severe adverse events have been observed following yellow fever vaccination, including anaphylaxis, neurotropic disease, and viscerotropic disease. With the later two conditions, the vaccine virus replicates either in the brain or other organs, such as the liver, to cause disease. Two possible risk factors for developing a severe reaction are advanced age and diseases of the thymus gland. Proper surveillance and support for adverse events following immunization should be part of any standard vaccine program or large vaccination campaign.

2) For urban yellow fever eradicate or control the vector; immunization when indicated.

3) Sylvan or jungle yellow fever, transmitted by *Haemagogus* and forest species of *Aedes*, is best controlled through immunization, which is recommended for all people in rural communities whose occupation brings them into forests in yellow fever areas, and for people who intend to visit those areas. Protective clothing, bednets and repellents are advised for those not immunized.

B. Control of patient, contacts and the immediate environment:

1) Report to local health authority: Events involving yellow fever cases are required to be assessed at the national level for potential notification to WHO under the *International Health Regulations*. See *Reporting*.

2) Isolation: Blood and body fluid precautions. Prevent access of mosquitoes to patient for at least 5 days after onset, by screening the sickroom, spraying quarters with residual insecticide, and using insecticide-treated bednets.

3) Concurrent disinfection: The homes of patients and all houses in the vicinity should be sprayed promptly with an effective insecticide.

4) Quarantine: Not applicable.

5) Immunization of contacts: Family and other contacts and neighbors not previously immunized should be immunized promptly.

6) Investigation of contacts and source of infection: Inquire about all contacts and all places, including forested areas, visited by the patient 3–6 days before onset, to locate focus of yellow fever; observe all people visiting that focus. Search patient's premises and places of work or visits over the preceding several days for mosquitoes capable of transmit-

ting infection; apply effective insecticide. Investigate mild febrile illnesses and unexplained deaths suggesting yellow fever.

7) Specific treatment: None.

C. Epidemic measures:

1) Urban or *Ae. aegypti*-transmitted yellow fever:

   a) Mass immunization, beginning with people most exposed and those living in *Ae. aegypti*-infested areas who have not been vaccinated against yellow fever in the last 10 years.

   b) Eliminate or treat all actual and potential breeding places.

   c) Spraying the inside of all houses in the community with insecticides has shown promise for controlling urban epidemics.

2) Jungle or sylvan yellow fever:

   a) Immediately immunize all people living in or near forested areas or entering such areas.

   b) Ensure that non-immunized individuals avoid those tracts of forest where infection has been localized, and that those just immunized avoid those areas for 7–10 days after immunization.

3) In regions where yellow fever may occur, a diagnostic post-mortem examination service should be organized to collect small specimens of tissues, especially liver, from fatal febrile illnesses of 10 days duration or less, provided biological safety can be ensured. Facilities for viral isolation or serological confirmation are necessary to establish diagnosis, since histopathological changes in the liver are not pathognomonic.

4) In Central and South America, confirmed deaths of howler and spider monkeys in the forest are presumptive evidence of the presence of yellow fever. Confirmation by the histopathological examination of livers of moribund or recently dead monkeys, or by virus isolation, is highly desirable. In Africa, monkeys are rarely symptomatic and rarely die from infections with yellow fever virus, and thus cannot be used to indicate the presence of yellow fever.

5) Immunity surveys through neutralization tests of wild primates captured in forested areas are useful in defining enzootic areas. Serological surveys of human populations are not useful where yellow fever vaccine has been widely used,

and can be difficult to interpret in places with other endemic flaviviruses.

D. Disaster implications: Mass vaccination may be considered if an epidemic is feared.

E. International measures:

1) Yellow fever cases are no longer required to be reported to the WHO under the newly updated *International Health Regulations* (IHR, 2005). However, if a case of yellow fever is felt to constitute a public health emergency, it should be reported to the WHO within 24 hours, by the most efficient means of communication available. To be considered a public health emergency, the event should meet at least two of the following criteria:
   • Public health impact of the event is serious.
   • The event is unusual or unexpected.
   • There is a significant risk of international spread.
   • There is a significant risk of international travel or trade restrictions.

2) Measures applicable to ships, aircraft and land transport arriving from areas with ongoing yellow fever transmission are no longer specified in the IHR (2005). There are, however, applicable guidelines listed in the IHR for any areas with ongoing disease transmission.

3) Animal quarantine: Due to the risk of nonhuman primates carrying zoonotic pathogens, such as yellow fever, the World Organisation of Animal Health (OIE) recommends in the Terrestrial Animal Health Code (2007) that in captive-bred nonhuman primates be held in quarantine for 30 days, and nonhuman primates captured from the wild be held in quarantine for 12 weeks.

4) International travel: A valid international certificate of immunization against yellow fever is required by many countries for entry of travelers coming from or going to recognized yellow fever zones of Africa and South America; otherwise, quarantine measures are applicable for up to 6 days. WHO recommends immunization for all travelers to areas other than major cities in countries where the disease occurs in humans or is assumed to be present in nonhuman primates. The *International Certificate of Vaccination against Yellow Fever* is valid for 10 years from 10 days after date of immunization; if re-immunization occurs within that period, it is valid 10 years from date of re-immunization.

YERSINIOSIS ICD-9 027.8

INTESTINAL YERSINIOSIS ICD-10 A04.6
EXTRAINTESTINAL YERSINIOSIS ICD-10 A28.2
[CCDM19: P. Griffin]
[CCDM18: E. Carniel]

1. **Identification**—Infection caused by enteropathogenic *Yersinia*, typically manifested by acute febrile diarrhea with abdominal pain (especially in young children). Other clinical manifestations (extraintestinal or otherwise) include acute mesenteric lymphadenitis mimicking appendicitis (especially in older children and adults) and systemic infections. The most common post-infectious complications are erythema nodosum (about 10% of adults, particularly women) and reactive arthritis. Bloody diarrhea occurs in up to one-fourth of patients with *Yersinia* enteritis; diarrhea may be absent in up to a third of *Y. enterocolitica* infections. Ileitis is the characteristic lesion induced by *Y. enterocolitica*. *Y. pseudotuberculosis* causes an acute mesenteric lymphadenitis, clinically characterized by an appendicitis-like syndrome, sometimes with diarrhea. Specific *Y. pseudotuberculosis* syndromes (Izumi fever, Far East scarlet-like fever) have been reported in Japan and the Russian Federation.

Diagnosis is usually made through stool culture. Cefsulodin irgasan novobiocin (CIN) medium is highly selective and should be used if there is reason to suspect infection with *Yersinia*; it permits identification in 24 hours at 28°C (78.4°F). The organisms may be recovered on usual enteric media if precautions are taken to prevent overgrowth of fecal flora. Cold enrichment in buffered saline at 4°C (39°F) for 2–3 weeks can be used, but this procedure usually enhances the isolation of non-pathogenic species. *Yersinia* can be isolated from blood with standard commercial blood culture media. Serological diagnosis is possible (agglutination test or ELISA), but availability is generally limited to research settings.

2. **Infectious agents**—Gram-negative bacilli. *Y. pseudotuberculosis* has 15 serotypes with 10 subtypes; over 90% of human and animal infections are due to O-group I. *Y. enterocolitica* has over 50 serotypes and 5 biotypes, many of them non-pathogenic. Strains pathogenic for humans are those of biotypes 1B, 2, 3 and 4; they are pyrazinamidase negative. Biotype 1A strains are non-pathogenic, whereas the very rare strains of biotype 5 have been isolated from hares. The distribution of pathogenic *Y. enterocolitica* varies in different geographic areas; biotype 4 (serotype O3) accounts for most of the cases in Europe, followed by bioserotypes 2 (serotypes O9 and O5, 27). Biotype 1B strains were responsible for most outbreaks in the USA, but bioserotype 4/O3 emerged in the 1990s and is now the most common type there.

3. **Occurrence**—Worldwide. *Y. pseudotuberculosis* is primarily a zoonotic disease of wild and domesticated birds and mammals, with

humans as incidental hosts. In some countries such as Japan or the Russian Federation, *Y. pseudotuberculosis* is the main cause of human yersiniosis. Globally, *Y. enterocolitica* is the species most commonly associated with human infection, causing up to 1%-3% of acute enteritis in some areas. This species has been recovered from a wide variety of asymptomatic animals. The most important documented source of *Y. enterocolitica* 4 (serotype O3) infection is pork, as the pharynx of pigs may be heavily colonized by *Y. enterocolitica*. Approximately two-thirds of *Y. enterocolitica* cases occur among infants and children; three-quarters of *Y. pseudotuberculosis* cases are aged 5 to 20. Human cases have been reported in association with disease in household pets, particularly puppies and kittens.

The highest isolation rates have been reported during the cold season in temperate climates, including northern Europe (especially Scandinavia), North America, and temperate regions of South America. Vehicles implicated in outbreaks attributed to *Y. enterocolitica* include soybean cake (tofu) and pork chitterlings (large intestines) in the USA, and the feeding of raw pork to infants in Europe. Contamination through milk (including pasteurized milk, where post-pasteurization contamination is more likely than resistance of the agent to the pasteurization process) is less common. Studies in Europe suggest that many cases are related to ingestion of raw or undercooked pork. Since 20% of infections in older children and adolescents can mimic acute appendicitis, outbreaks can sometimes be recognized by local increases in appendectomies.

4. Reservoir—Animals. The pig is the main reservoir for *Y. enterocolitica* 4 (serotype O3). Asymptomatic pharyngeal carriage is common in swine, especially in winter, and bioserotype 2 (serotype O9) has been isolated from ovine, bovine and caprine origins. *Y. pseudotuberculosis* is widespread among many avian and mammalian hosts, particularly rodents and other small mammals.

5. Mode of transmission—Fecal-oral transmission through consumption of contaminated food or water, or through contact with infected people or animals. *Y. enterocolitica* has been isolated from many foods; pathogenic strains most commonly from raw pork or pork products. *Y. enterocolitica* can multiply under refrigeration and micro-aerophilic conditions, and there is an increased risk of infection by *Y. enterocolitica* if uncured meat that was stored in plastic bags is undercooked. *Y. enterocolitica* (usually non-pathogenic strains) has been recovered from natural bodies of water. Nosocomial transmission has occurred, as has transmission by transfusion of stored blood from donors who were asymptomatic or had mild GI illness.

6. Incubation period—Probably 3-7 days, generally under 10 days.

7. Period of communicability—Secondary transmission appears rare. There is fecal shedding at least as long as symptoms exist, usually for

2-3 weeks. Untreated cases may excrete the organism for 2-3 months. Prolonged asymptomatic carriage has been reported in both children and adults.

8. Susceptibility—Gastroenterocolitis (diarrhea) is more severe in children, post-infectious arthritis more severe in adolescents and older adults. Male adolescents are particularly prone to infection with *Y. pseudo-tuberculosis*; *Y. enterocolitica* equally attacks men and women. Reactive arthritis and Reiter syndrome occur more often in people with the HLA-B27 genetic type. Septicemia occurs most often among people with iron overload (hemochromatosis) or immunosuppression (through illness or treatment).

9. Methods of control—

    A. Preventive measures:

        1) Prepare meat and other foods in a sanitary manner. Avoid eating raw pork, and pasteurize milk. Irradiation of meat is effective.

        2) Wash hands prior to food handling and eating, after handling raw pork, and after contact with animals.

        3) Protect water supplies from animal and human feces; purify appropriately.

        4) Control rodents and birds (for *Y. pseudotuberculosis*).

        5) Dispose of human, dog and cat feces in a sanitary manner.

        6) During the slaughtering of pigs, the head and neck should be removed from the body to avoid contaminating meat from the heavily-colonized pharynx.

    B. Control of patient, contacts and the immediate environment:

        1) Report to local health authority: Case reporting obligatory in many countries, Class 2 (see *Reporting*).

        2) Isolation: Enteric precautions for patients in hospitals. Remove persons with diarrhea from food handling, patient care, and occupations involving care of young children.

        3) Concurrent disinfection: Of feces. In communities with modern and adequate sewage disposal systems, feces can be discharged directly into sewers without preliminary disinfection.

        4) Quarantine: Not applicable.

        5) Immunization of contacts: Not applicable.

        6) Investigation of contacts and source of infection: A search for unrecognized cases and convalescent carriers among contacts is indicated only when a common-source exposure is suspected.

        7) Specific treatment: Organisms are sensitive to many antibiotics, but are generally resistant to penicillin and its semi-

synthetic derivatives. Treatment may be helpful for GI symptoms, and is definitely indicated for septicemia and other invasive disease. Agents of choice against *Y. enterocolitica* are the aminoglycosides (septicemia only) and trimethoprimsulfamethoxazole. Newer quinolones such as ciprofloxacin are highly effective. Both *Y. enterocolitica* and *Y. pseudotuberculosis* are usually sensitive to tetracyclines.

C. Epidemic measures:

1) Any group of cases of acute gastroenteritis or cases suggestive of appendicitis must be reported at once to the local health authority, even in the absence of specific causal identification.

2) Investigate general sanitation and search for common-source vehicle; pay attention to consumption of (or possible cross-contamination with) raw or undercooked pork; look for evidence of close contacts with pet dogs, cats and other domestic animals.

D. Disaster implications: None.

E. International measures: None.

ZYGOMYCOSIS
(Phycomycosis)
[CCDM19: M. Brandt]
[CCDM18: L. Severo]

Zygomycosis is a term that encompasses a wide array of infections caused by rapidly growing molds of the class Zygomycetes. The term usually refers to rapidly progressive, invasive infections due to fungi of the order Mucorales (also known as "mucormycosis"), although it can also be used to refer to infections caused by fungi within the order Entomophthorales. Infections due to Mucorales and infections due to Entomophthorales (conidiobolomycosis and basidiobolomycosis) present distinct epidemiological, clinical and pathological forms. The latter infections, for example, are typically subcutaneous and slowly progressive. Histopathologically, while infections due to Mucorales are characterized by fungal angioinvasion and tissue infarction, infection due to Entomophthorales usually results in a chronic, eosinophilic inflammatory response without angioinvasion. The Splendore-Hoeppli reaction may be seen around fungal hyphae in tissue infection due to Entomophthorales.

INFECTIONS DUE TO
MUCORALES   ICD-9 117.7; ICD-10 B46.0-B46.5

1. **Identification**—Infections caused by fungi of the order Mucorales result in disease that is typically rapidly progressive, destructive, and associated with high mortality. These fungi have an affinity for blood vessels, and cause thrombosis, infarction and tissue necrosis. The mycosis has an acute or sub-acute course. In debilitated persons it is the most fulminant fungal infection known. The 4 main systemic forms of the disease are the rhinocerebral, pulmonary, gastrointestinal and disseminated types. Cutaneous infection may also occur. The underlying disease influences the portal of entry of the fungus. Rhinocerebral disease represents one-third to one-half of all cases, and usually presents as nasal or paranasal sinus infection, most often in patients with poorly controlled diabetes mellitus. Necrosis of the turbinates, perforation of the hard palate, necrosis of the cheek or orbital cellulitis, proptosis and ophthalmoplegia may occur. Infection may penetrate to the internal carotid artery or extend directly to the brain and cause infarction. Pulmonary zygomycosis appears to occur most commonly among hematological malignancy patients with neutropenia and recipients of hematopoietic stem cell transplants. In the pulmonary form of disease, the fungus causes thrombosis of pulmonary blood vessels and infarcts of the lung. Gastrointestinal zygomycosis has been associated with severe malnutrition and has been reported to occur in pre-term neonates. In the gastrointestinal form, mucosal ulcers or thrombosis and gangrene of stomach or bowel wall may occur. Disseminated zygomycosis usually occurs in severely immunosuppressed patients, such as those with profound neutropenia and hematological malignancy. Deferoxamine therapy has been associated with disseminated zygomycosis. Nosocomial cases have been reported.

Establishing the diagnosis of zygomycosis can be challenging. Clinical manifestations in immunosuppressed hosts may be similar to those caused by other invasive mold infections, such as aspergillosis. Definitive diagnosis is usually made through microscopic demonstration of broad, "ribbon-like," non-septate or rarely septate hyphae in tissue or body fluids with an accompanying positive culture. Wet preparations and smears may be examined. Cultures alone are not diagnostic, because fungi of the order Mucorales are found in the environment. However, in an immunosuppressed patient with a compatible clinical syndrome, a positive culture for a Zygomycete should be taken very seriously. Similarly, the diagnosis may be difficult to establish based solely upon histopathology, since it may be difficult to appreciate the distinctive characteristics of Zygomycete fungal hyphae that differentiate them from those of other molds, such as *Aspergillus* spp., in tissue.

2. **Infectious agents**—*Rhizopus* is the genus most commonly implicated in human disease. One of the most common *Rhizopus* species causing zygomycosis is *R. arrhizus*. Other genera known to cause human

ZYGOMYCOSIS / 695

disease include *Mucor; Rhizomucor; Absidia; Cunninghamella; Apophysomyces; Saksenaea;* and *Syncephalastrum.*

3. Occurrence—Worldwide. Incidence may be increasing because of longer survival of patients with immunosuppression due to disease or medication, with diabetes mellitus and certain blood dyscrasias (especially acute leukemia and aplastic anemia), and who are treated with deferoxamine for aluminum or iron overload when receiving chronic hemodialysis for renal failure. Some institutions have reported increasing numbers of cases among hematopoietic stem cell transplant recipients in association with the use of voriconazole, a broad-spectrum azole antifungal that has potent activity against *Aspergillus* spp., but not against the Zygomycetes.

4. Reservoir—Members of the order Mucorales are common saprophytes in the environment.

5. Mode of transmission—Inhalation or ingestion of fungal spores by susceptible individuals. Direct inoculation in IV drug users and at sites of IV catheters and cutaneous burns may occur.

6. Incubation period—Unknown. Fungus spreads rapidly in susceptible tissues.

7. Period of communicability—No direct person-to-person or animal-to-person transmission.

8. Susceptibility—The rarity of infection in healthy individuals despite the abundance of Mucorales in the environment indicates natural resistance. Corticosteroid use, metabolic acidosis, deferoxamine and immunosuppressive treatment predispose to infection. Malnutrition predisposes to the gastrointestinal form.

9. Methods of control—

    A. Preventive measures: Optimal clinical control of diabetes mellitus to avoid acidosis.

    B. Control of patient, contacts and the immediate environment:

        1) Report to local health authority: Official report not ordinarily justifiable, Class 5 (see *Reporting*).
        2) Isolation: Not applicable.
        3) Concurrent disinfection: Ordinary cleanliness. Terminal cleaning.
        4) Quarantine: Not applicable.
        5) Immunization of contacts: Not applicable.
        6) Investigation of contacts and source of infection: Ordinarily not beneficial in sporadic cases, due to the ubiquity of these fungi in the environment. However, outbreaks due to contaminated medical supplies have occurred.

7) Specific treatment: Prompt initiation of a lipid formulation of amphotericin B and in some cases surgical resection of infected tissue are essential, given the high mortality rate. Control of the predisposing underlying condition (i.e. glucose control and treatment of acidosis in diabetics, reduction of immunosuppression) is also important. A newer antifungal, posaconazole, has been shown to be effective as salvage treatment in some patients who do not tolerate amphotericin B, or whose disease is refractory to amphotericin B. Hyperbaric oxygen has been used as adjunctive therapy, but its benefit has not been established.

C. *Epidemic measures:* Generally a sporadic disease. However, outbreaks have occurred in health care settings and have been linked to contaminated medical supplies.

D. *Disaster implications:* None.

E. *International measures:* None.

INFECTIONS DUE TO ENTOMOPHTHORALES

ICD-9 117.7;
ICD-10 B46.0-B46.5

Entomophthoromycosis includes two histopathologically identical entities: basidiobolomycosis and conidiobolomycosis. These two infections have been recognized principally in tropical and subtropical areas of Asia, Africa and Latin America. They are not characterized by thromboses or infarction, do not usually occur in association with serious pre-existing disease or cause disseminated disease, and seldom cause death.

BASIDIOBOLOMYCOSIS

Basidiobolus ranarum causes the subcutaneous form of entomophthoromycosis, presenting as a granulomatous inflammation. The fungus is ubiquitous, occurring in decaying vegetation, soil and the gastrointestinal tract of amphibians and reptiles. The disease presents as a firm, painless and sharply circumscribed subcutaneous mass, fixed to the skin, mainly in children and adolescents, more commonly in males. Common sites of infection are the buttocks, thighs and chest. The infection may heal spontaneously. Recommended treatment is oral potassium iodide.

CONIDIOBOLOMYCOSIS

Conidiobolus coronatus, occurring in soil and decaying vegetation, causes the mucocutaneous form of entomophthoromycosis. This usually originates in the paranasal skin or nasal mucosa, and presents as nasal obstruction or swelling of the nose or adjacent structures. The lesion may spread to involve contiguous areas, such as lip, cheek, palate or pharynx. The disease is uncommon, and occurs principally in adult males. Recommended treatment is oral potassium iodide or IV amphotericin B.

For both forms of entomophthoramycosis, incubation periods and modes of transmission are unknown. Person-to-person transmission does not occur.

A few cases of a rare primary visceral form of conidiobolomycosis due to *C. incongruus* have been reported in patients (immunocompromised or not) as lung infections spreading to contiguous organs.

Abbreviations and acronyms used in
Control of Communicable Diseases Manual

AAP	=	American Academy of Pediatrics
ACIP	=	Advisory Committee on Immunization Practices (CDC)
AFB	=	acid-fast bacilli
AFP	=	acute flaccid paralysis
AHC	=	acute hemorrhagic conjunctivitis
AIDS	=	acquired immunodeficiency syndrome
ALT	=	alanine aminotransferase (was SGPT)
aP	=	acellular Pertussis [vaccine]
AST	=	aspartate aminotransferase (was SGOT)
AZT	=	azidothymidine
BCG	=	bacille Calmette-Guérin
BPF	=	Brazilian purpuric fever
BSE	=	bovine spongiform encephalitis
BSL	=	biosafety level (i.e. BSL-1, -2, -3, -4)
ca	=	circa
CAT	=	computerized axial tomography
CCDM	=	Control of Communicable Diseases Manual
CD4	=	antigen of T-helper lymphocytes
CDC	=	Centers for Disease Control and Prevention
CF	=	complement fixation
CIE	=	counterimmunoelectrophoresis
CJD	=	Creutzfeldt-Jakob disease
cm	=	centimeter
CMV	=	cytomegalovirus
CNS	=	central nervous system
CRS	=	congenital rubella syndrome
CSF	=	cerebrospinal fluid
CTF	=	Colorado tick fever
DAEC	=	diffuse-adherence *Escherichia coli*
DAT	=	dried antigen test
DEC	=	diethylcarbamazine citrate
DFA	=	direct fluorescent antibody
DHF/DSS	=	dengue hemorrhagic fever/dengue shock syndrome
DIC	=	disseminated intravascular coagulation
DNA	=	deoxyribonucleic acid
DT	=	diphtheria/tetanus vaccine
DTaP	=	diphtheria/tetanus toxoids and acellular Pertussis vaccine
DTP	=	diphtheria/tetanus toxoids and whole cell Pertussis vaccine

EAggEC	= enteroaggregative *Escherichia coli*
EBV	= Epstein-Barr virus
EEE	= eastern equine encephalitis
EEG	= electroencephalogram
e.g.	= for instance
EHEC	= enterohemorrhagic *Escherichia coli*
EIA	= enzyme immunoassay
EIEC	= enteroinvasive *Escherichia coli*
EKC	= epidemic keratoconjunctivitis
ELISA	= enzyme-linked immunosorbent assay
EM	= electron microscopy—also erythema migrans
EMB	= ethambutol
ENL	= erythema nodosum leprosum
EPEC	= enteropathogenic *Escherichia coli*
EPI	= Expanded Programme on Immunization, WHO
ERIG	= equine rabies immune globulin
ESR	= erythrocyte sedimentation rate
ETEC	= enterotoxic *Escherichia coli*
FA	= direct fluorescent or immunofluorescent antibody test
FAO	= Food and Agriculture Organization, United Nations
FEE	= far eastern equine encephalitis
G6PD	= glucose-6-phosphate dehydrogenase
GBS	= Guillain-Barré syndrome
GI	= gastrointestinal
GSS	= Gertsmann-Staussler-Scheinker syndrome
HA	= hemagglutination
HAART	= highly active antiretroviral therapy
HAI/HI	= hemagglutination inhibition
HAV	= hepatitis A virus
HBV	= hepatitis B virus
HBcAg	= hepatitis B core antigen
HBIG	= hepatitis B immunoglobulin
HBsAg	= hepatitis B surface antigen
HCC	= hepatocellular carcinoma
HCV	= hepatitis C virus
HDCV	= human diploid cell rabies vaccine
HDV	= hepatitis D virus
HEPA	= high efficiency particulate air [filters]
HEV	= hepatitis E virus
HHV	= human herpesvirus
Hib	= *Haemohilus influenzae* type b
HIV	= human immunodeficiency virus
HPV	= human papillomavirus
HRIG	= human rabies immune globulin
HSV	= herpes simplex virus
HTLV	= human T-cell lymphotropic virus

HUS	= hemolytic uremic syndrome
ICD	= International Classification of Diseases
ID	= intradermal
i.e.	= that is
IEM	= immune electron microscopy
IF	= immunofluorescent testing
IFA/IFAT	= indirect immunofluorescent antibody/assay
IHR (2005)	= International Health Regulations (2005)
IG	= immune globulin (serum)
IgA	= immunoglobulin class A
IgG	= immunoglobulin class G
IgM	= immunoglobulin class M
IM	= intramuscular
IND	= investigational new drug
INH	= isoniazid
IPV	= inactivated poliovirus vaccine
IU	= international unit
IV	= intravenous
kg	= kilogram
kGy	= kiloGray
km	= kilometer
KFD	= Kyasanur Forest disease
KSHV	= Kaposi sarcoma-associated herpesvirus
l	= liter
LA	= latex agglutination
lb	= pound [weight]
LCM	= lymphocytic choriomeningitis
LD	= lethal dose
LTBI	= latent TB infection
mEq	= milliequivalents
mg	= milligram
mIU	= milli-IU (international units)
ml	= milliliter
mm	= millimeter
MDR	= multidrug resistant
MDT	= multidrug therapy
MOTT	= *Mycobacteria* other than tuberculosis
MMR	= measles-mumps-rubella [vaccine]
MR	= measles-rubella [vaccine]
MRI	= magnetic resonance imaging
MV	= Murray Valley [fever]
NAG	= non-agglutinable [vibrio]
NTM	= nontuberculous mycobacteria
NGU	= non-gonococcal urethritis
OHF	= Omsk hemorrhagic fever
OPV	= oral poliovirus vaccine
ORS	= oral rehydration solution

OspA	= outer-surface protein A
PAHO	= Pan American Health Organization
PCECV	= purified chick embryo
PCR	= polymerase chain reaction
PE	= Powassan encephalitis
PEP	= postexposure prophylaxis
PO	= oral (*per os*)
PPD-S	= purified protein derivative-standard
ppm	= parts per million
PVRVP	= purified vero cell vaccines
PZA	= pyrazinamide
q.v.	= see
RBC	= red blood cell
RDS	= respiratory distress syndrome
RIA	= radioimmunoassay
RIF	= rifampicin
RMSF	= Rocky Mountain spotted fever
RNA	= ribonucleic acid
rOspA	= recombinant OspA
RSV	= respiratory syncytial virus
RRV-TV	= rhesus-based rotavirus vaccine
RT-PCR	= retrotranscriptase PCR
RVA	= rabies vaccine, adsorbed
RVF	= Rift Valley fever
SARS	= severe acute respiratory syndrome
SARS CoV	= SARS coronavirus
SCBA	= self-contained breathing apparatus
SC	= subcutaneous
SI	= Système International d'Unités (International System of Units)
SLE	= St Louis encephalitis
sp.* or *spp.	= species
STEC	= shiga toxin-producing *Escherichia coli*
subsp.	= subspecies
STI	= sexually transmitted infection
TB	= tuberculosis
TCBS	= Thiosulfate-Citrate-Bile-Sucrose [medium]
Td	= tetanus and diphtheria toxoid
TIG	= tetanus immune globulin
TLTBI	= treatment of latent TB infection
TSS	= toxic shock syndrome
TT	= tetanus toxoid
TTP	= thrombobcytopenic purpura
UK	= United Kingdom
UNAIDS	= Joint United Nations Programme on AIDS
UNDP	= United Nations Development Programme
USA	= United States of America

USPHS	= US Public Health Service
UV	= ultraviolet
VAPP	= vaccine-associated paralytic poliomyelitis
VCA	= viral capsid antigen
vCJD	= variant CJD
VEE	= Venezuelan equine encephalitis
vs.	= versus
VSV	= vesicular stomatitis virus
VZIG	= varicella zoster immunoglobulin
VZV	= varicella zoster virus
WEE	= Western equine encephalitis
WBC	= white blood cell
WHA	= World Health Assembly
WHO	= World Health Organization
wP	= whole Pertussis [vaccine]
YF	= yellow fever
ZDV	= zidovudine

EXPLANATION OF TERMS
Technical meaning of some terms used in CCDM
(not binding definitions)

1. **Carrier**—A person or animal that harbors a specific infectious agent without discernible clinical disease, and which serves as a potential source of infection. The carrier state may exist in an individual with an infection that is unapparent throughout its course (such an individual is commonly known as **healthy** or **asymptomatic carrier**), or during the incubation period, convalescence and post-convalescence of a person with a clinically recognizable disease (commonly known as an **incubatory** or **convalescent carrier**). Under either circumstance the carrier state may be of short or long duration (**temporary** or **transient carrier**, or **chronic carrier**).

2. **Case-fatality rate** (synonyms: fatality rate, fatality percentage, case-fatality ratio)—Usually expressed as the proportion of persons diagnosed as having a specified disease who die within a given period as a result of acquiring that disease. In communicable disease epidemiology, this term is most frequently applied to a specific outbreak of acute disease in which all patients have been followed for a period of time sufficient to include all deaths attributable to the given disease. The case-fatality rate – where the numerator is "deaths from a given disease in a given period" and the denominator is "number of diagnosed cases of the disease during that period" – must be differentiated from the **disease-specific mortality rate**, where the denominator is "total population".

3. **Chemoprophylaxis**—The administration of a chemical, including antibiotics, to prevent the development of an infection or the progression of an infection to active manifest disease, or to eliminate the carriage of a specific infectious agent in order to prevent transmission and disease in others. **Chemotherapy** refers to use of a chemical to treat a clinically manifest disease or to limit its further progress.

4. **Cleaning**—The removal by scrubbing and washing, as with water, soap, antiseptic or suitable detergent or by vacuum cleaning, of infectious agents and of organic matter from surfaces on which and in which infectious agents may find favorable conditions for surviving or multiplying.

  • **Terminal cleaning** is the cleaning after the patient has been removed by death or transfer, or has ceased to be a source of infection, or after hospital isolation or other practices have been discontinued. See also **Terminal disinfection**.

5. **Communicable disease** (synonym: infectious disease)—An illness due to a specific infectious agent or its toxic products that arises through transmission of that agent or its products from an infected person, animal or inanimate source to a susceptible host; either directly or indirectly through an intermediate plant or animal host, through a vector, or through contact with the inanimate environment.

6. **Contact**—In the context of communicable disease, a person or animal that has been in association with an infected person or animal or a contaminated environment, and so has had an opportunity to acquire the infection.

7. **Contamination**—The presence of an infectious agent on a body surface, in or on clothes, bedding, toys, surgical instruments or dressings, or in other inanimate articles or substances including water, milk and food. Contamination of a body surface does not imply a carrier state. **Pollution** is distinct from contamination and implies the presence of offensive, but not necessarily infectious, matter in the environment.

8. **Disinfection**—Killing of infectious agents outside the body by direct exposure to chemical or physical agents. **High-level disinfection** may kill all microorganisms with the exception of high numbers of bacterial spores; extended exposure is required to ensure killing of most bacterial spores. High-level disinfection is achieved, after thorough detergent cleaning, through exposure to specific concentrations of certain disinfectants (e.g., 2% glutaraldehyde, 6% stabilized hydrogen peroxide and up to 1% peracetic acid) for at least 20 minutes. **Intermediate-level disinfection** does not kill spores; it can be achieved through pasteurization (75°C [167°F] for 30 minutes) or appropriate treatment with approved disinfectants.

- **Concurrent disinfection** is the application of disinfective measures as soon as possible after the discharge of infectious material from the body of an infected person, or after the soiling of articles with such infectious discharges; all personal contact with such discharges or articles should be minimized prior to concurrent disinfection.
- **Terminal disinfection** is the application of disinfective measures after the patient has been removed by death or transfer, or has ceased to be a source of infection, or after hospital isolation or other practices have been discontinued. Terminal disinfection is rarely practiced; terminal cleaning generally suffices (see **Clean-**

ing), along with airing and sunning of rooms, furniture and bedding. Steam sterilization or incineration of bedding and other items is sometimes recommended after a disease such as Lassa fever or another highly infectious disease.

- **Sterilization** involves destruction of all forms of microbial life by physical heat, irradiation, gas or chemical treatment.

9. **Disinfestation**—Any physical or chemical process serving to destroy or remove undesired small animal forms, particularly arthropods or rodents, present upon the person or clothing of an individual, or in the environment (see **Insecticide** and **Rodenticide**). Disinfestation includes delousing for infestation with *Pediculus humanus*, the human body louse. Synonyms include the terms **disinsection** and **disinsectization** when only insects are involved.

10. **Endemic**—A term denoting the habitual presence of a disease or infectious agent within a given geographic area or a population group; may also refer to the usual prevalence of a given disease within such an area. **Hyperendemic** expresses a habitual presence at all ages at a high level of incidence, and **holoendemic** (a term applied mainly to malaria) expresses a high level of prevalence with high spleen rates in children and lower rates in adults. (See also **Zoonosis**.)

11. **Epidemic**—The occurrence, in a defined community or region, of cases of an illness (or an outbreak) with a frequency clearly in excess of normal expectancy. The number of cases indicating the presence of an epidemic varies according to the infectious agent, size and type of population exposed, previous experience of or lack of exposure to the disease, and time and place of occurrence; epidemicity is thus relative to usual frequency of the disease in the same area, among the specified population, at the same season of the year. A single case of a communicable disease long absent from a population or the first invasion by a disease not previously recognized in that area requires immediate reporting and full field epidemiological investigation; 2 cases of such a disease associated in time and place are sufficient evidence of transmission to be considered an epidemic (see **Report of a Disease** and **Zoonosis**).

12. **Food irradiation**—A technique that provides a specific dose of ionizing radiation from a source such as a radioisotope (e.g., cobalt 60), or from machines that produce accelerated electron beams or X-rays. Doses for irradiation of food and material are: **low** - 1 or less kiloGrays (kGy), used for disinfestation of insects from fruit, spices and grain and for parasite disinfection in fish and meat; **medium** - 1-10 kGy (commonly 1-4 kGy), used for pasteurization and the destruction of bacteria and fungi; and **high** - 10-50 kGy, used for

sterilization of food as well as medical supplies (including IV fluids, implants, syringes, needles, thread, clips and gowns).

13. **Fumigation**—A process by which the killing of animal forms, especially arthropods and rodents, is accomplished by the use of gaseous agents (see **Insecticide** and **Rodenticide**).

14. **Health education** (synonyms: patient education, education for health, education of the public, public health education)—The process by which individuals and groups of people learn to behave in a manner conducive to the promotion, maintenance or restoration of health. Education for health begins with people as they are, with whatever interests they may have in improving their living conditions. Its aim is to develop their sense of their own responsibility for health conditions, as individuals and as members of families and communities. In communicable disease control, health education commonly includes an appraisal of what is known by a population about a disease, an assessment of habits and attitudes of the people as they relate to spread and frequency of the disease, and the presentation of specific means to remedy observed deficiencies.

15. **Herd immunity**—The immunity of a group or community. The resistance of a group to invasion and spread of an infectious agent, based on the resistance to infection of a high proportion of individual members of the group.

16. **Host**—A person or other living animal, including birds and arthropods, that affords subsistence or lodgment to an infectious agent under natural (as opposed to experimental) conditions. Some protozoa and helminths pass successive stages in alternate hosts of different species. Hosts in which a parasite attains maturity or passes its sexual stage are **primary** or **definitive** hosts; those in which a parasite is in a larval or asexual state are **secondary** or **intermediate** hosts. A **transport host** is a carrier in which the organism remains alive but does not undergo development.

17. **Immune individual**—A person or animal that has specific protective antibodies and/or cellular immunity as a result of previous infection or immunization, or is so conditioned by such previous specific experience as to respond in a way that prevents the development of infection and/or clinical illness following re-exposure to the specific infectious agent. Immunity is relative: a level of protection that could be adequate under ordinary conditions may be overwhelmed by an excessive dose of the infectious agent or by exposure through an unusual portal of entry; protection may also be impaired by immunosuppressive drug therapy, concurrent disease or the ageing process.

18. **Immunity**—A status usually associated with the presence of anti-

bodies or cells having a specific action on the microorganism concerned with a particular infectious disease, or on its toxin. Effective immunity includes both **cellular immunity**, conferred by T-lymphocyte sensitization, and **humoral immunity**, based on B-lymphocyte response. **Passive immunity** is attained either naturally through trans-placental transfer from the mother, or artificially by inoculation of specific protective antibodies (from immunized animals, or convalescent hyperimmune serum or immune serum globulin [human]). Passive immunity is of short duration (days to months). **Active humoral immunity**, which usually lasts for years, is attained either naturally through infection with or without clinical manifestations, or artificially through inoculation of the agent itself in killed, modified or variant form, or of fractions or products of the agent.

19. **Inapparent infection** (synonyms: asymptomatic, sub-clinical, occult, or unapparent infection)—See **Unapparent infection**.

20. **Incidence**—The number of instances of illness commencing, or of persons falling ill, during a given period in a specified population. The **incidence rate** is the ratio of new cases of a specified disease diagnosed or reported during a defined period of time to the number of persons at risk in a stated population in which the cases occurred during the same period of time (if the period is one year, the rate is the **annual incidence rate**). This rate is usually expressed as cases per 1 000 or 100 000 per annum, for the whole population, or specifically for any population characteristic or subdivision such as age or ethnic group (see **Prevalence rate**). **Attack rate**, or **case rate**, is a proportion measuring cumulative incidence for a particular group, over limited periods and under special circumstances, as in an epidemic; it is usually expressed as a percentage (cases per 100 in the group). The numerator can be determined through the identification of clinical cases or through seroepidemiology. The **secondary attack rate** is the ratio of the number of cases among contacts occurring within the accepted incubation period following exposure to a primary case to the total number of exposed contacts; the denominator may be restricted to the numbers of susceptible contacts when this can be determined. The **infection rate** is a proportion that expresses the incidence of all identified infections, manifest or unapparent (the latter identified by seroepidemiology).

21. **Incubation period**—The time interval between initial contact with an infectious agent and the first appearance of symptoms associated with the infection. In a vector, it is the time between entrance of an organism into the vector and the time when that vector can transmit the infection (**extrinsic incubation period**). The period between the time of exposure to an infectious agent and the time when the

agent can be detected in blood or stool is called the **prepatent period.**

22. **Infected individual**—A person or animal that harbors an infectious agent and who has either manifest disease or unapparent infection (see **Carrier**). An **infectious** person or animal is one from whom the infectious agent can be naturally acquired.

23. **Infection**—The entry and development or multiplication of an infectious agent in the body of persons or animals. Infection is not synonymous with infectious disease; the result may be unapparent (see **Unapparent infection**) or manifest (see **Infectious disease**). The presence of living infectious agents on exterior surfaces of the body, or on articles of apparel or soiled articles, is not infection, but represents contamination of such surfaces and articles (see **Infestation** and **Contamination**).

24. **Infectious agent**—An organism (virus, rickettsia, bacteria, fungus, protozoan or helminth) that is capable of producing infection or infectious disease. **Infectivity** expresses the ability of the infectious agent to enter, survive and multiply in the host. **Infectiousness** indicates the relative ease with which an infectious agent is transmitted to other hosts.

25. **Infectious disease**—A clinically manifest disease of humans or animals resulting from an infection (see **Infection**).

26. **Infestation**—For persons or animals, the lodgment, development and reproduction of arthropods on the surface of the body or in the clothing. Infested articles or premises are those that harbor or give shelter to animal forms, especially arthropods and rodents.

27. **Insecticide**—Any chemical substance used for the destruction of insects; can be applied as powder, liquid, atomized liquid, aerosol or "paint" spray; an insecticide may or may not have residual action. The term **larvicide** is generally used to designate insecticides applied specifically for the destruction of immature stages of arthropods; **adulticide** or **imagocide**, to those destroying mature or adult forms. The term insecticide is used broadly to encompass substances for the destruction of all arthropods; **acaricide** is more properly used for agents against ticks and mites. Specific terms such as **lousicide** and **miticide** are sometimes used.

28. **Isolation**—As applied to patients, isolation represents separation, for a period at least equal to the **period of communicability**, of infected persons or animals from others, in such places and under such conditions as to prevent or limit the direct or indirect transmission of the infectious agent from those infected to those

who are susceptible to infection or who may spread the agent to others.

- **Universal precautions** should be used consistently for all patients (in hospital settings as well as outpatient settings) regardless of their blood-borne infection status. This practice is based on the possibility that blood and certain body fluids (any body secretion that is obviously bloody, semen, vaginal secretions, tissue, CSF, and synovial, pleural, peritoneal, pericardial and amniotic fluids) of all patients are potentially infectious for agents such as HIV, HBV and other blood-borne pathogens. Universal precautions are intended to prevent parenteral, mucous membrane and non-intact skin exposures of health care workers to blood-borne pathogens. Protective barriers include gloves, gowns, masks and protective eyewear or face shields. A private room is indicated if patient hygiene is poor. Local and state authorities control waste management. Two basic requirements are common for the care of all potentially infectious cases:

  1) Hands must be washed after contact with the patient or potentially contaminated articles and before taking care of another patient
  2) Articles contaminated with infectious material must be appropriately discarded or bagged and labeled before being sent for decontamination and reprocessing.

Recommendations made for isolation of cases in section 9B2 of each disease may allude to the methods that have been recommended as category-specific isolation precautions, based on the mode of transmission of the specific disease, in addition to universal precautions. These categories are as follows:

- *Strict isolation*: To prevent transmission of highly contagious or virulent infections that may be spread by both air and contact. The specifications, in addition to those above, include a private room and the use of masks, gowns and gloves for all persons entering the room. Special ventilation requirements with the room at negative pressure to surrounding areas are desirable.
- *Contact isolation*: For less highly transmissible or less serious infections, or for diseases or conditions that are spread primarily by close or direct contact. In addition to the 2 basic requirements, a private room is indicated, but patients infected with the same pathogen may share a room. Masks are indicated for those who come close to the patient, gowns if soiling is likely, and gloves for touching infectious material.
- *Respiratory isolation*: To prevent transmission of infectious diseases over short distances through the air, a private room is indicated, but patients infected with the same organism may

share a room. In addition to the basic requirements, masks are indicated for those who come in close contact with the patient; gowns and gloves are not indicated.

- *Tuberculosis isolation (AFB isolation)*: For patients with pulmonary tuberculosis who have a positive sputum smear or a chest X-ray that strongly suggests active tuberculosis. Specifications include use of a private room with special ventilation and closed doors. In addition to the basic requirements, those entering the room must use respirator-type masks. The use of gowns will prevent gross contamination of clothing. Gloves are not indicated.

- *Enteric precautions:* For infections transmitted by direct or indirect contact with feces. In addition to the basic requirements, specifications include use of a private room if patient hygiene is poor. Masks are not indicated; gowns should be used if soiling is likely and gloves should be used when touching contaminated materials.

- *Drainage/secretion precautions:* To prevent infections transmitted by direct or indirect contact with purulent material or drainage from an infected body site. A private room and masking are not indicated. In addition to the basic requirements, gowns should be used if soiling is likely and gloves used when touching contaminated materials.

29. **Molluskicide**—A chemical substance used for the destruction of snails and other mollusks.

30. **Mortality rate** (synonym: death rate)—A rate calculated in the same way as an **incidence rate**, by dividing the number of deaths occurring in the population during the stated period of time, usually a year, by the number of persons at risk of dying during the period or by the mid-period population. A **total** or **crude mortality rate** refers to deaths from all causes and is usually expressed as deaths per 1 000. A **disease-specific mortality rate** refers to deaths due to a single disease and is often reported for a denominator of 100 000 persons. Age, ethnicity or other characteristics may define the population base. The mortality rate must not be confused with the **case-fatality rate**.

31. **Nosocomial infection** (synonym: hospital-acquired infection)—An infection occurring in a patient in a hospital or other health care facility in whom the infection was not present or incubating at the time of admission; or the residual of an infection acquired during a previous admission. Includes infections acquired in the hospital but appearing after discharge, and also such infections among the staff of the facility.

32. **Pathogenicity**—The property of an infectious agent that deter-

mines the extent to which overt disease is produced in an infected population, or the power of an organism to produce disease. Measured by the ratio of the number of persons developing clinical illness to the number of persons exposed to infection.

33. **Period of communicability/Communicable period**—The time during which an infectious agent may be transferred directly or indirectly from an infected person to another person, from an infected animal to humans, or from an infected person to animals, including arthropods. In diseases (e.g., diphtheria and streptococcal infection) where mucous membranes are involved from the initial entry of the infectious agent, the period of communicability starts at the date of first exposure to a source of infection and lasts until the infecting microorganism is no longer disseminated from the mucous membranes, i.e. from the period before the prodromata until the termination of a carrier state, if the latter develops. Some diseases (e.g., hepatitis A, measles) are more easily communicable during the incubation period than during the actual illness. In diseases such as tuberculosis, leprosy, syphilis, gonorrhea and some of the salmonelloses, the communicable state may persist—sometimes intermittently—over a long period, with discharge of infectious agents from the surface of the skin or through the body orifices. For diseases transmitted by arthropods, such as malaria and yellow fever, the periods of communicability (or infectivity) are those during which the infectious agent occurs in the blood or other tissues of the infected person in sufficient numbers to permit infection of the vector. For the arthropod vector, a period of communicability (transmissibility) is also to be noted, during which the agent is present in the tissues of the arthropod in such form and locus as to be transmissible (infective state).

34. **Personal hygiene**—In the field of infectious disease control, those protective measures, primarily within the responsibility of the individual, that promote health and limit the spread of infectious diseases, chiefly those transmitted by direct contact. Such measures encompass:

- Washing hands in soap and water immediately after evacuating bowel or bladder and always before handling food or eating
- Keeping hands and unclean articles, or articles that have been used for toilet purposes by others, away from the mouth, nose, eyes, ears, genitalia and wounds
- Avoiding the use of common or unclean eating utensils, drinking cups, towels, handkerchiefs, combs, hairbrushes and pipes
- Avoiding exposure of other persons to droplets from the nose and mouth expelled when coughing, sneezing, laughing or talking
- Washing hands thoroughly after handling a patient or a patient's

belongings, and keeping the body clean by frequent soap and water washing.

35. **Prevalence**—The total number of instances of illness or of persons ill in a specified population at a particular time (**point prevalence**), or during a stated period of time (**period prevalence**), without distinction between old and new cases. A **prevalence rate** (not to be confused with prevalence) is the ratio of prevalence to the population at risk of having the disease or condition at the stated point in time or midway through the period considered; it is usually expressed per 1 000, per 10 000 or per 100 000 population.

36. **Quarantine**—Restriction of activities for well persons or animals who have been exposed (or are considered to be at high risk of exposure) to a case of communicable disease during its period of communicability (i.e. **contacts**), to prevent disease transmission during the incubation period if infection should occur. The two main types of quarantine are:

- **Absolute or complete quarantine**: The limitation of freedom of movement of those exposed to a communicable disease for a period of time not longer than the longest usual incubation period of that disease, in such a manner as to prevent effective contact with those not so exposed (see **Isolation**).
- **Modified quarantine:** A selective, partial limitation of freedom of movement of contacts, commonly on the basis of known or presumed differences in susceptibility and related to the assessed risk of disease transmission. It may be designed to accommodate particular situations. Examples are exclusion of children from school, exemption of immune persons from provisions applicable to susceptible persons, or restriction of military populations to post or to quarters. Modified quarantine includes: **personal surveillance**, the practice of close medical or other supervision of contacts to permit prompt recognition of infection or illness but without restricting their movements; and **segregation**, the separation of some part of a group of persons or domestic animals from the others for special consideration, control or observation; removal of susceptible children to homes of immune persons; or establishment of a sanitary boundary to protect uninfected from infected portions of a population.

37. **Repellent**—A chemical applied to the skin or clothing or other places to discourage arthropods from alighting on and biting a person, or to discourage other agents, such as helminth larvae, from penetrating the skin.

38. **Report of a disease**—An official report notifying an appropriate authority of the occurrence of a specified communicable or other

disease in humans or in animals. Diseases in humans are reported to the local health authority; those in animals, to the livestock, sanitary, veterinary or agriculture authority. Some few diseases in animals, also transmissible to humans, are reportable to both authorities. Each health jurisdiction declares a list of reportable diseases appropriate to its particular needs (see the *Reporting* chapter). Reports should also list suspected cases of diseases of particular public health importance, ordinarily those requiring epidemiological investigation or initiation of special control measures. When a person is infected in one health jurisdiction and the case is reported from another, the health authority receiving the report should notify the jurisdiction where infection presumably occurred, especially when the disease requires examination of contacts for infection, or if food, water or other common vehicles of infection may be involved. In addition to routine reports of cases of specified diseases, special notification is required of most epidemics or outbreaks of disease, including diseases not listed as reportable (see **Epidemic**). Special reporting requirements are specified in chapters on the *International Health Regulations (2005)* and *Reporting of communicable diseases*.

- **Zero reporting** (synonym: null reporting) consists of the explicit reporting of "zero cases" when no cases have been detected by the reporting unit. This is a way of checking that the relevant data have not been forgotten or lost.

39. **Reservoir** (of infectious agents)—Any person, animal, arthropod, plant, soil or substance (or combination of these) in which an infectious agent normally lives and multiplies, on which it depends primarily for survival, or where it reproduces itself in such manner that it can be transmitted to a susceptible host.

40. **Rodenticide**—A substance used for the destruction of rodents, generally but not always through ingestion (see also **Fumigation**.)

41. **Source of infection**—The person, animal, object or substance from which an infectious agent passes to a host. **Source of infection** should be clearly distinguished from **source of contamination**, such as overflow of a septic tank contaminating a water supply (see **Reservoir**).

42. **Surveillance of disease**—In communicable disease control, surveillance consists of the process of systematic collection, orderly consolidation and analysis and evaluation of pertinent data with prompt dissemination of the results to those who need to know them, and particularly those who are in a position to take action. It includes the systematic collection and evaluation of:

    1) Morbidity and mortality reports

2) Special reports of field investigations of epidemics and of individual cases
3) Isolation and identification of infectious agents by laboratories
4) Data concerning the availability, use and untoward effects of vaccines and toxoids, immune globulins, insecticides and other substances used in control
5) Information regarding immunity levels in segments of the population
6) Other relevant epidemiological data.

A report summarizing the above data should be prepared and distributed to all cooperating persons and others with a need to know the results of the surveillance activities. The procedure applies to all jurisdictional levels of public health, from local to international.

- **Serological surveillance** identifies patterns of current and past infection using serological tests for antibody detection.

43. **Susceptible**—A person or animal not possessing sufficient resistance to a particular infectious agent to prevent contracting infection or disease when exposed to that agent.

44. **Suspect**—In the context of infectious disease control, illness in a person whose history and symptoms suggest that he or she may have, or be developing, a communicable disease.

45. **Terminal cleaning**—See **Cleaning**.

46. **Terminal disinfection**—See **Disinfection**.

47. **Transmission of infectious agents**—Any mechanism by which an infectious agent is spread from a source or reservoir to a person. These mechanisms are as follows:

- **Direct transmission:** Direct and essentially immediate transfer of infectious agents to a receptive portal of entry through which human or animal infection may take place. This may be by direct contact such as touching, biting, kissing or sexual intercourse, or through direct projections (droplet spread) of droplet spray onto the conjunctiva or onto the mucous membranes of the eye, nose or mouth during sneezing, coughing, spitting, singing or talking (risk of transmission in this manner is usually limited to a distance of about 1 meter or less from the source of infection). Direct transmission may also occur through direct exposure of susceptible tissue to an agent in soil, through the bite of a rabid animal, or trans-placentally.
- **Indirect transmission:**

· **Vehicle-borne**—Contaminated inanimate materials or objects (fomites) such as toys, handkerchiefs, soiled clothes, bedding, cooking or eating utensils, surgical instruments or dressings; water, food, milk, and biological products including blood, serum, plasma, tissues or organs; or any substance serving as an intermediate means by which an infectious agent is transported and introduced into a susceptible host through a suitable portal of entry. The agent may or may not have multiplied or developed in or on the vehicle before being transmitted.

- **Vector-borne**

 (1) **Mechanical:** Includes simple mechanical carriage by a crawling or flying insect through soiling of its feet or proboscis, or by passage of organisms through its gastro-intestinal tract. This does not require multiplication or development of the organism.

 (2) **Biological:** Propagation (multiplication), cyclic development, or a combination of these (cyclopropagative) is required before the arthropod can transmit the infective form of the agent to humans. An incubation period (extrinsic) is required following infection before the arthropod becomes infective. The infectious agent may be passed vertically to succeeding generations (**transovarian transmission**); **trans-stadial transmission** indicates its passage from one stage of the life cycle to another, as from nymph to adult. Transmission may be by injection of salivary gland fluid during biting, or by regurgitation or deposition on the skin of feces or other material capable of penetrating through the bite wound or through an area of trauma, often created by scratching or rubbing. This transmission is by an infected nonvertebrate host and not simple mechanical carriage by a vector as a vehicle. An arthropod in either role is termed a vector.

 • **Airborne transmission:** The dissemination of microbial aerosols to a suitable portal of entry, usually the respiratory tract. Microbial aerosols are suspensions of particles in the air consisting partially or wholly of microorganisms. They may remain suspended in the air for long periods of time, some retaining and others losing infectivity or virulence. Particles in the 1-to 5-micrometer range are easily drawn into the alveoli of the lungs and may be retained there. Not considered as airborne are droplets and other large particles that promptly settle out (see **Direct transmission**).

- **Droplet nuclei**—Usually the small residues that result from evaporation of fluid from droplets emitted by an infected host (see above). They may also be created purposely by a variety of atomizing devices, or accidentally as in microbiology laboratories, abattoirs, rendering plants or autopsy rooms. They usually remain suspended in the air for long periods.

- **Dust**—The small particles of widely varying size that may arise from soil (e.g., fungus spores), clothes, bedding or contaminated floors.

48. **Unapparent infection** (synonyms: asymptomatic, inapparent, subclinical, or occult infection)—The presence of infection in a host without recognizable clinical signs or symptoms. Unapparent infections are identifiable only through laboratory means such as a blood test, or through the development of positive reactivity to specific skin tests.

49. **Universal precautions**—See **Isolation**.

50. **Virulence**—The ability of an infectious agent to invade and damage tissues of the host; the degree of pathogenicity of an infectious agent, often indicated by case-fatality rates.

51. **Zoonosis**—An infection or infectious agent transmissible under natural conditions from vertebrate animals to humans. May be **enzootic** or **epizootic** (see **Endemic** and **Epidemic**).

INDEX

M

Maculatum infection, 528
Malaria
  blood donations and, 388–391
  communicability of, 378
  disaster implications of, 392
  drug resistance and, A49
  epidemic measures for, 391
  humanitarian emergencies and,
    A61
  identification of, 373–374
  incubation period for, 377–378
  infectious agents, 374
  methods of control, 378–387,
    392–393
  mode of transmission, 376–377
  occurrence of, 375–376
  susceptibility to, 378
  treatment, 386–387
Malignant neoplasms, 393–402
Mammals, fish-eating
  as a disease reservoir, 201
Mammals, small
  as a disease reservoir, 70, 273,
    286, 297, 370, 480, 509, 528,
    672, 674
Manchuria
  hantaviral disease in, 270–271
Marburg disease, 206
Marsupials
  as a disease reservoir, 40, 685
Mass gatherings
  counseling, A34
  dead body management, A33
  health services, A32
  infection control, A32–A33
  laboratory support, A31
  outbreak alert, A31–A32
  outbreak communication, A33–
    A34
  quarantine, A33
  risk assessment, A28–A30
  risk management and planning,
    A30–A31
  standard operating procedures,
    A34

  surveillance, A31–A32
Mass vaccination
  for arthropod-borne viral
    encephalitides, 45–46
  for cholera, 125
  deliberately caused outbreaks
    and, A54
  for diphtheria, 196–197
  disease education and, A56–
    A57
  disease eradication and, A56–
    A57
  displaced persons and, A53–
    A54
  infectious disease outbreaks
    and, A51–A55
  for maternal and neonatal
    tetanus, A57
  for meningitis, 420–421, 424–
    425
  measles and, A57
  new vaccines and, A55–A56
  for poliomyelitis, 190–491
Mayaro virus, 40
Measles
  epidemic measures, 408
  humanitarian emergencies and,
    A60
  identification of, 402–403
  methods of control, 405–408
  occurrence of, 403–404
  susceptibility to, 404
  vaccination and, A57
Mebendazole, 17, 102, 212, 612–
  613
Melarsoprol, 634
Melioidosis, 409–412
Meningitis
  bacterial, 414–415
  hemophilus, 421–423
  humanitarian emergencies and,
    A61
  mass vaccination and, A51–A52
  meningococcal, 415–421
  neonatal, 426
  pneumococcal, 423–425
  viral, 412–414